PLIGHT OF HIV INFECTED WOMEN

PLAN OF ACTION FOR PREVENTION AND CONTROL

is not taken into consideration for this study. Therefore, purposive sampling technique is adopted to contact the respondents by resorting to snowballing procedure. Accordingly, 200 women living with HIV positive in Chennai city were interviewed with the structured interview schedule to collect required information on the line of objectives formulated for the study. Apart from interview with the respondents, discussion was also held with Government officials and NGOs working in AIDS intervention programmes. Available data had been subjected to process statistically leading to analysis and interpretation. Based upon the analysis and findings, a specific action plan has been evolved to provide care and support for the women infected with HIV and to create AIDS free society.

The present study is comprised of seven chapters. The First chapter presents an introduction to women infected with HIV with brief account of causes and consequences of HIV on women and the theoretical frame work. The Second chapter presents a review of literature related to the study in order to establish research gap. The Third chapter deals with the methodology adopted which includes objectives, operational definition of concepts, sampling procedure and sample size, tools of data collection and method of analysis. A comprehensive view on the global scenario of HIV/AIDS is presented in Fourth chapter. The Fifth chapter deals with analysis and discussion of primary data with a view of derive findings based on the objectives designed for the study. The Sixth chapter contains the major findings, suggestion and conclusion. The implication of research in the form of Action Plan towards prevention and control of HIV/AIDS and care and support and relief and rehabilitation of infected people with the goal of creating AIDS free society is presented in the Seventh chapter.

"Let's arm our children with opportunity and hope.
Our slogan is 'parents to work and children to school'"

Aditya Kumar Patra

Sakthi S.

Acknowledgements

I express my profound gratitude to my guide Dr. S. Gurusamy, Professor and Head, Department of Sociology, Gandhigram Rural Institute for providing me guidance and encouragement to complete the research work in time. I am deeply indebted to his family members for showing concern towards me.

My sincere thanks are due to Dr. T. Karunakaran, Vice-Chancellor, Dr. Sundaravadivelu, Registrar, Dr. Susila Kirubaharan, Deputy Resistrar, Gandhigram Rural Institute for permitting me to pursue my research work in the Department of Sociology under Faculty Improvement Programme. At this juncture, the help extended by Dr. Dwaraki, the former Professor and Head, Department of Sociology is deeply remembered.

I am thankful to Dr. Kubendaran, Professor and Head, Department of English for editing my work. I am also indebted to Dr. Ramachandran, Professor and Head, Department of Economics and Dr. Sumangala, Professor, Department of Economics, Gandhigram Rural Institute for providing valuable suggestions to strengthen my Action Plan.

I express my deep sense of gratitude to Malini Subramani, former Principal of Queen Mary's College, Mrs. Saraswathi Govingdaraj, Dr. Ananthi, Dr. Prema Gopinath, Mrs. Anusuya, Mrs. Rajalakshmi, Mrs. Prabha and Mrs. Kalavathi, my beloved professors and friends, Department of Sociology, Queen Mary's College for their encouragement and help throughout my study and permitting me to avail F.I.P. to pursue my research work.

I am deeply indebted to my friends Mrs. Uma, Lecturer, Department of Physical Education, Ms Kala Devi, Lecturer, Department of Geography, Mrs. Sumathi Lecturer, Department of English and Mrs. Asha, Lecturer, Department of Commerce, Queen Mary's College, Dr. Lakshmana Singh, Professor and Head, Department of Sociology, Bharathiar University, Coimbatore, Dr. Karupaiah, Reader in Sociology, Madras University and Dr. Alphonse Raj, Reader in Sociology, Loyola College, Chennai for their valuable guidance and support throughout my study.

I express my due gratitude to Dr. Kannan, Reader in Sociology, Manonmaniam Sundaranar University, Tirunelveli and Dr. Ani, Professor and Head, Department of Sociology, Mother Theresa University, Kodikanal for helping me by providing literature related to women and HIV/AIDS.

My heartfelt thanks are due to Mr. Christudas Gandhi, I.A.S, Dr. Gobal, I.A.S and Mr. Viajakumar, I.A.S, the Directors of Tamil Nadu State AIDS Control Society for helping me to collect statistics and the list of NGOs working in AIDS Intervention Programmes in Chennai.

I also deeply indebted to Dr. Krishnamurthy, Director of AIDS Prevention and Control Project (APAC), Dr. Manorama, Director of CHESS, Dr. Hariharan, Director of Indian Community welfare Association, Dr. Dhanikachalam, former NGO Advisor of Tamil Nadu State AIDS Control Society and the members of World Vision, Chennai for supporting me to collect primary Data and to shape Action Plan, the part of research work.

I am happy to extend my profound thanks to Mr. Arulmoni, Madurai Meenakchi Mission Hospital, Mrs. Sasikala, Family Planning Association of India, Madurai, Mr. Raja and Prassana Raja, the Director and Secretary of Mother Saratha Devi Social Service Society, Ottenchatram for extending their support during my pilot study.

I sincerely acknowledge the support of Ms. Kausalya, President, Indian Positive Net Work, Chennai, Mrs. Varalakshmi, Mrs. Seethalakshmi, staff of Tamil Nadu State AIDS Control Society, Mr. Pitchamani, President, Positive Net Work, Theni. I am also deeply indebted to all my respondents for providing valuable information and suggestions.

I am extremely thankful to my friends Mr. Mani, Mr. Jayaseelan, Ms. Thirukani and Ms. Shilpa, the Research Scholars, Department of Sociology, and Mr.Sabesh Manikandan, Kubendran Gandhigram Rural Institute for their encouragement and assistance in computerizing thesis.

I am always remembering my father Mr. G. Shanmugam Pillai, who is blessing me from the heaven for all my success in life.

I place on record my deepest appreciation to my mother Mrs. Ponnammal Shanmugam, brothers S. Govindaraj, S. Guru and S. Mohan and my beloved G. Karthiha and G. Dinesh Kumar and G. Iswarya and Mrs. Anitha Guru. I am highly indebted to my mother-in-law Mrs. Gomathi Alwar, sister in-law

Dr. Lalitha, Mrs. Rani Alwar Ramanujam, and my borther Dr. Alwar Ramanujam for their affectionate interest in my health and studies which helped me to provide deep concentration on research. I am extremely thankful to my sister Mrs. Raji Muth, my brother-in-law Lr. Muthu, Mr. Mani and all my family members and my friends Mrs. Padma Vasu and Mr. Vasu for providing moral and psychological support during my critical period which helped me to recover my physical strength to speed up my research work.

I am highly proud of my husband Mr. A.V Ravi Prakash, Asst. Professor, Pondicherry Engineering College, Pondicherry. Without his moral and psychological support it is very difficult for me to complete this research work. I am also highly indebted to my son Goutham R Prakash for tolerating my absence in home. I am very grateful to my son Mr. Prabu for heart warming encouragement throughout my study period.

Finally, I extend my thanks to each and everyone who have helped me in some way or other in this endeavour.

Sakthi, S.

Contents

Contents

LIST OF ABBREVIATIONS

AIDS	-	Acquired Immuno Deficiency Syndrome
APAC	-	AIDS Prevention and Control Project
ART	-	Anti Retroviral Therapy
ARV	-	Antiretroviral Drug
CAPACS	-	Chennai Corporation of AIDS Prevention and Control Society
CSW	-	Commercial Sex Worker
ESI	-	Employees State Insurance
FHAC	-	Family Health Awareness Campaign
FSW	-	Female Sex worker
GIPA	-	Greater Involvement of People living with HIV/AIDS
GOs	-	Government
Govt.	-	Government
HIV	-	Human Immuno Virus
IDU	-	Injecting Drug User
IUD	-	Intra Uterus Device
MSM	-	Men Seeking Men
NACO	-	National AIDS Control Organisation
N.G.Os	-	Non-Governmental Organisations
PFA	-	Parliamentary Forum on AIDS

PHC	-	Primary Health Centre
PLWHA	-	People Living with HIV/AIDS
PPTCT	-	Prevention of Parent to Child Transmission
PTCT	-	Parent to Child Transmission
RTI	-	Reproductive Tract Infection
STD	-	Sexually Transmitted Disease
SHG	-	Self Help Group
TNSACS	-	Tamil Nadu State AIDS Control Society
UNAIDS	-	United Nations Programme on HIV/AIDS
UNDP	-	United Nations Development Programme
UNFPA	-	United Nations Fund for Population Activities
UNIFEM	-	United Nations Development Fund for Women
VCCTC	-	Voluntary Confidential Counseling and Testing Center
WHO	-	World Health Organisation

1

Introduction

> "Every human being is the author of his own health or disease."
>
> —*Buddha*

Human beings are affected by a number of diseases caused by germs, bacteria, viruses, fungi and parasites. But epidemic produced by bacteria and other viruses are controllable and preventable and we have controllable vaccines and medicines to safeguard the population from these epidemics. There is no discrimination or stigma with the diseases caused by bacteria, germs, virus and parasites. But as far as Human Immuno-Deficiency Virus (HIV) and Acquired Immuno Deficiency Syndrome (AIDS) are concerned, it is entirely different from other diseases which society is faced today.

The first documented case of AIDS in the United States was identified in 1980s by a young immunologist, Dr. Michael S. Gottlieb at the University of California, Los Angeles. HIV-1 was identified in 1983 by Dr. Robert Gallo and other medical scientists at the National Cancer Institute in Bethesda, Maryland. At about the same time, Dr. Luc Montagnier of the Pasteur Institute in Paris isolated HIV-2 from AIDS patients (Singhal *et al.*, 2003: 46-49).

HIV/AIDS have a peculiar character of affecting the immune system of the body and make body susceptible to a number of infections leading to AIDS – a fatal stage of the body. Unlike other epidemics there is no vaccine for prevention and no medicine for the cure of the diseases. It affects the entire demographic and economic structure of the society by increasing mortality rate among the youth and children who are considered as the back bone of the development of any nation.

For AIDS, the transmission routes are clear and it is closely associated with individual behaviour. Therefore, it is hundred per cent preventable if the behaviour of individual is very much in line with societal expectations.

Certain behaviours such as sex outside matrimonial life, homosexuality, drug addiction, prostitution are unapproved behaviours and these are stigmatized in the society. The spread of HIV has its route in these stigmatized behaviours. Therefore, those who got AIDS/HIV are socially neglected, economically isolated and psychologically deprived by the society in general and by their family members in particular. As a result of social discrimination many infected people are generally out of the mainstream of social life. The social stigma makes them to develop mental strain and stress and unbearable fear about their future

In the beginning of the epidemic it was said that it is the disease of gay men or homosexuals and confined only to the western countries where these behaviours are not considered as abnormal behaviours. But now the disease is more and more identified with general population and it made us to feel that every one is under risk. The epidemic encircled the whole globe with out leaving any country with AIDS free status. The disease has no compromise with the people based on their caste, class, religion sex, age, power etc.

If there is no control on the rapid spread of the disease, it will threaten the entire survival of the society. Therefore, HIV/AIDS should be treated not only as major public health problem but also a social problem. Because, it has all the characteristics of social problems which affect larger sections of population to produce adverse impact on the society (Horton and Leslie 1970: 4).

Immune System

The immune system is a complex assembly of organs, cells, and proteins that defend the body against potentially harmful foreign substances. The co-ordinate action of these components against such substances is called immune responses. The immune system is involved in various major activities within the body. It defends the body against invasion by pathogens, which are disease-causing micro organisms such as viruses, bacteria, fungi and parasites. It identifies and destroys abnormal or mutant cells and thus defends the body against the growth of cancerous tumor cells. It also eliminates worn out dead and damaged cells and rejects cells from other organisms.

The immune system accomplishes many of its activities by the action of white cells, which are technically called leukocytes. The leukocytes are divided into three sub groups called 'T' cells, 'B' cells and natural killer cells. Specific immunity is carried out by 'T' cells and 'B' cells. The 'T' cells also called CD4+ cells.

When HIV entered into the body it not only replicates at enormous speed but also cause the death of the host cells by selectively targeting CD4+ cells. The CD4+ cells become its virus factory. Although the body wages a battle against HIV from the first day of infection–replacing upto 1 billion 'T' cells killed by HIV very day. But over a period of years the immune system gradually wears out and loses its ability to regenerate immune system cells killed during battle. This leads to a steadily widening gab between the number of cells killed each day and the number replaced. Once the gap widens the point that immune function is compromised, an individual with HIV is open to the opportunistic infections and cancers characteristics of AIDS (Kimberly *et al.* 1998: 13).

HIV – A Description

Acquired immunodeficiency syndrome (AIDS) is a disorder caused by the human immunodeficiency virus (HIV), which like all viruses is a submicroscopic parasite that can only survive and reproduce inside the cells of a host organism. HIV is a particular type of virus, a retrovirus, and more specifically, a lentivirus. HIV is able to infect CD4+ cells, a component of the immune system. The losses of CD4+ cells largely devastate the immune system in individuals with AIDS. HIV's sole activity is the production of new copies of itself. HIV infection persists for many years and attrition of the immune cells needed to fight infection gradually leads to an inability to generate new immune responses required to suppress HIV, and the replication rate of the virus increases to very high levels. The loss of CD4+ cells and a rise in the amount of HIV circulating in the blood stream (called the viral load) are the hall mark of AIDS (Harry W. Kestler *et al.*, 1998: 5).

Definition of AIDS

AIDS case definitions are established by the Centers for Disease Control and Prevention (CDC) in the United States. In 1981, after reports of Pneumocystis carinii pneumonia, Kaposi's sarcoma and other opportunistic infections in young gay men in San Francisco, New York and Los Angeles, the CDC began surveillance for a newly recognized disease to be called AIDS. In 1982, CDC developed a surveillance case definition for this syndrome focusing on the presence of opportunistic infections. AIDS case definition was expanded in 1985 by including the total of 20 conditions. Four of these conditions were cancers, kaposi's sarcoma and three distinct types of lymphoma. The remaining conditions were opportunistic infections – those caused by bacteria, fungi, protozoans and other infectious agents. The CDC has made another revision in 1987 by including three additional conditions. One of the new conditions was an opportunistic infection called tuberculosis (TB), but only the extra pulmonary (outside the lungs) type. The other conditions were nct opportunistic infections, but rather conditions resulting from the direct effects of infection by HIV in the digestive system (wasting syndrome) and the central nervous system. These conditions were found among heterosexual African American and Latino individuals. These new cases also included high number of injecting drug users. In 1992, the CDC has again taken steps to expand the surveillance definition to address certain populations, namely women, injecting drug users and communities of color. In November 1994, the CDC announced that it was expanding the surveillance definition with effect from January 1, 1993.

According to this definition any HIV-positive individual with a CD4+ cell count of 200 or less or whose CD4+ cells represented less than 14 per cent of all lymphocytes are called AIDS patients. Two additional illnesses are also included in the case definition that is AIDS – defining in children but not in adults. (*Theresa et al.*, 1998: 11).

Historicity of HIV/AIDS

The sudden appearance of AIDS in early 1980s prompted studies of the origin of this apparently new, fatal human disease. Sabatier (1988: 34-35) has given three explanation of the origin of the HIV virus. The first explanation is that it may originate from an old human disease unknown to science for the long time. The second assumption is that it has originated from species other than human beings like apes, monkeys. The third explanation is that it may accidentally originated in labouratories while conducting experiments.

The early theory believes that the virus has spread through homosexual contact of men. This syndrome therefore was initially called guy-related immunodeficiency or GRID (Parvi, 1992: 2). The spread of the syndrome soon identified as contagious agent which transmitted through sexual contact, transfusions of contaminated blood, and use of contaminated hypodermic needles. A new retrovirus was identified in 1983 and was subsequently demonstrated to be the cause of AIDS. This virus was named human immuno deficiency virus, or HIV.

The cross species theory reveals that the virus was already existed in animals and transmitted to human beings (Sahmi 1993: 2). The first evidence to support the cross over theory for HIV came in 1985, when an HIV-like virus was discovered in rhesus monkeys (macaques) that had developed Simian Acquired Immuno Deficiency Syndrome (SAIDS). The virus was named Simian Immunodeficiency Virus of macaques, or SIV mac. SIV mac was shown to be related to both HIV-1 and HIV-2 but was more closely related to HIV-2. Since those first studies, the SIV family tree has expanded to five branches representing five different simian species, all from Africa. The SIVs have been detected in sooty mongabeys in West Africa; in African green monkeys in East, Central and West Africa; in the Sykes monkey in Kenya; in a mandrill colony in Gabon; and finally in chimpanzees, also from Gabon.

The sooty mongabeys were kept as household pets in West Africa and the Africans may be infected with SIV in the past through the contact with house hold pets or monkeys hunted for food. Inadequately sterilized needles or contaminated blood products may have played a role in spreading SIV among humans. Needles that could be reused were widely introduced into rural African clinics after world war second and this widespread needles use coincides with the emergence of HIV. Needle reuse may have resulted in SIV being rapidly transmitted from person to person, allowing SIV to adopt humans through mutation. SIV became HIV when it was able to cause disease in human beings and be sexually transmitted. Once SIV had adapted to humans and was capable of being spread by sexual contact, the virus spread worldwide through international travellers (Mark 1998: 17).

The virus HIV-1 and HIV-2 are believed to have had a common ancestor in Africa. Very recently new HIV, which is more dangerous than HIV-1 and HIV-2 is detected in New York in America among homosexual men. This new HIV is more susceptible to opportunistic infection very quickly than other two HIVs. Researches are going on to study further details about the virus (*Sun News*, 1.30 PM on 17-2-05).

The medical condition, which was later to be called AIDS, began to be noticed in the late 1970s and early 1980s in several widely spreaded locations, including Belgium, France, Haiti, the United States, Zaire and Zambia (Tinker, 1988: 33-35). The first medical reports of the syndrome were published in the United States in June 1981 (US Centre for Disease Control, 1981: 250-252). For few years preceding these reports, a small but growing number of homo sexual men and their physicians in New York city, Los Angeles and San Francisco were noticing rare or unusual disease symptom –pneumocystis pneumonia, kaposi's sarcoma in young men. These ailments seemed to be related to inexplicable deterioration in the men's immune systems (Randy Shills, 1987: 630). Doctors began to suspect the existence of a new, sexually transmitted infection. Doctors at the US Centre for Disease Control (CDC) in Atlanta, Georgia, began to suspect that blood transmission could be a factor and similar symptoms were also recorded among intravenous drug users. By the end of 1981, doctors in Zaircan capital of Kinshasa had also begun to documents dozens of cases where their patients multiple infections seemed to relate to a collapse of the body's immune infection (Lamey and Malemeka, 1982: 507-11). It prompted the physicians to observe the similarity between the symptoms of Zambian patients and those which had broken out among American homosexual (Bayley, 1983: 1318-1320).

During 1970s cases of AIDS had been seen by Belgian doctors in Africans. The first seems to have been a 34 year old *Zairian airline* secretary (Vandepitte. *et al.*, 1983: 925-926). Late 1980s and early 1981 doctors at a Parisian clinic identified a case of pneumocystis pneumonia in a Portuguese man, in a Zairian women and in a French woman who came from Zaire (Offenstadl. *et al.*, 1983: 775). Of the two hundred patients affected by the new disease in Europe, fifty two were Africans (Biggar, *et al.*, 1984: 157-173). In Haiti, the combination of kaposis sarcoma and uncontrollable opportunistic infections has appeared in 1978-79 (Pape, *et al.*, 1983: 945-950). Haitian refugees with immunodeficiency disease were seen in increasing numbers in New York City and Miami during 1980-81. By mid 1982, the CDC had documented thirty four such cases. By October 1982, researchers in Haiti had diagnosed sixty one cases (*Morbidity and Mortality Weekly Report*, 1982: 353-361). Since 1982 the similar symptoms of cases were reported from various parts of the world and HIV/AIDS became the global problem.

The Unique Feature of HIV/AIDS

AIDS epidemic is vastly different from epidemics of yester-years for the following reasons:

- Primarily it is a sexually transmitted disease. Sexual activity is not something that can be banned morally, socially or legally.
- The new infection is rapidly increasing in every country. The moment the AIDS virus HIV enters a person's blood stream he/she is capable of infecting the next person he/she has sex with.

- Social stigma is attached with the AIDS since it has its roots with sexual behaviours. Therefore infected people have lack of courage to face the reactions of the society.
- Majority of the people are ignorant about the spread of HIV and its preventive mechanism.
- Limited facilities for testing and lack of affordability increases the spread of HIV/AIDS even without the knowledge of the infected people.
- The causative organism of AIDS is a virus and these viruses are not affected by antibiotics at all. It is not easy to find a curative agent for AIDS. Vaccines are not yet available, treatments are limited and a cure is still a vision for the future.

Therefore AIDS will create severe damage to our society. The increasing trends of HIV infection and deaths due to AIDS would not only produce adverse impact on individual, households and communities but also on the benchmarks of human development like infant survival, life expectancy, per capita income, school enrolments, health, and loss of trained human resources and so on.

Routes of HIV Transmission

HIV may be found in the cells, bodily fluids and secretions of infected persons and the presence of virus in the bodily fluids and secretions have different degrees of transmission risk. HIV can be easily isolated in semen, vaginal secretions and blood and breast milk. It is not easy to isolate the virus from tears, saliva, perspiration and urine. Therefore, it is currently accepted that the virus is transmitted to others only through blood, semen, vaginal secretions and breast milk (Digumarti Baskara Rao, 2000: 6).

According to Thomas *et al.* (1997: 26) the HIV can pass on to an individual mainly through the following three routes:

1. *Sexual exposure*: It is most commonly transmitted through sexual contact: from women to men, from men to women, between men seeking men.

2. *Contact with contaminated blood and blood products*: HIV is also transmitted through infected blood. People have become infected by blood transfusion, infected blood products including donated organs and by sharing of syringes and hypodermic needles. In many parts of the world, donated blood is now screened for antibodies to HIV, making this form of transmission is rare. However, in places where blood is not systematically tested and where many people are infected with the virus, transmission in this way may still be common. The virus has been also transmitted by recycling needles that have not been properly sterilized.
3. *From parent to child through pregnancy and birth*: This is known as pre-natal transmission. Before, birth it may be transmitted across the placenta to the developing foetus. During birth, the virus may be transmitted via the mother's blood or bodily secretions. A small number of cases of transmission through breast milk have been recorded in some regions.

HIV can also be transmitted through some innocuous routes like ritual tonsuring of the head at religious places where mass ritual tonsuring is taking place, common razor used in hair-cutting saloons and by village barbers who shave customers without changing disinfecting blades and piercing the ears, tattooing and ritual circumcision, if done in group (Sahami, 1993: 19).

The Groups Vulnerable to HIV Infection

Though every one is under the risk of acquiring HIV infection, certain groups are more vulnerable to HIV based on their life on high risk situation. These groups are called high risk groups. The high risk groups identified by the UNAIDS are past and present intravenous drug users, prostitutes, devadasis and their sexual partners, homosexual and bisexual men, Eunuchs involved in sexual activities particularly with homosexual men, prison inmates involved in homosexuality, multi-sexual partners, drug addicts, street children involved in sex and drug abuse, truck drivers who involved in sexual activity in the highway. Defense personnel who are engaged in sex with prostitutes, children of HIV positive women, sexual partners of HIV infected people, thalassemia patients who often receive blood from the donors, migrants who are away from their home for a long time and are involved in extra marital sex, construction workers etc. (Thomas *et al.,* 1997: 29).

Implications of HIV/Aids

The dreaded disease caused by HIV not only produces adverse impact on the individual but it also threatens existence of the basic social institutions of family and community and nation at larger level. HIV/AIDS is not only a health problem, but it is also a societal problem with important social, cultural and economic dimensions (Ahuja, 1999: 415).

Implication on the individuals

If the person is infected by HIV, immediately his/her character is assassinated by the public even without considering the mode of infection. The individual with HIV is subjected to criticism, boycott, segregation and dissociation, by their family members, friends, neighbours and fellowmen in the community.

Still the people have the fear that the virus can be transmitted even by touching or sharing of articles with the infected persons. The fear of death and the socially unapproved behaviours linked with the transmission of HIV resulted in stigmatization and discrimination towards the people infected with HIV positive.

The HIV positive people are looked down and they are isolated and rejected by the members of the society from the normal day to day life. In majority of the cases the individuals are blamed for their infection and they are treated like strangers who are involved in spreading HIV into general population. As a result they are denied proper care and support to lead a positive life with HIV positive status. The societal isolation creates psychological depression and mental stress and strain which affect the health of the people infected with HIV positive and invite the opportunistic infection without giving opportunity to prolong their life span. Loss of courage to face the society leads them to feel themselves as inefficient persons to continue or to take up work. Besides, the people with HIV positive also face lot of discrimination in their work places. In many cases they are thrown out of employment due to fear of contracting infection. Loss of hope on peaceful and dignified future questioned them about the meaning of life and resulted in alienation which forces them to end their life by committing suicide. The discrimination and stigmatization forced many people infected with HIV positive to get away from their own location to far away places where their infected identity can be hidden. And also the individuals who cannot cope up with their positive result normally get scared to face the friends and family members. These persons will try to hide their HIV status from the society in general and family members in particular.

Implication on the family

The whole family will get affected if any of its members is infected by HIV. The stigma associated with HIV not only affects the individual but also the entire family. If the infection is known to the public, the total family will be criticized and they may be excluded from the social activities of the society/community. In many cases the education, employment and marriage of the sibling is affected to a larger extent and force them to change their residence from their original place. The burden is heavy on the women. Because she has to bear the economical responsibility due to loss of employment and income of the infected persons. The early death of the economically productive youth leads to loss of income to the family. The expenditure incurred to treat the opportunistic infection forces them to lose all their resources and lead them towards indebtedness. The children are also affected for none of their faults. Significant per centage of children have been orphaned due to the loss of their parents.

Implication on Community

High prevalence of HIV infection in the community will leads to shortage of labour force which is highly essential for the development of any community. The increasing rate of women infection will definitely question the morality and ethics of particular community/society and it will strengthen the stigma associated with HIV/AIDS.

Implication at National level

The impact of the epidemic is visible in the demographic structure of the society. The morbidity and mortality rate is high among the youth–the most productive age groups. As a result children and old population will be found more in the region where the HIV and AIDS prevalence is high. South Africa is adversely affected by the increasing proportion of mortality and morbidity (Carael *et al.*, 1998: S1). The large increase in adult mortality and moderate increase in child mortality lead to dramatic falls in life expectancy (Boerma *et al.*, 1998: S3). The infection is high among the women. Around 25% of the women infected with HIV positive in the world are at their reproductive age. The higher infection rate among the women of reproductive age will affect the fertility rate of country (Stover and Way, 1998: S29). Since there is no cure for AIDS, the epidemic produces adverse impact on the economic structure of the country. The loss of human resource and loss of labour forces due to sickness also create adverse impact on the growth of national income. The growth of per capita income depends on the growth rate of healthy labour and capital that can be invested by the country towards the development activities. Sub-Saharan Africa has the lowest levels of per capita income of any developing region and it has faced lot of economic problems since 1980 due to AIDS (Ainsworth and Over, 1994: 232-233). The treatment for HIV/AIDS is very costly and the Government has to divert a major portion of its resources to distribute medicines either at subsidiary cost or free of cost like India. At national level the costs are incurred primarily through testing blood and blood products, improving treatment for sexually transmitted diseases, implementing precautions in health care settings, tracking the diseases and educating the public about the risk of the diseases. Besides, the medical researches require huge money to develop vaccine to prevent HIV/AIDS and drugs for the treatment of people infected with HIV/AIDS. At present the developed drugs are very expensive and beyond the reach of an average man (Ramamurthy, 2000: 1-21.

Women's Vulnerability To HIV/AIDS

HIV/AIDS is projected as women's epidemic. There is a common belief that the women in sex work are the major cause for spreading the virus in the society. The tendency of feminizing the disease is found among the general population in almost all countries without considering the real risk of women to acquire infection through their sexual partners. The disease becomes women specific by blaming the sex workers and women are perceived as virus carriers in many developing countries.

According to UNAIDS Global Epidemic 2004, majority of the women were infected through their single sexual partners especially in their marital life. Women usually have a faith that they will not get infection since they have sex with their single sexual partner/husband. Therefore, majority of the women will not be aware of their infection till their pregnancy or the death of her faithful partner. The negative attitudes towards HIV/AIDS by the society make her sexual partner to hide his HIV status with his family members. As a result, when men's infection is known to their family members, they blame their innocent wives/sexual partners for transmitting infection. The women's behaviours and character are questioned rather than analyzing real fact for men's infection. Many infected women have been abandoned by their family members as a result of such baseless blame.

In reality women are particularly vulnerable to infection and increasing numbers of women are becoming infected. Among the people infected with HIV/AIDS 57% are women and in many countries women outnumbered men as in the case of Africa.

Women's vulnerability to HIV/AIDS has different dimensions due to the following factors:

Social status of women in the society

Throughout the world irrespective of the development of the nations the women enjoy only secondary social status in the society. Globally around 60 per cent of women live below poverty line with illiterate status. They have inadequate access to property and other infrastructural facilities related to health care services (Usha, 2000: 12). The lower status of women within the family and society is heightening by their economical dependence on males. This makes women to feel less power to control their reproductive health. The feeling of powerlessness both in the personal relationship and in the society has resulted in keeping silent in sexual interaction and changing their traditional role by demanding the use of condom for safe sex. If a woman demands these she will be treated as of bad woman or thought to be inferring the infidelity of her husband and in the case of sex worker she has to face the risk of violence or lose clients and income if she advocates the use of condom (United Nations Commission on the Status of Women, 1998: 3). Therefore the powerlessness as a result of lower social status increases the risk of getting HIV infections.

Economic Subordination

Economic factors, such as poverty increases the risk of HIV for poor women mainly in two ways: 1. Poverty and lack of better resources lead many unmarried women to exchange sexual favors for economic survival. 2. Struggle for economic survival coupled with personal autonomy may lead many to form relationships with many partners and consequently increase the risk of HIV infection. Significant proportions of unmarried women are driven to become sex-workers due to destitution. There is a growing trend among poor married women living along the busy inter-State routes on national highways to take up prostitution as a means of coping with poverty. They mainly have truck drivers as their clients who now have emerged as the major high risk group. In the cross-border areas of the nations, the poor women have engaged in sex work with professional groups like armymen and other security personnel who have very high incidence of HIV. (Usha, 2001). They will be less successful in negotiating protection, and it is less likely that they will leave a relationship where they perceive more risk. Malnutrition, uncontrolled fertility, complications of childbirth, poorly performed abortion, predisposes women to intrapartal hemorrhages. This directly increases the risk of HIV through unmonitored transfusion of blood). The groups of young women most vulnerable to HIV infection are those who are homeless or living in poverty. UNICEF estimates that over 40 million young people in the world are living on the streets. Many of those have left home because of sexual abuse or poverty (Digumarti Bhaskara Rao, 2000: 122).

Cultural and Traditional Factors

Power imbalance is found in all societies and it is supported by socio-cultural system and controlled by men. As a result culture of silence is found around sex. It prevents the open discussion of sexual matters not only with men but also with women. The culture of silence dictates that the women should be ignorant about sex and passive in sexual interactions. Therefore, it is very difficult to reach the women with the message of safe sex practices. Even when the women are informed about safe sex, it is very difficult for them to negotiate its practices with their sexual partners. (Carovano, 1992: 131-142). The traditional norm of virginity for women that exists in many societies increases the risk of infection for young women. Because, it creates fear and it restricts their ability to ask for information about sex. The concept of virginity also puts young girls at risk of rape and sexual coercion in high prevalence countries because of the erroneous belief that sex with a virgin can cleanse man's infection. In addition, in cultures where virginity is highly valued, some young women practice alternative sexual behaviours, such as anal sex, in order to preserve their virginity, although these behaviours may place them at increased risk of HIV. (Weiss *et al.* 2000: 233-245). The strong norms of virginity and the culture of silence that surrounds sex prevent women to take treatment for sexually transmitted diseases which is highly stigmatized in the society (Weiss *et al.*, 2000).

In the Indian context, sex is highly sensitive, confidential and purely related to the private life of the individual and it forces people not to discuss any aspects of sex in the public sphere. Therefore, culture itself acts as a stumbling block to access knowledge about sex and sexuality and its related issues including STD, HIV/AIDS etc.

Cultural practices

In many societies sex is considered as taboo, not for discussion. Women are ill-informed on sexual matters and their sexual desire and decision on sex is controlled by men. Women have no negotiating powers and the societies have double standards on the sexual behaviour of its members. It imposes **rule of chastity** on women but accept men's multiple sexual partners. The use of contraceptive measures depend on the willingness of the male partners and women's social status depends on bearing children and the uses of condom is opposed to the cultural tradition of having children. Males are expected to initiate relationships, and sexual assertiveness in women is often stigmatized or even punished. **Age differences for sex** is strictly maintained by culture of many societies like India. In such countries women usually have sex with older men who have been sexually active for longer period and have had more chances for sexually transmitted infection. Certain cultural practices of the regions increase the risk of HIV infection for women. In some parts of the world, women use herbal and other agents in the vagina to cause dryness, heat and tightness. This practice is referred to as **"dry sex"** in which women feel like virgins and because they think that female secretions are unclean. The material used by women may include pieces of cloth, leaves, ground stone, herbs or western medications and their use has been reported in Nigeria, Zaire, Zamba, Malawi, Zimbabwe and South Africa (Sandala *et al.*, 1995: S61-S68). The substances used can cause inflammation and erosion of the vaginal mucosa, making it easier for HIV to enter. **Female genital mutilation (circumcision)** is practised in various African countries (Jones *et al.*, 1999: 219). Infibulations leads to extensive tearing and bleeding when sexual intercourse is attempted. It may also cause couples to practice riskier anal sex. The procedure itself could be risk if unsterilized instruments are used for several patients in succession (UNAIDS 1998: 11).

Early marriage of women is another important cultural practice which increases the risk of sexually transmitted infections for women. Most of developing countries like India, Pakistan, Sri Lanka, Bangladesh, etc. are practising both child marriage and early marriage. In these countries women are withdrawn from the school soon after they attained puberty. The girls are forced into marriage with men who are elder than her age. Most of these girls are entering into marriage without knowing anything about sex and sexuality and reproductive health. Along with other social norms their age at marriage becomes a barrier for them to discuss or to learn the matters related to sex. In this context, they accept the domination of their husbands on their body as well as on their day to day life. Poor knowledge on reproductive health increases the risk of HIV infection. The knowledge on reproductive health is either poor or lacking among the age groups of 15-40 years. At these ages both men and women are sexually active and many a times their unsafe sexual activity increases the chances of infection. There are lots of discussions throughout the world about reproductive health, but the message has not reached the vulnerable group of 15-40 years and the women become innocent victims in the context of HIV/AIDS.

In recent years, in various parts of the globe **male circumcision** is getting more popular since the people believe that circumcision may reduce the risk of HIV infection (Kim Best, 2001). There is evidence that male circumcision protects against HIV infection in Africa and the uncircumcised men in Africa are twice as likely to be infected as circumcised men (Singhal, 2003: 48).

Male circumcision is considered as a ritual practice by many communities especially Muslims. It is also a traditional ritual practice for the Christians in the continent of Africa. Similarly, circumcision is the common cultural and traditional practice in North America. The rate of infection identified here is only less than one per cent. But in South Africa, the rate of infection ranges from 15 to 25% where less per centage of men have undergone circumcision (Halperin, 1999). Male circumcision provides significant protection against HIV infection and other sexually transmitted diseases such as syphilis and gonorrhea. The circumcised males are two to eight times less likely to become infected with HIV (*AIDS Update*, 2000). The specific cell called 'Langerhans cells' are found in the foreskin of the male. These cells are the major receptors of HIV primary infection (Best, 2001). Therefore, the removal of specialized cells in the penis reduces the risk of HIV infection (Szobo, 2000). But if it performed in an unsterilized situation it will increases the risk of all HIV. **Lack of male circumcision** is found in many countries such as India. Many women are getting infected through their faithful male partners. If men had undergone circumcision, they may not get infected with HIV and in turn the women may not get infected with the dreaded diseases.

In many developing countries including India, sons are preferred over daughters. The concept of **son preference** is the principal determinant of high fertility in most regions. In the regions where son is given more importance, the women never come forward to use condom as safe sex to prevent them the STDs. Their attitude towards giving birth to male child may increase the risk of HIV infection in their marital life.

Female Biological Vulnerability to HIV

Women are biologically more vulnerable than men to HIV infection and other sexually transmitted diseases. The major factors responsible for differential transmission are the larger mucosal surface areas exposed to virus in women and the semen having high concentration of virus compared with vaginal secretions. Young girls are particularly vulnerable. Their immature cervix and relatively low vaginal mucus production presents less of barrier to HIV, making them biologically more vulnerable to infection than older pre-menopausal women (Digumarti Bhaskara Rao, 2000: 281).

Many women get HIV infections by a single sexual contact. The chances of a woman being infected by one act of sexual intercourse with an HIV positive man are about one in 100. The chance of a man being infected by one act of sexual intercourse with an HIV positive woman are about one in 1000, but this probability may increase considerably if one of them has STD (Moses *et al.*, 1991: 407-11)

Women are disproportionately the recipients of blood transfusions and other blood products (e.g. for anemia or child birth complications). In the absence of adequate blood screening, women's vulnerability to blood-borne HIV transmission increases.

Marriage increases the women's vulnerability to HIV

Marriage may be viewed as a social and economic commitment between individuals and families. Sexual access, procreation, child rearing and other services are universal to social expectation of marriage. Because of this and as well as lower social status and economic dependence, married women may be unable to challenge their husband's extra-marital affairs or insist on condom use for themselves. The magnitude of HIV transmission in stable/monogamy relationship in the event of disloyalty is high inspite of vigorous and purposive intervention programmes. The infection among women in monogamy relationships are current problem in all regions of the world in general and India and Thailand in particular. In these regions the men who visit sex workers also have wives or other stable partners (Isabella de Zoysa *et al.*, 1996: S197-S203). Marriage provides no protection against HIV. Across the world millions of women infected through heterosexual sex were infected by their husbands. Double standard of culture with regard to virginity keeps silence when men have multi sexual partners or engage sex with sex workers. If the men are infected through their behaviours of multisexual contact, they will pass the infection to their wives or stable partners. The women in monogamy relationship never emphasized the need of using condom with the faith that they will not get infected through their husbands or stable partners. The married women have higher rate of infection than their unmarried, sexually active peer (Isabella de Zoysa *et al.*, 1996: S197-S203).

Most of the men who got infections are highly ignorant about their infections. Because they never relalised the need for taking HIV test before getting married or whenever they had sex with sex workers. Some men will get married with the ignorance of their own infections and they will pass the infections to their wives. On the other hand some men are hiding their infections from others and transmit the virus to their wives. Therefore, many women are not aware of the risk of getting infection from their malc partners. They are also not aware that their husbands have HIV/AIDS (Baingana *et al.*, 1995: S21-S30).

It is very difficult to implement HIV prevention among the married women. The factors which act as barriers to the prevention of HIV transmission in the stable relationships are: First, there is a widespread belief that sex with a stable partner carries few risks. Second, communication between stable partners about protective behaviours is compromised by prevailing norms about partner and gender relations. Third, condom use and other risk-reducing behaviours are problematic in long-term unions, because it prevents procreation. Many seem unable or unwilling to recognize that they may be exposed to HIV infection in their stable relationship, even when they are aware of their partner's past or current risk behaviours. Most people believe that the "normal" sex with a stable partner is safe and sex "outside" the marriage and with "promiscuous" partners is risky. Many preventive messages, such as "stick to your partner", "love faithfully", or "love carefully" reinforce the notion that HIV infection only strikes "others" who deviate from the norm of loving, being faithful and having trusting relationships. Thus, monogamy is somehow constructed as a protection against HIV (Isabelle de Zoysa *et al.*, 1996, S197-S203).

Sexually transmitted diseases and HIV/AIDS to women

Sexually transmitted diseases have challenged the control measures even in the most developed countries. It acts as a co-factor in HIV transmission by increasing susceptibility to HIV. The diseases are multi dimensional and their prevalence in any community depends on various socio-economic factors (Nair *et al.,* 1973: 1967). The presence of sexually transmitted diseases (STDs), particularly ulcerative conditions, increases the likelihood of infection in both men and women. STDs are common amongst young women, particularly in Africa, the Caribbean and Latin America and Asia. They are not easy to detect in women and so most women remain unaware of their presence. World Health Organisation estimates that about 330 million cases of treatable STDs exist worldwide at any time and 50-80% of STDs in women are asymptomatic or go unnoticed because they are internal (UNAIDS, 2000: 11).

STDs—especially those, such as chancroid and syphilis, which cause ulcerative lesions—greatly facilitate both the acquisition and transmission of HIV. However, women with STDs are often asymptomatic and fail to recognize any infections. As a result, women are more vulnerable to HIV infection because they are more likely to have untreated STDs. Often their vulnerability to STDs is the result of their partners' behaviour rather than their own.

Preventing and curing the STDs may reduce the incidence of HIV infection. But the women, who know their infection, tend to avoid STD clinics for fear of being recognized and stigmatized. Women normally used to visit primary health centers and family planning and maternal and child health clinics to seek medical services. But unfortunately, the facilities to treat STD are often less equipped to diagnose and treat STDs. Further, women's inaccessibility to STD clinics, economic dependency and house hold responsibilities, negative attitudes of health workers towards the women with STD prevent them from getting treatment. Lack of sex education also increases the risk of STD among youth. Biological and psychological changes associated with marked desire for sexual adventures during adolescence have put the teenagers in the "high risk" group. Urbanization and industrialization have not only broken down the established class structure but also shattered the social and religious constraints which prevented promiscuous sexual behaviour (Dutta, 1998: 16). The prevalence of STD is higher among the women involved in prostitution.

Innocent women never discuss any STD due to cultural constrains and the infection is tolerated by the women.

Female sterilization increases the risk of women's infection on HIV/AIDS

In many countries young women and adolescent girls were very much conscious about preventing pregnancy rather than getting infected from sexually transmitted infections. The women who involved in pre marital sex are often familiar with oral pills rather than condoms (Blanc and Way, 1998: 114). The magnitude of condom use is found to be less among the women at younger age. In a thickly populated country like India, Family Planning is an official policy. In these countries both men and women are motivated to undergo terminal methods of male and female sterilizations. Once any one of the spouses has undergone sterilization they never think about safe sex to avoid sexually transmitted infections (Biddlecom *et al.*, 1997: 108). In a country like India more and more women are enthusiastic about female sterilizations and their number is increasing by leaps and bounds. As a result of permanent method of birth control, these women were liberalized from procreation rather than sexually transmitted infection through their male sexual partners. The permanent family planning methods act as a barrier for both men and women to use condom for safe sex and increases the risk towards HIV and other sexually transmitted infections.

Lack of awareness on reproductive health enhances the vulnerability to HIV/AIDS

Many women have poor understanding over their own bodies, mechanisms of HIV/STD transmission and their level of risk in unprotected sex. Many men also have inadequate information about their own bodies and women's reproductive health. A time of growing sexuality and identity consolidation, adolescence is also at greatest risk of contracting sexually transmitted diseases (STDs) and the HIV virus. The women in general and adolescent girls in particular are ignorant about their reproductive health. The culture of silence prevents them from gaining information with regard to the problems associated with their reproductive health. In many developing countries women's education is compromised with the tradition and culture. Therefore, the illiteracy or poor education has not allowed them to acquire knowledge on their reproductive health and the information related to their own risk of getting sexually transmitted infection and HIV/AIDS. The women's inaccessibility to the reproductive health education has resulted in adolescent childbearing in developing countries. The proportion of birth to unmarried adolescents is increasing in the countries of North Africa, Asia, Latin America and Sub-Saharan Africa (Singh, 1998: 117). The increasing pattern of high pre marital pregnancy appears to reflect a low incidence of contraceptive use, especially condom (Garenne *et al.*, 2000: 47). The exposure to media and the influence of modernization and peer pressure has made many girls from the educated community to get involved in non-marital sexual activity without insisting on condom use for intercourse. Their involvement in unprotected sex is based on their insufficient knowledge and distorted judgments of the risks of becoming pregnant and acquiring sexually transmitted infections (Gage, 1998: 154).

Ineffective health programmes implemented by the government on the reproductive health is one of the major causes in Sub-Saharan Africa for the exposure of young girls into risky sexual behaviours (Zabin and Kiragu, 1998: 210). The regions of Ghana and the regions of Western Countries have open social environment. Such free social environment influences boys and girls to experiment with sex without giving much importance to the implication of reproductive health and the diseases associated with the risky behaviours (Mensch *et al.*, 1999: 95). The adolescent unproductive sexual behaviours increase the vulnerability to HIV infections both in rural and urban areas.

Attitude towards parenthood increases women's vulnerability to HIV infection

In most societies, women's primary role is to bear and nurture children. The status of women in the society is directly related to her capacity to become a mother. The childless women are looked down by the society and they are sidelined in all social and cultural ceremonial celebrations. Number of children given birth by the women is the rating scale to perceive the women's position is the family as well as in the society. The norms related to parenthood have two broad implications on women in relation to HIV/AIDS and STDs. One is that women are expected to concentrate more on their reproductive role rather than productive role as earning members to the family. The second consequence is that the childless woman used to try to become pregnant with unprotected sex without getting treatment for her/his infertility. In such cases if men are infected, the woman will also get infection without her knowledge.

Violence against women and HIV infection

Violence against women is an important factor which increases the risk of women's vulnerability to HIV infection. Rape is high risk factor which is inadequately recognized or addressed. In developing countries many poor and underprivileged women are subjected to sexual harassment like rape, molestation, and kidnapping and abduction either by the members known to their family or by the members of affluent community in work place. Drunken behaviour of the youth is reported as a major cause for the sexual harassment of women in the developing countries India (Sangmeswaran, 2004). Sexual harassment is a crime against women which increases the risk of HIV infection. Marital violence is more tolerated by the society than the violence outside the marriage. The rape within the marriage is not recognized as offence in many parts of the world and it is the privilege given to the men in the male dominated patriarchal society. Physical and sexual violence against women are intensified during wars and armed conflicts. Sexual violence can also occur against children, homosexuals, and transgendered people. The myth prevailing everywhere among the men in the society is that the sex with the children or young girls may cure or prevent all sexually transmitted infection including HIV/AIDS. As a result of this myth many girl children are trafficked and forced into prostitution. The sex under the condition of force or violence never think to use condom and it increases the risk of HIV and STDs infection to women.

Migration of male increases women's vulnerability to HIV infection

Male migrants are away from their home for a longer period. For example, transport workers, military and armed force workers, traders, seasonal agricultural labourers, are highly mobile and they have to leave their spouses and families for longer periods. Sex impulsion, separation from spouses, and stress and strain owing to their work influence male migrants to seek sex with sex workers and to use drugs with their peer groups in order to get relief from their personal problems. Thus, poor migrants are not in a position to value one's own life or to take steps to protect one's own health. Generally, the migrants are not much aware of the use of condom. The lack of or poor usage of condom increases the risk of HIV infection. These migrants were not coming forward to test their HIV status though they know their risk behaviours. As a result, they were unaware of their infection. If the men are infected due their risky behaviours, they well pass the infection to their wives or other sexual partners when they returned home. The impact of prevailing power imbalance and its associated gender inequality and women's faith on their male sexual partners do not permit the women even to suggest safe sex. The risky behaviour of men and their ignorance of their HIV infection increases women's vulnerability to HIV infection.

Migration of women increases their vulnerability to HIV

Generally the migrant women have least power to protect themselves from sexual exploitation. Many women migrants have ended up in prostitution to earn more money to improve the standard of living of their family members. Geographic mobility to young girls would lead to increased risk. Migration among the young girls under the age of 15 is predominant in rural areas in many Latin American Countries, in some African countries such as Ghana and Morocco and in Asian countries such as Bangladesh, India, Indonesia and the Philippines. They migrate to urban areas for seeking schooling and employment. A large proportion of the young women migrating to European countries from Asia and Africa end up in prostitution. Many sex workers move from place to place either voluntarily or involuntarily. For example, women from Cambodia, Laos, Myanmar and Vietnam work in brothels in Thailand. Sex workers from Thailand and Philippines work in Japan. Thai women became sex workers in Singapore and Nepalese women work in India. Sex workers may spread HIV from cities to rural areas when they returned home (UNDP, 2004: 1).

The process of increasing feminization of migration is found through out the world. It is estimated that roughly 48% of all migrants in the world are women (UNDP, 2004: 5). Women migrants from Asia constituted the largest number of unskilled workers in labour receiving countries. Rampant gender inequalities, low social status and lack of understanding of their sexuality and reproductive health and lack of access to information and service make migrant women especially vulnerable to HIV/AIDS. Large number of migrants face an acute risk of exploitation, physical violence, sexual abuse and socio-political marginalization. Sexual abuse and sexual exploitation will also increase women migrant's vulnerability to HIV infections (UNDP, 2004: 6).

Parent to Child Transmission of HIV

Parent-to-child transmission (also called PTCT, or "vertical transmission") is common today, resulting in millions of pediatric AIDS cases. The chances of a baby born to an HIV positive mother being infected are 40 per cent (Singhal *et al.*, 2003: 49).

Throughout the world hundreds of babies are born with HIV positive every day and there is no sign of decreasing trend in the world. Such increasing trend is mainly because of the failure of recognizing child's rights which is guaranteed under the United Nations Conventions of the Child Rights.

The HIV-infected mother can pass virus to her baby in the womb itself or during pregnancy, labour, delivery or after birth through breast feeding. The vertical or prenatal transmission is the major cause for the infant to get infection. The risk of transmission from mother to child is around 15-30% if the mother does not breast feed the child. But it can rise as high as 30-45% with prolonged breast feeding (Khurana, 1998: 103). Therefore, WHO has recommended bottle feeding for the children of HIV infected mothers (Thomas *et al.*, 1997: 42). In developing countries, the infection rate is increasing among the women at child bearing age. The increasing rate of infection among the women will increases the infection rate in infants (UNAIDS Briefing paper, 1997). The viral load of the mother is an important factor which influences the prenatal transmission. If the viral load is high, the risk of infection is also high (UNAIDS, July, 2004).

In 2004, around 640,000 children under 15 became infected with HIV mainly through mother to child transmission and 90% of these children are living in developing countries (UNAIDS, 2004). It is estimated that by the year 2010, if the spread of HIV is not controlled, around 75% of the infant mortality and under-five child mortality in the world will be due to AIDS (UNAIDS Briefing paper, 1997).

Since the beginning of the pandemic, over 5 million infants have been infected with HIV. Among them 90% were born in Africa and the worst affected region is Sub-Saharan Africa. In this region, the HIV infection rates of 10-30% are common among the pregnant women. At the same time the number of cases also increasing in Eastern Europe, India, and South East Asia (UNAIDS, 2002: 1-8). In these regions the infection rate among pregnant women ranges from 1% to 5% and it increases the vulnerability to infant infection (Gangakhedkar, 1999: 125-136).

HIV infection is a major contributing factor to childhood diseases and mortality in developing countries. It will threaten the survival of the child. The risk of transmission can be reduced up to 50% with the administration of anti retroviral drugs to mother and baby at the time of delivery, in conjunction with replacement of breast feeding (UNAIDS, 2002: 1).

In 1994, French and American researchers found that a two-month course of the antiviral drug AZT (Zidovudine) administered to HIV positive women in pregnancy during labour and delivery and after birth to their newborns reduced the rate of mother-to-child transmission by two-thirds in the absence of breast feeding. This preventive regimen is impossible to apply in many developing countries. Because, AZT is a very expensive drug and it is only available for the wealthy (UNAIDS Briefing Paper 1997). In Western countries the mother to child infection is found to be less due to effective voluntary testing and counseling, access to anti retroviral therapy, safe delivery practices and the widespread availability and safe use of breast milk substitutes (UNAIDS, August, 2001).

Poverty is the key reason for increasing pediatric transmission in developing countries. The women who are infected by HIV in developing countries are identified as poor and they are not in a position to avail anti retro viral drugs to prevent mother-to-child transmission. Besides, breast feeding is the common norm in most of the developing countries. Lack of awareness on supplementary feedings and lack of financial sources to avail such supplementary feeding force the women to depend only on breast feeding to their child. Therefore, the nursing mother has an increased risk of transmitting the virus to her infants.

The important factor which is responsible for mother to child transmission is lack of awareness and ignorance about the status of HIV infection. Most of the people are not interested to take up voluntary testing to know their HIV status owing to their risk behaviour. Therefore, many pregnant women are ignorant about their own infection and the need of taking anti-retroviral drug to prevent their babies from infection.

Stigma and Discrimination Associated with HIV/AIDS

Goffman (1963: 3) described stigma as "an attribute that is deeply discrediting within a particular social interaction". His explanation on stigma focuses on the public attitude toward a person who possesses an attribute that falls short of social expectations.

"Stigma" is a powerful tool of social control used to marginalize people. It can exclude people and can have great power over their lives with regard to social interaction. Generally, the public have a belief that they can get HIV by any kind of physical contact with the people infected with HIV positive. They also have a belief that the promiscuous individual alone can get HIV. The negative conception on HIV forces the public to treat the people infected with HIV very badly and indifferently. This problem of stigmatization is found all over the world. When people with HIV are treated as outcasts or as morally bad people, it is discrimination (PFA, 2004: 1).

HIV related stigma refers to all unfavorable attitudes, beliefs, and policies directed towards people perceived to have HIV/AIDS as well as towards their significant others and loved ones, close associates, social groups and communities. Patterns of prejudice, which include devaluing, discounting, discrediting and discriminating against these groups of people will strengthen the existing inequalities related to gender, sexuality and race.

Causes for HIV Related Stigma

According to Goffman (1963), diseases associated with the highest degree of stigma share following common attributes:

1. The person with the disease is seen as responsible for having the illness.

2. The disease is progressive and incurable
3. The disease is not well understood among the public
4. The symptoms cannot be concealed.

HIV infection has all these common attributes and attracts high level of stigmatization. First, people infected with HIV are often blamed for their life style and many people believe that HIV could be avoided if individuals made better moral decisions. The behaviours associated with HIV, for example, sex outside the marriage, sex between men, injecting drug use, and prostitution are already stigmatized in the society. Therefore, people infected with HIV positive are often thought of as responsible for infection. Second, although HIV is treatable, it is a progressive and incurable and life threatening disease. Third, HIV transmission is poorly understood by some people in general population. As a result of the poor knowledge and misconception, they scared of contracting HIV by accepting the presence of the people infected with HIV positive. Finally, although asymptomatic HIV infection can often be concealed, the symptoms of HIV related illness cannot be concealed. HIV related symptoms may be considered by the people as repulsive, ugly and disruptive to social interaction (Herek, 1999).

Impact of Stigma on the People Infected with HIV Positive

The stigma associated with HIV/AIDS prevents the high risk groups from taking up HIV test voluntarily. The delay in testing further increases the transmission of HIV. The discrimination and social stigma has made many people to be ignorant about their disease. The ignorance on the status of HIV leads to the spread of virus into the general population. Early detection of HIV infection is important. Knowledge of one's own HIV seropositivity can lead to earlier treatment and improved outcomes. Knowledge of seropositivity can also lead to changes in risk behaviours that can reduce or eliminate the risk of HIV transmission.

The nature of stigma also prevents the infected people by disclosing their HIV status in the society. Even after testing

HIV positive, many people have denied their seropositivity and many have not accepted their seropositivity status. The denial and hiding of the disease from others again aggravates the situations by spreading the disease to their sexual and needle injecting partners.

Delay in testing, denial and non-disclosure of the infection are major causes for the increasing rate of infection in the general populations.

Impact of Stigma on Women

Women's social and economic vulnerability and gender inequality make women to find difficulties in coping with the stigma and discrimination associated with HIV infection. HIV positive women bear a double burden: they are infected and they are women. HIV testing is a critical ingredient for receiving treatment or for accessing drugs to prevent the transmission of HIV from a woman to her child. But the woman is ostracized, marginalized and even killed as consequences of exposing her HIV status (*Hindu*, July 18, 2003). Since women are sexually, economically and biologically vulnerable to HIV/AIDS and other STDs, they are often stigmatized and blamed for "causing" HIV/AIDS and other STDs. Women are frequently identified as "reservoirs of infection" or as "vectors for transmission" to their male partners and their offspring. This inaccurate view on women by the public will neglect the focus on men's equal responsibility in preventing HIV/AIDS. It will also prevent the development of programmes to meet the needs of women to protect themselves from all sexually transmitted diseases including HIV/AIDS.

Generally, the people assume that if a woman has HIV infection, she has engaged with multiple sexual partners or engaged in prostitution. As a result, the infected woman's character is under the threat of assassination and such women are treated as "bad women". Many of such infected women have been dismissed from their jobs or not hired for jobs, evicted from their homes, abandoned by their husbands or other long-term partners, and denied the custody of their children, denied shelter and share of household property, refused access to treatment and care and often blamed for their husbands' HIV diagnosis. In addition, women perceived to be at risk of HIV infection have been denied health insurance.

Some countries have implemented mandatory testing schemes targeting women. Women who test positive or who are suspected of being infected suffer from increased discrimination, random and institutional violence, arrest, incarceration and deportation. Most often such testing is without the woman's informed consent, and without appropriate pretest and post test counseling (Digumarti Bhaskara Rao, 2000: 284).

In all regions women are expected to assume care giving responsibilities to the children and other family members who are sick. In the case of HIV/AIDS also women are expected to take care of their infected partners and it gives more stress and strain. Owing to sickness, loss of employment of the male partner forces her to take up employment outside the home to cope with loss of income of the male partners. When she becomes ill she will not get any one support to take care of herself.

Often women are blamed for husbands' HIV status. If the man is diagnosed HIV first, automatically the woman's fidelity is questioned by the husband and by her in-laws (Bharat, 2001). In case where the man has admitted his relationship with the sex workers, the burden of blame still falls on the wife for failing to "satisfy" her husband's sexual impulsions. These women were often isolated, shunned by family and friends, and become the target of abuse or gossip. Therefore, women infected with HIV positive tend to be more stigmatized than men due to social expectations of moral integrity. As a result, many women infected with HIV positive are experiencing violence in the homes (Sathiamoorthy and Suniti Solomon, 1997).

THEORETICAL FRAME FOR THE STUDY

Structural Functional Theory

Social structure refers to the recurrent and patterned relationship that exists among the components of social system. The social structures have interrelated and inter dependent parts in the form of institutions. Each institution or parts serves the function to maintain stability and equilibrium in the society at larger level for the existence of society and its members. The consequences which permit the adoption or adjustment of a system is called functions (Zanden, 1990: 29).

The social structure consists of invisible rules and institutional arrangements like family, religion, education, etc, to guide the behaviours of the individuals. The major assumption behind structural functionalism is to maintain stability, harmony in the society and to adopt changes according to new needs and demands through evolution. If any institution or parts of structure fails to perform its function, it will result in imbalance or disequilibrium in the society.

The social structure has two basic components – status and roles. Status refers to the individual's position and power in the society. It may be achieved or ascribed status. A status carries with it a set of culturally defined rights and duties. It is called roles. The norms of the structure specify the appropriate and inappropriate behaviour for the occupant of particular status.

According to functionalist perspectives, unequal distribution of social rewards is necessary to get the essential task of the society from its member to maintain harmony and equilibrium. Kingsley Davis and Wilbert Moore argued that social stratification is both universal and necessary, and hence no society is ever totally classless. In their view, all societies require stratification to fill all the statuses composing the social structure and motivate people to perform the duties associated with these positions (Zanden, 1990: 242).

For a functionalist, society is system, a combination of things or part that forms a larger whole. All the parts of the society are related to one another. Institutions such as family, religion, the economy, the state, education are among the crucial parts of any society. Changes in one institution have implication for other institution and for the society as a whole.

Robert K. Merton argues that the institutions and other parts of the society can contribute to the maintenance of the social system. But at the same time they can also do the opposite to other parts of the social system. The consequences that lessen the adoption or adjustment of the system are termed by him as dysfunctions. Merton also distinguishes between manifest and latent functions. Manifest functions are consequences that are intended and usually recognized by the participants in a system. Latent functions are consequences that are unintended and often not recognized (Turner, 2002: 87-97).

Durkheim argues that the social structure is made up of norms and values. It regulate the behaviour of the people which is considered as appropriate and worthy in different settings. According to him the individual can learn the normative behaviours through socialization. Socialization is a process which makes individuals become the members of society and makes social life possible. For Durkheim social solidarity is ensured by socialization. Durkheim's conceptualization of social systems in terms of "normal" and "pathological" states exclusively depends on the adoption and practices of culturally expected norms and values (functional needs) by the individual in the society (Jones, 2005: 37-40).

Talcott Parsons defined "social structure as a stable system of social interaction". Parsons takes "action" as the building block of the system. The term action refers to the behaviour of the individual. For Parsons, the cultural institutions of the society consist of cognitive beliefs, systems of expressive symbols and private moral obligations. The main function of the cultural system is the legitimation of the society's normative order. Cultural value patterns provide the most direct link between the social and cultural systems in legitimizing the normative order of society. They define what is appropriate and what is not, not necessarily in a moral sense but in accordance with the institutionalized order (Francis Abraham. M. 1982: 63). According to him the social system has the following characteristics (Turner, 2002: 58-65):

1. It involves a process of interaction between two or more individual
2. Each one of the individuals influences the another individual

3. Their interaction is mainly based on collective goal orientation or common value and of a consensus of normative and cognitive expectations.
4. The actor is confronted with a variety of situational conditions as societal environment t and ecological constrains
5. The actors' orientation to the situation is both motivational and value oriented.

It is evident from the structural functionalist perspectives, that members of society are expected to do their duties according to the norms and cultural values of the society.

For Weber, the society is existed because of social action. People do things because they decide to do so in order to achieve ends they desire. Having selected their goals, and taken account of the circumstances they find themselves in, they choose to act. Social structure is the outcome of such action; ways of living are the product of motivated choice. Existing action created social circumstances exercise constraint as structural forces but action is nonetheless still mental in origin – chosen in the light of the actor's perception of these structural constraints (Jones, 2003: 82)

Application of Structural functionalist theory to the present study

The individual has to act according to the norms and rules of the various institutions of the society. To fit in as a member of the society, the individual is learning all the culturally expected norms, values and rules from the childhood through various institutions like family, school, religious institutions, government etc. The individual is socialized in such a way as to act according to the norms and values of the society. The individual should not think of deviating from the laid norms and values of the society.

Indian society is highly a culture-bound society. The individual behaviours are encircled by the rigid norms, values, rules, moral codes, mores and traditions of the society. The Indian culture and traditions have a belief that the adoption of culturally expected norms and values alone help to maintain harmony and equilibrium in the society. It also has a fear that if the individual is allowed to act according to his own choice without giving importance to values of the culture, the Indian society will lose is credibility, reliability and integrity.

Family, marriage, religion and community are the important institutions which serve to socialize the individual in accordance with the cultural expectations of the society. Gender-related behaviours status and roles and sex and sexuality are learned by the individual due to the influence of these institutions. The society's norms regulate sexual behaviour by specifying who may engage in sexual behaviour with whom and under what circumstances. The Indian society is very rigid in regulating the sexual activities of the individual with the cover of silence around the sex. Discussing sexual matter is considered as taboo in India. The people are not allowed to discuss sex and sexuality with any one including spouse. As a result, fear is created among the people to learn or collect information related to sex and sexuality.

In India, family and marriage are highly valued. The individuals are expected to engage in sex only after marriage. Sex outside wedlock is highly devalued in the society. The pre marital and the extra marital sexual relationship will entirely damage the life of the people who engage in such activities. If such relationship is known to others, the particular individual has to face stigma and discrimination in the society. Murders due to extra or pre marital relationship are frequently reported in the local newspapers and magazines of India.

Indian society is patriarchal. Men are the dominant figures in the family. The women are expected to have the character of ideal wifehood. It means the husband must be considered as God and the wife should be faithful to him even if the husband has deviant behaviour and seek pleasure outside the marriage. The good wife must never do anything that would displease her husband. According to Manu – the Hindu code maker–"Women must particularly be guarded against evil inclinations. If they are not guarded, 3they will bring sorrow on both the families" (Kapadia, 1966: 254). Manu therefore wants woman to be under the surveillance of her father in her childhood, her husband in her youth and her sons on the death of her husband. "A woman should never think of independence from the father, the husband or the sons because by so doing she will make both the families contemptible." Her status is determined only through her reproductive capacity. She is expected to bear children, that too male children. As per social norms male has to take decision with regard to family matters. The male has to decide the contraception to control the birth.

But normally, the safe sex is not a rule in family among the spouses. Therefore, in the era of HIV/AIDS infection, women are subjected to the infection as a result of unsafe sexual behaviour.

With regard to marriage, age difference between bride and bridegroom is strictly maintained in the society. The bride must be younger than the bridegroom. This age gap further strengthens the inequality and low status of women. As a result of younger age, the woman can not raise her voice against her husband's sexual domination on her body. The hidden aspect of sex and sexuality which is deep rooted in the culture prevents the woman to gain knowledge on her reproductive health. According to the traditional norms of good woman, she cannot practice it in her life if she knows little knowledge about reproductive health.

Even the friendship between male and female is not encouraged in the society. The girl must be away from the boy. As far as sex is concerned, men are also not encouraged to involve or experience sex outside wedlock. As per religion and culture it is immoral. Sex is related to morality in India. If any one deviates from this norm he will be treated as an immoral person. Therefore, the secret behind sex influence the weak minded men as a result of poor socialization to experience it with the sex workers. The same secrecy prevents men to use condom to safeguard from sexually transmitted diseases. Once he is infected he will take the virus to his innocent wife and children through his wife.

In Indian society irrespective of regions, cultural taboo is associated with sex and it is not a open topic for discussion in the family and society. Religion also promotes the culture of silence around sex and it imposes virginity on women rather than men. Such kind of cultural notion and peer pressure encourages men to have an experience with sex outside their marital bond. Besides in every society the individual have certain status and accordingly roles. The society is expected value-oriented action or use of value rationality to satisfy their sexual urge. The individuals' irrational action is responsible for acquiring HIV infection for both men and women who have sex outside marriage. The infection among the spouse and children affect the institution of the family. It will question the socialization of the individual in the family with regard to morality and moral values of the stability of the family. If the institution of family is affected it will bring adverse changes in the institution of economy, government, politics, education etc. In turn it affects the social health and social fabric of whole society by bringing imbalance and disequilibrium among the different parts of the social structure.

Therefore, the structural functional aspects of society are responsible for acquiring as well as spread of HIV infection in India.

Theories of anomie and alienation

According to Durkheim, the mechanical solidarity is achieved in the traditional society where the simple division of labour and the feeling of togetherness exist. But in modern society there are so many different roles to be played and so many different ways are possible. Durkheim believed that human beings are not naturally consensual. He believed that if it is left to our own devices, we are anti-social. He pointed out that during time of rapid social change people become unsure of what is expected of them, and they find it difficult to fashion their actions in terms of conventional norms. Old norms do not seem relevant to current conditions and emerging norms are too ambiguous and poorly formulated to provide effective and meaningful guidelines for behaviours. Under these circumstances, Durkheim believed, an upsurge in deviant behaviour could be expected. The individual has unlimited desires and it can be regulated by a moral force. The moral power is superior to the individual and he must accept the social and moral expectation to maintain social solidarity. But any abrupt transition such as economic disorder, industrial crisis or sudden prosperity can cause a deregulation of a normative structure. As a result the mechanism of solidarity breaks down and normlessness ensures. Durkheim called this situation as **anomie.**

For Merton, social structure consists of culturally approved goals and institutionalized means to achieve the goals. Merton defined anomie as the disjunction between cultural goal and institutionalized means. The process where by exaltation of the end generates a literal demoralization and de-institutionalization (Francis Abraham, 1981: 181). Merton identified the following five responses to the end-means dilemma and the violation of which culturally adopted means leads to anomie (Zonden 1990: 210-211).

1. **Conformity**: It exists when people accept both the cultural goals and the culturally approved means to achieve the goal. Such behaviour is the bed rock of stable society.
2. **Innovation**: The individual accepts the cultural goals but rejects the approved means.
3. **Ritualism**: It involves the abandoning or scaling down of the lofty cultural goals but accept the cultural means.
4. **Retreatism**: Rejection of both cultural goals and cultural means and without substituting new norms for them.
5. **Rebellion**: Rejection of both cultural goals and cultural means and substitute new norms for them.

According to Merton anomie refers to a property of a social system, not to the state of mind of this or that individual within the system.

The concept of **alienation** was first used by Karl Marx. For Marx, the history of mankind is not only a history of class struggle but also the increasing alienation of man. In the capitalist society, the estranged or alienated labour involves four aspects: the worker's alienation from the object he produces, from the process of production, from himself and from community of his fellow men. Marx felt that when the labours are devalued and sink to the level of commodity, he/she will *get* *al.*ienated. Marx has identified two "hostile power" which render labour and its product alien. One is the capitalist who commands production and the other is the economic system which governs the behaviour of capital and the process of production (Marx, 1964: 124).

Treating alienation from the personal standpoint of the actor Melvin Seeman found five basic ways in which the concept of alienation has been used:

1. Powerlessness,
2. Meaninglessness,
3. Normlessness,
4. Loneliness and
5. Self-estrangement (Francis Abraham, 1982: 199).

Scnacht argued that the individual may *get al.*ienated due to loneliness, exclusion from social and cultural participation, lack of identification with other's views, interests and tastes, dissatisfaction in social relations, lack of job satisfaction, feeling of powerlessness, dissociation from popular culture, dissociation from societal values, rejection of societal behavioural norms and incomprehensibility of events (Abraham, 1982: 199).

Application of theory of anomie and alienation to the present study

The contemporary society is a highly complex society. Unlike traditional society the individuals are expected to perform different roles to meet the challenges of life. As a result of urbanization, industrialization, modernization and globalization, the present society is witnessing frequent changes. Thc rapid changes taking place in the society increase the inequality with unequal distribution of wealth and means to meet the ends. It has the characteristics of materialism, consumerism, exploitation and dehumanization. Modernity eroded the faith in ethics. It has given farewell to God and its related religious faith and moral values and norms. The society became fit for the person who knows the tactics of extracting the benefit without evaluating its morality.

The people, especially the migrants, illiterates, marginalized groups including women and poor, unemployed, and the rich who always have the intention of enjoying all worldly affairs find very difficult to satisfy their needs by using conventional norms. For them, the old norms are unsuitable to earn for their livelihood and/or to satisfy their needs. The emerging new norms are too confusing and it has not helped them for their empowerment and modifies their behaviour. As a result of normlessness the individual gives more importance to fulfill his desires rather than societal expectations.

HIV/AIDS emerged and spread nook and corner of the world as a result of the risk behaviour of individual. These individuals have not given importance to culturally accepted norms in the society. Poverty and other economical crises forced some women to fulfil their goal of survival by violating culturally approved means of earning and taken prostitution as a means for survival. Their sexual involvement with different customers increases the chances of getting HIV infection.

For sex, marriage is the only means which is approved by the society. Sex outside the marriage is considered as deviant behaviour. But the migrants and the others who have sexual impulsion find prostitution as an easily available source to satisfy their sexual urge. It increases the chances of getting and spreading HIV infection. The prevailing normlessness in the society created number of deviants including drug addicts and criminals. They find lot of confusion to match their life with the new norms emerging as a result of modernization.

The survival strategy makes them frustrated and to become addicts either by using heroin or using injecting drugs. They have a false hope that it will help to forget their problems to some extent in subconscious mind. As a result of frustration, the injecting drug users often seek sex with sex workers without realizing their risk and the need for safe sex. Their unsafe sexual behaviour increases the risk of getting HIV infection not only for them but also for the sex workers. If the infected people have other sexual partner/wives or if they get married they will infect the innocent women.

The individual is not the only person responsible for the spread of HIV infections in the world. The society is responsible for individual's risk behaviour. Because the rapidly changing society has increased the gap between rich and poor and it has not distributed the resources equally to all people. The people who have more resources and who have the capacity to control the flow of resources are more powerful and they try to exploit the powerless by devaluing their rights. The present economic system also favours only to the growth and benefit of economically, socially, politically and intellectually wealthy people. The sense of powerlessness, meaninglessness, normlessness, isolation and self-estrangement of the individual causes alienation not only from himself but also from his goal, means and community and the world to a larger extent. The conflict with the present situation forces alienated individual to take another option as means to survival. The poor, poverty stricken and under privileged women who are alienated as a result of their economic suppression and domination of economically powerful people and have chosen prostitution as a alternative means for their survival. Similarly are the exploited, low skilled, unskilled and unemployed people who are involved in migration as a result of the alienation due to their devolution in the local areas. Their separation from the spouses influences them to satisfy their sexual urge through sex workers and get infection.

The infected individuals are isolated from the society. They will not get support and care from their primary relationship and they are excluded from social and cultural participation. They loose their identity with others. The infected individuals also normally develop the feelings of powerlessness and inability to influence others to get support and help. They develop the sense of feeling that their rights are denied and their life is made meaningless by the non infected and so called conservative people in the society. Their disassociation from the normal social network as a result of their infection make them to *get al.*ienated and forces them even to the extent of committing suicide.

The stigma and discrimination affects different segments of population in different ways. The revelation is based on the nature of infection. The women who got infection through their husbands will easily reveal their status to their family members rather than sex workers and who got infection through their promiscuous relationship and pre marital sex. Though the discrimination have no bond, the house wives may get little support from their parents and sympathy from their relatives, friends and neighbours.

The spread effect is more in India due to the severity of anomie among the infected individual and non-revelation of HIV status in the society.

Jurgen Habermas Neo-Conflict theories or Critical theories

Habermas argued that expecting revolution from the proletariat class in the contemporary society is meaningless. They are now a pampered class of people within the trap of the capitalist class. In such situation, Habermas puts his critical theory of communication and domination. According to Habermas, we must talk to each other in order to find common ground and establish a consensus with the others over meaning. It is because we are capable of being rational and reasonable to co-exist with others in our every day social encounters. So long as the parties to a communicative exchange have an equal opportunity to state their views, so long as they treat each other as equals and honest, the agreement on the issues can be easily obtained. In other words, so long as an encounter is approached rationally with reason, the differences can be overcome (Jones, 2005: 171).

In order to solve the problem of domination, Hebermas suggests the construction of an ideal speech community. His main point is that purposive rationality penetrates every day practices, especially every day communications. His ideal speech community has the features of

(i) all individuals capable of speech can participate in the debate,

(ii) all individuals have equal right to give their reasons for their stated position and

(iii) no individual can be denied the right to participate in the debate (Doshi, 2003: 475-76).

Application of Habermas Neo-conflict theories/ critical theories in the present study

Women are the marginalized segments in the institution of family under the domination of patriarchal culture. The domination of male over the female is also supported by the religion and the commercial economic system of the country. The women are not given much opportunity to express their opinion related to the issues which affect them adversely. As far as sexual relationship is concerned, they are denied the rights of communication with their sexual partners. The lack of communication is the major factor for the spread of infection among the women in India. The communication/information disseminated through various print and visual media has created sufficient knowledge and awareness about AIDS and its implication on the society. No doubt, the women and men have some knowledge about AIDS and its prevention. The communication between spouses or between sexual partners with regard to safe sex is essential to prevent the infection between them. Women should be given equal opportunities to state their views with regard to sex and sexuality. If male partner treat the women as equal and honest they can easily arrive consensus with regard to the use of condom as preventive method for all sexually transmitted infections.

The stigma based hidden status of HIV infection affects not only the infected individual but also their family. The infected individual undergoes traumatic experiences due to non-communication of their feelings and inflectional status either to their marital partners or to their family members. The implication of non-communication with regard to HIV infection at level of individual, family and community may bring adverse impact in the spread of infection to the larger society.

Therefore, communication at all level is the urgent need to prevent and control the rate of HIV infection in all societies.

Significance of Present Study

Women become the epicenter of HIV/AIDS epidemic in India and in almost all parts of the country, the epidemic is feminized without realizing the circumstances leading to infection. The infected women are subjected to discrimination, abuse and violence. The stigma and discrimination may affect their social interaction in the social system. The present study is undertaken to fulfill the research gap by identifying the circumstances leading to HIV/AIDS, socio-economic conditions of women infected with HIV positive, circumstances leading to prostitution, sexual behaviour after infection, changes taken place in the social interaction of the women infected with HIV positive and attitude of infected women towards pregnancy and child birth.

Chapterisation

The present study is comprised of seven chapters arranged in systematic sequence. The First chapter presents an introduction of women infected with HIV positive with a brief account of causes and consequences of HIV on women. The Second chapter presents review of literature related to the study. The Third chapter deals with the methodology adopted to conduct the present study, which includes objectives, operational definition of the concept, sampling procedure and sample size, tools of data collection and method of analysis. A comprehensive view on the global scenario of HIV/AIDS is presented in the Fourth chapter. The Fifth chapter analyses the primary data with a view to derive findings based on the objectives designed for the study. The Sixth chapter contains major findings, suggestions and conclusion of the study. The implication of research in the form of Action Plan towards prevention and control of HIV/AIDS, care and support and relief and rehabilitation of HIV/AIDS affected people with the goal of creating AIDS free society is presented in the Seventh chapter.

2

Review of Literature

It is important to mention various studies and surveys related to HIV/AIDS for making a modest attempt towards greater understanding of the issue focused. The review of literature is focused on the issues related to socio-economic factors and HIV/AIDS, high risk behaviour and HIV/AIDS, stigma and discrimination, violence against women and HIV/AIDS, reproductive health and HIV/AIDS, women's knowledge on HIV/AIDS, impact of HIV/AIDS and intervention taken by both government and non-governmental organizations.

Social and Economic Factors and HIV/AIDS

Prakasa Rao and Nandini Rao (1982: 11-37) described that in India, marriage was treated as an alliance between two families rather than a mere union of two individuals and the traditional normative patterns did not provide any opportunity to the prospective spouses to participate in the decision making process of their own marriage and it is largely arranged by parents on the basis of matching of horoscope.

Ramasamy *et al.* (1988: 179-187) have discussed the relationship between promiscuity and family pathology. They have concluded that promiscuity is deeply ingrained in the personality of the individual and is a product of early life experiences. Thus the family and its impact on the individual are very vital in determining the activities of a person.

Ryder *et al.* (1989: 1637-42) study based in Kinshasa indicates that the deprivations caused by poverty itself lead to faster development of AIDS among women, even increasing the likelihood of that their new born children will be HIV positive.

Luciano Sandala *et al.* (1994: S61-68) studied the relationship between "dry sex" practices and HIV infection in Lusaka, Zambia. A cross sectional study was carried out in a sexually transmitted diseases clinic in Lusaka among 329 women aged 15-50 years. The study identified 58% of seroprevalence among the sample but no practice was statistically significantly associated with HIV.

Alessandro Cozzi Lepri *et al.* (1995: 1151-55) have conducted a study among 854 HIV infected women and men in Italy to evaluate the influence of gender in HIV disease progression. Their findings were:

1. The risk of CD4 lymphocyte count declining below 200 was not significantly different between women and men.
2. Progression to AIDS was slightly slower among women than men. The cumulative mortality from AIDS tended to be lower in women than in men but the difference is not significant.

Gangakhedkar *et al.* (1997: 2000-92) studied the risk of HIV infection among the monogamous married women attending sexually transmitted clinics in Pune, India. The study has compared the incidence of HIV and other STDs among 525 female sex workers with 391 other women (almost all of whom were married and reported only on sexual partner) and identified that 50 per cent of sex workers and 14 per cent of other women were HIV positive. Over all, 43 per cent of the sex workers and 65 per cent of the other women were diagnosed as having one or more genital infections. The study also found that among the sex workers, HIV seropositivity was associated with inconsistent condom use, genital ulcers and genital warts. Among the other women, only having a partner who had been diagnosed with an STD predicted HIV infection. The investigators of the study reported that the married women have a belief that they are at low risk because they have only one partner. The authors concluded that an increasing proportion of women and infants in India will become infected with HIV if we have not heightened efforts to disseminate information about HIV and other STDs.

Schoultz, Ksristan Kay (1998: 1327) have undertaken an exploratory study to understand the ways in which fundamental social structures and cultural factors contribute to different levels of Sexually Transmitted Infection vulnerability in Hausa society in Niamey, Niger. The study results suggest that those Hausa men and women who express the strongest social ties to the systems and beliefs of the modern world are best equipped to protect themselves and are therefore least socially vulnerable to sexually transmitted infections, while those who maintain more traditional beliefs and practices have fewer effective resources upon which to rely for protection from infection and are therefore more socially vulnerable. Within this evolving social stratification, there are important differences between men and women which ultimately place women at an overall disadvantage relative to men in terms of social vulnerability to sexually transmitted infections. The data collected for the study suggest that until efforts are made to address the effects of the social structural and cultural factors which contribute to gender differentials in sexually transmitted infection risk, and individual-action (or "lifestyle") approach to sexually transmitted infection risk reduction is unlikely to be successful.

Rwabukwali, Charles Barwogeza, (1998: 3976) have studied the "Gender, poverty and AIDS in Kabarole, in Western Uganda" to understand and unravel the complex interaction between cultural norms and women's social and economic dependency, and how these limit Batoro women's ability to reduce their risk of HIV infection through safer sexual practices. Specially, the study aims to identify the socio-cultural and sexual behavioral pasterns that influence the vulnerability of Batoro women to increased risk of HIV infection. The study found that most of the women in the sample were complying with government advice to reduce the number of sexual partners, and to be faithful to one's spouse in order to avoid AIDS. However, a range of cultural, economic, and social factors, including gender inequality and male sexual behaviour combine to maintain women's vulnerability to HIV infection. Most women believe that their best chance of avoiding AIDS is to become economically independent of men. Therefore, the author suggested taking socio-cultural and economic factors into account when introducing AIDS control programs, and the need for co-ordination at all levels with regard to service delivery for AIDS control.

Hirve and Sathe (1999: 17) have identified that increased mobility owing to increased urbanization and industrialization is the major cause for higher vulnerability of HIV infection in the regions of Maharasthra and the increased mobility of men and their unsafe sex with sex workers increases women's vulnerability to HIV and other sexually transmitted diseases.

Martin S.L *et al.* (1999: 417-426) studied the domestic abuse in five districts of Uttar Pradesh and found that 18-45 per cent of husbands were physically abused their wives due to poverty and lack of education. Economical backwardness is taken as a tool for men to discriminate the women. The condition become worst if they are infected with HIV/AIDS.

Karen Hardee *et al.* (1999: 52-59) have studied reproductive health policies and programmes in eight countries – three in Asia (Bangladesh, India and Nepal), three in the Middle East and Africa (Jordan, Ghana and Senegal) and two in Latin America and the Caribbean (Jamaica and Peru). It is found from this study that India is targeting on specific method called female sterilization as a family planning programme since 1967. As of 1992-1993, 41 per cent of married women aged 13-49 used a method, with female sterilization accounting for 75 per cent of all modern methods of birth control. It is evident from this study that the Indian women were very conscious to avoid birth rather than infection and once they undergone sterilization they were not bothered about using condom to safeguard themselves from sexually transmitted diseases. Such behaviour among women is also one of the causes for increasing HIV infection among women in India.

Karuppaih (2000) has studied the Socio-cultural and economic correlates of HIV/AIDS in Madras City. His analysis indicated that the economically poor and illiterate and primary school educated people were more vulnerable to HIV/AIDS infection due to high risk behaviour and lack of or poor knowledge on HIV/AIDS and prevention and control measures.

Digumarti Baskara Rao (2000: 101-105) has studied the women's susceptibility to HIV epidemic. His study revealed that the most of the women who are infected by HIV are wives and other partners and these women are becoming infected through sexual transmission at a significantly younger age than men and most of the girls and young women are in their teens and early twenties. The direct function of power relations between men and women and, in particular, or men's sexual identity, illiteracy and lack of access to information are the major factors for the infection of women identified from the study.

Elizabeth Reid (2000: 120) studied the factors affecting the lives of young women which make them vulnerable to HIV infection. According to the study, the prevalence patterns of HIV infection are known to be a factor of poverty, social and geographic mobility, commerce, tourism, social disruption and civil unrest.

Myo Thani (2000: 148) argued that the poor women are severely affected by the AIDS epidemic in Southeast Asia. He says that the AIDS epidemic is becoming a women's disease for two reasons. One is, as the epidemic spreads to more areas and progresses from being a disease of a few subgroups to that of the larger population, more and more women become infected. The second is, the epidemic affects women, especially poor women due to biological, sociological and economic reasons. According to him, epidemiologically, the virus is more easily transmitted from men to women than the other way round and women frequently lack control over their own sexual lives or those of their husbands outside the marriage, even though extra marital relations, as well as intravenous drug abuse or bisexual behaviour, are possible routes for the entry of the HIV into the marital union.

The author also reported that the women's ability to insist on protected sex is affected by socio-cultural barriers to women as decision makers, limited literacy, mobility and access to information and cultural and moral attitudes towards sexuality. According to him women may not be able to discuss sexual matters in public, or even with their husbands and social and sexual passivity make insistence on the use of condoms as protection against HIV infection difficult.

Syamala Nataraj (2002: 36-40) has studied the women in prostitution in Chennai, Tamil Nadu. According to her study a prostitute does not earn only for herself; she sells sex for her children, for her family. A study conducted by her shows that over 60 per cent of the women in prostitution are dalits and 50 per cent maintain independent households. The author has concluded that continuing gender discrimination and the failure of the State to provide opportunities for women to ensure education and economic independence is the single largest factor that fuels the entry of women into prostitution.

Naomi Rutenberg (2002: 3) explored that HIV prevalence is high in communities where early age of child bearing is common. Adolescent boys and girls may place themselves at risk of HIV to realize their child bearing preference.

Kelly and Gray (2003: 446-451) studied the "age differences in sexual partners and risk of HIV-1 infection in rural Uganda" and identified the positive relationship between age of the partners and HIV infections. The study found that the risk of HIV infection doubles for adolescent women with male partners ten or more years older.

Ann E. Biddlecom, (2004: 66-67) explained that certain social, cultural and economic factors are attributed with women which make more vulnerable to HIV/AIDS. Their study shows that sexual activity tends to start earlier for women, particularly because women marry at younger ages (and therefore have more regular sexual intercourse) than men and many young women are married to much older men (often a decade or more older), who are likely to have had sex with several different partners in the past. Some of them will therefore have and STI, including HIV, and may transmit it to their young wives. Their study also reveals that women experiences sexual abuse and rape more than men and poverty push women, especially young women to risk their lives by accepting money or goods in exchange for unsafe sex.

They also stressed the importance of recognizing social constraints in combating the spread of HIV/AIDS. According to them HIV/AIDS is not a disease that individuals can prevent alone and married women have to bear much of the HIV/AIDS burden in many parts of the world, so the ABC approach (Abstain, Be faithful, use of Condom) is generally ineffective for them. Therefore, abstinence does not make sense within marriage, while monogamy and condom use require both partner's cooperation.

The Hindu (2004: November 30) has published the article of David C. Mulford, U.S Ambassador to India. The article argued that HIV/AIDS is the most serious public health a challenge facing India today and India is at critical juncture in the epidemic. The article also revealed that in India 36 per cent of the people estimated to be infected with HIV are women, and it has the potential to have much higher number in future. The same issue also shares that in sub-Saharan Africa, the proportion is 57 per cent. Young girls are particularly vulnerable and in some African communities, as many as 20 per cent of girls aged 15-19 years are infected, compared to just 5 per cent of boys the same age. World wide, almost 50 per cent of HIV positive people are women.

The report further revealed that HIV is spreading rapidly among females for many reasons. The lower status of women and girls and practices such as male infidelity, prostitution, child sexual abuse, and ex trafficking are factors. In addition, male-to-female HIV transmission during sex is twice as likely to occur as female-to-male transmission. The report also indicated that the rate of female injecting drug use, another common way HIV/AIDS is transmitted, is increasing.

The Hindu (2004: December 1) in its editorial on "Women at Risk" argued that women are being infected at an alarming rate primarily because of ignorance, socio-cultural biases, poverty and sexual abuse and violence. The report says that the vulnerability of women to HIV/AIDS is a huge challenge to the societies which have severely discriminatory attitudes towards women. It quoted the *AIDS Epidemic Update 2004* released by the Joint United Nations Programme on HIV/AIDS

(UNAIDS) and the World Health Organistions and reveled that the rise in infection is at its peak in East Asia, Eastern Europe and Central Asia and half of the infected adult population of 37.2 million people (aged 15-49) are women, marking a steady rise from 47 per cent in 1998.

The editorial further revealed that in India, 25 per cent of all newly infected are women and the increasing trend is mainly because of some states inadequate prevention efforts which allowed men to engage in high-risk behaviour to transmit the virus to women with whom they have a regular relationship. These women are often unable to negotiate safe sex, within marriage or outside, for variety of reasons including the transmission from drug injectors. According to the editorial, Chennai has on of the highest HIV prevalence rates among pregnant women in the country, and 64 per cent of drug injectors in the city were also found to be positive in 2003.

The editorial also revealed that the World AIDS Day on 2004 has been dedicated to the concerns of women. The idea is to highlight the links between gender inequality and the epidemic.

The Hindu (2004: December 5) has given an insight with regard to HIV/AIDS epidemic in India. It has revealed that the epidemic in India is no longer confined to high-risk groups or urban populations but is gradually spreading into rural areas and the general population and the younger women are most vulnerable to infection. According to the report, the number of women infected is steadily rising in India and one in every four AIDS reported is a women and 37 per cent of the cases is found among the sexually active age group of 15-29 years. Rural women are particularly vulnerable to being infected as they have less access to health care and information on HIV/AIDS. The report further says that it is the marriage, not promiscuity or other high risk behaviour makes the vast majority of the Indian women vulnerable to HIV.

National Institute of Social Defence (2004: 8) claims that married women in India are more susceptible to HIV/AIDS as they have no control over the sexual behaviour of their husbands. It further reported that increasing levels of HIV infection is found among Indian women, who, are largely in monogamous relationship. It says that these women have virtually no control over their husbands' sexual behaviour and the disease is spreading to rural areas through migrant labourers and truckers. As a large number of women become infected, the number of children infected through vertical transmission is also likely to increase, says the same report.

Kalpana Sharma (2005: 3) studied the contraceptive option available for women to avoid pregnancy and abortions in Uttar Pradesh. The study says that in theory, women are supposed to be given a choice in contraception methods, but in reality, the only choice before them is sterilization through tubectomies. According to the study the total number of sterilizations performed in U.P, 97 per cent are done on women and these sterilized women were never thinks about the need of safe sex.

Thinamalar (2005: January 1) has published that one-fourth of the new infection in India is occurred among women and 90 per cent of these women had sex only with their husbands. Therefore, majority of the married women in India have got infection through their husbands.

High Risk Behaviour and HIV/AIDS

Jeff Goodwin (1978: 17) studied cause for high risk social movements in the Huk Rebellion in Philippines during 1946-54. The study has documented "sex opportunism", which is often described as "sex problem", as a cause for high risk behaviour for the men involved in Huk Rebellion. He described that the men were unhappy without women and the substantial number of married men within the Huk movement were engaged in extra marital sexual relations with women in the Huk camps in the Sierra Madre. It shows the ground reality of men's sex and sexuality in the context of HIV/AIDS.

Potterat (1985: 329) examined the concept of susceptibility and exposure for explaining women's reasons for entering the sex industry. The susceptibility model contends that psychological characteristics (e.g. alienation, feeling of worthlessness) in conjunction with traumatic events (e.g. incest), predispose some women to the lure of prostitution. The exposure model predicts that interpersonal contact with and inducement from significant others involved in the sex industry (eg. friends, family members), lead to personal involvement.

John *et al.* (1987) has described that HIV infection has become rampant among high-risk groups in the coastal states of Maharashtra and Tamil Nadu and among injecting drug users in northeastern India including Manipur and Nagaland. Their report also showed that the spread of infection to the general population is mainly due to the unsafe behaviour of high risk groups.

Hospedales (1988: 32) study explain that heterosexual contacts could become the main source of infection and that it could therefore spread to the general population of Europe and United States. This study also revealed that many homosexuals are often also bisexual and the wives of these men are not aware of these customs and of their risk of infection.

Bongaarts (1988: 4-6) identified that the probability of infection depends on the frequency of sexual contact, prevalence of infection in the contact group, and the rate of partner change. The infectiousness of partner is a function of gender (male-to-female transmission is more efficient), stage of disease (individuals with AIDS or symptomatic HIV disease are most infectious), and the use of condoms.

Schneider (1989: 74) study showed that in the United States and Western Europe intravenous drug users (IVDU) represent a considerable fraction of all AIDS cases. In Italy 62 per cent of all HIV positive cases are found among IVDUs. In the Federal Republic of Germany the relative proportion of female AIDS cases is increasing mainly due to intravenous drug use. Of the AIDS cases among women, 57 per cent had a history of intravenous drug use. In the United States, 8 per cent of diagnosed AIDS cases are among women. Half of these are caused by drug use and 21 per cent of them were sexual partners of drug users.

Bhave *et al.* (1992) report revealed that the seroprevalence is raising among high risk groups, particularly among sex workers. Her survey showed the increasing trend of seropositivity among sex workers by one per cent of infection among sex workers in 1987, 18 per cent in 1990 and 34 per cent in 1992. The survey result revealed the potential risk of spreading HIV infection among general population by increasing the infection rate among women attending antenatal clinics.

Elford *et al.* (1993) has said that the predominant mode of infection in India is heterosexual intercourse. Their article also revealed that India has to face severe impact due to HIV/AIDS as a result of its population growth.

Thomas Cox and Bal. K. Suvedi (1994: 7) have studied the sexual networking in five urban areas in the Nepal Terai. Epidemiological evidence suggests that the principal route of AIDS transmission is heterosexual with commercial sex fueling the current spread of HIV in Nepal. According to their study, high prevalence of sexually transmitted diseases (STDs) and low rates of condom use facilitates HIV transmission in Nepal. In addition, lack of public awareness, related to the country's low rate of literacy, a shortage of appropriate AIDS education message, and strong cultural prohibitions against the public discussion of sex further contribute to the problem. This study also identified that the transport workers are the major clients of sex workers and because of their mobility they became the core group of potential transmitters of HIV.

Jeanette J. Rodrigues *et al.* (1995: 723-25) have studied the risk factors for HIV infection in people attending clinics for sexually transmitted diseases in India among 2800 patients in Pune, India. The study has concluded that in India the prevalence of HIV infection is alarmingly high among female sex workers and men attending clinics for sexually transmitted diseases. It also found high prevalence of HIV infection in monogamous, married women who denied any history of sex working. The study also revealed that high risk sexual behaviour, including lack of condom use and high number of sexual partners are the main cause for the infection of STDs. The dramatic increase in prevalence of HIV-1 in these high risk groups suggests there is an urgent need for comprehensive and national efforts in India to control sexually transmitted diseases and to provide intensive education on HIV and AIDS targeted at changing high risk behaviour.

Hardman (1997: 20) argued that economic vulnerability force women into streets and he also stated that because of women's restricted access to financial and material resources, some women may resort to prostitution as a resistance or response to poverty. In other wards, according to the author, prostitution may be viewed as an active coping strategy in the face of privation.

APAC (1998: 25) has studied the community prevalence of sexually transmitted disease in Tamil Nadu among 2000 people (both male and female) in three districts of Tamil Nadu. The study has concluded that (i) the prevalence of any STD condition in Tamil Nadu was 15.8% and this fell in the high endemic rate for the community and the classical STD remains 9.7% in the study community. (ii) The age group maximum at risk for any STD was 30-39 years. (iii) Prevalence of HIV among women was higher than men. (iv) While all STD were widely prevalent in both rural and urban population, HIV appear to be more prevalent in the rural areas than in urban. (v) Genital discharge and sexual complaints were very common and were reported in upto 38% of the population.

Pottert (1998: 333-40) examined the sequences and timing of prostitution entry and drug use among the women involved in prostitution. The study showed that among the regular drug users, 66 per cent use drug prior to entering prostitution, for 18 per cent drug use and prostitution occurred concurrently and 17 per cent take drug following their entry into prostitution.

APAC (1998) report on third wave surveillance survey among 558 respondents of various risk groups in Tamil Nadu revealed the marital status of the people who had multiple sex partners. The report shows that the majority of the sex workers are married and the level of illiteracy was high among sex workers. Majority of the commercial sex workers are engaged in full-time sex trade. Women engaged in occupation like vegetable/ fruits vendors, house-maid, construction workers, workers in film industry, person in other petty trades also practises commercial sex and they constituted 53% of the commercial sex workers respondents. Majority of the unmarried female factory workers (44.8%), male factory workers (48%), truckers

(42.8%) and helpers 42.8%) are found to be unmarried in this survey. These high risk groups are the potential sources for spreading the dreaded virus HIV into the general population.

APAC report on Sixth Wave with regard to HIV Risk Behaviour Surveillance Survey among 6195 high risk population in Tamil Nadu and 4980 in Pondicherry has captured certain salient findings in which the truckers and helpers perceive that sex with casual partners is not risky and there is an emotional relationship with casual partners and sex becomes more enjoyable without condoms. They also perceive that AIDS is curable as lot of advertisements in the recent days are promoting on remedies. Besides, as far as commercial sex workers are concern that they have perceived that having sex without condom with regular partners is not risky. The intravenous drug users perceived that their involvement in drug decrease their sexual potency and therefore they involved in paid sex. The men seeking sex with men perceived that sex with men is not risky and it is safe and no need of using condom

Krishnamurthy *et al.* (1998: 39-48) study on HIV/AIDS and Safe Sex Practices among Female Sex workers in India is an exploratory study and it explored the profile of female sex workers and their sex practices. As per the study result the female sex workers had a mean age of 31.23 years and more than 60 per cent of them were married. The number of respondents married and living with their husband was almost equal to those respondents were unmarried. Illiteracy is the common features and they had no sources of income other than commercial sex. The study also revealed that the commercial sex workers are part of the floating population in many towns, especially where commercial sex activity is seasonal. Many commercial sex workers go to tourist centers, places of pilgrimage and large towns. The commercial sex workers interviewed for this study engage in different patterns of soliciting as all of them move around in different places. The brothel based commercial sex workers reportedly used public places for direct soliciting. However, 52 per cent of the commercial sex workers reported that soliciting is done at bus stands, 36.3 per cent from the streets and 33.4 per cent from other public places like railway stations, parks beaches, temples and cinema theatres. Indirect soliciting was through pimps, 16.3 per cent through brothel keepers, three per cent through auto drivers, clients, friends and relatives and through phone calls 18.4 per cent. It was found that most of the commercial sex workers did not feel it necessary to use condoms with regular partners and they used to have a sexual intercourse with clients though they have symptoms of infections.

Lakshmi Bai *et al.* (1998: 59-64) study on "High Risk Behaviour" stated that many men knowingly or out of sheer ignorance pursues such risks unmindful of the consequences. Hetero-sexuality is one such risky activity where man indulges for temporary pleasure. This illicit or extra marital indulgence is an open invitation to a dreaded scourge, may be STD or AIDS or it may be both, which would ruin him physically and mentally. These groups are not only exposed to this risk but are also spreading these diseases to their wives and children and other sexual partners. This group consists of truck drivers and their associates who stay away from the warmth of their family for week operating goods transport services from one end of the country to another.

Benedict B.B. Naanen (1999) has studied the women involved in prostitution in "Itinerant Gold Mines" of Cross River Basin of Nigeria. He concluded that colonialism, under-development, class kinship and sexual exploitations, and a tradition of sexual freedom contributed in varying degrees to increase cross river prostitution in Nigeria. He identified very poor knowledge on safe sexual practices among the women involved in sex work in Nigeria. According to Naanen, the unsafe sexual practices among the women in prostitution and their sexual partners increase the chance for spreading the sexually transmitted diseases like STD/HIV/AIDS through the river basin of Nigeria.

Vijaya Srinivasan (1999: 5) summerised the risk factors predisposing individuals to STD infections including HIV infections. The major factors are female gender, age at first intercourse, number of sex partners, sex with low paid sec workers, high level of partner mixing through a core group of infected transmitters and heavy petting and foreplay. Besides, low socio-economic status, drug abuse and presence of other intercurrent STD conditions, poor treatment seeking behaviour of the STD patients also increases HIV positive status and reinfection among STD core groups. According to the author, the asymptomatic groups are an independent cohort which poses special threat to the community in spread of STD infections.

Jagatheeswary, *et al.* (2000) have studied the relationship between HIV and STD. They have conducted the study among patients attending the STD clinic at the Governmental Central Hospital in Chennai between January 1993 and September 1997. The study revealed that the incidence of HIV among STD patients has been increasing since 1992 (from 8% to 14.2%). This study also revealed that the incidence is higher in male than in female.

Sivaramamurthy *et al.* (2000) have studied the sexuality, sexual behaviour and awareness about HIV/AIDS among rural men near Salem, Tamil Nadu. This study found that most of the men are enjoyed paid sex and among them many have the perception of having sex with virgin girl will cure AIDS. It also revealed that the men have first sexual experience with women other than their wife and pre marital and extra marital affairs are prevalent among the rural men in Salem. It is also identified from the study that as the educational level increases, the age at which the first sexual encounter also increases and even though 99% of men are aware of AIDS, only 18.2% know all methods of transmission and 37.9% do not know anything about modes of transmission.

Panda *et al.* (2000) studied the transmission of HIV from injecting drug users to their wives in Manipur in India in 1996. HIV status was determined by ELISA test and found that positive association between injecting drug users and HIV positive status of their wives. The study identified 45% of the injecting drug users wives were HIV positive and only 15% of the couples reported regular usage of condoms during intercourse. The researcher suggested improved control of STDs, condom promotion, and improved blood screening in Manipur to control the spread of HIV among the wives of injecting drug users.

Praveen Sethi (2000) has studied the relationship between tourism and prostitution. According to Praveen Sethi sex tourism is a major component of International travel to South-east Asia and has been given both overt and covert encouragement by government as a source of foreign exchange. His study explored that many tourist from western countries are visiting to South-east Asian countries just to enjoy sex and the control of sexuality is vested with the men of foreign travellers. The women in sex work have no power and the controlling mechanisms on sexuality are dominated by masculinity. It lead to unsafe sexually practices which is the main route cause for the transmission and the spread of HIV/AIDS. The sex tourism is the main cause for the spread of HIV in South-east Asian countries, especially in Thailand.

Joyce V. Lyons (2000: 79) studied the behaviour patterns of Thai long-haul truck drivers and identified that they use to take amphetamines (in pill form) and alcohol and engage in sex with sex workers to release the amphetamine effect. These long-hauls truck drivers have belief that sleeping with prostitutes in brothels is perfectly natural and their habits of drinking alcohol make the prostitutes find very difficult to convince the truckers to use condoms. The study has concluded that long-haul truck drivers behaviour exposed them to a significant risk of contracting the HIV and they are the core group to transmit the virus to their wives and to the general population.

Richa Singh (2001: 1944) has identified that marginalized groups, living in economically unstable/disadvantageous social settings have been particularly vulnerable to HIV/AIDS infection. He has studied one such vulnerable group workers in Wazirpur Industrial area, New Delhi. He identified that the most of the workers are migrants, particularly from Bihar, Uttar Pradesh, Madya Pradesh, Orissa, Nepal and West Bengal and they are working as a casual labourers in temporary jobs. Among them majority of them were from rural areas and they stay far away from their families, living with friends and relatives or kins from their village. They often speak about their loneliness and anxieties of being away from their families. The author has argued that social identities are important determines of sexual behaviour and the notion of masculinity, i.e., "being man" forces the workers to involve in instable sexuality–sex with multiple sexual partners which heightens not only their vulnerability to HIV/AIDS infection and also their womenfolk.

Dinesh Varma (2004) has reported the Behaviour Surveillance Survey (BSS) conducted by AIDS Prevention and Control Project (APAC) run by Voluntary Health Service in Chennai, Tamil Nadu. The survey covered a sample of 1,600 men students and 6,000 women students in schools and colleges of Madurai, Coimbatore, Salem, Vellore and Nagercoil. According to the survey, though the urban youth seemed to have a clear idea of the risk of paid sex, they have low risk perception of having sex with casual partners. The survey also found that the school drops and youth in urban slums are engaged in "high-risk" behaviour by spending money on commercial sex workers.

Rochelle Dalla (2004: 190) has identified the positive relationship between childhood sexual abuse and prostitution in her study entitled "I fell off (the mothering) track: Barriers to effective mothering among prostituted women". The study revealed that childhood sexual abuse results in separating emotions from sexual activity on the victims begins to view herself as debased, the process referred to as "mortification of self". It facilitates her identification with prostitution.

Krishnamuthy (2005: 5) has conducted a study with AIDS Prevention and Control (APAC) to assess the prevalence of sexually transmitted infections in Tamil Nadu and identified the prevalence rate of 10.6 per cent in the State. The study shows that the prevalence of sexually transmitted infection among men was 9.2 per cent and women was 11.5 per cent. Asymptomatic infections were high among both sexes. The infection rate among two high risk groups – prostitution and truckers and helpers showed that the STI prevalence in the first group was 56 per cent and it was 15 per cent in the latter group. The study showed the need to track emerging misconceptions and counter them through multiple channels of communication.

Ramya Kannan (2005: 8) has reported the outcome of the research conducted by Chennai Corporation AIDS Prevention and Control Society between April 2002 and March 2005. It has surveyed 3,699 street children in Chennai, of whom 409 had to be treated for STD. It also identified two children (one boy and one girl) as HIV positive. According to the study, living on and off the streets is the biggest risk factor for children to acquire sexually transmitted infection. It also revealed that children sleeping on the streets at night are sexually abused periodically by strangers which led to the infection of STD.

Stigma and Discrimination

Jacob *et al.* (1987: 412-413) have indicated that the social stigma not only affectthe life of the patient profoundly but also cause serious problems for those with whom the patient has personal, intimate, familial and occupational ties.

Richard W Goodgame (1990: 383-389) has explained some important cultural factors which made hindrance in revealing HIV status to the infected persons in Uganda. This is due to the feeling that providing this information is cruel in the cultural context. Africans are averse to talk about death or dying. Another cause for concern about informing patients of their diagnosis is the fear of an adverse reaction such as suicide or a decision to spread the infection purposefully. Therefore, according to him considering cultural factor is important in dealing with the social dimension of any disease.

Young *et al.* (1991: 777-986) have studied the effect of family structure on the sexual behaviour of adolescents and they found significant relationship between parents / single parent family and the adolescent sexual behaviour such as age at first sex experience, frequency of intercourse and the level of sexual activity. It is commonly noticed that the influence on the child by both the parents is greater and stronger when compared with that of a single parent.

McEwan (1992: 577-584) and Jemmolt *et al.* (1993: 41-53) have investigated sexual behaviour under the influence of alcohol and the relationship between drinking habits and unsafe sex. They have shown in their study that alcohol and drug users during sexual activity are predictors of the HIV risk related behaviour. Their study revealed that there is a significant relationship between alcohol and unprotected coitus and failure to use condoms. Therefore, in the socio-cultural context, it is observed that the various habits formed during different stages of one's life influence the total attitude of a person including his /her inclination to sex.

Francois-Xavier Bagnoud Center for Health and Human Rights (1995: 10-36) has given many conditions under human rights perspectives which can influence a person's well-being. Such conditions include access to medical services and access to healthy physical, biological and social environment. According to this center, discrimination and lack of respect for human rights and dignity are the root cause of the HIV/AIDS pandemic. Therefore, the center has suggested perceiving the health action programmes under human right perspectives in the context of HIV/AIDS. It also stated that HIV prevention and care for HIV infected people and people with AIDS are closely related activities. So, caring for HIV infected people includes counseling and support to help to prevent further transmission of HIV.

Machika TANNO, *et al.* (1997: 223) have conducted a case study to identify the agony of a family of AIDS patients. From the experiences of the study, the agony of the family was summarized as below:

1. Fear of Infection.
2. Fear of being known to others.
3. Damage to family bondage.
4. Fear of being neglected by nurses.

Reid and Jeanette Brown (1998: 971) studied the emotional impact of two young women whose mothers are HIV- infected. The researcher say that because of the stigma and prejudices attached to HIV/AIDS, it appeared that young people who lived in families affected by HIV/AIDS were susceptible to psychological distress and may have been in need of special services. The study came out with the finding that young peo0ple affected by HIV/AIDS were significantly emotionally impacted. Some of the more imposing manifestations of the emotional impact were anger, depression, withdrawal, anxiousness, fear, shame, helplessness, and hopelessness. The emotional impact was also manifested in behaviour problems such as violent behaviour, combativeness and non-compliance with authority figures and truancy from school. The narrative analyses of the study revealed five distinct themes or patterns that reflected these young women's life experiences. The themes that emerged were: emotional distress, wall of silence, mother/daughter relationship issues, physical problems and school problems. The major recommendations from this study were for mental health services such as family counseling, support groups for HIV-infected parents, and peer support groups for the young people affected by HIV/AIDS to be provided through a community mental health clinic.

Francis Lobo (1999: 3) argued that the stigma of HIV/AIDS is intensified because of the behavioural actions (example, sexual and drug activities linked to morality and sin) and the illness progression (example, debilitating, disfiguring and fatal manifestations) associated with the disease. According to him these conditions lead people who are diagnosed with HIV/AIDS or who are significant others of people with the illness to experience severe social distancing. In the case of multiple stigma, social distance is added with each successive stigma which led to feelings of emotional and social isolation.

Jocop K. John (2000) from Christian Medical College, Vellore, Tamil Nadu has studied the problems faced by the infected people in the society. The study identified many personal and social implications due to HIV/AIDS. The issues such as death, sex, drug abuse etc. have been associated with significant psychological and social distress. It is found from the study that most individual with HIV/AIDS consider suicide is a best means to escape from the societal discrimination and stigma.

Meena Gopal (2000: 7-8) has studied gender and disease in India. Her study concluded that because of gender implication women who are diseased has to undergo greater suffering both in the house and in the community. In the case of communicable diseases, the women were more stigmatized and they were isolated often from all activities within the household such as cooking, child-care etc.

Tokunbo Simbowale Osinubi (2003: 32) studied the people attitudes towards the prevalence of HIV/AIDS and their perception towards AIDS victims in Ibadan, Southwestern Nigeria. The study was carried out among 2,500 household and revealed that most of the respondents do not believe in the existence of the HIV virus or AIDS. Most of them do not have adequate knowledge on how the virus is contracted, spread and how to avoid it. Most of them believe that the AIDS or HIV virus can be contracted through social contact like eating, conversing and associating with an AIDS patient. This belief has an adverse impact on the sexual relations in families with AIDS victims.

Ann E. Biddlecom *et al.* (2004: 66-67) expresses that women who test for HIV infection may face serious consequences from husbands and partners – stigma, rejection, domestic violence and economic reperc-ussions, including those related to inheritance and divorce. They also reported that fear of these consequences my keep women from seeking testing and thus help the virus to spread and many women are still on the short end of the ARV receiving line.

The Hindu (2004: December 5) published the study on discrimination against women with HIV/AIDS which is sponsored by UNIFEM and jointly conducted by CFAR and a Positive Women's Network, Chennai in 2002 in three districts of south India – Kerala, Karnataka and Tamil Nadu. The study revealed that the stigma and discrimination appeared on top of the list of problems with women facing harassment and violence within and without family. The study also revealed that the women are negatively impacted by humiliation at both individual level – within the marital and natal homes – and lack of programmatic responses from the States have driven women to destitution. According to the study, torture by in-laws, rejection by parents and denial of property rights to positive women worsened the situation.

Besides, outside the family, the reluctance of the community to let positive women rent property or use community property while performing last rites were listed out as most commonly faced problems by the women infected with HIV positive in this study.

Meena Menon (2005: 13) argued that the poor services provided by the hospitals influenced higher suicidal rate among the HIV positive patients in Mumbai hospitals. She says that there are two reasons for these suicides. One is people feel that they will not be cured and there is a feeling of neglect by the hospital staff. Another one is that there is a psychological breakdown to induce the people with HIV positive to get suicide.

George Paul (2005) described that the HIV/AIDS patients are discriminated by the doctors due to the most outrageous attitude of refusing treatment on the perception that they are going to die anyway. He also described that the discriminatory practices in the health care sector leads to hiding of HIV status by the patients while taking treatment in the hospitals.

Violence Against Women and HIV/AIDS

Friedlan *et al.* (1991: 144) studied the survival status of AIDS patients in United States and found poor survival of women than men due to poor use of antiretroviral treatment.

Fleming *et al.* (1993: 61) reported that the half of the HIV cases in the developing world are women and most of them are belong to ethnic and racial minorities. Social, economic and cultural discrimination against the minority groups facilitated the infection of HIV/AIDS.

Deepa Punia *et al.* (1996: 17) described the sexual victimization of women, young girls and female children. In their article they argued that the female children are abused and discriminated at every step and as a result they their physical, social and psychological developments were adversely affected in several ways. According to them, in every day many women were subjected to rape, kidnap, abduction, eve-teasing, molestation etc. and many women face such sexual atrocities from their men either within the family or close to their family.

Risa Deneberg (1997: 2-4) found strong association between sexual abuse including abuse in childhood and risk of HIV infection for women. According to the author, childhood sexual abuse was significantly associated with: use of intravenous drug use, exchange of sex for drugs, money or shelter, higher number of sexual partners and have a sexual relationship with a person at high risk for HIV. The report further revealed that the HIV positive women have to face increased risk of domestic violence as a result of her HIV status.

Martin (1999: 1967) studied the relationship between the domestic violence and reproductive behavioural health variables in five districts of Uttar Pradesh. The data on spousal abuse were collected in 1995-96 from 6,695 married men aged 15-65 years. Significant bivariate associations were found between abuse and reproductive health and behaviour variables. It is found that the variables of men who had pre and extra marital sex, STD symptoms, not practicing condom and experienced an unplanned pregnancy have strongest association with nonconsensual sex followed by physical abuse and then by forced sex.

Martin (1999: 44) studied the cause for physical and sexual abuse of women in the marital life in five districts of Uttar Pradesh and data on spousal abuse were collected in 1995-96 a part of a survey on male reproductive health that included 6,695 married men aged 15-65 years. The study has identified significant association between wife abuse and reproductive health behaviour of husband. The study also found significant association between poverty, low education and abuse of women by their husbands.

News Today (2002: February 10) reported that violence against women is increasing in India in the form of rape including custodial rape and trafficking of women. The report also says that custodial offence is increasing in India and sex workers are the main victims.

Nahid Tobia, *et al.* (2004: 19) studied female genital mutilation/cutting (FGM/C) and described that it is a traditional social practice that involve cutting or removing parts of the external genitalia of girls or young women. They reveal that the purposes of the practices of FGM are cultural: a rite of passage to womanhood and of curbing female sexuality and it is practiced predominantly and in various forms in at least 25 African countries and some Asian communities. According to them FGM is associated with both long term and short term health complications. The short term effects can includes great pain, excessive bleeding, infection and shock, most due to unsanitary conditions, failed procedures by inexperienced circumcisers and inadequate medical services afterward. Long term complication includes urinary tract infections and painful sexual intercourse and its related problems including STD and HIV/AIDS.

Anandhi Subramanian (2004: 4) argued that one in three women throughout the world will suffer violence in her lifetime. She will be beaten, raped, assaulted, trafficked, harassed or forced to submit to harmful practices such a female genital mutilation and in majority of the cases, the abuser will be a member of the woman's own family or someone known to her. According to her violence against women is pandemic that knows no boundaries of culture, geography, age or wealth and the abuse of women stems from a multiplicity of cultural circumstances influenced by power relations which is inherent in social structure and is reinforced by politics.

Ranjita Biwas (2005: 4) found that trafficking of women and girls is a major problem in eastern India. Her articles reveal that feminization of poverty has blurred the line between what is right and what is wrong even for the women involved and in majority of the cases the girls are trafficked by known persons, relatives, lovers, and even family members. Her report found that 75 per cent of the trafficked women have direct link with the traffickers and it explored that the main method of coercion which includes kidnapping, promises of jobs in cities and false marriage. Natural disasters will also increases trafficking of women and girls due to poverty and death of parents and these women have no voice to insist safe sex.

Reproductive Health and HIV/AIDS

Frances A. Althaus (1997: 130-39) has discussed the female circumcision, which is practiced in 28 countries in North Africa in the context of human rights and reproductive health.

According to his study, female circumcision is practiced in male dominated society with a view to control female sexuality and fertility.

Laurie Schwab Zabin and Karungari Kiragu (1998: 210-32) have reviewed the literature on health consequences of adolescent sexual behaviour and child bearing in sub-Saharan Africa, and the social and cultural context in which they occur. Their article has explained the most reproductive health problems experienced by adolescents. They argued that because of age related customs (for example, female circumcision and early marriage) or age-related vulnerability (for example, to economic pressure and to male domination), the health problems are often exacerbated among adolescents. The article also reveals that the biological and social factors often create excess risk for adolescence. Declining ages at menarche are likely to contribute to increase reproductive health risk for young women, whether in the context of traditional early marriage and childbearing or in the context of growing rates of out-of-wedlock sexual activity, sexually transmitted diseases and abortion.

Young Mi Kim (1998: 4-11) have studied the women's ability to take decision with regard to the adoption of contraception in 25 service deliver sites in Kenya. The study has adopted structured observation techniques followed by counseling sessions. The result of the study revealed that many of the women in marital life have very poor knowledge on their reproductive health and they have little choice to choose contraceptive methods to avoid birth. The study also revealed that these women have better knowledge on oral contraception rather than condom which is suggested both for family planning and prevention of sexually transmitted diseases.

John C. Caldwell *et al.* (1998: 149) studied the adolescent sexuality and reproduction in the changing world. The study results revealed that the adolescent women's sexual behaviour has changed from the traditional sexual behaviour as a result of massive economic, institutional and social changes in the context of global economy and society. The Western concept of companionate heterosexual relations before and during marriage is getting more popular as a result of globalization which brought easy movements of films, magazine, novels and girls are more affected by these influences than the boys, and wives more than husbands.

Karen Hardee *et al.* (1999: S2-3) evaluated the reproductive health policies and programmes in eight countries such as Bangladesh, India, Nepal, Jordan, Ghana, Senegal, Jamaica and Peru. The evolution report revealed that while all countries have adopted the ICPD definition of reproductive health and all have initiated policy reforms to reflect a new focus, less has been accomplished in implementing integrated reproductive health programmes. Several challenges are faced by all countries including improving knowledge and support among stakeholders, planning for integration and decentralized services, developing human resources, improving quality of care and maintaining a long-term perspective regarding the implementation of the Cairo agenda.

Susheela Singh *et al.* (2000: 21-28) have studied the gender differences in the timing of first intercourse in 14 countries throughout the world. According to the authors, early initiation of intercourse and the context within which sexual activity begins are key indicators of adolescents' potential risk for unplanned pregnancy, abortion and sexually transmitted diseases. The study has collected data from nationally representative surveys of reproductive behaviour of 15-19 year old boys and girls. The result of the study showed that in most countries, roughly one-third or more of teenage women have had sexual intercourse, in four countries (Ghana, Mail, Jamaica and Great Britain) about three in five are sexually experienced. Between about one-half and three-quarters of adolescent males in seven countries have ever had intercourse, but the proportion is one-third or less in Ghana, Zuimbabwe, the Philippines and Thailand. In most countries, sexual intercourse during the teenage years occurs predominantly outside marriage among men but largely within marriage among women.

Evasius K. Bauni *et al.* (2000: 69-80) studied the adoption of family planning and sexual behaviour of women at the age group of 18-39 years through focus group discussion in Nakuru district,

Kenya. The researcher argued that the twin risks of unwanted pregnancy and HIV/AIDS infection remain central concerns of reproductive health programmes. The findings of the study reflected that:

(i) The presence of STDs is increasing in the study area and the study groups have estimated that the prevalence of STDs within the range of three to seven persons infected out of every ten residents.

(ii) Many infected men seek treatment without their partners' knowledge.

(iii) It is estimated that every ten homes, seven will have a girl or woman who has experienced an unwanted pregnancy.

(iv) Although knowledge of condoms is widespread in the study area, their acceptability and use is not so widespread.

(v) Most married couples are not using condom due to opposition by spouse.

(vi) The women in the study area believed that condoms are known and used by men in their extra marital affairs and if they insist it in the marital life, the person would be considered promiscuous.

(vii) Condom use and disposal is embarrassing for many married women.

(viii) Many women have no idea to protect them from the risk of HIV/AIDS and they have justified their passive response with their husbands.

Nancy L. Sloan *et al.* (2000: 55-58) studied the STD and the ability of women to understand the symptoms of STD in developing countries. The result of the study showed that they women are less able to recognize the symptoms of STD and its risk factors.

Kim Best (2001: 8-10) has analysed the reproductive behaviour of women in some African countries including Zimbabwe and Yaounde. The analysis showed that about third of the HIV infected mothers passes the virus to their newborns without taking treatment. Because, most HIV infected women do not know their HIV status before they conceive and some prepare pregnancy even if they know their HIV status due to their desire to have children which is rooted in social system with regard to motherhood. The analysis also revealed the antiretroviral drug is beyond the reach of many women during pregnancy to prevent mother to child transmission and they also depend breast feed for their babies which provide another root of transmission for children.

Kim Best (2001: 12) studied the fertility status of HIV infected women in sub-Saharan Africa and identified lower fertility rate among the HIV infected women than the uninfected women. The study revealed that many women, due to their HIV status, may abstain from sexual relations, use contraception or have abortions to avoid giving birth to children.

The Hindu (2002: November 17) reported the Behavioural Surveillance Survey (BSS) carried out by the Central Government of India in 2000-01. The report revealed that overall awareness about HIV/AIDS among young people in the reproductive age group (15-49 years) was 76.1 per cent, higher among men than among women and also better known in cities than villages. The same report further revealed that only around one-third of rural women in Bihar, Gujarat, Uttar Pradesh, Madhya Pradesh and West Bengal ere aware of the disease.

ICPD–The International Conference of Population and Development (2004: 11) defined reproductive health as a state of complete physical, mental and social well being and not merely the absence of disease or infirmity, in all maters relating to the reproductive system and to its functions and processes. According to ICPD, reproductive health therefore implies that people are able to have a satisfying and safe sex life and that they have the capability to reproduce and the freedom to decide if, when and how often to do so. "Implicit in this last condition are the right of men and women to be informed and to have access to safe, effective, affordable and acceptable methods of family planning of their choice, as well as other method of their choice for regulation of fertility which are not against the law, and the right of access to appropriate health-care services that will enable women to go safely through pregnancy and child birth and provide couples with the best chance of having a healthy infant.

ICPD also defined reproductive health care in the line of above definition. It defined reproductive health care as the constellation of methods, techniques and services that contribute to reproductive health and well-being by preventing and solving reproductive health problems. It also includes sexual health, the purpose of which is the enhancement of live and personal relations, and not merely counseling and care related to reproduction and sexually transmitted diseases.

Any Coen and Geeta Rao Gupta (2004: 15) described that gender equality cannot be achieved without honoring reproductive rights. According to them, gender inequality compromises women's sexual and reproductive autonomy. They also felt that women must depend on men for food or shelter because they have no property or inheritance rights under law and the resulting power imbalance makes it impossible to demand safe sex or make other reproductive choice for women.

Feffrey O'Malley (2004: 60-62) has stressed the importance of integration of Sexual and Reproductive Health and Rights (SRHR) services and HIV/AIDS issues and its related programmes. The author projected that the overwhelming majority of HIV infections are sexually transmitted or associated with pregnancy and breastfeeding, so both HIV prevention and SRHR efforts must focus on sexuality and reproduction. He also expressed that both sexual and reproductive ill health and HIV are rooted in the same social pathologies, including unequal gender relations, sexual violence, and discrimination against sexual minorities, conflict and poverty.

Amanda Kolburn Kawal and Lynn Blinn Pike (2004: 377) examined the role of older siblings in protecting adolescents from engaging in unsafe sexual practices. The study has included 297 participants with the age of 17 years from Midwestern high school. The result of the study showed that siblings discussion about safe sex in conjunction with parental discussion predicted better attitude towards safe sexual practices for adolescents which include safe sex, self-efficacy for refusing sex, self-efficacy for communication about condom use and self-efficacy for buying and using condom.

Women's Knowledge on HIV/AIDS

Singh and Malavia (1990: 103) has conducted a survey among female sex workers in Delhi in 1998 and identified very low per centage (5%) of awareness on AIDS and usage of condom (20%). The same study also identified increased awareness on AIDS (70%) and usage of condom (70%) after intervention programmes.

Chuttani (1991: 20-22) conducted a survey among 669 men and 829 women in the villages in and around Delhi and Haryana. The study identified very less awareness (12%) on HIV/AIDS among the women than men (50%).

National Family Health Survey (1993: 2-3) explains the Knowledge of AIDS among the women of Tripura State, India. The report shows that the knowledge of the existence of Acquired Immuno Deficiency Syndrome (AIDS) is limited in Tripura. Only 13% of the ever married women age 13-49 have heard about AIDS, the per centage of misconceptions about different ways of getting AIDS ranges from 35% who think that it can be contracted from shaking hands with some one with AIDS, 82% have thought that AIDS can be contracted thought mosquito , flea, or bud bug bites. 41% of women have thought it is curable and 3% have believed that and AIDS vaccine exists. Only 30% correctly thought that AIDS can be avoided by using condoms during intercourse and 35% have thought that it can be prevented by practicing safe sex. Others modes of avoidance of AIDS such as checking blood prior to transfusion, sterilizing needles and syringes for injections and avoiding pregnancy when infected with AIDS are mentioned by only 13% of fewer women who have heard about AIDS.

McGrath (1993: 55) study on AIDS and the urban family showed that many women were not aware of their sexual partner's HIV infection. This lack of knowledge may be attributed partly to reluctance in AIDS patients to acknowledge their illness themselves or disclose it to their wives.

Gladys Baingana *et al.* (1995: S32) have assessed the knowledge of a partner's AIDS diagnosis, perceived risk of HIV infection, need for HIV testing and future support plans among women partners of male Ugandan AIDS patients. They have conducted a cross-sectional descriptive survey at New Mulago Hospital, Kamala, Uganda among wives of 177 male AIDS patients in 1992. The study revealed that many women are not aware of the risk of getting infection from their male partners. Their survey also identified that an overwhelming majority of subjects (88%) were not aware of their husbands or main sexual partner's infection status. The study also identified the significant relationship between women's financial independence and their knowledge about their sexual partner's HIV infection status. The findings suggested that the women's economic liberation of women should be considered as an important factor for HIV prevention.

Geeta Bhave *et al.* (1995: S21-25) have studied the level of knowledge on HIV and use of condoms among the sex workers in Bombay with a view to develop and test HIV intervention programmes targeting sex workers and madams in the brothels of Bombay. In a controlled intervention trial, with the measurements before and after the intervention, 334 sex workers and 20 madams were recruited from an intervention site, and 207 and 17, respectively from a similar control site, in red light areas of Bombay. The study found that the base line level of knowledge about HIV and experience with condoms was extremely low among both sex workers and madams. But after intervention, the use of condom level has increased and they were willing to refuse clients who would not use them. But in the same time they were concerned about losing business if condom use was insisted upon. This study also confirmed high rate of HIV prevalence among female sex workers in Bombay. They stressed the strengthening the intervention programmes with regard to condom use to prevent and control the transmission of HIV and sexually transmitted diseases.

Banatuvala (1995: 104) studied the causes for increasing the risk of HIV infection among heterosexual men and women. According to the study, lack of awareness with regard to infection status of the infected people increases the risk of spreading infection to the general population.

Rajkumar (1996: 13) carried out a survey to assess the awareness about HIV/AIDS among women in different population sub groups and identified low level of knowledge in Tamil Nadu and Maharastra were the infection is high.

Thomas William (1996: 33) studied the HIV/AIDS awareness among 80 college students of North Arcot Ambedkar District of Tamil Nadu. The study has revealed that the male students have good knowledge on the general aspects of AIDS (prevention and control) and the female have insufficient knowledge both on the basic preventive aspects of the disease.

Hirve and Sathe (1997: 17) have surveyed 4976 women of currently married and in the age group of upto 47 years in the rural areas of three rural coastal districts of Western Maharashtra, an area with a high potential for spread of HIV/AIDS. According to their study only 35% of women were aware about AIDS, and among them knowledge about sexual route of transmission was the most common (75%) followed by the use of contaminated needles and blood transfusion (40%). Mother to child transmits was mentioned only by about 15%. This study showed that age had an inverted 'U' shaped statistically significant relationship with AIDS awareness, with awareness of AIDS being lower in the younger and the higher in the higher age group. A statistically significant increasing trend in awareness about AIDS was seen with increasing literacy levels. According to the study, television played a major role in conveying information about AIDS to the public in general and women in particular.

Suresh K Anjum (1998: 21) has cited the survey conducted by the U.S. based East-West Center with regard to knowledge of HIV/AIDS among Indian women. According to the article, 30,000 married women were interviewed by the organisations and the report of the survey showed that most rural women were not even aware of the disease. The report revealed that only 19.1 per cent between 25-29 years of age had heard about AIDS and only 20.4 per cent between 30-34 years and 14 per cent between 45-49 years knew about the hazards of AID. Among the communities, 40.2 per cent are Christians, 16.5 per cent are Hindus and 10 per cent are Muslims.

Arrow for Change (2000: 3) has conducted a research on among young Filipinas in Australia in order to examine the interplay between young women's knowledge and attitudes about sex and sexuality, the influence of culture and the social context in which sex occurs. The study found low level of knowledge on sexually transmitted diseases among majority of the young women and the women have adjust between two sets of cultural values – their native culture and the culture of the country where they live. The research has suggested the need of health education specifically migrant women who face this conflict.

The Hindu (2004: November 30) has reported the women's awareness on HIV/AIDS in India. According to the report, in India, awareness of HIV/AIDS among women is distressingly low – only 20 per cent of women in some areas have correct knowledge about the disease.

Sharma. K. (2005: 3) has argued that in majority cases, the woman would not have known about the possibility of contracting the diseases through sexual relations with her husband and even if she knew, and was aware of the precautions that ought to be taken, she would not have been in a position to insist due to her subordinate position as a woman and as a wife.

Impact of HIV/AIDS

Berkley *et al.* (1990: 1237) has conducted a survey in Uganda during 1997-98 to identify the impact of HIV on women. The survey concluded that the women are increasing infected by HIV mostly through their AIDS affected sexual partners and they are struggling to cope not only with their spouse's illness but also with her own potential risk of HIV infection and with her family future well-being.

Wendy Ledger (1997: 3-24) has described AIDS as a national calamity of Kenya. He described that the virus is affecting the society in a variety of interrelated ways and it has generated worst impact on the national economy and development by taking the lives of economically productive youth, increasing the expenditure on identifying vaccine for AIDS and giving treatment for the infected, and implementing intervention programmes for prevention, control and care.

Pushpa Khurana (1998: 80) explored the social and economic impact of HIV/AIDS on women. She argued that the women should bear the double burden in the family by taking the care of the entire household and the sick who are affected by HIV and other illness. In addition the infected women give birth to 30-40 per cent infected babies and the babies and they will be orphaned due to the narrowing life expectancy of their parents as a result of AIDS.

Basia Zaba and Simon Gregson (1998: S41-50) have measured the impact of HIV on fertility in Africa. The study has identified the lower fertility among HIV infected women in all age groups. Lower fertility amongst HIV positive women cause a population attributable decline in total fertility of the order of 0.4 per cent for each per centage point of HIV prevalence in the general female population. The study argued that in populations that do not use contraceptives, HIV positive women have lower fertility principally as a result of fetal losses consequent to infection with HIV and co-infection with other sexually transmitted diseases and behaviour factors with regard to avoiding pregnancy to prevent infants from HIV infection enhance this differential.

Syed V. Naveed (1998: 133) has studied the interpersonal relationships among the relatives/friends of HIV/AIDS patients in a metropolitan city - Hyderabad in India. He also examined the process of change in relations with reference to personal factors. The study revealed that the large number of respondents have very poor interest to have an international relationships with the HIV/AIDS patients. Besides, the nature of change of interpersonal relations is positively related to the level of misconception about transmission of disease. When a person's level of misconception is high he/she is likely to have a negative change in his/her relations with the patients.

UNDP (1999: 4) has described AIDS as development issue. According to the report, HIV/AIDS presents major challenges to human survival, human rights and human development, with implications far beyond the health sector and the social and economic consequences of the epidemic are one of the most serious threats to sustainable human development.

Inn Mackinnon and Adam Piore (2001: 5-8) argued that the HIV infected women are more stigmatized and discriminated in India than the men. According to the author, most of the infected women are innocent victims and they have to face more violence both in husbands' family and her own natal family.

UNAIDS (2002: 1-19) report says that the HIV/AIDS epidemic is the fourth biggest global killer and it is now the leading cause of death in sub-Saharan Africa. The report also revealed that in many countries, AIDS is erasing decades of progress made in extending life expectancies. The impact on life expectancy signifies a major blow to a society's development. The UNAIDS has projected that in the 45 most affected countries, between 2000 and 2020, 68 million people will die earlier than they would have in the absence of AIDS.

UNAIDS report further explained that the impact of HIV/AIDS is severe on households by leaving the children as orphaned due to the death of their infected parents, and lose of income and increased expenses for medical treatment and giving care to the infected persons push the affected household deeper into poverty. Besides, the government has to deal the problem of additional/huge expenses on the health sectors. In addition to this, AIDS weaken economic activity by squeezing productivity, adding costs, diverting productive resources and depleting skills. The epidemic's potential impact on the rule of law has challenged the social cohesion in many countries in which the stability and progress of country depend.

The Hindu (2004: July 12) has reported the U.N. Secretary-General Kofi Annan in the International AIDS Conference. The report revealed that the world leaders have not done enough to combat the history's biggest epidemic and the Asian countries, including India and China stand to lose more than 18 million workers to AIDS over the next decade including huge losses of households and business and stifling economic growth.

The Hindu (2004: July 11) has published the ILO's ominous estimates in the impact of HIV/AIDS on the globe. According the report of ILO (International Labour Organisation) 35.7 million people between the ages of 15 and 49 years could be affected with HIV, 26 million of who are workers. While tens of millions of workers have already died, millions more are dropping out of the labour force. The ILO estimates that in 2005, two million workers globally will be unable to work-up from 500,000 in 1995. By 2015, the number will double to four millions.

The same report also revealed the study carried out by four organisations of people infected with HIV/AIDS in India (the Delhi, Manipur and Maharashtra Network of Positive People, and the Positive Women's Network of South India). The study found that about one-third of respondents were unemployed because of ill-health and a third still worked but had disclosed their HIV status (38 per cent) fearing job loss and only about a third has revealed their status.

National Institute of Social Defence (2004: 1) stated that the rate of increase of HIV/AIDS is on the rise and, as per an estimate, there could be 100 million people testing HIV positive by the year 2010 and lack of proper and adequate medical facilities in the developing world makes the survival of infected people very lean. The news letter of National Institute of Social Defence also revealed that the largest spread of HIV/AIDS is found among the mot sexually active population in the age group of 15-49 year and out of 14,000 new HIV infections occurring daily, a whopping 12,000 persons are from this age group alone. Unprotected sex and injecting drug use are the two chief modes of transmission of this disease in the Asia Pacific regain. The news letter suggested considering the issue of adolescent sexual and reproductive health as central theme of HIV/AIDS prevention and controlling intervention programmes.

Intervention

World Health Organisation (1988) reports on the social aspects of AIDS stress that persons suspected or known to be HIV positive should remain integrated within the society and help to assume responsibility for preventing HIV transmission to others.

Foley M *et al.* (1994: 1483-1487) have emphasized on the importance of family support to HIV/AIDS patients in their paper on family support for heterosexual partners suffered from HIV infection. They found that awareness and family support were associated with gender of the family members, HIV sero-positivity and sex education. Further, they suggested that family support is very essential to arrest the spread of sexually transmitted diseases as well to discourage the people without HIV/AIDS.

Asian Red Cross and Red Crescent Regional AIDS Task Force (1997: 18) has organized Regional workshop on Home and Community Care for people infected with HIV/AIDS (PLWHA) in Thailand. The workshop has stressed the importance of providing family and community care to PLWHA to prevent and control the spread of HIV. According to the report of the workshop, the discrimination and stigma associated with AIDS can be overcome if the public are motivated to accept the PLWHA by providing care and support.

Riedel, Marion C (1998: 4813) have explored the relationships between family role tasks and the mental health and custody plans of AIDS-affected youth. They interviewed women with AIDS and their adolescent children in New York city. In this study most of the women were contracted HIV through sexual contact with an IV drug-using partners. The study found that the women were experiencing g relatively high rates of AIDS-related physical distress and less than a third of the mothers had formal custody plans for their adolescent children, but almost all had made some informal arrangements. Prospective guardians were mostly maternal kin-mothers and sisters. The infected women's mental health distress was associated with higher role task performance toward siblings, in the household and overall, though only the first relationship was significant. These relationships were moderated by the youths' gender, mothers' level of illness, residential stability, the age of the adolescent, and number of siblings.

Tamil Nadu State AIDS Control Society (1998: 41) expressed that HIV infected persons can live upto ten years or more without developing AIDS, if provided they are cared for and given support, not just medical but emotional too.

Michal C Latham and Elizabeth A Preble (2000: 525) have described that HIV and AIDS have seriously affected women of reproductive age in sub-Saharan Africa and it increases mother to child transmission mainly through breast milk. Therefore, the researchers have suggested formula milk instead of breast milk for the infants. According to the authors, the infected mothers living in poor households in developing countries prepared the breast milk to feed the infant due to the expensive cost of formula methods. They have stressed the importance of exploring the possibility of alternative feeding methods to safeguard the infant from infections.

Lawyers Collective (2000: 3) has expressed that the best way of preventing the spread of HIV/AIDS infection is to promote and protect the right of affected populations, so that they are empowered to protect themselves. Promoting the protecting of the HIV infected with help them to choose safer behaviours and to access services like information, counseling and healthcares, without the fear of discrimination or penal sanctions. It is more important in the control of the epidemic. According to them, exclusionary approaches to single out the vulnerable population may motivate them to move underground and they may not observe changes in their behaviour for preserving the social health of the society. It makes the control of epidemic impossible and it increases the vulnerability and it affects all intervention programmes.

Indian Express (2001: May 29) has reported that there is no time scale to say when a person could become sick and it depends on the body's immune power-how long it can fight against opportunistic diseases. According to the report, an HIV positive person can live for a long period, as long a the person takes responsibilities for self, that is, leading a quality life, avoiding stress and strain, taking proper medicines, avoiding smoking and consumption of alcohol, ensuring adequate sleep and exercise with proper emotional supportive counseling.

Thinathanthi (2003: January 1) has reported the marriage between HIV infected man and women in Ernakulam in Kerala, India. This news indicates that the infected persons should be denied to get marriage, but they should be advocated to choose partners among HIV infected persons.

The Hindu (2003: December 1) reported the decision taken by the government with regard to free antiretroviral drugs to the HIV/AIDS patients at free of cost through government hospitals and antenatal clinics. According to the report, Tamil Nadu, Andhra Pradesh, Karnataka, Maharashtra, Manipur and Nagaland have given priority for free antiretroviral drugs scheme. The report also further revealed that the supply would be initially to be three categories of patients: children of parents infected with HIV, women having the infection and men who suffer from full-blown AIDS.

The Hindu (2004: November 30) reported that NGOs are playing a vital role in providing care and support of people infected with HIV/AIDS and creating attitudinal changes with regard to positive people in the public. It has cited the work rendered by the CHESS (Community Health Education Society), a Chennai based NGO in providing care to the pregnant woman who was negated by the hospital for delivery and isolated by the neighbours. The CHESS has admitted her in their hospital and helped to deliver a baby and the baby was given sufficient care by the staff which made the neighbours to change their mind and accommodate the positive women to live along with them.

The Hindu (2004: December 1) published that the HIV positive patients are not receiving adequate medical care and support after they are discharged from hospitals and they are abandoned by relatives. In order to provide them good care, the State Government of Tamil Nadu is launching the project in which the village Health Nurses will visit patients' homes to render personal care with the objective of follow-up care.

The Hindu (2004: December 6) reported the six significant concerns identified by the positive women to safeguard their right and lives and it includes health care and treatment, property succession and inheritance within natal and marital homes, access to reproductive rights and health, livelihood opportunities, decision-making powers and access to state-sponsored benefits.

The New Indian Express (2004: 7. December 1) has reported the movement of People Infected with HIV in India (INP+) in Chennai for promoting care and support of the affected community. The net work has stressed to facilitate and improve the access to treatment and information for people infected with HIV. It also advocated the promotion and protection of human right of people infected with HIV with active involvement of affected people at all levels of decision making. The positive net work also demanded social acceptance and life free from stigma and discrimination.

Thinamalar (2005: June 14) reported the 'team sex' which influence the girls who are studying in various colleges of Salem in Tamil Nadu. The report revealed that the girls who are in need of money for their lavish life are influenced by the prostitution net work and they take these girls for paid sex in team like a tourist.

Robert Szabo and Roger V Short (2000: 1592) studied the relationship between male circumcision and risk reduction of HIV/AIDS. According to the study, no new infection occurred among any of the 50 circumcised men over a period of 30 months, whereas 40 of 137 uncircumcised men became infected during the same period. The study revealed that the inner surface of the foreskin, which is rich in HIV receptors, and the frenulum, a common site for trauma and other sexually transmitted infections, must be regarded as the most probable sites for viral entry in primary HIV infection in men. He argue in the light of his evidence of the study, advocating male circumcision may be treated as new preventive strategies to prevent and control the spread of infection both for male and female.

Grosskurth *et al.* (2000: 1981) critically evaluated the findings of two studies carried out in Mwanza and Rakai with regard to the control of sexually transmitted diseases as a means for decreasing the incidence of HIV-1 infection. These studies reported a statistically significant 38% reduction in HIV-1 infection among the patients who have treated for syphilis. The authors assert that the results from these studies are complementary to each other, and provide important insights into current thinking on the management of STD in the context of AIDS prevention.

WISE Words (2000: 1) argue that women are not only biologically more susceptible to contracting HIV, but they also face social barriers that prevent their access and use of available prevention methods and the recognition of gender-related constraints for HIV prevention has led for female controlled and initiated methods of protection including female condom. The article revealed that the female condom is generally accepted and used by the women in Brazil, Thailand, South Africa and Zimbabwe. But the cost of female condom prohibits many women, especially poor women, around the world from using them.

Peter Piot (2000: 1), the Executive Director of the Joint Nations Programme on HIV/AIDS in UNAIDS stressed the addressing of gender inequality in HIV/AIDS prevention programmes. According to him women's economic dependence on men makes women less able to protect themselves while social norms limit their access to information about sexual matters. He also expressed that the greater social acceptance of high-risk male sexual behaviour can expose both men and their partners to infection.

William R. Finger (2001: 14) stressed the importance of encouraging the young women to use condom and to develop skills to refuse unwanted sex. He stated that the young women are often inexperienced with condoms and also feel invulnerable to risk and these factors challenges the intervention programmes which are targeted on adolescent girls. The article also revealed that in addition to condom use, the women and girls should be given knowledge on the early detection of sexually transmitted infections and its cure and prevention. The author has suggested the integration of family planning programmes with HIV/AIDS intervention programmes to make the people to receive condom without the fear of stigma.

The Hindu (2004: April 22) expressed the article of The United Nations' General Assemble global response for combating HIV and AIDS. The news revealed that about $9 billion is required annually to combat HIV and AIDS and half of which would be needed in sub-Saharan Africa. According to the article, about $4.8 billion would be required for prevention, including interventions focusing on youth, workplace programmes, mother-to-child transmission and condom distribution and another $4.4 billion would be needed for treating opportunistic infection to which HIV patients become susceptible. The article further revealed that since 15,000 new infections occur each day, the annual resources needed for an expanded global response would increase from $3.2 billion in 2002, $4.7 billion in 2003, $6.8 billion in 2004 to $9.2 billion in 2005.

According to the article, the level of spending by 2005 would provide prevention services for over 22 million, and voluntary counseling and testing for nine million. An additional 35 million women would receive testing at prenatal clinics and 9, 00,000 would receive antiretroviral drugs to prevent mother-to-child transmissions. Special prevention programmes would reach almost sex million sex workers, 28 million men who have sex with men and three million injecting drug users. These costs would include funds for over six billion condoms.

The Hindu (2004: December 2) reported that the main challenge for India is to break down the barriers of denial and the denial of epidemic has led to inaction. It has an view that the AIDS pandemic is one where the media has an important role, and may even save more lives, than doctors.

Ramyakannan (2004: 5) report in Hindu says that the members of the positive community throughout the state have brought several complaints of harassment and discrimination by medical and para-medical personnel in both the government and private health sectors. Her report also reveals that stigma over HIV/AIDS still exists in the medical community and doctors are often hesitant to treat patients, who reveal their HIV status.

The Hindu (2004: July 12) published the talk of the Union Minister for Health and Family Welfare, Anbumani Ramadoss at the second Asia-Pacific Ministerial meeting on HIV/AIDS in Bangkok. According to the report, India has taken political commitment to control the spread of HIV/AIDS. The report also revealed that India had identified cases of 5.1 million HIV infections, accounting to less than one per cent of the population and anti-retroviral therapy (ART) had been introduced in India in April 2004 at free of cost, through the public sectors.

The Hindu (2004: December 1) says that economic dependence has rendered millions of women vulnerable because they are unable to set the terms of their relationship with men. Violence and coercion within marriage, and lack of access to property, basic education and employment opportunities are important factors that subjugate women. Therefore, it has suggested reviewing the laws to empower women and liberal approach in funding employment ventures on the line of health education on HIV/AIDS. The report also stressed that the 'APC' approach to prevention–Abstinence, Being faithful and reducing the number of sexual partners, and Condom use–will have only a limited impact if the underlying socio-economic and cultural cause are not addressed.

National Institute of Social Defence (2004: 8) published press clippings with regard to the survey conducted by ORG-MARG (Operation Research Group-Marketing and Research Group) to assess the condom usage among the couples in urban India (*India Today*, 2004: Oct. 4). The survey identified the drastic decline of condom use in Urban India due to the barrage of publicity surrounding condoms and HIV/AIDS prevention. According to the survey, many people have a feeling that condom is only for high-risk groups and not for non-risk groups.

The Hindu (2005: February 8) quoted the Union Health and Family Welfare Minister, Anbumani Ramadoss statement and reported that India has began human clinical trial of an investigational vaccine designed to prevent Human Immunodeficiency Virus infection and Acquired Immunodeficiency Syndrome at the Pune-based National AIDS Research Institute and if the trial is successful, a vaccine against the disease would be available within eight years.

The Hindu (2005: February 10) reported that the senior Vatican official has supported the use of condoms to fight Africa's AIDS pandemic, contradicting the Catholic Church's official position. According to the statement given by the Cardinal Georges Cottier, though contraception is officially forbidden by the Catholic Church, the use of condom in some situations can be considered morally legitimate. He also warned that sex with condoms is not safe.

Prasad (2005: 13) revealed that there has been a positive correlation between circumcision and reduced risk of HIV infection. He has quoted the trial carried out among 3000 heterosexual male volunteers in South Africa and revealed that the incidence of HIV infection in circumcised volunteers was three times lower compared with uncircumcised men. He suggested that inclusion of male circumcision in intervention strategy may help to prevent infection through sexual contact.

Research Gap and Present Study

Review indicates the issues involved in HIV/AIDS infection and its transmission to vulnerable groups in terms of socio-economic factors, high risk behaviour and HIV/AIDS, stigma and discrimination, violence against women, reproductive health, women's knowledge on HIV/AIDS, impact of HIV and intervention. However, these revelations and expositions are inadequate to understand comprehensively the various problems of HIV infected women. Accordingly a comprehensive attempt focusing on the various circumstances leading to HIV positive for women, influence of socio-economic factor leading to the infection of women, discrimination due to HIV infection, sexual behaviour of women after infection, impact of HIV/AIDS on social relationship of women and their attitude towards pregnancy and child birth after infection with sociological overtone was felt and found as research gap with special reference to women in larger cities.

Accordingly, to fulfil this research gap the present study is formulated to conduct the same in Chennai City, the Capital of Tamil Nadu with a strong methodological support and also specific research questions of:

1. What is the socio-economic background of women infected with HIV positive?
2. Why the infection rate is high in monogamy relationship?

3. Whether HIV infection increases the rate of widowhood?
4. Is there any change in the sexual behaviour of sex workers and housewives after infection?
5. Why the sex workers remain in sex work even after knowing their infection?
6. What is the impact of HIV on social relationship of women after infection?
7. Are the infected women revealing their HIV status to others?
8. Is there any gender discrimination in treatment?
9. Is there any economic change in the life of women after infection?
10. How women perceive pregnancy and child birth after infection?

3

Research Methodology

Over View of HIV/AIDS as Social Problem

HIV/AIDS is not an individual problem. But it is the problem of entire society. It affects the public at large. If it is an individual problem, we can find solution very easily within the framework of individual's life style. Since it affects larger society, HIV/AIDS should be treated as social problem. Therefore, controlling the situation is always beyond the ability of one or few persons. This responsibility should be placed upon society at large. Collective efforts are needed to restore social ethics which describes human conduct as right and wrong in group relations.

Social disorganisation is the major factor for the infection and spread of HIV virus into the general population. Social disorganisation is a condition of society, community or group in which there is a break down of social control, or of social order, or of formal and informal norms that define permissible behaviours. It is characterized by impersonal secondary relations, anonymity, loneliness, high mobility and extreme specialization, contradictions in social systems, malfunctioning of economic systems, defective functioning political systems, lack of co-operation, breakdown of social values, lack of unity, indiscipline, unpredictability, lack of consensus and integration of institutions and inadequate social control.

Social problem will emerge when there is a change in the equilibrium forces of the social structure. The traditional norms and values and practices become ineffective due to the intervention of new life style as a result of modernization, westernization and globalization. The disruption in the traditional values brought changes in the social and economic life of the people. Many become impoverished as a result of technological transformation and modernization. The technological transformation in the field of economy and modernization in all sphere of the structure led to migration and unemployment of unskilled, semi skilled labourers. Prostitution and paid sex, drug abuse are the direct impact of migration and unemployment which is identified as major risk factor for infection and the spread HIV/AIDS.

The phenomenon of cultural lag is another important factor which prevents the practice of intervention programmes implemented by the government and non-governmental organisations to control and prevent further spread of infection. With the influence of various mass media, the people are exposed to sex and safe sex knowledge. But the conservative attitude of the people creates fear among them to use condom as a means of safe sex whenever they have heterosexual experiences. The conservative thought and its related fear act as barriers to practice the intervention programmes in their life style.

The prevailing value conflict between male and female with regard to breaking the silence surrounding the sex and suggesting and adopting condom during sexual encounter is another important cause to increase the women' vulnerability towards HIV/AIDS. A value is a generalized principle of behaviours to which the members of a group feel a strong, emotional, positive commitment. The values provide a standard for judging specific acts and goals. Each member of the group is expected to remain committed to the values accepted by the group. The value of Indian culture expects women to be submissive and men to be aggressive in sex and sexuality. Such expectation made Indian women to be ignorant about sex and safe sex and its related implication on their life.

Personal deviation and peer group pressure is another important variable for the behaviours of injecting drug use, prostitution, promiscuous relationships, pre and extra marital behaviours. Deviation is non-conformity to social norms.

Personal deviancy develops because of either an individual's inability to follow generally accepted norms or an individual's failure to accept generally accepted norms. A deviant behaviour of the individual is either directly or indirectly related to deficiency in socialization. The deviants, though they have learnt norms and values of the society, they are unable to put them into practice. The deviants as a result of their peer group pressure used to engage in high risk activities which bring all infections including HIV. These deviants also act as carrier as well as transmitter of virus to their innocent sexual partners.

Risky behaviours in the context of AIDS refer to behaviours that increase the chances of getting infected by HIV or transmitting the virus. Such behaviours include having sexual intercourse without condom (male or females), practicing anal sex, sex with several partners, having sex with sex workers, injecting drug use and using unclean equipment, and if HIV positive going through pregnancy, child birth and breast feed with voluntary counseling and testing and other interventions. Vulnerability to HIV infection arises from circumstances that are beyond the direct control of the people involved. Such circumstances include poverty, low social status, gender discrimination, social discrimination, marginalization and criminalization. These circumstances also reduce or deny a person's access to HIV information, services, means of prevention and support. Gender inequality increases the vulnerability of both men and women to HIV infection.

Women and children, injecting drug users, poor people, refugees, migrants, prisoners, homosexual men, injecting drug users, sex workers are considered as vulnerable population. These vulnerable populations may face increased stigma and discrimination as a result of their HIV status.

The AIDS epidemic claimed 2.9 million lives in 2003, and an estimated 4.8 million people acquired HIV virus in 2003. As on December 2003, 37.8 million (range 34.6-42.3 million) of people are globally living with HIV positive. Among the global total one-third of the people living with HIV are young people between

15-24 years. The UNAIDS Global report on HIV/AIDS 2004 reveals that half of all people infected with HIV/AIDS are women. As on December 2003, of the total 37.8 million of people living with HIV positive, 17 million are female. The new infection included 800,000 children. Among them more than 90% have infected through parent to child transmission (PTCT). About 90% of the infection through PTCT occurred in Sub-Saharan Africa, but the number of such infection is increasing in other regions, particularly South-East Asia.

No country is free from HIV infection. South Africa remains the world's worst affected region of the world. It has 10% of world's population, but is the home for 70% global infection. Women in Africa are being infected at an earlier age than men. Asia has 60% of the world's population. Now it becomes the home for fastest growing AIDS epidemic in the world. In Asia, an estimated 7.4 million people (range 5.0-10.5%) are living with HIV. Around half a million (range 330 000-740 000) are believed to have died of AIDS in 2003, and about 1.1 million (range 610 000-2.2 million) become newly infected. In Asia HIV/AIDS is concentrated more in India, China, Philippines, Thailand, Myanmar, Indonesia, and Nepal.

India has the largest number of people living with HIV next to South Africa. It is estimated that 5.1 million people living with HIV in 2003. Most infections acquired sexually, but injecting drug use dominates in the north-east of the country. In this area, infection level of 60-75% has been found among injecting drug users using non-sterile injecting equipment. In India's southern states of Andhra Pradesh, Karnataka, Maharashtra and Tamil Nadu, HIV is transmitted through heterosexual sex, and is largely linked to sex work. In many states infection level among pregnant women in sentinel antenatal clinics have found to be more than 1 per cent. This suggests that sex workers' clients may have passed HIV to their wives. In many parts of India, HIV transmission through sex between men is also a major concern. The homosexual men may also have sex with women - wives or other female sexual partners.

The Government of India has taken tremendous efforts through NACO and State AIDS Control Societies to disseminate the knowledge related to HIV/AIDS to the public in general and high risk groups in particular. But the level of knowledge is still inadequate and incomplete. The people of India have not taken the issue as serious social problem. The information with regard to HIV/AIDS, safe sex, preventive mechanism, its impact has not reached many parts of rural India where the epidemic has taken its entry through rural to urban and urban to rural migration. As a result of cultural constrains, women, girls and adolescents have limited access to gain knowledge about sex, safe sex, reproductive health, condom use, antiretroviral therapy, voluntary testing, treatment etc. The poor knowledge and increasing risk behaviours among youth and risk groups further fuel the epidemic in India.

Statement of the Problem

In India, the HIV infection has engulfed all parts of the country irrespective of its socio-economic developments. HIV/AIDS is no longer a problem restricted to specific groups with high risk behaviours in India. The epidemic has reached to the level of infecting non-risk groups including women and children. In India women are increasingly at greater risk of getting infection due to cultural constraints in the male dominated patriarchal society.

The ratio of infection between male and female is 3 :1. The majority of the infection occurs in young women with the age group of 15-24 years. Heterosexuality is identified as major risk factor for women's infection in India. Many women have infected with the risk behaviours of others especially from their husband in the marital life. Discrimination, poverty, gender based violence and conservative culture and traditional norms, attitude towards parenthood are the important factors which fuel the epidemic among the women and now it is feminized in India. The Indian women either know nothing or too little about HIV and various mechanisms to protect themselves from infection. Even if they know some thing about HIV and safe sexual practices, it is often rendered useless by the discrimination and violence they face in the society.

The 'ABC' approach – Abstain, Be faithful and use Condom has not produced significant impact in the control and prevention of HIV among women and adolescent girls. This is mainly because the success of the approach entirely depends on the behaviours of the men in Indian social context. The persisting gender inequality has taken the dreaded disease called AIDS into a socio-economic crisis.

In India, women living with and affected by HIV/AIDS have to face lot of consequences including taking care of ill and AIDS related stigma and discrimination throughout their life. In many cases they are blamed by their husband and in-laws for being the "vectors" or "carriers" of HIV. Though they are shouldering the responsibility of taking care of other infected persons in the family, for example husband and children, they find no one to take care of them when they fell ill and the society has no care and support mechanisms for the victims of HIV/AIDS.

The socio-cultural values and religious norms in India prevent women to use female control protection method. They have no right to get free from these harmful traditional practices, violence and to exercise control over their own bodies. In the Indian context, women's sex and sexuality is controlled by men due to the rights given to them in the patriarchal family system.

The violence against women is major human right and public health problem in India. It increases female vulnerability to HIV. Rape, sexual abuse, trafficking, sex trade and exploitation of women are frequently reported by various media (print and visual). The sexual abuses increase women's vulnerability towards HIV.

The Indian women suffer with restricted economic option. Illiteracy, ignorance, lack of skill and limited or lack of opportunities to acquire skill pushes them into the trap of poverty, violence and homelessness. The Indian social structure never encouraged women to possess and inherit property. Her economic insecurity increases her personal insecurity in the form of domestic violence, unsafe sex and other HIV related risk factors. The feminization of poverty as a result of rapid economic changes and introduction of mechanization forced marginalized women to engage in unsafe sex for money and other survival needs which increases their vulnerability to the infection sexually transmitted infections including HIV/AIDS.

Tamil Nadu has highest number of infection in India. The infection rate is steadily increasing among the STD patients and pregnant women. Young girls are under the threat of infection due to the prevailing myth that the sex with virgin can cure the infection. As a result of increasing migration from rural to urban the increasing number of innocent housewives are getting infection from their husbands with risky behaviour. The people in general and risk group in particular are hesitant to undergo HIV test. They have a fear that if they take up HIV tests they will be labeled as promiscuous. The stigma and discrimination associated with HIV/AIDS also enable women to become the victim of HIV/AIDS.

There is no legal mechanism in India, to know the HIV status of the individual before marriage. Since most of the marriages are arranged based on the horoscope in the Indian families, the marrying partners have no chance to know their own HIV status which increases the risk of both men and women in the marital life.

In this context the present study makes an attempt to expose the plight of women living with HIV positive in Chennai city, Tamil Nadu.

Objectives

The objectives of the present study are as follows :

1. To study the social and economic background of women living with HIV positive.
2. To analyse the marital status of women and vulnerability to HIV infection..
3. To examine the circumstances leading to HIV infection and related behaviour on women.
4. To investigate the sexual behaviour of women after infection.
5. To analyse the impact of HIV status on social relationships of women.

6. To expose women's attitude towards pregnancy and child birth after infection.
7. To suggest suitable measures and prepare a plan of action leading to prevention and control of HIV in society in general and women in particular.

Significance of the Study

Many studies have revealed the causes and social and economic implication of HIV/AIDS in general. Many studies have not examined the problems of women living with HIV positive in the patriarchal society like India where women have limited access to gain reproductive knowledge, less control over their body and more subjected to sexual abuse and violence. It is a social responsibility to protect women from the dreaded disease of HIV/AIDS and its related stigma and discrimination. It is more essential to identify the plight of women living with HIV positive in the Indian society which give more importance to moral values and family ethics so that positive measures can be initiated to ensure HIV free society.

Operational Definition of the Terms used in the Topic

Women living with HIV positive

The term refers to the female who are living with HIV status.

Chennai

Chennai is the City which is in the capital of Tamil Nadu State.

Tamil Nadu

Tamil Nadu is one of the southern States in peninsular India.

Research Design

The nature of the present study is diagnostic. The study is diagnostic because it exposes the important problems experienced by the women living with HIV in various social and economic spheres. There is no need for specific hypothesis for this study, since the objectives are conceptually clear.

Selection of the Study Area

Table 3.1. Aids Cases in Tamil Nadu
(Districtwise - cumulative)
(Reported up to September 2001by Tamil Nadu State AIDS Control Society, 2001)

Sl. No.	*Name of the District*	*Male*	*Female*	*Total*
1.	Chennai	2876	867	3743
2.	Thiruvellore	436	132	568
3.	Kancheepuram	335	95	430
4.	Vellore	513	176	689
5.	Thiruvannanmalai	387	120	507
6.	Villupuram	603	205	808
7.	Cuddalore	480	129	609
8.	Dharmapuri	354	112	466
9.	Salem	774	241	1015
10.	Namakkal	703	200	903
11.	Erode	619	183	802
12.	Coimbatore	271	61	332
13.	The Nilgiris	24	1	31
14.	Perambalur	212	78	290
15.	Trichy	596	203	799
16.	Ariyalur	23	15	38
17.	Karur	238	54	290
18.	Pudukkottai	92	29	121
19.	Thanjavur	152	54	206
20.	Tiruvarur	39	9	45
21.	Nagapattinam	54	14	68
22.	Dindigul	312	95	407
23.	Madurai	521	168	689
24.	Theni	170	37	207
25.	Sivagangai	69	24	93
26.	Virudhunagar	64	11	75
27.	Ramanathapuram	38	12	50
28	Tirunelveli	165	33	198
29.	Thoothukudi	128	27	155
30.	Kanyakumari	23	5	28
	Address not known	272	40	312
	Other States	60	17	77
	Total	11601	3453	15054

Chennai city in Tamil Nadu is purposively selected on the basis of reported AIDS statistics available in the Tamil Nadu State AIDS Control Society. The prevalence of HIV in Chennai is also confirmed by survey of literature, pilot studies and interaction with Government and Non-Governmental Organisations. Besides, homosexual activities are increasing in Chennai and the report of the Indian Community Welfare Organisation revealed that there are 7,000 homosexuals identified among the estimated 65,000 people in Chennai City. Since homosexual men are often functionally heterosexual, the risk of STD and HIV spreading to males as well as females is very high (*Indian Express*, 1999. Oct. 14). Chennai Corporation of AIDS Prevention and Control Society (CAPACS) is established in 1998 with the objectives of strengthening the activities related to awareness, accessibility and action. The Organisation was established as per the direction of National AIDS Control Organisation (NACO) exclusively for Chennai in view of the high density of floating population which the city attracts regularly.

Besides, being the capital city, Chennai is a well known place for multi sectoral activities with increasing urbanization, modernization, industrialization and commercialization. Floating and migratory population from various parts of the state, country and world are the common feature of Chennai. The city oriented life encouraged multisexual activities, both pre-marital and extra marital sex. Many attractive tourism spots including Mahabalipuram and Kanchipuram are located close to Chennai. The well organized road transport, air ways and sea port influences tourists from all over the world. As a result of population growth and movements, the sex industries have well organized underground net work to encourage prostitution which are responsible for the spread of sexually transmitted diseases including HIV/AIDS.

So, Chennai is purposely selected for the study. As for the respondents are concerned, purposive sampling is adopted to select 200 women living with HIV positive by applying snowball technique with the support of Non Governmental and Governmental agencies.

Pilot Study

The pilot study has been conducted by the researcher in the districts of Chennai, Dindigul and Madurai in order to obtain general view with regard to women living with HIV. In addition to interaction and focused discussion with HIV infected women, the researcher also referred the relevant articles and annual reports related to the prevalence of high risk groups and sexual behaviours of those groups in their respective working areas.

Universe

According to AIDS cases surveillance report by Tamil Nadu State AIDS Control Society, as on October 2001, the total number of samples screened for HIV in Tamil Nadu was 8,15,922 and among them number of persons found seropositive were 20,051 with 2.45 seropositivity rate per thousand. The estimation of State wise HIV prevalence report of the NACO from 1998-2003 reveals the HIV prevalence rate in Tamil Nadu during 2001 is high based on the prevalence rate of various risk groups including patients attending STD clinics (12.60%), Women attending antenatal clinics (1.13%), Intravenous drug users (24.56%) and men seeking men (MSM) with 2.40%.

High secrecy is maintained by the Government of Tamil Nadu in keeping the records of reported cases as well as revealing their address to the public. The current prevalence rate of HIV is an estimated figure based on the sentinel surveillance data on the selected sites according to UNAIDS/WHO criteria, it is highly difficult to obtain exact number of people living with HIV/AIDS in general and women in particular for all districts of Tamil Nadu. Therefore due to this limitation, universe is not taken into consideration for this study.

Sample Design

The available data based on Tamil Nadu AIDS control Society on the reported cases of AIDS in various districts in Tamil Nadu suggested that the HIV prevalence rate is high in Chennai. Therefore, purposive sampling technique is adopted to contact the respondents by resorting to snowballing procedure. Accordingly 200 HIV infected persons representing cross sections living in Chennai city were interviewed for the purpose of empirical investigations. The respondents were identified with the support of Governmental and Non-Governmental Organisations (NGOs) in Chennai city.

Sources of Data

The present study has used both primary and secondary sources of data. The primary data were collected directly from the respondents (women living with HIV positive) by the researcher.

The main instrument for the collection of primary data was the interview schedule which was structured in order to collect relevant data. Though the interview schedule was constructed in English, the interview was conducted in Tamil, which is the regional language of Tamil Nadu. The interview schedule administered with the women living with HIV positive consisted the questions intended to elicit information regarding personal data, family particulars, socio-economic status, marital details, circumstances leading to HIV positive, circumstances leading to commercial sex work, sexual behaviour after HIV infection, details about HIV testing and pre and post test counseling, social relationship of the respondents in the family, in neighbourhood, in work place, and among relatives and friendship, the discrimination experienced in treatment and in work place and their perception of pregnancy after infection.

The secondary data were collected from sources like journals, magazine, newspapers, books, articles, pamphlets, reports, web sites etc.

Tools for Data Collection

Personal interview was carried out with the structured interview schedule in order to collect required information from the respondents in consonance with the objectives formulated for the study. Observation techniques (both participatory and non-participatory), and focused group discussion with the women living with HIV positive also used to supplement and strengthen the primary data.

Discussion was also held with the Government Organisation especially with the officials of Tamil Nadu State AIDS Control

Society in Chennai, Non-governmental Organisations working in AIDS Prevention and Control Activities and Funding Agencies like AIDS Prevention and Control Project (APAC).

Pre-test

The constructed interview schedule was put to field test with few women living with HIV positive in order to test its suitability and relevance. Later, the schedule was edited and standardized based on the results of the pre-test.

Data Editing, Coding and Analysis

After collecting data from the respondents, the interview schedule was scrutinized and edited for checking the errors and omissions. After editing, the collected data were coded to enter into the master table for classification of data for tabulation. Conventional statistical tools such as average and per centages were employed for data processing and analysis.

Scope and Limitations

As the present study is based on the sample of women living with HIV positive, it is bound to be limited in its scope and applicability. As far as scope is concerned, it is mainly focused on the discrimination faced by the women in various socio-economic spheres in terms of comparison with their male infected partners. The study also focused on the perception of infected women towards their pregnancy and transmission of HIV to the infants. The research also further focused on the possible ways and means to prevent and control the spread of HIV infection in the form of suggestion of an action plan.

Reluctance, hesitation, fear, anger and sickness to cope with the interview on the part of the women living with the HIV positive are the major limitations of the study while collecting sensitive and crucial information. However, the researcher has taken a number of visits to meet the respondents in order to persuade and motivate to collect reliable data.

Reference Period

The reference period of the present study was 2001 to 2005.

4

HIV/AIDS: A Global Scenario

Tracing the History of HIV/AIDS

The Human Immuno Deficiency Virus (HIV) started threatening the entire world since early 1980s. It is a retrovirus that infects the immune system, mainly CD4 cells and macrophages, which is the key components of immune system. It destroys or impairs the functions of immune system, leading to "immune deficiency" called AIDS – "Acquired Immune Deficiency Syndrome". The word acquired was chosen because the illness was neither genetically determined nor, the result of other conditions. In other words, it was acquired during the normal life and the term AIDS is used when the disease has progressed and the person develops one or more serious infections or conditions (Thomas, 1997: 2). The majority of people infected with HIV, if not treated, develop signs of AIDS within eight to 30 years. Symptoms of AIDS generally appear when the numbers of CD4 white blood cells decreases to 200 per cubic millilitre (ml^3) of blood (UNAIDS, Q&A, 2004: 3).

A century ago, that is in 1884 itself, the German bacteriologist Robert Koch in his key paper on tuberculosis he spelled out the three criteria for proving a microbe guilty of causing a disease. First, the germ must be found growing abundantly in every patient and every diseased tissue; second, the germ must be isolated and grown in the laboratory; and third, the purified germ must cause the disease again in another host. Together, these came to be known as Koch's Postulates (Ellison and Duesberg, 1994: 21). The scientists agreed that the evidence on the link between HIV and AIDS passes this test. There is a clear correlation of clinical findings of AIDS and the identification of HIV in the blood (UNAIDS Q&A, 2004: 3). Search for tracing the virus followed the Robert Koch's postulates.

Biologists estimated that the first HIV cases occurred in Africa in the 1930s and then for many unknown reasons, it burst out of its African origins and transmitted throughout the world without leaving any place with AIDS free status (Zhu *et al.*, 1998: 94-99).

Chronologically speaking, the origin of HIV may be traced from 1950s where the similar appearance of AIDS is noticed in some African region after World War II (Thomas, 1997: 26). AIDS like symptom in patient was identified as early as 1959 (Sabatier, 1988).

In 1959 a British sailor with Kaposi's Sarcoma and pneumocystis died in Manchester. In 1969, a 15-year old black US boy died with Kaposi's Sarcoma and opportunistic infections in St. Louis (Thomas, 1997: 26). In the late 1970, the first clue of a strange new disease began to turn up in certain European hospitals. A 47-year old Danish doctor, Dr. Grethe Rask, had practised medicine in a remote hospital in Zaire, died in Denmark in 1977. A biopsy showed that the cause of death was the rare Pneumocystis Carinii Pneumonia (PCP) (Singhal: 2003: 48). In 1978, a 27-year old Rwandan mother developed the immunodeficiency symptoms and died. In the same year a 34-year old Zairean women died due to opportunistic infection in Kinshasa. In 1979 a 44-year old homosexual man died with Kaposi's Sarcoma in New York city (Thomas, 1997: 26). Kaposi's Saracoma is a kind of cancer found very common among AIDS patients in the West.

A dozen AIDS cases were retrospectively identified in the United States and Haiti between 1972 and 1976 (Korber *et al.*, 2000: 1789-96). An Air Canada flight steward called Gaetan Dugas who was identified as homosexual frequently visited Paris and played a vital role in transmitting the virus in the United States (Shilts and Randy, 1987).

In 1980 the first unusual immune system failure was documented by Dr. Michael S. Gottlieb, a young immunologist at University of California, Los Angeles in the United States. His first patient sought medical care because of weight loss, candidiasis (Singhal, 2003: 49), yeast infection, and Pneumocystis carinii pneumonia which is the disease rarely struck anyone but cancer patients (Ellison and Duesberg, 1994: 103). The report on the new symptom of disease made the local physicians in Los Angeles to refer several similar cases to Gottileb and it was found that all were active homosexuals (Ellison and Duesberg, 1994: 103).

The opportunistic infections of these patients led Gottlieb to suspect problems with their immune systems, and he found that the men had a deficiency of T lymphocytes (Arvind Singhal, 2003: 49). In 1981 the Centre for Disease Control's (CDC) weekly medical surveillance report called Morbidity and Mortality Weekly Report cited a cluster of cases of Karposi's Saracoma, a rare type of skin cancer usually found among elderly men of Mediterranean ancestry. All of the individuals in the cluster were young gay men. Similar cases were also reported gay men from New York, San Francisco and Los Angeles (Maclure, 1998: 467-73).

The epidemiologist of the CDC started to search the causes and means of transmission of this strange new disease of immune suppression. They assumed that a virus was being transmitted through sexual contact among gay men and it caused immune deficiency in the human body which allowed to acquire various opportunistic infection. In the beginning, the disease did not have an official name and it was called by "Gay Related Immune Deficiency Syndrom" (Singhal, 2003: 50). By July of 1982 the CDC decided to call it the Acquired Immune Deficiency Syndrome (AIDS) (Ellison and Duesberg, 1994: 105).

By 1983, scientists in France discovered virus which caused AIDS and showed that it was undeniably a new virus. At first, different names were given to the AIDS virus by the French and the American workers and ultimately, the International Committee on the Nomenclature of Viruses intervened and the name 'human immunodeficiency virus or HIV' was accepted

(Pavri, 1992: 4-5). HIV-1 was identified by Dr. Robert Gallo at the National Cancer Institute in Bethesda, Maryland and HIV-2 by Dr. Luc Montagnier of Pasteur Institute in Paris in 1983 (Singhal, 2003: 46).

These two human HIV viruses are distinguishable by their genome makeup but are believed that it had a common ancestor in Africa. Scientist believed that HIV-2 was transmitted to humans from a simian source, probably the sooty mongabeys that are hunted for food in Senegal, Guinea, the Ivory Coast, and Gambia. HIV-1, which is more lethal, is closely related to Simian Immunodeficiency Virus and it was transmitted from the Central African Chimpanzee called 'Pan troglodytes. HIV-1 mutates very rapidly, and Simian Immunodeficiency virus crossed over to humans as Human Immunodeficiency Virus (Arvind Singhal, 2003: 46). While HIV-1 is found worldwide, HIV-2 is mostly found in West Africa and now the cases have been reported from East Africa, Europe, Asia and Latin America (*The Week*, 2001: 6).

In the course of the year, three modes of transmission–contaminated blood and blood products transfusion including contaminated needles, sexual intercourse, and mother to child transmission were described (UNAIDS, Q & A, 2004: 1).

The Current Feature of HIV/AIDS

HIV is currently spreading at the rate of one new infection in every fifteen seconds, according to Dr. Michael Merson, head of the Global Programmes on AIDS at the World Health Organisation. The virus is also spreading geographically beyond the urban areas and reaching deeper into the countryside. No country is exempted from infection and it has covered all directions of the world -East and West, North and South. Every day, throughout the world, an estimated 16,000 people become infected with the HIV (UNAIDS REPORT, 1999)

Young male and female are increasingly affected by HIV and every day, 7000 people between the ages of 10-24 worldwide acquire the virus. This means 2.6 million new infections a year (Avert Organisation, 2005). Approximately one-quarter of those living with HIV/AIDS are men under age 25. More than 70% of HIV infections worldwide are estimated to result from sex between men and women. Ten per cent can be traced to sexual transmission between men, and 5 per cent of infections are due to needle-sharing by people who inject drugs and four out of five injecting drug users are men (Parliamentary Forum on HIV/AIDS, 2004)

Another disturbing trend is the growing proportion of women infected with HIV, over 15,000 women become infected every week and in many countries women surpassing the rate of men's HIV infection, according to Merson. HIV is also spreading into the general population in many parts of the world, and is no longer linked to groups with high risk behaviours.

Global Patterns of HIV Infection

Three categories of global pattern and the countries are given below: (Pavri, 1992: 16).

Table 4.1. Global Pattern of HIV Infection

Pattern I	Extensive spread of HIV began in the late 1970s/ early 1980s. Homosexual male and intravenous drug users have been predominantly affected populations, but heterosexual transmission is increasing. Western Europe, North America, some areas in South Africa, Australia, New Zealand.
Pattern II	Extensive spread of HIV began in the mid-to-late 1970s/early 1980s. Heterosexual transmission has continues to predominate. Africa, Caribbean, some areas in South America.
Pattern III	Introduction and/or extensive spread of HIV did not occur until mid-to-late 1890s. Extensive spread of HIV is now being documented in several countries in South East Asia, but the prevalence of HIV, in most countries classified within this pattern, remains relatively low. Countries in Asia are included in Pattern III, where HIV was introduced late. Asia, the Pacific region (minus Australia and New Zealand), the Middle East, Eastern Europe and some rural areas of South America.

Trends of Global HIV Infection

The following estimated figures reflect the increasing trends of HIV infection in the world (Table 4.2):

Table 4.2. Global Summary of AIDS Epidemic (1996-2004)

	1996	*1999*	*2000*	*2001*	*2002*	*2003*	*2004*
No. of infection (in million)	29.4	33.6	34	35	37	38	39.4

Source: UNAIDS Global summary of the *AIDS Epidemic Update*, December 2004.

It was estimated that around 29.4 million HIV infection in 1996 and the current estimates of 2004 shows that around 39.4 million people were living with HIV through out the world. It is almost an increase of 10 million within eight years that is from 1996-2004 (UNAIDS, 2004: 6). It shows that the number of people living with HIV continue to rise, despite the fact that all countries have effective prevention strategies.

Mode of Transmission of HIV/AIDs

Table 4.3. Hiv/AIDs – Region wise mode of Transmission

Regions	*Epidemic Started*	*Mode of Transmission*
Sub-Saharan Africa	Late 70s and early 80s	Heterosexual
South and South East Asia	Late 80s	Heterosexual
Latin America	Late 70s and early 80s	Male to male, Intravenous drug use, and Heterosexual
America, W. Europe, Australia/New Zealand	Late 70s and early 80s	Male to male, Intravenous drug use, and Heterosexual
Caribbean	Late 70s and early 80s	Heterosexual
Central/Eastern Europe, Central Asia	Early 90s	Intravenous drug use, Male to male
East Asia, Pacific	Late 80s	Male to male, Intravenous drug use, and Heterosexual
South Africa, Middle East	Late 80s	Intravenous drug use, heterosexual

Source: Digumarti Bhaskara Rao, (2000: 211)

Worldwide, between 75 and 85 of every 100 HIV infection in adults have been transmitted through unprotected sexual intercourse including oral, vaginal or anal sex. Heterosexual (male-female) intercourse accounts for more than 70 per cent of global adult HIV infections and homosexuals (male-male) intercourse accounts for 5-10 per cent. HIV is more likely to be transmitted through intercourse when either one or both partners have a classic Sexually Transmitted Disease (STD). Around 25-35 per cent of all infants born to HIV infected women themselves become infected with the virus before or during birth, or through breast-feeding. This mother-to-child (vertical) transmission accounts for more than 90 per cent of global infections in infants and children (Digumarti Bhaskara Rao, 2000: 209).

The sharing of HIV infected injection equipment by drug users resulting in blood borne HIV transmission, which accounts for 5-10 per cent of all adult infections. This proportion is growing in many areas of the world. Transfusion of HIV infected blood or blood products accounts for 3-5 per cent of all adult HIV infections. In many parts of the world HIV transmission through the transfusion of infected blood has been reduced by the use of voluntary blood donors, the routine screening of donated blood for HIV, and more rational use of blood aimed at reducing the number of transmission (Digumarti Bhaskara Rao, 2000: 209).

A Global Overview of the AIDS Epidemic

Table 4.4. Regional HIV and Aids Statistics and Features, end 2002 and 2004

Regions	*Adult and children living with HIV (in million)*	*Adult and children newly infected with HIV (in million)*	*Adult prevalence %*	*No. of women (15-49) living with HIV (in million)*	*Percent of adult (15-49)women living with HIV*	*Adult and children death due to AIDS (in million)*
			Sub-Saharan Africa			
2004	25.4	3.1	7.4	13.3	57	2.3
2002	24.4	2.9	7.5	12.8	57	2.1
			North Africa and Middle East			
2004	540 000	92 000	0.3	250 000	48	28 000
2002	430 000	73 000	0.2	200 000	48	20 000

South and South East Asia						
2004	7.1	890 000	0.6	2.1	30	490 000
2002	6.4	820 000	0.6	1.8	28	430 000
East Asia						
2004	1.1	290 000	0.1	250 000	22	51 000
2002	760 000	120 000	0.1	160 000	21	37 000
Oceania						
2004	35 000	5000	0.2	7100	21	700
2002	28 000	3200	0.2	5000	18	500
Latin America						
2004	1.7	240 000	0.6	610 000	36	95 000
2002	1.5	190 000	0.6	520 000	35	74 000
Caribbean						
2004	440 000	53 000	2.3	210 000	49	36000
2002	420 000	52 000	2.3	19 000	49	33000
Eastern Europe and Central Asia						
2004	1.4	210000	0.8	490 000	34	60 000
2002	1.0	190000	0.6	330 000	33	40 000
Western and Central Europe						
2004	610 000	21 000	0.3	160 000	25	6500
2002	600 000	18 000	0.3	150 000	25	6000
North America						
2004	1.0	44000	0.6	260 000	25	16 000
2002	970000	44000	0.6	240 000	25	16 000
Total						
2004	39.4	4.9	1.1	17.6	47	3.1
2002	36.6	4.5	1.1	16.4	48	2.7

Source : UNAIDS *AIDS Epidemic Update*, December (2004 :7-9).

The number of people living with HIV has been rising in every region and no country in the world remains unaffected. The epidemic is not homogeneous within and between the countries. The epidemic has steepest increase in Sub-Saharan Africa, Caribbean, East Asia and in Eastern Europe and Central Asia. In other regions of the world the epidemic is gradually increasing not only among risk groups but also among general population.

UNAIDS and WHO have divided the globe into 10 epidemic zone in order to obtain easy estimation of HIV/AIDS in different regions of the globe. These zones are Sub-Saharan Africa, East Asia, South and South East Asia, Oceania, Eastern Europe and Central Asia, Western and Central Europe, North Africa and Middle East, North America, Caribbean and Latin America.

It is evident from Table 4.4 that the Sub-Saharan Africa has the largest number of people living with HIV positive followed by South and South East Asia. Latin America, Eastern Europe and Central Asia, East Asia and North America. Western and Central Europe, North Africa and Middle East, Caribbean and Oceania regions have low level of infection rate in 2004. But the comparison of rate of infection in 2004 with the 2002 and 2001 shows that these regions will also soon comes under the heavy epidemic regions.

Women and Aids

The women are increasingly infected in many regions. AIDS is affecting women more severely where heterosexual is the dominant mode of transmission. Globally, half of all people living with HIV positive are female. UNICEF survey says that above 50% of young women in high prevalence countries did not know the basic facts about AIDS (UNAIDS AIDS Epidemic Update, December 2004: 8). Women's HIV infection has its roots not only from women's ignorance about HIV/AIDS and sex and sexuality but also from their disempowerment. Most women around the world become HIV infected through their partners' high risk behaviours where women have either little or no control.

In 1996 it was estimated that 42 per cent of the 21.8 million adult living with HIV/AIDS are women, and the proportion has increased to 47 per cent in 2004 (UNAIDS AIDS epidemic update, 2004: 5).

Socio-economic inequality, gender discrimination, poverty, illiteracy and lack of skills, multiple partner relationships, transactional sex, intergenerational sex, violence against women, cultural backwardness are some of the major causes for increasing infection among women in all parts of the world.

The prevalence of HIV infection among women is concentrated more in Sub-Saharan Africa, Caribbean, Latin America, Eastern Europe and Central Asia and Asia.

The Trends of Adult Women (15-49 Years) Living with HIV in High Concentrated Regions

Table 4.5. Percentage of Infection among Adult Women from 1985-2004 in High Prevalence Regions

Regions	*1985*	*1990*	*1995*	*2000*	*2004*
Sub-Saharan Africa	49	54	56	57	57
Caribbean	45	50	47	48	49
Latin America	18	22	30	34	36
Eastern Europe and Central Asia	0	23	28	32	34
Asia	0	19	22	27	30

Source: *UNAIDS AIDS Epidemic Update, 2004: 7.*

Table 4.5 reflected that the HIV prevalence among women is rapidly increasing year by year in the above mentioned regions. Hetero sexual contact is the major mode of transmission in Sub-Saharan Africa and Caribbean. Three quarters of all women with HIV worldwide live in Sub-Saharan Africa. Adult women in Sub-Saharan Africa are upto 1.3 times more likely to be infected with HIV than their male counterparts and the infection is greatest among young women aged 15-24 years. In South Africa, Zambia and Zimbabwe the young women (aged 15-24) are three to six times more likely to be infected than young men. Women constitute nearly half of the 420 000 adults living with HIV in the Caribbean, where young women 15-24 years of age are almost twice as likely to be infected than are young men (*UNAIDS AIDS Epidemic Update*, 2004: 8).

Women represent 36% of the 1.7 million adult living with HIV in Latin America. In this region the epidemic is centered largely among men who have sex with men and injecting drug users. The risk groups normally have sex with sex workers and they also mostly have wives or other sexual partners. In Eastern Europe, the AIDS epidemics are spreading within and between particular population groups such as sex workers or injecting drug users and then into the general population. In these regions women and girls are increasingly affected. In East Asia women comprise 22% of all adults living with HIV and 28% of young people (aged 15-24 years) living with HIV. In South and South-East Asia, 30% of adults and 40% of young people living with HIV are women and girls. Women accounted for more than one quarter of new HIV infections in India and HIV transmission between spouses has become a more prominent cause of new infections in countries such as India, Cambodia, Myanmar and Thailand (*UNAIDS AIDS Epidemic Update*, 2004: 8).

In the industrialized countries of Western Europe and North America, one quarter of people living with HIV are women and the infection is increasingly lodged among women of marginalized sections of populations, including minorities, immigrants and refugees. African American and Hispanic women represent less than one quarter of all women in the United States of America, but accounted for 80% of AIDS cases reported among women at the turn of this century (*UNAIDS AIDS Epidemic Update*, 2004: 9.).

Sub-Saharan Africa

Sub-Saharan Africa is located in the south of the Sahara desert, in Africa. It is the worst-affected region in the world by the AIDS epidemic. The region has just over 10% of the world's population, but is home to over 60% of all people living with HIV. In 1996 14 million people were estimated as HIV positive. However, in 2002, 24.4 million adult and children and in 2004, 25.4 million were estimated as HIV positive. It has almost 11 million of increased infection from 1996. The per centage of adult infection rate in 2002 is 7.5 where as it was found to be stable (7.4%) in 2004. Less than one million (783,700) AIDS deaths were estimated during 1996. But the death rate of adult and children due to AIDS has increased to 2.3 million in 2004 from 2.1 million in 2002. An estimated 3.1 million adults and children became infected with HIV during the year 2004. This brought the total number of people living with HIV/AIDS in the region to 25.4 million by the end of the year 2004.

Many African countries are experiencing generalized epidemics. This means that HIV is spreading throughout the general population, rather than being confined to populations at higher risk, such as sex workers and their clients, men who have sex with men, and injecting drug users.

All the countries in Sub-Saharan Africa have prevalence rate about 17% with Botswana and Swaziland having about 35%. In West Africa HIV prevalence is much lower and no country in this region have prevalence rate above 10%. Adult prevalence rate in central and East Africa is estimated as 4-14 per cent (*Report on the Global Epidemic*, 2004: 7-8).

Women at greater risk in Sub-Saharan Africa

Sub-Saharan Africa ranks first in Women's HIV infection. In the beginning of the era of AIDS epidemic, which was in 1985 the per centage of adult women's (15-49 years) was estimated as below 50%. But it has increased to 57% in 2004 (*UNAIDS AIDS Epidemic Update*, December 2004: 11). Among them 76% of young people are aged between 15-24 years. African women are being infected at an earlier age than men, and the gap in HIV prevalence between them continue to grow. At the beginning of the epidemic in sub-Saharan Africa, women living with HIV were vastly outnumbered by men. But today there are, on average, 13 infected women for every 10 infected men when compared to 12 infected women for every 10 infected men in 2002.

The difference between infection levels is more pronounced in urban areas, with 14 women for very 10 men, than in rural areas, where 12 women are infected for every 10 men. Adult women in Sub-Saharan Africa are 1.3 times more likely to be infected than their male counterparts (*UNAIDS Report on the Global Epidemic*, 2004: 11-12).

The difference in infection levels between women and men is even more pronounced among young people aged 15-24. Today, there are 13 infected women for every 10 infected men in Sub-Saharan Africa. It has its ranges from 20 women for every 10 men in South Africa, to 45 women for very 10 men in Kenya and Mali (*UNAIDS Report on the Global Epidemic*, 2004: 7-8). In Sub-Saharan Africa, heterosexual transmission is by far the predominant mode of HIV transmission. Unsafe injections in health-care settings are believed to be responsible for around 2.5% of all infections.

HIV has spread rapidly among people with high-risk behaviours and widely among those assumed to be at lower risk. Prevalence among urban sex workers ranges from 20 per cent to 50 per cent in various countries of Sub-Saharan Africa. Infection rates among women attending antenatal clinics have grown rapidly to high levels in some areas, have stabilized at lower levels in others and appear to be declining in some areas like Kampala and Uganda. An estimated two-thirds of all new cases of mother-to-child transmission worldwide occur in sub-Saharan Africa (Ramamurthy, 2000: 111).

Median HIV prevalence in Pregnant women attending antenatal clinics in Sub-Saharan Africa from 1998-2003

The prevalence of HIV among antenatal women in different countries of Sub-Saharan Africa shows that the rata of infection is rapidly increasing among the women in African countries (Table 4.6).

In Southern Africa, the epidemic is rapidly increasing among the antenatal women whereas in Eastern Africa the epidemic remain constant and it shows certain declining trends in Uganda. The low prevalence is found in Western Africa, especially in the regions of Ghana, Nigeria and Senegal. But the region of Cameroon and Cote d'ivoire has higher prevalence of infection in Western Africa. In these regions, the median HIV prevalence levels have reached to 10% among pregnant women.

Table 4.6. Percentage of HIV Prevalence Among Pregnant Women from 1997-2003

Regions	*1997-98*	*1999-2000*	*2001*	*2002*	*2003*
		SOUTHERN AFRICA			
Botswana	37	38	40	40	39
Mozambique	No data	10	15	15	—
South Africa	20	23	25	27	30
		EASTERN AFRICA			
Ethiopia	13	10	10	10	9
Kenya	13	14	10	9	9
Uganda	10	5	6	5	—
		WESTERN AFRICA			
Ghana	3	3	6	5	—
Cote d'ivoire	10	9	10	10	—
Nigeria	—	5	6	4	5
Senegal	0	0	4	0	—

Source: *UNAIDS AIDS epidemic update*, 2004: 20.

Causes for Women's HIV infection in Sub-Saharan Region

Poverty, lower status of women, female circumcision, involvement in sexual activities at early ages, pre marital sex to overcome financial strain are the major factors for women to get infected by the dreaded virus HIV. The culture of silence surrounding sexuality, exploitative transactional and intergenerational sex and violence against women within the relationship are the other important causes for African's women's vulnerability towards HIV/AIDS.

Impact of HIV/AIDS on Africa

HIV/AIDS has a widespread impact on many sections of society.

- In many countries of Sub-Saharan Africa, AIDS has reduced the life expectancy of the people. Millions of adults are dying at young or in early middle age. Average life expectancy in Sub-Saharan Africa is now 47 years, when it could have been 62 without AIDS.

- The toll of HIV/AIDS on households can be very severe. Many families are losing their income earners. Many of those dying have surviving partners who are themselves infected and in need of care. They leave behind children grieving and struggling to survive without a parent's care. HIV/AIDS strips the family assets further impoverishing the poor.
- In all affected countries, the HIV/AIDS epidemic is bringing additional pressure to bear on the health sector.
- A decline in school enrolment is one of the most visible effects of the HIV/AIDS epidemic on education in Africa.
- HIV/AIDS dramatically affects labour, setting back economic activity and social progress. The vast majority of people living with HIV/AIDS in Africa are between the ages of 15 and 49 - in the prime of their working lives.

Caribbean

The Caribbean is the second most affected region in the world with regard to women's infection with the adult prevalence rate of 2.3 per cent. It was estimated that 270,000 people were living with HIV AIDS in 1996 (Digmarti Bhaskara Rao, 2000: 217), but the infection has almost doubled in 2004. Among adult in the age group of 15-44, AIDS has become the leading cause of death (*UNAIDS Global Epidemic Update*, 2004: 35). Among young people 15-24 years of age, an estimated 3.1% of women and 1.7 of men were living with HIV in 2004. In five countries such as **Bahamas, Belize, Guyana, Haiti and Trinidad** and **Tobago** the national prevalence exceeds 2%. The adult prevalence is almost stabilized in Caribbean.

In this region, 12 countries face a generalized epidemic, with 1% prevalence among pregnant women. Heterosexual transmission is the main mode of transmission and it is only in Puerto Rico that injecting drug use drives the epidemic. **Haiti** is the most affected country, with 30,000 AIDS related deaths a year and 120,000 orphans due to AIDS. Its adult prevalence rate remains stable at 5% to 6% (WHO, 2003: 7).

HIV infection among Women in Caribbean

The highest infections among women in the Americas are in Caribbean countries. Women constitute nearly half of the adult living with the HIV positive. Young women are 2.5 times more likely to be infected than young men in the Caribbean island. The women in several countries like Barbados, Bermuda, Dominican Republic, Jamaica and Trinidad and Tabago and territories which depend on tourism are severely affected by HIV infection (*UNAIDS Global Epidemic Update*, 2004: 11).

In 2002-2004 around 49% of all people living with HIV positive in Caribbean are women. In 1985 the rate of infection among women was identified as 45%. But now it has increased to 49%. The ratio of infection between men and women is 2: 1. Women younger than 24 years in the Dominican Republic were almost twice as likely to be HIV infected than their male counterparts. In Jamaica teenage girls are 2.5 times more likely to be infected than boys in the same age group of 10-19 years.

Haiti continues to have the largest number of people living with HIV in Caribbean. It has 280 000 (range 120,000-600,000) people living with HIV in 2003. The median HIV prevalence among women (25-49 years) attending antenatal clinics has fallen from 4.5% in 1996 to 2.8% in 2003-2004. HIV prevalence among pregnant women aged 15-24 years appears to have declined from 3.6% to 2.8% in 2003-2004. The over all infection among pregnant women varies between 1.8% and 7.0% in different parts of Haiti.

Jamaica has an estimated 22000 (range 11 000-41 000) people living with HIV in 2003. HIV prevalence among pregnant women attending antenatal clinics is found to be at 1.4% in 2002. But it has increased to 2.7% in St. James and 1.9% in Kingston and St. Andrews. High HIV prevalence is also observed among patients at sexually transmitted clinics in 2002. Almost 8% of men and 5% of women in sexually transmitted clinics are infected by HIV.

In **Bahamas** where an estimated 5000 people were living with HIV in 2003 and the HIV prevalence among pregnant women fall from 4.8% in 1993 and 3.6% in 1996 to 3.0% in 2002 due to stronger preventions techniques.

In **Barbados** region, declining trend in HIV infection is observed. HIV infection among pregnant women dropped from 0.7% in 1999 to 0.3% in 2003. Mother-to-child transmission also reduced due to the expansion of voluntary counseling and testing services and the provision of anti retroviral treatment. In Bermuda, the number of AIDS cases decreased by almost half (19 to11) between 2000 and 2002.

HIV prevalence in **Guyana** was the second highest in this region (2.5%) in 2003. The epidemic is serious in Dominican Republic with HIV prevalence among pregnant women higher than 2%. Most of the infections are due to unprotected sex. HIV prevalence is very low in Cuba .But now it has observed rising trends in HIV infection as a result of sex between men.

Factors influencing Women's HIV Infection in Caribbean

The causes for their infection are due to the fact that some girls have sexual relationship with older men who are more likely to be HIV infected. The same trend has also been documented in several countries of Caribbean regions. This trend is due to large proportion of men who have sex with men, also have sex with women. This is partly responsible for the increasing feminization of the epidemic.

Latin America

All the main modes of transmission exist in most countries of Latin America along with significant levels of risky behaviours–such as early sexual entrance, unprotected sex with multiple partners and the use of unclean drug-injecting equipment. HIV prevalence rate is increasing in many Latin American Countries.

Around 1.7 million people are living with HIV in Latin America in 2004 compared with 1.5 million in 2002 and 1.3 million in 1996. In 2004 it is estimated that 95 000 people have died due to AIDS. The mortality rate is higher when compared to the mortality rate of 2003 (84 000) and 2002 (74000) and 1996 (70,000). Among young people 15-24 years of age, 0.5% of women and 0.8% of men were living with HIV in 2003. The adult's prevalence rate is 0.6% in 2004.

Several Central American countries, such as **Belize, Honduras, Guyana and Suriname** have an estimated HIV prevalence of 1% or more among pregnant women. The infection among Latin American women was estimated around 15-20% in 1985 and it was increased to 35% in 2002 and 36% in 2004. The ratio of men with HIV infections to women with HIV infections has narrowed considerably to about 3 to1. This is partly because a large proportion of men who have sex with men, also have sex with women.

National HIV prevalence is now estimated to be 1% in Belize, Guyana, Honduras and Suriname. In most countries HIV infection is not generalized but is highly concentrated in populations at particular risk. Despite a national prevalence below 1%, Brazil has 40% of people living with HIV in Latin America. In some Brazilian cities, more than 60% of drug users are HIV positive.

In most **South American countries**, almost all infections are caused by contaminated drug-injecting equipment or sex between men. **In Puerto Rico,** more than half of all infections in 2002 were associated with injecting drug use, and about one-quarter were heterosexually transmitted (UNAIDS report on the global epidemic, 2004).

In **Central America**, injecting drug use plays less role, and the virus is spread predominantly through sex. HIV prevalence among female sex workers ranges from less than 1% in **Nicaragua,** 2% in **Panama,** 4% in **El Salvador** and 5% in **Guatemala,** to over 20% in **Hondura** (UNAIDS report on the global epidemic, 2004).

Unsafe sex among men who have sex with men is common across the whole region. The 13% of HIV prevalence in **Honduran** and the 8 to 18% of infection in Central America was among men who have sex with men. In Honduras 7% of male prisoners were infected with HIV infection. Unsafe sex is the major cause for the infection in the **Andean countries** of South America. In these places, prevalence rates have ranged from 14% in Lima, Peru to 20% in Bogotá in **Colombia** and 28% **Guayaquil** in **Ecuador.** In these regions, the large per centages of men who have sex with men also have unsafe sex with women which ultimately increase women's vulnerability to HIV/AIDS.

The spread of HIV through the sharing of drug injecting equipment is of growing concern in several countries, notably **Argentina, Brazil, Chile, Paraguay, Uruguay** and the northern part of **Mexico.** Injecting drug use accounts for an estimated 40% of reported new infections in **Argentina** and 28% in **Uruguay**. In both of these countries a growing number of women with HIV are injecting drug users or the sexual partners of men who are injecting drug users.

The increasing infection in Latin America is mainly due to low rates of condom use, and high numbers of sexual partners and low perceptions of risk.

Provision of anti-retroviral

Countries in Latin America for example Brazil, Argentina, Chile, Mexico and Uruguay, Colombia, Costa Rica and Paraguay are making efforts to provide antiretroviral drugs to patients with HIV/AIDS related illnesses. The Brazilian government has estimated that antiretroviral treatment has contributed to a 50% fall in mortality rates, a 60-80% decrease in morbidity rates and a 70% reduction in hospitalizations among HIV-positive people. Argentina reported decreasing numbers of deaths between 1999 and 2004 with stabilization over the last two years (Rob Noble, 2004: wp1).

East Europe and Central Asia

The infection is drastically increasing in East European and Central Asian countries. The infection was estimated as just 50,000 in 1996. But it has increased to 1.4 million in 2004. Around 210 000 people were newly infected with HIV during 2003 and 60 000 people have died due to AIDS till 2004 as against 1000 people in 1996. Like other countries, in these regions also the infection is found in higher per centage among the young people with the age of 15-24 years. Among them, the estimated rate of infection for women is 0.8% (0.4-1.6%) and for men it is found to be around 1.7% (0.8-3.7%). In both the regions, the women's HIV infection was estimated as 20% in 2001. But it has increased to 21% in 2002 and 34% in 2004 (UNAIDS Global Epidemic Update, December 2004: 52-60).

Eastern Europe

In the Eastern Europe, Ukraine is the worst affected region and Russian Federation is the home to the largest epidemic in the entire region. In 2001, the Russian Federation has 55% of infection in the Eastern European countries. But it has increased to 70% in 2004 mainly due to the activities of commercial sex and injecting drug use. In other regions of Eastern Europe, the epidemic is in its early stage (*UNAIDS AIDS Epidemic Update*, 2004: 52).

Across the continent, HIV infections through heterosexual contact are increasing steadily and women account for a rising proportion of HIV diagnoses. Most of the infections are among adult below the age of 30 years. In Ukraine 25%, in Belaras 60% are aged between 15-24 years. Most of the drug users are under the age of 19 years of age (30% in St. Petersburg, 20% in Ukraine, and 12% in Moscow). The use of unclean equipment, sharing of drug injecting equipment is the common norm among the drug users (Avert Organisation.2004: 1).

Social and economic transition forced large number of youth towards injecting drug use and commercial sex activities. Around 81% of women entered into prostitution at their younger age of 15-39 years. Therefore, the rate of infection is higher (64%) among the women at the age group of 20-24 years. Around 30% infection in Ukraine among women is heterosexual in 2003. It is three times higher than the documents of 1997 (11%). In Eastern Europe, 40% of infected women were at their reproductive age and 60% are under the age of 25 years. Nearly 1% of pregnant women were tested HIV positives in these regions. The increasing trend of infection among women shows the increasing trend of mother-to-child transmission. In 2001 around 27% of child infection is through mother-to-child transmission. But it has decreased to 12% in 2003 as a result of effective intervention programme (*UNAIDS AIDS Epidemic Update*, 2004: 52-60).

Central Asia

Kazakhstan, Kyrgyzstan, Tajikistan, Turkmenistan and Uzbekistan are the five countries associated with Central Asian Republics (Jawahar, 2004: 1). The number of reported cases of infection is still low in Central Asia. But the infection is dramatically increasing. Officially reported cases in the five countries of Central Asia jumped from about 500 in 200 to over 12000 in 2004. Unreported cases are higher in these regions. The Centre for Disease Control and Prevention in Central Asia has estimated that around 90000 people are living with HIV in these regions. One third of all identified cases were detected only in 2003. The rapid increase is between 2000 and 2003 is three fold in Kazakhstan, nine fold in the Kyrgyz Republic, 17 fold in Tajikistan and 16 fold in Uzbekistan. The male-female ration was greater than 4: 1 in all countries. The rate of infection is higher among the prisoners (8%). The infection among pregnant women in the entire region is found to be below 1% and among drug users is around 2% (The World Bank Group, 2005: 1).

In Central Asia, the epidemic is driven by injecting drug use and unsafe sex and it is concentrated among young people. Therefore, drug users and prostitutes forming the largest risk groups. According to World Health Organisation, 70% of all new infection in Uzbekistan are among injection drug users. The impact of stigma with regard to HIV/AIDS is higher in Central Asian Countries. The prevailing stigma reduces the harm reduction programme for drug users, prostitutes and other higher risk groups. The stigma also prevents high risk people from taking HIV test (Naz Nazar, 2004: 1).

Central Asian countries are located on both the sides of major drug trafficking routes into the Russian Federation and Europe. Young people particularly economically marginalized are more vulnerable. In Kazakhstan, for example, three quarters of people diagnosed with HIV were unemployed. In Kazakhstan and Kyrgyzstan 70% of all HIV positive persons are under 30 years of age. Condom use is generally low among the young people in Eastern Europe and Central Asia and it increases the rate of infection among the general population in general and women in particular (Avert Organisation, 2004: 1).

Asia

The Asian continent comprises of South and South East Asia and East Asia. In East Asia 22% of the adults living with HIV/AIDS are women. Among them 28% are young people aged between 15-24 years. In South and South East Asia more than a quarter of adults and 40% of young people living with HIV/AIDS are women. Until now the mode of infection in Asia is mainly through injecting drug use and sex work. Factors affecting the spread of HIV/AIDS among women and girls in the regions are poverty, early marriage, trafficking and sex work, migration, lack of education, gender discrimination and violence. HIV transmission between spouses has become a more prominent cause of new infection in countries such as Cambodia, Myanmar, Thailand anu India. Injecting drug use is the major mode of transmission in countries such as Indonesia, Nepal and Bangladesh.

Table 4.7. HIV and AIDS Statistics and Features end of 2002 and 2004

Year	*Adult & Children living with HIV (in million)*	*No. of Women living with HIV (in million)*	*Adult & Children newly infected with HIV (in million)*	*Adult prevalence (%)*	*Adult & Child death due to AIDS (in million)*
2004	8.2 (5.4-11.8)	2.3 (1.5-3.3)	1.2 (720 000-2.4 million)	0.4 (0.3-0.6)	540 000 (350 000-810 000)
2002	7.2 (4.6-10.5)	1.9 (1.2-2.8)	1.1 (540-2.5 million)	0.4 (0.2-0.5)	470 000 (300 00-690 000)

Source: UNAIDS Global Epidemic Update, December 2004: 36-49.

National HIV infection level in Asia is low compared with some other continent like Africa. The latest estimate shows that 8.2 million people are living with in 2004. Among them 2.3 million are adult women. The new infection during 2004 is 1.2 million. AIDS claimed 540 000 lives in 2004. Among young people 15-24 years of age, 0.3% of women and 0.4% of men were living with HIV by the end of 2004.

Classification of Asian regions

Asian countries can be divided into several categories according to the epidemic they are experiencing (UNAIDS AIDS

Epidemic Update, (2004: 36). They are classified as:

Table 4.8. Classification of Regions Based on Prevalence of HIV

Early Hit countries	Cambodia, Myanmar and Thailand
Low prevalence countries	Bangladesh, East Timor, Laos, Pakistan and the Philippines
High prevalence countries	Indonesia, Nepal, Vietnam, China and India

Early Hit Countries

Early hit countries are located close to "Golden Triangle" which is known for drug trafficking. Sex industry flourished in these regions due to widespread poverty. Ignorance, gender inequality, lower status, poor knowledge on AIDS, and poor education causes for the spread of epidemic in early hit countries.

Cambodia

The UNAIDS statistics of global over view of AIDS epidemic states that the Cambodia's national HIV prevalence is around 3% — the highest rate of infection in Asia (UNAIDS, 2002). According to UNAIDS statistics of 2003, there were 170 000 people between the age group of 15-49 are living with HIV. Among them women and children accounted for 51,000 and 7300. The adult prevalence rate is 2.6% and the AIDS death in 2003 is 15,000. The women attending anti natal clinics accounted for 2.2% (http: /hivinsite.ucsf.edu/global).

HIV was first detected in 1991 during serological screening of donated blood in 1991 and the first cases of AIDS were diagnosed in late 1993 (Arvind Singhal *et al.*, 2003: 111). Active commercial sex and "bridging" networks played a major role in the rapid spread of HIV, with a large portion of HIV incidence comprising transmission from sex workers to their male clients (Ramamurthy 2003: 13). HIV Sentinel Surveillance (HSS) data of Cambodia reveals that the sexual contact, both homo (14%) and hetero sexual is the major cause for the spread of epidemic followed by injection drug use. HIV prevalence rate is suspected to be high on the Thai border. The results provided the first evidence of a highly disseminated HIV epidemic, with prevalence of HIV upto 38% among female sex workers, 8% among police and the military and about 2.5% among women attending antenatal clinics (WHO, 2003: 26).

A survey of female sex workers by the Government of Cambodia in 1995 revealed that 38% were HIV positive. Therefore, Cambodia has borrowed the idea of 100 Percent Condom Programme and implemented in all regions of Cambodia. As a result condom use by brothel-based commercial sex workers has increased from 53% in 1998 to 78% in 1999 the increased condom use reduced the infection among brothel-based sex workers from 43% in 1998 to 29% in 2002. There have also been sustained declines in prevalence among their customers, who include urban policemen, military conscripts and motorcycle taxi riders (Singhal *et al.*, 2003: 112).

Table 4.9. Percentage of HIV Infection among Different Risk Groups from 1999-2002

Risk groups	*1999*	*2000*	*2001*	*2002*
Direct Sex Workers	13	9	8	6
Indirect Sex Workers	5	5.5	4	3
Police men	2.5	2	1.5	1
Pregnant women	1	2	1.5	1

Sources: UNAIDS AIDS epidemic update, 2004

The above table shows that the rate of HIV prevalence is decreasing among female sex workers, both direct and indirect due to the impact of various intervention programmes with regard to safe sex by using condom.

Myanmar

Geographical mapping of officially reported AIDS cases show that the eastern states/divisions have been the hardest hit by the epidemic. The central and delta regions have moderate rates of infection, with the lowest found on the western borders. The UNAIDS global report of 2003 reveals that an estimated 320,000 adult with the age of 15-49 are living with HIV positive in 2003 with the adult prevalence rate of 1.2%. Among them the women with the age of 15-49 living with HIV positive in 2003 is found to be 97,000. The children infected with HIV are estimated as 7600 in 2003. AIDS mortality is accounted for 20,000 in 2003 (UNAIDS, 2004).

HIV/AIDS situation in Myanmar is 'explosive' and it becomes a major contributor to the erosion of the well being of the general population. The infection has moved towards general population from most vulnerable sub -populations, such as injecting drug users and sex workers. HIV in Myanmar is mostly spread by injecting drug use and risky sex, both heterosexual and between men. The prevalence among injecting drug users is found in large area- from Yangon to the Shan State (Taunggyi, Lashio and Muse), bordering India, and Myitkyina in Kachin State.

The first HIV positive case in Myanmar was found in 1988 and the first AIDS case in 1991. UNAIDS (2002) data shows that the infection rate among commercial sex workers is (CSW) 33.5%, blood donors accounted for 1.1%, new military recruits have 2.2% and pregnant women's infection is around 2.2%. The official reported HIV cases show 30% are due to injecting drug use and 68% are due to unprotected heterosexual transmission (Myanmar Business Coalition of AIDS, 2002: 1). In some places, 78% of drug injectors tested positive in 2003. Each year the infection rate among injecting drug users are found to be around 45% to 80%. HIV infection among the patients attending sexually transmitted clinics have increased from 6% to 9% in 2003 (UNDIAD, December, 2004: 43).

The epidemic has been able to spread quickly throughout Myanmar due to several reasons. These include low awareness of HIV/AIDS amongst the general population' improper STD care, irregular HIV testing, low use of condoms, and large commercial sex business hidden from public life which makes it harder to control HIV/AIDS among commercial sex workers.

Thailand

Thailand has around 570,000 people living with HIV/AIDS including 200 000 women and 12,000 children. The estimated adult prevalence rate in 2003 is 1.5% (0.8-2.8%). The number of people died due to AIDS in 2003 is accounted for 58,000 (UNAIDS, Dec 2004: 44). Hetero sex, much of it between commercial sex workers and their customers (Celentano *et al.*, 2000: 535-40) and sharing needles among the injecting drug users are the main mode of HIV transmission in Thailand.

The first case of AIDS was reported in Thailand in 1984, (Phanuphak *et al.*, 1985: 195-199, Limsuwan *et al.* 1986: 164-169). In 1988-89 in the first major wave of the epidemic exploded among injecting drug-users, and found 40% in 1989. The second wave of infection spread among sex workers. In 1989, it was found that 44% of sex workers in Chiang Mai, in the north, were infected with HIV. The third waves of the epidemic identified among male clients of sex workers, their wives and partners, and their children (Weniger, 1991: S71: S85).

An estimated 200,000 of Thailand's 63 million people are commercial sex workers. During 1989 to 1995, 600,000 Thai men became HIV positive and the figure gone upto 984,000 in 2002 (Singal *et al.*, 2003: 103). At present it is estimated that one fifth of all new HIV infection is occurring among injecting drug users and in Northern Thailand 30% of drug injectors are infected with HIV and in other parts it was around 51%. The HIV prevalence is found to be 17% among men who have sex with men. Most of the men who are visiting brothel based sex workers, homosexuals and injecting drug users have wife and girl friends. Therefore, increasing number of women is infected by their husbands and the infection levels among pregnant women remain high in many parts of the country including the South, where they exceeded 2% in 2002 (UNAIDS, Dec. 2004: 44).

A massive intervention programme with strong political commitment (through mass media and other Government and non-governmental agencies) to control HIV has reduced men's visits to commercial sex workers by half, raised condom usage, and decreased STDs (Sexually Transmitted Diseases) and achieved substantial reductions in new HIV infections (World Bank, 2000: 1) from 140,000 in 1991 to 29000 in 2001 (Ramamorthy, 2000: 115) to 21,000 in 2003 (UNAIDS, July 2002: 31-32).

The main routes of HIV transmission occurred through commercial sex has been changed due to Thailand's massive 100% condom programme with the aim of 100% condom use for all commercial and casual sex. As a result by 1992, condom use in brothels had claimed to 90% and the rate of sexually transmitted diseases among males dropped to 90% and the infection rate among conscripts in the Royal Thai Army has decreased from 4% in 1993 to 1.3% in 1999 (Ainsworth et, 2000: 6).

But steady transmission of HIV from the infected male clients of female sex workers, and from infected male injecting drug users to their regular sex partners (wives and girlfriends) is observed in Thailand (World Health Organisation, 2001: 21-23). Now half of the newly identified infections are occurring among the wives and sexual partners of men who got infected several years ago (UNAIDS 2002: 10).

Though the rate of HIV infection among commercial sex workers was reduced from 50% in 1991 to 20% in 2001 still there is evidence that HIV prevalence is on the rise among sex workers in some parts of the country, particularly in Bangkok (World Bank, 2000: 2). The unsafe sexual behaviour is increasing among young people in Thailand and the rates of infection among teenagers have increased to 17% from 11% (WHO, 2001: 21-23). Still one-in 100 Thais are infected with HIV, and AIDS has become the leading cause of death (Ramamorthy, 2000: 115). Poverty, injecting drug use and a flourishing sex industry provided fertile conditions for rapid spread of the virus in Thailand.

Low Prevalence Countries

The rate of HIV/AIDS is found to be less in some of the Asian countries which are given in Table 4.10:

Table 4.10. Low Prevalence Countries

	Bangladesh 2002	*East Timor 2003*	*Mongolia 2003*	*PDR Lao 2003*	*Pakistan 2003*	*Philippines 2003*	*Sri Lanka 2003*
Female Sex workers	0-07%	3%	0	0-1.1%	0	<1%	0-02%
Men who have sex with men	0-0.2%	0.9%	—	—	—	0	—
High risk men	0	0	0	0	—	0	0
STI clinic clients	0	—	0	—	—	—	0-1%
Drug injectors	0.4%	—	—	—	0	0	—

Source: UNAIDS Epidemic. Update: December, 2004: 45

High risk men include truck drivers, launch workers, boyfriends of sex workers, taxi drivers and soldiers, military recruits, transport workers and male military.

Hetero sex and injecting drug use are the main mode of HIV transmission in low prevalence countries. Female sex workers are infected more in these regions when compared to other risk groups. HIV/AIDS is not yet documented properly in Maldives and Buttons. The threat of continued growth in HIV prevalence in these regions depends on the proportion of people engaging in unprotected sex with infected partners, its spread to pregnant women and their babies, and the proportion exposed to unsafe blood-related procedures. Sri Lanka, Maldives, Philippines, Malaysia, Bangladesh and Japan are encouraging tourism to increase its national income. In these regions sex work is flourishing and the culture of injecting drug use is increasing as a result of tourism. It also increases rural to urban migration (Ramamurthy, 2003: 236).

Sex work is the predominant cause for the spread of HIV in Bangladesh and Philippines. Malaysia's HIV infection is largely derived from injection drug users. In Malaysia 55% of people detected with HIV between 1998 and 2001 were drug injectors. Migration is identified as the major cause for the spread of HIV infection in East Timor and Pakistan. In Japan, HIV prevalence is steadily raised among male blood donors and men who have sex with men. These men might also be transmitting the virus to female sex workers (*UNAIDS, AIDS epidemic Update*, December, 2004: 45-46).

The low prevalence countries the adult prevalence rate varies from 0.1% to 0.4%. The number of HIV infection also varies from 500 to 38,900. The highest number of women living with HIV/AIDS is found in Pakistan (38,900) and Malaysia (8500). The lesser number of infected women is identified in Sri Lanka (600) and PDR Lao (<500) (UNAIDS report 2003).

Poverty, gender inequalities and low level of education and literacy contribute to HIV vulnerability to women. In low prevalence countries women in general have lower socio-economic status, less mobility and less decision making power. Women in these regions have low awareness on HIV/AIDS, its implications and safe sex practices. Besides, safe sex matters are not discussed at interpersonal level. It increases their HIV vulnerability. Illiteracy makes an obstacle for HIV/AIDS prevention in general and much harder to reach women than men with information about how they can protect themselves from HIV infection. The economic and social dependency on men and social restriction on their mobility often make it difficult for women to obtain access to health and social services and access to basic reproductive health care. Their restricted decision making power in the family again make an obstacle to negotiate with their partners for safer sexual practices. These marginalized people enter into prostitution for their livelihood and they are more vulnerable to HIV infection and condom use among them is relatively low. Their low awareness of the implications of unsafe sex increases their vulnerability to HIV (Ramamurthy, 2003: 123-240).

High Prevalence Countries

High prevalence countries in Asia are identified as China, Nepal, Indonesia and India.

China

China is experiencing one of the most rapidly expanding HIV epidemics in the world. It has 30% of annual rate of increase since 1999. Based on this calculation it is estimated that the number of people living in China will exceed 10 million by 2010, if there is no sufficient control on epidemic. The most frequent mode of HIV transmission has been injecting drug use in Southern and Western China and unsafe practices paid blood donors in other regions. Hetero sexually transmitted HIV is occurring primarily in the Eastern provinces of China, fueled by an increasing commercial sex trades and by large number of migrants moving to other provinces in search of labour. The per centage of female prostitute not using condom is identified as 66.7% in 1999 and 37.4% in 2001. HIV prevalence among injecting drug users is found to be 35-80% in Xingjian and 20% in Guangdong. The estimated injecting drug users in China range from a low of about less than half million to three million. These infected injecting drug users have transmitted and can be expected to transmit their infection to a large proportion of their sex partners (WHO, 2003: 53) In rural areas, where people earned money by donating blood plasma in early 1990s, infection level of 10 to 20 per cent have been found, rising to 60% in certain communities (Rob Noble, September, 2004).

In China, its 31 provinces, autonomous regions and municipalities are witnessed the rapid spread of HIV transmission. China has a larger population than any other country in the world at 1.3 billion, 720 million of whom are aged between 15 and 49, the period of greatest sexual activity and drug use. China has become more of a market-lead economy in the last decade, and these economic changes have had social repercussions. Sex before marriage is now more socially acceptable, especially to young people, and there has been a rapid rise in commercial sex. As a result of the increase in sexual freedom, STDs have risen at a rate of about 30% each year for the past ten years.

According to UNAIDS statement, the estimated number of HIV/AIDS in China is 2003 is 840 000. Among them the adult with the age 15-49 years accounted for 830 000 and the estimated adult prevalence of HIV/AIDS in 2003 is 0.1%. The women living with HIV/AIDS accounted for 190 000 in 2003. The estimated number of AIDS death in 2003 is found to be 30 000.

Nepal

In Nepal, the topography, environmental degradation, poverty and economic migration are linked together and they combine with other factors to increase vulnerability to HIV. The predominant mode of transmission is sexual contact, most likely heterosexual. Highest rates of HIV have been identified in injecting drug users (IDUs), commercial sex workers, their clients, labour migrants and youth and young people. The rate of infection is high among the adult population between the ages of 15-49. Increasing levels of sexually transmitted diseases and limited information about homosexual and bisexual transmission facilitate the rapid spread of infection in all regions of Nepal.

The first cases of AIDS were reported in Nepal in 1988. But the Government of Nepal has identified only 0.5% of HIV prevalence among general population in June 2002. . The infection among adult with the age group of 15-49 is found to be 16000 in 2003 (UNAIDS 2004) and the number of adult and child mortality due to HIV/AIDS is 3100 in 2003. Among the people living with HIV, the IDUs accounted for maximum per centage (68%) in 2002. The report published by the Nepal Government in 2000 says that the HIV prevalence among the sex worker was 17.3%, among the people affected by sexually transmitted diseases accounted for 0.7-6.6%, followed by the blood donors (0.28-0.48%) and the infection found among the anti natal care women was only 0.2%. (Ramamurthy, 2003: 174).

One in 200 adult in Nepal is living with HIV positive and nine people a day died of AIDS in 2003 (Mennonite Central Committee, 2005). It shows that HIV is increasing in Nepal as a result of unemployment, migrant labor, civil unrest, drug use and prostitution. Intravenous drug users have highest risk of contracting HIV infection in Nepal followed by commercial sex workers, their clients and migrant labourers.

Nepali Capital, Kathmandu, is host to a great influx of of people from various parts of the country for seeking employment in industries, such as carpet, transport, stone quarries and constructions. The use of commercial sex is high among men who come to the city alone. Many women coming to the city fall into prostitution as a way to earn money for basic survival (Mennonite Central Committee, 2005)

The rate of HIV prevalence is high among the general population in Kathmandu Valley due to widespread commercial sex work and larger per centage (40.4%) of youths involvement in taking intravenous drugs. In 2000, it is found that among intravenous drug users in Nepal, 40% are HIV positive. It is also estimated that as many as 70 per cent of commercial sex workers returning from India are HIV positive. Estimates of the number of Nepali men working in India are around 1 million and above. Many of these men are contracting HIV/AIDS in

India and bringing it back to their wives in Nepal. It is estimated that 10% of HIV infection is found among the men returning from Mumbai to Nepal. Many of these infected people do not know that they are infected and many of them may be engaging in unsafe sexual practices. Such kind of unsafe sexual behaviours and intravenous drugs using habits among the youth has taken the country to the "concentrated epidemic" zone where HIV/AIDS prevalence consistently exceeds 5% in one or more subgroups. (Ramamurthy. V, 2003: 175-178)).

Due to their highly marginalized status in society, sex workers have little access to accurate information about reproductive health and sexually transmitted infections. Truckers and migrant workers are their main customers and it is found that 10.2% of truckers are infected with sexually transmitted infections and 1.5% is infected with HIV. Condom usages are very limited among these marginalized segments (Ramamurthy, 2003: 186).

Indonesia

It is estimated that about 110 000 (0.1%) of HIV infection is found in the age group of 15-49 years. HIV/AIDS data collect in Indonesia from all sources indicated that HIV prevalence rates were higher among female sex workers and it ranges from 1% to 5% in several areas of Indonesia. HIV prevalence is also increasing among injecting drug users in Jakarta (over 35% in 2000). During 1990s, most HIV infections in Indonesia could be attributed to infections acquired outside the country and to a pocket of epidemic heterosexual transmission in areas such as Merauke. Since the late 1990s, there has been an explosive HIV epidemic in injecting drug use populations in Indonesia. As of 2003, the most common pattern of HIV transmission in Indonesia has been from HIV infected persons to their spouses or regular sex partners and this will continue tc be the predominant pattern of HIV transmission in Indonesia. Indonesia is now classified as a country with a concentrated HIV epidemic, primarily among injecting drug use population (WHO, 2003: 60).

Indian Scenario on HIV/AIDS

Table 4.11. Important Landmarks of HIV Infection in India

Year	*Events*
April 1986	First cluster (ten prostitutes) of HIV seropositives detected in Madras, Tamil Nadu.
May 1986	First patient of final stage disease detected in Bombay, Maharashtra (recipient of unscreened blood transfusion during cardiac surgery in USA).
Dec. 1986	First seropositive male detected from STD clinic in Tamil Nadu.
July 1987	First seropositive blood donor in Vellore, Tamil Nadu (retrospective detection subsequent t to the recipient's illness).
July 1987	Spouse to spouse transmission is identified (the same donor's wife).
Oct. 1987	Detection of a seropositive infant (born to the abovementioned parents).
June 1988	First AIDS death (sex workers in Kamathipura, Mumbai.
April 1988	First indigenous case of full-blown HIV disease in an Indian.
Jan. 1989	Evidence of HIV antibodies in indigenously produced blood products.
Jan. 1989	Evidence of exposure to HIV among a high proportion of donors used by commercial manufacturers followed by a government ban on production.
July 1989	Government gazette notification for mandatory screening of blood donors for freedom from HIV antibodies.
Jan-Feb. 1990	Recognition of a cluster of seropositives in IV drug users in north-east India.
July 1992	Constitution of the National AIDS Control Organisation (NACO); at state levels also.
Oct. 1992.	Establishment of the National AIDS Research Institute, Pune by Indian Council of Medical Research (ICMR).

Year	*Events*
Dec 2004*	Free Antiretroviral drugs are given to the people living with HIV positive in the high prevalence states
July 2005*	India has begun human clinical trial of an investigational vaccine designed to prevent Human Immunodeficiency Virus (HIV) and Acquired Immuno-deficiency Syndrome (AIDS).

Sources: Khorshed M. Pavri, (1992: 17).
**The Hindu*, December 2004 and July 2005.

Like most countries in Asia, India is included in the Pattern III distribution of HIV disease. Although HIV begins in late 1980s, all the known modes of viral spread have been identified within the short period. There is not "one" single HIV epidemic in India. The spread of HIV in India is diverse and many states of India have low rate of infection. The epidemic is extreme in Southern states. As of December 2004, 92% of all nationally reported AIDS cases have been found in 10 of the 28 states and 7 Union territories. The greatest numbers were in Maharasthra and Gujarat in the West; Tamil Nadu and Andhra Pradesh in the South; Manipur and Nagaland in the North East (NACO, March 2005). In Southern States, the epidemics are mostly due to hetero sexual contract, while infections are mainly found amongst injecting drug users in Manipur and Nagaland (UNAIDS/WHO, 2004) and one-fourth of the HIV positives throughout the world may live in India (Sinha, 1999: 81).

India has a population of one billion, and around half of this population is in sexually active age group of 15-49 years (NACO, 1998: 15). The first AIDS patient in India was diagnosed by Dr. Suniti Soloman, a microbiology professor at the Madras Medical College in Chennai in 1986. The initial cases of HIV was identified among the sex workers in Chennai while the police involved in sending their assigned quota of 100 commercial sex workers per month to the city prison. Dr. Suniti Soloman has collected the blood sample from one month's batch of 100 sex workers. Among them six were identified as HIV positive in the test Enzyme Linked Immunosorbent Assay (ELISA) at the

Christian Medical College in Vellore and the result rechecked with the Western Blot analysis in the United States. All the six are confirmed HIV positive and none of them have non-Indian customers. This shows that HIV was already circulating within India (Arvind Singhal *et al.*, 2003: 115).

From 1986 to mid 1990s the Indian government proclaimed that AIDS was a foreign disease, and that the epidemic could never spread in a family-centered society like India. However, in 1999, 1400 Indian citizens were being infected each day and by 2002 this figure had jumped to 5000 (Arvind Singhal *et al.*, 2003: 115).

Within a short period AIDS has emerged as one of the most public health problem in the country. During the recent years the occurrence and spread of HIV/AIDS in the country has shown the following trends and shift in paradigm (NACO, 1998: 15):

1. HIV is prevalent in almost all parts of the country.
2. HIV/AIDS is spreading from urban to rural areas.
3. HIV/AIDS is also spreading from high risk behaviour groups to general population.
4. One in every four cases reported is a woman.
5. More and more women attending antenatal clinics are sero-converting to HIV positive, leading to the added risk of prenatal transmission.
6. Highest per centage of infection is reported to occur through the sexual contact.
7. About 89 per cent of the reported cases are from sexually active and economically productive age groups of 15-49 years.
8. Migration and mobility has increased the chances of the disease spreading to other areas/persons.
9. The social stigma attached to sexually transmitted infection also hold good for HIV/AIDS with more disastrous consequences.

(A) Causes for the rapid spread of HIV/AIDS in India

(a) India is believed to be moralistic society as a influence of religion. Due to various reasons, the gradual decline in moral value increased pre-marital sex and in turn it has increased the rate of sexually transmitted infection.

(b) For economical reasons, mobility and migration has increased among migrant labour, truckers, helpers, uninformed personnel from rural area to urban area which lead to lack of spousal sex. Most of the migrant workers are highly mobile and often live in unhygienic conditions in urban slums. Long working hours, relative isolation from the family and geographical mobility may foster casual sexual relationships and make them highly vulnerable to STDs and HIV/AIDS (Ekstrand M *et al.*, 2003: 56). Migrant workers tend to have little access to HIV/STD information, voluntary counseling and testing and health services.

(c) Flourishing sex industry and its extension beyond red light areas is another important reason for the spread of HIV infection. In Mumbai alone have 15,000 sex workers (Gomare *et al.*, 2003), and 70% of the sex workers in Mumbai are HIV positive (Shankaran, 2002).

(d) Increasing culture of using drugs among the youth also yet another cause for the spread of infection into the general population. Injecting drug use is a major problem in northeastern states, Mumbai, Kolkata, Delhi and Chennai (Reid G. and Costigan G, 2002: 81).

(f) The most vulnerable groups are known for their illiteracy/poor education and low socio-economic conditions. They have very poor knowledge of safe sex and condom use.

(b) Mode of spread of HIV infection in India

The predominant mode of transmission of HIV in India is hetero sexual contact (85.7%), followed by injecting drug use (2.2%), blood transfusion (2.6%), prenatal transmission (2.7%) and other route which is not able to specify the people living with HIV positive (NACO, July 2004: 14).

Table 4.12. Routes of HIV Transmission, end of December 2004 and 31 March 2005

Transmission Categories	*2004 (in %) **	*2005 (in %) ***
Sexual	85.83	85.76
Blood and blood production	2.07	2.03
Intravenous drug users	2.70	2.55
Prenatal	3.45	3.58
Unidentified	5.95	6.08

Sources: * Monthly update on AIDS, NACO, 31 August 2004
**Monthly updates on AIDS, NACO, 31 March 2005.

(c) Pattern of HIV epidemic in India

India's epidemic seems to be following the Type 4 pattern, like in Thailand. In the **first wave,** HIV infection is seen amongst sex workers or intravenous drug users (IDUs) that are also known as the **core transmitters or core groups.** In the **second wave,** the epidemic spreads from these groups at highest risk to bridge populations (clients of sex workers, patients of sexually transmitted infections, partners of drug users, mobile populations such as truck drivers, single male member migrants etc.). When evidence suggests affliction of spouses and children of the clients of sex workers, the HIV epidemic is understood to have reached its **third wave.** Recently a **fourth wave** comprising of adolescents has been proposed to indicate the severity of the epidemic.

(d) HIV/AIDS prevalence in India

The HIV prevalence in adult population can be broadly classified into three groups of States/Union Territories in the country (Ramamurthy.V, 2003: 51).

Group I (High prevalence/generalized epidemic): States like Maharasthra, Tamil Nadu, Karnataka, Andhra Pradesh, Manipur and Nagaland where the HIV infection has crossed 1 per cent or more in antenatal women.

Group II (Moderate prevalent/concentrated epidemic states): States like Gujrat, Goa and Pondicherry where HIV infection has crossed 5 per cent or more among high risk groups but the infection is below 1 per cent in antenatal women.

Group III (Low prevalent states): Remaining states and Union Territories where the HIV infection in any of the high risk groups is still less than 5 per cent and is less than 1 per cent among antenatal women.

(e) HIV Estimate in India

Richard Feacham, head of the Global Fund to Fight AIDS, Tuberculosis and Malaria made a statement that India is surpassed South Africa in the number of HIV infected people, and HIV/AIDS epidemic was growing very rapidly in India and it was out of control (The Hindu, 2005: 14). Table 4.13 reveals the seriousness of the epidemic in India by showing increasing trend every year.

Table 4.13. HIV Estimates: India from 1990—2005

	No of HIV infection – year wise								
Year	1990	1994	1998	1999	2000	2001	2002	2003	2005*
In millions	0.2	1.75	3.5	3.7	3.86	3.97	4.58	5.106	5.134

Source: NACO, annual report (2004: 15).
*NACO monthly update on HIV/AIDS, March. 2005.

India is categorized as a low prevalence nation. But in a view of large population, a mere 0.1% increase in the prevalence rate would increase the number of living with HIV by over half-million (NACO, July 2004: 14). HIV prevalence across the country is about 0.98% in the age group of 15-49 years, just below the "tipping point' of 1% where the disease will become much more difficult to control. The UNAIDS/WHO estimated that 5,100,000 people are living with HIV in India. Among them 5,000,000 are adult, 1,900,000 are women and 120,000 are children (UNAIDS/WHO, 2004).

In India, every day approximately 1500 people become infected with HIV and of that number, young people below 25 years of age account for over 50% of the infections. About 90 per cent of the infected people themselves are not aware of their HIV status and may therefore be transmitting the virus to their partners. Low awareness is the main causes for the rapid spread of HIV infection in India (Parliamentary Forum on HIV/AIDS, 2004).

According to the latest (May 2005) data released by the Ministry of Health and Family Welfare and the National AIDS Control Organisation (NACO), the number of new infection for the year 2004-05 has increased by only about 28,000 as against 5.2 lakhs in 2003-04. The total infection figure now stands at 5.134 million in comparison to 5.106 million reported in 2003-2004. In absolute numbers, India continues to have the most number of cases after South Africa, which has 5.3 million HIV infected persons. In terms of per centage, India has an HIV prevalence of 0.91 per cent among the adult population as compared to 21.5 per cent in South Africa (Aarti Dhar, 2005: 15).

While 1,114 HIV/AIDS related deaths were reported in 2004-05, 1514 deaths were reported in 2003-04. The decrease in the number of fresh cases can be attributed to major steps taken by the Government in creating awareness and introducing the Anti-Retroviral Therapy (ART) treatment. The trends across the country show that there is no galloping HIV epidemic in India as there is no evidence of an upsurge in HIV prevalence. However, there are regional epidemics in various parts, with high prevalence of HIV among both the Sexually Transmitted Diseases (STD) clinic attendees and antenatal clinic attendees (Aarti Dhar, 2005: 15).

The surveillance data on 2004 reveals that 69.3 per cent of the new cases were from six "high prevalence" States, 28 per cent were from "low prevalence" States and the remaining were from "medium prevalence" States. Of the 1.3 lakhs "known HIV positive cases", 8000 were receiving treatment in government hospitals. "About 44,000 causes are reported from Tamil Nadu alone because of better treatment facilities and greater awareness in the State (The Hindu, 2005: 15).

(f) Recorded AIDS cases in India

The data published by Tamil Nadu AIDS Control Society in June 2003 reveals the following reported AIDS cases by NACO from 32 States of India. The following table reveals that the prevalence of AIDS cases is high in Tamil Nadu, Maharashtra, Andhra Pradesh, Gujarat, Karnataka and Manipur.

Table 4.14. AIDs Cases in India (Reported by NACO) from May 1986-June 2003

Sl. No.	State	1996	1997	1998	1999	2000	2001	2002	2003	2005	HIV % 2003
1.	Tamil Nadu	199	521	532	2730	3866	7354	21813	24667	48180	0.75
2.	Maharashtra	520	930	824	64	279	6454	9234	9234	12963	1.25
3.	Karnataka	12	55	39	47	541	1261	1654	1707	2343	1.25
4.	Manipur	55	147	0	61	344	1033	1238	1238	2866	1.25
5.	Madya Pradesh	6	68	76	116	279	759	972	996	1314	0.00
6.	Gujarat	104	6	2	1	245	1259	2474	2660	5406	0.40
7.	Delhi	27	90	13	0	64	642	766	807	950	0.13
8.	Uttar Pradesh	48	53	16	41	93	461	845	983	1383	0.00
9.	Chandigarh	0	0	0	124	93	427	684	733	1119	0.50
10.	Kerala	26	3	1	0	56	267	267	267	1769	0.33
11.	Rajastan	0	51	25	27	53	248	666	751	1153	0.13
12.	Pondicherry	24	8	9	0	0	141	157	157	302	0.13
13.	Punjab	0	0	48	52	31	135	231	248	292	0.00
14.	Assam	0	9	3	11	62	125	149	171	225	0.00
15.	Nagaland	0	6	0	19	43	211	319	331	736	1.25
16.	West Bengal	11	7	0	0	0	725	930	930	2397	0.50
17.	Orissa	0	0	0	0	49	82	82	82	128	0.00
18 .	Andhra Pradesh	19	15	7	2	0	1265	3341	3707	11,280	1.25
19.	Haryana	0	0	0	0	47	189	271	271	440	0.25
20.	Himachal Pradesh	0	0	0	15	16	91	109	112	223	0.00
21 .	Bihar	1	1	0	0	36	92	148	152	155	0.00
22.	Goa	0	0	0	7	10	75	155	194	508	0.50
23 .	Mizoram	0	5	0	7	3	20	47	50	106	1.38
24.	A & N Islands	0	0	0	0	9	17	24	27	33	0.00
25.	Meghalaya	0	8	0	0	0	8	8	8	8	0.00
26.	Jammu & Kasmir	0	0	0	0	0	2	2	2	2	0.00
27.	Sikkim	0	1	1	0	0	4	6	8	8	0.13
28.	Daman & Diu	0	0	1	0	0	1	1	1	1	0.50
29.	Dadra & Nagar Haveli	0	0	0	0	0	0	0	0	0	0.13
30.	Arunachal Pradesh	0	0	0	0	0	0	0	0	0	0.38
31.	Lakshadweep	0	0	0	0	0	0	0	0	0	0.00

Sl. No.	State	1996	1997	1998	1999	2000	2001	2002	2003	2005	HIV % 2003
32.	Tripura	0	0	0	0	0	0	6	6	5	0.00
33.	Uttrakhand									0	0.00
34	Ahemdabad Mun.Corp.	–	–	–	–	–	–	–	–	520	–
35	Chennai M.C.	–	–	–	–	–	–	–	–	–	–
36	Mumbai M.C	–	–	–	–	–	–	–	–	7042	1.25
	Total	*1052*	*1984*	*1597*	*3325*	*6218*	*31336*	*46599*	*50500*	*1,03,857*	

Source: *Monthly updates on AIDS, NACO, 31 August 2004: 1.
**Monthly updates on AIDS, NACO, 31 March 2005: 2

As per standard AIDS case definition, only 1052 cases were reported to NACO from all over the country during 1996. It has increased to 96,978 in December 2004 which include 69,559 male and 27,419 female (NACO, August 2004). But in March 2005, the NACO has recorded the higher number of AIDS cases (1,03,857) with the infection of 74,020 males and 29,837 females. The year wise reported AIDS cases clearly indicate the increasing trends of HIV infection in India.

(g) Age and sex-wise distribution of AIDS cases in India

Table 4.15. Age and Sex-wise Distribution of AIDs Cases in India end of March 2005

Age group	*Male*	*%*	*Female*	*%*	*Total*	*%*
0-14	2,651	3.6	1,836	6.3	4,487	4.3
15-29	20,665	27.9	13,211	44.2	33,866	32.6
30-49	45,024	60.8	13,215	44.3	58,239	56.1
>50	5,690	7.7	1,575	5.2	7,265	7.0
Total	74,020	100	29,837	100	103,857	100

Source: *Monthly updates on AIDS*, NACO, 31 March 2005: 2.

The epidemiological analysis of reported AIDS cases reveals that AIDS is increasingly affecting young people in the sexually active age group of 15-49 years including 68.7% of male and 27% of female. Around 89% of the reported cases are occurring in sexually active age and economically productive age group of 15-44 years (Parliamentary Forum of HIV/AIDS, 2004). Children accounted for 4.3% of total AIDS cases in India.

(h) HIV prevalence among various risk groups

Table 4.16. HIV Prevalence among various Risk Groups - State-wise in 2003

Sl. No.	*State / Union Territories*	*Percentage of HIV prevalence*					
		FSW	*MSM*	*IDU*	*STD*	*ANC-Urban*	*ANC-Rural*
1.	Andhra Pradesh	19.4	13.2	—	19.6	1.25	0.75
2.	Arunachal Pradesh	—	—	—	0.0	0.00	0.00
3.	Assam	—	—	—	1.20	0.00	0.00
4.	Bihar	4.8	1.6	—	0.40	0.00	0.00
5.	Chhattisgarh	—	—	—	2.27	0.25	0.00
6.	Delhi	2.0	—	14.4	7.20	0.13	0.00
7.	Goa	30.1	—	—	14.30	0.50	0.19
8.	Gujarat	—	—	—	4.50	0.40	0.00
9.	Haryana	—	—	—	1.20	025	0.33
10.	Himachal Pradesh	0.4/8	—	—	0.80	0.00	0.50
11.	Jammu & Kashmir	—	—	—	1.86	0.00	0.00
12.	Jharkhand	—	—	—	0.13	0.00	0.00
13.	Karnataka	14.4	10.8	2.8	10.40	1.25	1.00
14.	Kerala	2.29	—	—	4.00	0.33	0.00
15.	Madhya Pradesh	—	—	—	1.20	0.00	0.00
16.	Maharashtra	—	—	—	10.00	1.25	0.00
17.	Mumbai	54.9	18.8	24.8	18.40	1.25	N.A
18.	Manipur	12.4	29.2	24.4	13	1.25	0.40
19.	Meghalya	—	—	—	0.40	0.00	0.00
20.	Mizoram	—	—	6.4	3.80	1.38	0.00
21.	Nagaland	4.4	—	12.9	0.90	1.25	1.20
22.	Orissa	—	—	—	2.40	0.00	0.00
23.	Punjab	—	—	—	1.60	0.00	0.13
24.	Rajasthan	—	—	—	3.70	0.13	0.12
25.	Sikkim	—	—	—	0.00	0.13	0.00
26.	Tamil Nadu	8.8	4.4	—	9.20	0.75	0.50

Sl.	State/Union Territories	Percentage of HIV prevalence					
		FSW	MSM	IDU	STD	ANC-Urban	ANC-Rural
27.	Tripura	—	5.26	—	0.00	0.00	0.00
28.	Uttar Pradesh	—	—	—	0.55	0.00	0.00
29.	Uttrakhand	—	—	—	0.00	0.00	0.00
30.	West Bengal	6.45	—	2.70	1.45	0.50	0.50
31.	A & N Islands	—	—	—	1.60	0.50	0.25
32.	Chandigarh	1.20	—	—	1.66	0.50	0.00
33.	D & N Haveli	—	—	—	—	—	0.00
34.	Daman & Diu	—	—	—	—	—	0.00
35.	Lakshadweep	—	—	—	0.00	0.00	0.00
36.	Pondicherry	—	—	—	2.60	0.13	0.14

Source: NACO – Facts and Figures, 2004.

Table 4.16 reveals that the Female sex workers (FSW) and Injecting Drug Users (IDU) are the major transmitter of HIV virus to the general population. The table also reveals that STD patients are getting infected by HIV in many States. Ante-natal women, both in urban and rural areas are also under the threat of HIV infection almost in all states.

(i) State wise distribution of AIDS cases

Table 4.17. Distribution of Reported AIDs Cases by State at the End of December 2003

States	*Percentage*
Tamil Nadu	44.7
Maharashtra less Mumbai	16.7
Andhra Pradesh	7.9
Gujarat	6.5
Mumbai	4.7
Karnataka	3.2
Manipur	3.2
Madhya Pradesh	1.9

States	*Percentage*
West Bengal	1.7
Delhi	1.5
Nagaland	0.6
Others	8.4

Source: NACO, Annual Report, 2004: 24.

In India Tamil Nadu has higher per centage (44.7%) of reported AIDS cases followed by Maharashtra (16.7%). The numbers of AIDS cases are increasing in Andhra Pradesh, Gujarat, Mumbai, Karnataka, and North Eastern States.

(j) Women living with HIV/AIDS in India

The estimates by UNAIDS/WHO shows that the number of women infection is steadily rising. One in every four AIDS cases reported are woman (Sinha, 1999: 89) and 90% of women with HIV having only one sexual partner in their lives (Parliamentary Forum of HIV/AIDS, 2004). Every year HIV infection among married women is increasing as a result of marital partner's unsafe sexual contact with sex workers and use of injecting drug use. Cultural degradation is witnessed as influence of western culture. Many married women are exposed to extra marital relationship and are subjected to HIV infection. Many of these women have no knowledge about HIV and its implication and the necessity of safe sex (Break-through organisation, 2005: wp13).

For millions of Indian women, sexual intercourse is not a question of choice but rather one of survival and duty. Fertility and her relationship to her husband are often the source of an Indian woman's social identity. HIV/AIDS epidemic in India as inextricably tied to the social and cultural values and economic relationships between men and women and within communities. While social inequalities facilitate its spread in the country, the virus, in turn, reflects and reinforces these inequalities. Women are the least powerful because Indian society praises patriarchy and male sexuality and mourns the births of daughters. In addition, there is an absence of choice at the individual and systemic levels, whether it is the choice to use a condom or even to have sex.

For women, low economic and social status, abuse and violence, as well as limited legal and social protection increase their vulnerability to HIV/AIDS. Knowledge of HIV/AIDS continues to be surprisingly low. The National Family Health Survey, 1998-99 shows that only four out of 10 women of reproductive age have heard of AIDS. Awareness is much lower among rural and less educated women. Only 18 per cent of illiterate women have heard of AIDS, compared with 92 per cent of women who had at least completed high school (Population Reference Bureau, 2005: wp1)

The virus has expanded the boundaries of high-risk groups to adolescent girls (married and single); married women of reproductive age; sexually active single women; sex workers; college and university students; pregnant women; and women survivors of sexual abuse and rape. Women constitute 25 per cent of known AIDS cases in the country, and seven of 10 women affected by HIV are from poor rural and poor urban communities (Population Reference Bureau, 2005: wp1)

Women with HIV are subjected to various forms of violence and discrimination based on gender. They could be refused shelter, denied a share of household property, refused access to treatment and care, or blamed for a husband's HIV diagnosis. In cases, where a man has admitted he had sexual relations with sex workers, the burden of blame still falls on the wife for failing to "satisfy" her husband.

(k) Rural and Urban distribution of HIV/AIDS

In India, the epidemic is moved towards rural areas. Increasing number of rural population is getting infected by HIV with the influence of increased migration and unsafe multi-sexual behaviour and low/lack of awareness on HIV/AIDS and safe sex practices.

HIV Sentinel Surveillance data on 2003 revealed that the infection rate is increasing in rural areas. According to the HIV Sentinel Surveillance data on 2003, the total number of infection estimated in urban areas is 20.46 lakhs (40.1%) and among them 12.97 lakhs are male and 7.49 lakhs are female. The estimated number of infection in rural areas is 30.60 lakhs (59.9%) with

19.22 lakhs male and 11.35 lakhs female (NACO – Facts & Figures 2003: 4). The surveillance data on 2004 suggests that 21.27 lakhs (42.43%) people from urban areas and 30.07 lakhs (58.57%) of people from rural areas were infected with HIV (Dhar, 2005: 15).

About 28% of rural people in India and 11% of urban people have never heard of AIDS (Parliamentary Forum of HIV/AIDS, 2004). The Behaviour Surveillance Survey (2001), reveals that the overall per centage of condom use in last sex with non-regular partner is 49.3%. Condom usage among the rural population is considerably low (45%) when compared to urban masses (63%) and it is also found to be low among women (urban-52%, rural-35%) than men (urban - 65%, rural - 48%) (NACO, 2004: 25). The same survey also reveals that the greater per centages (12-13%) of both rural and urban men have non-regular sexual partners than women of rural and urban areas (3-5%).

(l) HIV INFECTION IN HIGH-RISK AND GENERAL POPULATION

Table 4.18. Distribution of HIV Infections in various Sub-population

Group	*STD Patients*	*General population*	*FSWs*	*IDUs*	*Children*	*Total*
No. in lakhs	14.93	34.77	0.103	0.71	0.55	51.06

Source: NACO, Facts and Figures, 2003: 4.

In India, high risk groups are considered as the patient attending STD clinics, MSM (men seeking men) clinics and drug de-addiction centers while mothers attending antenatal clinics are considered as a proxy for the general population. The HIV/AIDS estimate by NACO reveals that the general population is increasingly infected with HIV (34.7 lakhs) followed by patients with STD (14.9 lakhs). Among the STD population two-thirds are females (6.20 lakhs).

(m) SEXUALLY TRANSMITTED INFECTION AND HIV/AIDS IN INDIA

Sexually transmitted infection (STD) and HIV are behaviourally and epidemiologically linked. An individual with sexually transmitted infection is eight to ten times more vulnerable to contracting HIV. Many infected people do not seek treatment due to stigmatization with the diseases. HIV/AIDS intervention programme involved in providing awareness related to increasing treatment seeking behaviour for STD. In India, the STD clinic is increasing year by year. During 2000-2001 it was only 504, but it is raised to 735 in 2003-2004 (NACO, 2004: 41). The annual report of the National AIDS Control Organisation (NACO, 2004: 45) reveals that the STD is increasing in the states of Uttar Pradesh (22.5%), Andhra Pradesh (12.7%), Madhya Pradesh (12.3%), Tamil Nadu (8.1%), Maharashtra (6.5%), Chattisgarh (5.7%), Karnataka (4.3%), Gujarat (4.3%), Orissa (3.1%) and Mumbai (2.8%).

(n) Regionwise distribution of HIV/AIDS in India

(i) Southern Region

Southern regions are called as high prevalent States. Southern regions include Tamil Nadu, Andhra Pradesh, Karnataka, Kerala and Goa. In these regions the epidemic is crossed from high risk population to general population and HIV infection has crossed more than one per cent in antenatal women. Distribution of reported AIDS cases by states cumulative figures till 2003 shows that Tamil Nadu rank first in India in HIV/AIDS with the per centage of 44.7%. HIV infection in Tamil Nadu is increasing year by year. It was reported that 17.30% of HIV infection among patients attending STD clinics (16.30%) and women in antenatal clinics (1.0%) in 1998. But in 2003 higher per centage of infection was recorded among intravenous drug users (63.8%), STD patients (9.20%), and men seeking men (4.40%), female sex workers (8.8%) and women in antenatal clinics (0.75%). It is also recorded that 0.75% of urban and 0.50% of rural women attending antenatal clinics are infected with HIV

The per centage of reported AIDS cases in Andhra Pradesh is 7.9% in 2003. It has higher per centage of HIV infection among patients attending STD clinics. In 1998, HIV infection among STD patients was reported as 24.90% and it has increased to 30.40% in 2002. But during 2003 the infection rate among STD patients was reduced to 19.60% as a result of awareness created by Andhra Pradesh Government. The infection rate among women in antenatal clinics also reduced from 2.25% in 1998 to 1.25% in 2003. The state also observed higher per centage of infection among female sex workers (19.4%) and men seeking men (13.2%) in 2003. In Andhra Pradesh 1.25% of urban and 0.75% of rural women attending antenatal clinics are recorded as HIV positive (NACO, Statewise HIV Prevalence 2004: 1-9).

Karnataka accounted for 3.2% of AIDS cases in 2003 (NACO, July 2004: 24). HIV infection in Karnataka is found to be high among female sex workers (14.4%), men seeking men (10.8%) and patients of STD clinics (10.40%). The State witnessed lower per centage of HIV infection among intravenous drug users (2.8%). HIV infection among women attending antenatal clinics is found to be 1.25% in both rural and urban areas.

In Kerala HIV infection is found to be in increasing trend as a result of large number of its workforce in the Gulf or in other metropolises of India such as Mumbai, Delhi, Kolkata, Chennai etc. HIV infection in 2003 is recorded among female sex workers (2.29%), patients attending STD clinics (4.00%) and women attending antenatal clinics (0.33%) of urban sites.

(ii) Western Region

Western region include Madhya Pradesh, Maharashtra, Rajasthan and Gujarat. In these regions HIV infection is high in Maharashtra and Gujarat. At the end of December 2004, it is estimated that HIV infection in western region is caused by increasing number of STD patients. HIV prevalence among STD patients higher in Maharashtra (10.00%) followed by Gujarat (4.50%) and Rajasthan (3.70%). Low rate of HIV prevalence is estimated among the STD patients in the state of Madhya Pradesh (1.20%). Increasing number of women attending antenatal clinics in the urban sites of Maharashtra (1.25%), Gujarat 0.40%), Madhya Pradesh (1.20%) and Rajasthan (0.13%) are infected with HIV/AIDS (NACO, Statewise HIV Prevalence 2004: 1-9).

In Mumbai, HIV prevalence among female sex worker is estimated as 54.29% in 2003. Higher rate of infection is also estimated among injecting drug users (24.8%), patients attending STD clinics (18.40%) and the clinics of men seeking men (18.8%). It is also estimated that 1.25% of women attending antenatal clinics in Mumbai are infected with HIV (NACO, State wise HIV Prevalence 2004: 1-9).

(iii) Northern Region

In India, the northern region has low rate of infection than southern and western regions. Female sex workers are the primary contributors for the spread of HIV infection in Bihar (4.8%), and West Bengal (6.45%). HIV infection is slowly picking up as a result of increasing number of infection among the patients attending STD clinics in Haryana (1.20%), Himachal Pradesh (0.80%), Jammu and Kashmir (1.86%), Orissa (2.40%), Punjab (1.60%) and Uttar Pradesh (0.55%). The infection rates among women attending antenatal clinics in northern regions are comparatively less and it ranges from 0.13%-0.50% (NACO, State wise HIV Prevalence 2004: 1-9).

(iv) Northeastern region

Injecting drug use is the primary cause for the rapid spread of HIV infection in Northeastern region. Northeastern region include Arunachal Pradesh, Assam, Manipur, Meghalaya, Mizoram, Nagaland and Tripura. HIV infection is less in Arunachal Pradesh, Assam and Tripura and it is high in Manipur, Meghalaya, Mizoram and Nagaland (NACO, State wise HIV Prevalence 2004: 1-9).

The major factors which facilitate for the increase of HIV infection in the State of Manipur is recorded as sex between men (29.2%), injecting drug use (24.8%), STD (13.00%) and female sex works (12.4%). The increasing rate of STD is primary cause for the spread of HIV infection in Assam (1.20%) and Meghalaya (0.40%). Injecting drug use is identified as important contributing factor for rapid spread of HIV infection in Nagaland (12.9%) and Mizoram (6.4%). Sex between men is recorded in Tripura (5.28%) for the spread of infection.

HIV prevalence among women attending antenatal clinics also found to be higher in north eastern regions of Arunachal

Pradesh (0.38% in urban areas), Manipur (1.25% in urban and 0.40% in rural areas), Mizoram (1.38% in urban areas), and Nagaland (1.25% in urban and 1.20% in rural areas).

(v) Union Territories

HIV/AIDS is recorded in Union Territories expect Dadra and Nagar Haveli and Daman and Diu. Among all Union Territories, HIV prevalence is high in Goa. Sex tourism is the unique feature in Goa. Sex tourism causes increased HIV infection among female sex workers (30.1%) in 2003 followed by the patients attending STD clinics (14.30%). The HIV infection among antenatal women in Goa is comparatively less (0.50% in urban and 0.19% in rural areas) in southern regions (NACO, Statewise HIV Prevalence 2004: 1-9).

Increasing rate of STD is identified as major cause for the spread of HIV infection in 2003 in Pondicherry (2.60%) and Andaman and Nicobar Islands (1.60%) and Chhattisgarh (2.27%). HIV infection rate is rapidly increasing in Delhi, the capital of India as a result of increasing number of infection among injecting drug users (14.4%), patients attending sexually transmitted diseases clinics (7.20%), and female sex workers (2.0%). The rates of HIV infection among women attending antenatal clinics are estimated between 0.13% to 0.50% (NACO, State wise HIV Prevalence 2004: 1-9).

HIV Prevalence in Tamil Nadu

The State Tamil Nadu is situated in the extreme south off India with the population of 62.11 million (Census 2001). According to Tamil Nadu State AIDS Control Society, for the year 2004, the projected mid-year population was 64.09 million of which the rural population accounts for 34.86 million (56.12 per cent) while the urban population accounts for 27.25 million (43.88 per cent) Tamil Nadu has 30 districts with 201 Taluks, 385 blocks, 832 towns, 6 corporations, 102 municipalities, two cantonments, 611 Panchayats, 111 census towns and 16,317 villages (Census 2001).

The first HIV positive case was detected in Tamil Nadu in 1986 among the female sex workers. HIV prevalence among the sex workers is also proved in 1990 when the State Government of Tamil Nadu forcibly tested hundreds of sex workers for HIV, and locked up 800 HIV positive women (Dube, 2000: 27). The epidemic today challenges the present social system and safe future of the individual in the State. Earlier, it was believed that the commercial sex workers and truck drivers are at the risk of contracting HIV infection. Today, many other groups have been identified. They are migrant labour, industrial workers, refugees, fisherman, slum-dwellers, hotel and lodge workers, domestic helpers, street children and men seeking men (Tamil Nadu State AIDS Control Society).

According to UNAIDS report, the greater danger for India is the fact that the infection rate in some states, like Tamil Nadu is "three times higher in villages than the cities" (Sinha, 1999: 89). People living with AIDS is high in Tamil Nadu with the per centage of 44.7 and among the 49 HIV high prevalence districts in India, seven are in Tamil Nadu including Madurai, Trichy, Salem, Coimbatore, Namakkal, Tirunelveli and Chennai (NACO: 2004: 15). AIDS cases reported to NACO from Tamil Nadu till March 2005 is 48, 180, the highest in India (NACO, 2005) and the HIV prevalence rate is estimated as 0.75 per cent in 2003 (NACO, 2004).

It is estimated from Sentinel Surveillance data (2003) of the Tamil Nadu State AIDS Control Society, the people living with HIV positive in the State is about 4.32 lakhs. Though the common mode of HIV transmission is heterosexual, the sentinel surveillance between the periods 1993-2004 indicates that intravenous drug users rank first with a HIV prevalence of 39.92 per cent followed by STD patients (8.40 per cent) and antenatal women (0.63 per cent).

HIV rates among antenatal women declined from 1.13 per cent in 2001 to 0.63 per cent in 2004. But, HIV prevalence rate among the antenatal women of 15-24 age groups has increased to 1.25% in 2004 from 0.25% in 2002. The sentinel surveillance also shows that the HIV infection rate is also declined among STD patients from 14.80 per cent in 2002 to 8.40 in 2004. It is also recorded that the infection rate is started decreasing among men seeking men (4.00% in 2000 to 2.40% in 2002) and sex workers 8.8% in 2003 to 4.0% in 2004. But according to NACO 2004 report, the HIV prevalence is increasing among truckers (2.65% in 1994 to 9.43% in 1997), and intravenous drug users (26.70% in 2000 to 39.92% in 2004).

The Department of Health, Government of Tamil Nadu has recorded the highest number of HIV cases in Namakkal and Salem where the lorry movements is high. The HIV cases have been increasing at an alarming rate in Dindigul district. Blood transfusion, pre marital sex, vertical transmission and heterosexual transmission are cited as causes of the infection. The number of cases coming for treatment or preliminary tests at private hospitals and laboratories at Ottanchatram, Palani, Natham, Vedasandur, and Dindigul towns have been steadily growing year after year. Though the officials identify Palani and Kodaikanal vulnerable as both attracted tourists from all over the country, in reality, the number of patients coming to the private laboratories and clinics at Natham, Vedasandur and Ottanchatram and hundreds of peripheral villages is high. A survey conducted by a NGO confirmed that pre marital sex was on the rise among the youth in Dindigul and Ottanchatram towns. About 85% of the cases among the heterosexuals were in the age group of 18-35 years and among them 67% were from rural areas (*The Hindu*, Dec. 5, 2002).

(a) *AIDS Cases in Tamil Nadu*

Table 4.19. District-wise AIDs Cases in Tamil Nadu (Up to June 2003)

Sl. No.	*Name of District*	*Up to 1996*	*1997*	*1998*	*1999*	*2000*	*2001*	*2002*	*2003*
1.	Chennai	96	195	210	497	1237	4128	7012	7656
2.	Thiruvellore	—	—	25	140	216	623	875	933
3.	Kancheepuram	81	46	27	75	106	453	627	650
4.	Vellore	23	51	37	80	205	778	1241	1348
5.	Thiruvannamalai	28	22	39	83	179	547	790	839
6.	Villupuram	40	38	35	109	347	873	1228	1317
7.	Cuddalore	24	30	42	110	223	675	941	1003
8.	Dharmapuri	17	13	19	66	187	527	851	922

Sl. No.	*Name of District*	*Up to 1996*	*1997*	*1998*	*1999*	*2000*	*2001*	*2002*	*2003*
9.	Salem	45	45	75	162	363	1098	1465	1578
10.	Namakkal	—	—	46	201	388	973	1469	1602
11.	Erode	14	13	45	189	259	865	1165	1251
12.	Coimbatore	30	4	21	92	108	364	450	498
13.	Nilgiris	2	4	2	7	9	32	39	29
14.	Perambalur	3	13	31	42	125	309	561	595
15.	Trichy	33	25	44	174	252	885	1267	1340
16.	Ariyalur]	—	—	—	—	1	53	—	—
17.	Karur	1	19	15	48	94	312	547	595
18.	Pudukkottai	5	1	8	16	30	144	214	229
19.	Thanjavur	29	7	14	31	54	227	425	488
20.	Tiruvarur	—	—	1	10	16	55	95	99
21.	Nagapattinam	10	5	10	8	15	71	109	119
22.	Dindigul	19	4	7	66	54	450	1172	1336
23.	Madurai	58	1	7	93	45	932	1576	1682
24.	Theni	—	—	5	41	55	226	299	314
25.	Sivagangai	10	—	1	16	16	97	138	144
26.	Virudhunagar	5	—	5	13	17	90	136	138
27.	Ramanathapuram	—	—	2	9	16	53	62	63
29.	Tirunelveli	5	5	7	17	36	241	335	244
30.	Thoothukudi	2	—	9	24	42	169	212	227
31.	Kanyakumari	2	1	2	6	8	30	41	44
32.	Address not known	297	3	10	—	2	312	312	312
32.	Other States	—	—	—	—	2	83	98	99
	Total	879	545	801	2391	4707	16677	25779	27794

Source: Tamil Nadu AIDS Control Society, June 2003

Table 4.19 reveals that AIDS cases are increasingly reported from all districts of Tamil Nadu from 1998 onwards. Chennai rank first in AIDS cases followed by Madurai, Namakkal, Salem, Vellore, Trichy and Dindigul.

(b) Causes for the spread of HIV in Tamil Nadu

1. Widespread gender inequality coupled with poverty, dependence, exploitation, discrimination are the major cause for the spread of infection among women in particular and people in general (Kannan, 2003).
2. Poverty and illiteracy influences prostitution and encourages bootleggers and drug traffickers. Prostitution in major cities of Tamil Nadu is well organized and networked by mercenary gangs comprised hardened criminals though there are individual operators and streetwalkers, who fetch clients from the roads. Well organized prostitution is brothel dens. At the helm of affairs in these brothels is a 'madam', often a woman who is the in-charge or manager of the brothel house (*The Hindu*, March19, 2002).
3. Irrespective of high awareness on HIV/AIDS, the youth in general and women in particular are lacking access to right information on sexual health issues (Varma, 2004).
4. Tamil Nadu is progressing in industrial, marketing activities and it also invites multinational companies to establish its enterprises in Tamil Nadu. The development on the economic activities increases lorry transport in Tamil Nadu from various parts of the country. The truck transport facilitated the growth of highway prostitution and unsafe sex (Dev, 2005: 59-62).
5. The orthodox Tamil Culture created fear in the minds of women to choose contraception and to discuss safe sex practices with their sexual partners. The only choice before them is sterilization through tubectomies (Sharma, 2005: 3). Once the women get sterilization, they never think about either to use or to suggest condom for safe sex with their husband. The lack of safe sex in the marital life increases women's vulnerability to HIV/AIDS in Tamil Nadu.
6. Poverty and inequality in health care deliveries is a common phenomena in all states of India and especially,

the rural India has poor health care facilities. It prevents women to take treatment for their reproductive health problems (*The Hindu*, Editorial, 2005: 10). Therefore many sexually transmitted infections are unnoticed by women.

7. The prevalence of sexually transmitted infection among general population is high in Tamil Nadu (3.3 million). Asymptomatic infections were high among both sexes and the rate was similar in both rural and urban areas (Krishnamurthy, 2005: 5). The higher rate of sexually transmitted infection in the state is the reflection of unsafe high risk behaviours among the people of Tamil Nadu.

8. Insufficient awareness on HIV/AIDS, its implication and safe sex practices among rural population increases HIV infection in southern parts of Tamil Nadu (Thinamalar, 2005).

9. Atrocities and sexual violence against women and girl children is rapidly increasing in Tamil Nadu. In 2002, 1766 sexual harassment cases were registered in Tamil Nadu and an official analysis of various cases reveals that rape and molestation were most prevalent in Villupuram, Thirunelveli, Chengalpattu, Thanjavur and 557 rape cases were reported in 2003 in Tamil Nadu (Sangameswarm, 2004). Atrocities and violence against women are rampant in homes rather than at public places (Devi, 2004: 4). Violence against women increases women's HIV infection in Tamil Nadu.

10. HIV related stigma is high in Tamil Nadu than any other States of India. The people living with HIV/AIDS are discriminated, harassed and ill treated by medical and para-medical personnel in both the government and private health sectors (Kannan, 2004). Such discrimination prevents people at high risk group to take HIV test to know their HIV status and to adopt sex practices.

11. Due to drought and unemployment in rural areas, the rural people in Tamil Nadu is involved in migration towards urban and sub-urban areas and lives in the environment which provides the ground for multisexual and unsafe sexual behaviour.

(c) HIV/AIDS intervention programmes in Tamil Nadu

Tamil Nadu State AIDS Control Society (TNSACS) - the first in the country, an autonomous organisation, was created in 1994 to implement AIDS intervention programmes more vigorously across the State with non-government organisations (NGOs) partners who conducted intervention programme aimed at various target populations (Singhal *et al.* 2003: 118).

The main components, strategies and intervention under the AIDS Control Programmes includes Blood safety, training and voluntary blood donation activities, Targeted Intervention Programmes through NGOs, Institutional and Infrastructural strengthening, Training and Capacity building activities, Control of Sexually Transmitted Diseases and Reproductive Track Infection care and also Out-reach services, Condom Promotion activities, Information, Education and Communication, Care and Support for AIDS patients, Training, Sentinel Surveillance, Programme Management, and Advocacy, Social mobilization and Sensitization Programmes, Legal and General Counseling and also Help line Services, Voluntary Counseling and Testing Centres to identify HIV affected and to provide counseling and Prevention of Parent to Child Transmission (Finance and Budget, TNSACS, 2004: wp1).

The HIV prevention programme in Tamil Nadu was two-pronged, with a specialized effort, mainly through one-on-one peer communication, aimed at high-risk groups like sex workers, coupled with an intensive mass media campaign aimed at the general population. Sex workers were persuaded to use condoms with their customers by the specialized communication programmes, and their customers were urged to use condoms with sex workers by the general media campaign. Advertising and public relations firms in India were hired to mount the media campaign in Tamil Nadu. As a result, public awareness of AIDS jumped from 23 per cent in 1994 to 98 per cent in 2000 and condom use had increased among sex workers, truck drivers and factory workers (Singhal *et al.*, 2003: 119-20).

TNSACS initiated several measures to strengthen HIV prevention, care and support programmes. The sentinel surveillance survey and behavioural surveillance survey is undertaken among the selected groups in the population known as "sentinel groups" at regular intervals at regular sentinel sites to monitor trends in HIV infection.

(i) Awareness creation Programme

Information, Education and Communication (IEC) interventions have also been launched to reduce the stigma and discrimination associated with HIV/AIDS and also to safeguard and protect the human rights of People Living with HIV/AIDS (PLWHA). The massages of faithfulness and safe are being used as a part of the awareness campaign through the electronic and print media and through outdoor publicity campaigns both in rural and urban areas in Tamil Nadu. Red Ribbon Clubs are formed in colleges to promote awareness about HIV/AIDS, mode of transmission and prevention among adolescent and young adults. (TNSACS, 2004: wp2).

(ii) School AIDS Education Programme

School AIDS Education Programme is conducted with the objectives of creating an awareness of HIV/AIDS among school students and teachers. All the students studying in 9th and 11th standard are covered under the School AIDS Education Programme. During 2003-2004, 5216 Government and Government aided High Schools and Higher Secondary Schools and 3201 Matriculation Schools were covered under the School AIDS Education Programme and 15 lakhs students were benefited out of this programme (Finance & Budget, TNSACS, 2004: wp7).

Tamil Nadu is a pioneering State in introducing HIV/AIDS information in regular school curriculum during the year 2003-2004. All the 8417 High Schools and Higher Secondary Schools including matriculation schools both in the public and private sectors have been brought under this programme with the support of UNICEF and USAID assisted APAC (AIDS Prevention and Control) Project (Health and Family Welfare Department, 2004: wp2).

(iii) Targeted interventions programme

TNSACS is presently implementing 75-targeted interventions, of which 20 are aimed at sex workers, 15 at truckers, 31 at industrial and migrant workers and 2 at men seeking men. The targeted interventions are implemented through non-governmental organisations, which play a crucial role in combating the HIV/AIDS epidemic (TNSACS, 2004: wp2).

(iv) STD Clinics

High burden of sexually transmitted diseases in the society makes it highly vulnerable to HIV/AIDS. The TNSACS extends support, through provision of infrastructure facilities, equipments and drugs to 57 STD clinics in Tamil Nadu in various institutions including Medical College Hospitals (11), District Headquarter Hospitals (26) and Taluk Hospitals (20). Specialist treatment is provided in all the STD clinics free of cost. In addition HIV/AIDS cases are treated as in-patients in Government Hospitals of Thoracic Medicine, Tambaram, and Government General Hospitals and also in Medical College Hospitals for all opportunistic infections at free of cost (TNSAC, 2004: wp1). Measures have also been taken to bring about appropriate attitudinal changes among medical and para-medical staff in the STD clinics to make them patient friendly

(v) Legal Cell

Legal cell is established in Tamil Nadu AIDS Control Society with the objectives of providing counseling for those infected and affected by HIV/AIDS, protecting and promoting Human Rights of those living with HIV/AIDS, mobilizing lawmakers to adopt effective laws and to take legal and establish committees to address legal and ethical issues, establishing effective liaison with People living with HIV/AIDS, NGOs, Academic Institutions, Corporate Sectors and Government Institutions and publishing concept papers on issues and policies.

(vi) Care and Support

Care and support–medical and emotional, can help people living with HIV/AIDS to lead a fulfilled live with free from discrimination. The government accords high priority for making quality medical care and treatments available to the people living with HIV/AIDS in the state. TNSACS extended financial support for the purchase of drugs for opportunistic infections and for Poor Exposure Prophylaxis (PEP) drugs. It also assists the association of People Living with HIV/AIDS towards running day care centers and community care centers. It extended support to 13 private institutional care centers, five community care centers and seven drop-in-centers and seven networks by people living with HIV positive. Further, the government has waived sales tax on ART drugs with a view to help the People Living with HIV/AIDS (TNSACS – Care and Support, 204: 1-wp9). TNSACS employs positive people and it insisted the NGOs working with HIV/AIDS to appoint at least one positive person in their organisations. Special wards have been set up for HIV/AIDS patients for giving treatment for various opportunistic infections in the Government Hospital of Thoracic Medicine in Tambaram, Chennai.

(vii) Family Health Awareness Campaign (FHAC)

The Family Health Awareness Campaign (FHAC) is an important strategy to identify and treat Sexually Transmitted Diseases and Reproductive Track diseases (RTI) and to treat them with syndromic management, basically to eliminate aggravating factors such as STD and RTI which contribute for faster spread of HIV/AIDS. The campaign was concentrated on general public, both in rural and urban areas. FHACs have been conducted in Tamil Nadu from 1999 to 2003 every year and with the support from National AIDS Control Organisation, Government of India. During 2003, FHAC camps were conducted in 14,889 locations across the state with adequate multimedia publicity and as a result, the number of persons with STD identified and treated in these camps went up from 6,63,330 in 2002 to 11,05,047 in 2003, of which 8,31,988 were women (Policy Note - Health and Family Welfare Department, 2005: wp2).

(viii) Condom Promotion

Top priority has been given to promote condom usage among people, both high risk and low risk, to prevent transmission of HIV through sexual route of transmission. NGOs have been involved in social marketing of condoms. At present condoms are available in the fair price shops in the state. Condom at free of cost is distributed to the people through health care institution, STD clinics, outreach camps and also through NGOs. Subsidised or low priced condoms are distributed among the people in targeted intervention areas an non-intervention areas with the support of NGOs.

(ix) Blood Safety

The Tamil Nadu State Blood Transfusion Council closely monitors the activity of the Blood Banks with the association of the Directorate of Drugs Control. Government has taken various efforts to increase the share of voluntary donation and as a result, the share of voluntary donors went up from 59.40% to 64.05% during 2004 and the zero prevalence among the blood donors went down from 0.21% t 0.18% in 2004.

(x) Prevention of Parent to Child Transmission Programme

To prevent the vertical transmission of HIV from the mother to child, Prevention of Parent to Child Transmission of HIV (PPTCT) Programme is being implemented in 65 centers Tamil Nadu including 14 Government medical Colleges, six Private Medical Colleges, 28 District Government Headquarters Hospitals, eight Private hospitals and nine Corporation Mother and Child Health Centers (Finance and Budget, TNSACS, 2004: 6-wp7). The special features of the PPTCT programme are counseling to all the pregnant women and their husbands attending antenatal clinic centers, testing for HIV, administration of ART prophylaxis to the identified positive pregnant women and their children and improvements in general antenatal clinic practices (Policy Note - Health and Family Welfare Department, 2005: wp3).

(xi) Voluntary Confidential Counseling and Testing Centers (VCCTC)

The VCCTC function as a bridge between prevention and care and support intervention. It has the objectives of (i) drawing and counseling the high-risk groups, (ii) bringing about desired changes in their behaviour, (iii) identification of sero positive persons, (iv) extending psychological support to HIV positive persons and (v) referring HIV positive persons for appropriate medical treatment wherever necessary (Policy Note - Health and Family Welfare Department, 2005: 3). There are 43 VCCT Centers established in all government head quarters hospital and government medical colleges. In 2004, 85,801 persons availed testing facilities and among them 20,590 were identified as HIV positive (Finance & Budget, TNSACS, 2004: wp6).

(xii) Anti Retroviral Therapy (ART)

The Government of India has taken a policy decision to make Anti Retroviral drugs available in the public health system in the country. Under this initiative, the ART programme was launched as the first phase in Government hospital for Thoracic Medicine, Tambaram in Chennai with effect from 1st April 2004 (Policy Note - Health and Family Welfare Department, 2005: wp3).

(xiii) Greater involvement of people living with HIV/AIDS (GIPA)

The government is committed to the concept of greater involvement of people living with HIV/AIDS programmes. The positive networks are actively involved in the decision making process of TNSACS at various levels. The government has issued orders to include a women member of Positive Networks in all the Hospital Advisory Committees in the state.

(xiv) Partnership with NGOs to reach high risk groups

The TNSAC had coordinated with NGOs in the implementation of HIV/AIDS prevention Programmes among marginalized and vulnerable population who are at high risk and creating awareness among general public. Now it has shifted its focus towards bringing behavioural changes through Targeted

Interventions involving grass root level NGOs and peer educators/outreach workers/counselors. The TANSAC funds 621 NGOs and currently 107 programmes are implemented in the state for different risk groups such as sex workers, truckers, industrial workers, prisoners, men seeking men, migrant workers, networking with people living with HIV/AIDS, youth and adolescents, tribal and research studies. Awareness, condom promotion and demonstration, STD care, counseling are the important sub-components of these interventions (Finance & Budget, TNSACS, 2004: wp3).

(xiv) Training and Capacity Building

In order to have better service delivery system and to have institutional strengthening in private and public sector, training activities has been given due importance by making adequate provision in Action Plan to impart training on HIV/AIDS to medical, para-medical and personnel of different sectors and departments. During 2003-2004, 930 officials from various medical and para-medical departments were given training on various aspects related to HIV/AIDS.

(xv) Positive net work by the people with HIV positive

TNSACS has provided funds to organize people with HIV positive by establishing positive net work. There are seven net works functioning in Tamil Nadu and recently, the TNSACS has constituted an advisory committee in every Government hospital in the state to monitor and prevent discrimination in treatment and care of persons living with HIV/AIDS and women living with HIV positive are included in all advisory committee (Kannan, 2004: 5).

In spite of all these intervention programmes the rate of HIV infection is increasing among high risk groups in general and women in particular in Tamil Nadu.

5

Analysis and Discussion

This chapter is devoted to analysis and discussion of primary data collected from the study area. It is divided into six sub-sections focusing on a specific aspect of the study.

The first sub-section deals with socio economic status of respondents which includes respondents' personal, family particulars and economic condition of respondents. The second sub-section is directly related to marital status of respondents. The third sub-section deals with circumstances leading to HIV positive both for housewives and sex workers. The fourth sub-section explains about the sexual behaviour of respondents after infection. The fifth sub-section represents the social relationship of respondents with their family members, neighbours, friends and relatives. This section also gives elaborate view about the discrimination faced by the respondents in hospitals and work place. The sixth sub-section evaluates the attitude of respondents towards pregnancy after infection.

Tables are presented logically by merging relevant variables in consonance with the objectives of the study. Percentage and averages are widely used to analyse the available data and accordingly interpretations are made.

SOCIO-ECONOMIC STATUS OF RESPONDENTS

Table 5.1. Age-wise Distribution of Respondents

Sl. No.	*Age (in years)*	*No. of Respondents*	*Percentage*
1.	15 – 19	16	8.0
2.	20 – 24	47	23.5
3.	25 – 29	86	43.0
4.	30 – 34	28	14.0
5.	35 – 39	23	11.5
	Total	200	100

Table 5.1 reveals the age wise distribution of respondents in the study area. It shows that all (100 %) HIV infected respondents fall in the reproductive and economically active age group of 15-39 years. This study also reveals the high (66.5%) concentration of HIV infection in the sexually active age group of 20-29 years.

The inference drawn from the table is that the majority (66.5%) of respondents with infection belong to the hyper sexual active age group of 20-29 years.

Table 5.2. Community-wise Distribution of Respondents

Sl. No.	*Community*	*No. of Respondents*	*Percentage*
1.	S.C	52	26.0
2.	S.T.	3	1.5
3.	M.B.C.	22	11.0
4.	B.C.	93	46.5
5.	F.C.	30	15.0
	Total	200	100.0

The analysis of data on communitywise distribution of respondents indicates that 46.5% respondents belong to backward community (B.C.). The respondents belong to schedule caste (S.C.) is found to be 26%. The respondents belong to forward caste (F.C.) constitute 15%. It is found from the analysis that 11% respondents and 1.5% of respondents belong to most back ward community (M.B.C.) and schedule tribes (S.T.) (Table 5.2).

As regards this study, the higher percentage (57.5%) of respondents belongs to the socially Backward Class (B.Cs) and Most Back Word Class (M.B.Cs) in view of their husbands' involvement in multi sexual behaviour leading to transmission of HIV to their wives (Table 5.2).

Table 5.3. Education-wise Distribution of Respondents

Sl. No.	*Educational Status*	*No. of Respondents*	*Percentage*
1.	Illiterate	28	14.0
2.	Primary	49	24.5
3.	High School	54	27.0
4.	Higher Secondary	35	17.5
5.	Graduation	31	15.5
6.	Technical Education	3	1.5
	Total	200	100

Table 5.3 shows the educational status of the respondents. The analysis of data shows that out of 200 respondents, only 14% were illiterate and the remaining 61.5 per cent were literate. Among the literate groups, 27 per cent respondents have completed high school, 17.5 per cent respondents have studied upto higher secondary, 15.5 per cent have obtained graduate degree and 1.5 per cent were professionally qualified.

The inference drawn from the table is that literate women are highly prone to infection than the illiterate women.

Table 5.4. Religion-wise Distribution of Respondents

Sl. No.	*Religion*	*No. of Respondents*	*Percentage*
1.	Hindu	170	85.0
2.	Muslim	14	7.0
3.	Christian	16	8.0
	Total	200	100

Table 5.4 explains the religion wise distribution of respondents in the study area. It is observed from the table that out of 200 respondents, 85% were Hindus, 8% were Christians and 7% were Muslims.

Since majority (85%) of the respondents were Hindus, the inference drawn from the table is that there is a change in the moral and traditional attitude of younger generation.

Table 5.5. Social Status of the Respondents

Sl. No.	*Social status*	*No. of Respondents*	*Percentage*
1.	Housewives	131	65.5
2.	Sex workers	62	31.0
3.	Students	7	3.5
	Total	200	100

As far as the social status of the respondents is concerned, 65.5% are wives. The sex workers accounted for 31.0%. The remaining 3.5% are students studying in various colleges of Chennai (Table 5.5).

The inference drawn from the table is that wives are highly vulnerable to HIV/AIDS.

Table 5.6. Causes for Migration of Respondents to Chennai

Sl. No.	*Causes*	*No. of Respondents*	*Percentage*
1.	Marriage	54	27.0
2.	Employment	26	13.0
3.	HIV infection	27	13.5
4.	Education	6	3.0
5.	Prostitution	12	6.0
6.	Non-migrants	75	37.5
	Total	200	100

Table 5.6 explains the causes for migration of respondents to Chennai. Of the total, 62.5% of respondents were migrated to Chennai from various parts of Tamil Nadu as well as from various States of India.

Marriage constituted the major (27%) cause of migration to Chennai. HIV infection influenced 13.5% respondents to migrate to Chennai. Employment is the primary cause for 13% respondents' migration. Involvement in prostitution made 6% respondents to migrate to Chennai and education is the important cause for 3% respondents' migration.

It is also identified from Table 5.6 that the higher percentage (61.6%) of respondents migrated to Chennai from different parts of Tamil Nadu. Among outside Tamil Nadu migrants, the women from Andhra Pradesh were dominant (20.8%) followed by Kerala (8.8%), Karnataka (6.4) and Gujarat (2.4%).

The conclusion drawn from the table is that the majority (62.5%) under study is the migrants of different parts of Tamil Nadu for various reasons. The marriage constitutes the major cause for the migration of many women to Chennai. To hide HIV infection from the relatives, friends, neighbours, to avail treatment facilities, etc. also lead many women to migrate to Chennai.

Table 5.7. Family Size of the Respondents

Sl. No.	*Size of the family*	*No. of Respondents*	*Percentage*
1.	Small (> 4 members)	45	22.5
2.	Medium (4 – 6 members)	86	43.0
3.	Large (< 6 members)	69	34.5
	Total	200	100

The analysis of the data on "family particulars of the respondents" have identified that 43% of the respondents have medium size family with the members of 3 to 4. Significant 34.5% of respondents also has large family size with the members above five. The small family of the respondents accounted for 22.5 % with the family members of less than four (Table 5.7).

The inference drawn from the analysis is that the infected women's families have the characteristics of medium and large size families.

Table 5.8. Structure of Family of Respondents

Sl. No.	*Structure of the family*	*No. of Respondents*	*Percentage*
1.	Joint	154	77.0
2.	Nuclear	46	23.0
	Total	200	100

As far as the structure of the family is concerned, the nuclear family is dominant (77%) than the joint family (23%). The conclusion drawn from the table is that HIV infection is high (77%) in the nuclear family than the joint family (Table 5.8).

Table 5.9. Dependent and Non-dependent Family Members of Respondents

Sl. No.	*Family members*	*No. of Respondents*	*Percentage*
1.	Dependent - Children	126	63.0
2.	Dependent - Old age	44	22.0
3.	Non Dependent	30	15.0
	Total	200	100

The study also found that the great proportion (63 per cent) of respondents have dependent children within the age of less than 17 years and also a significant proportion (22 per cent)of respondents have an old age dependents with the age ranging from 58 and above. The respondents who have non-dependent family members constituted only 15 per cent.

The inference drawn from the analysis is that majority (63 per cent) of the respondents have dependent family members that increased the burden of the HIV infected women.

Table 5.10. Educational Status of Respondents' Family Members

Sl. No.	*Education of Family members*	*No. of Respondents*	*Percentage*
1.	Illiterate	34	17.0
2.	School educated	128	64.0
3.	Graduation	38	19.0
	Total	200	100

The educational level of the family members varies from illiterate to graduation. Majority (64%) of the respondents' family members have school education and 19% of the respondents' families have graduates. Besides 17% of respondents family members were illiterate (Table 5.10).

It is explored from the analysis that the majority (82%) of the respondents' family members are literates.

Table 5.11. Employment Status of Family Members

Sl. No.	*Employment status of family members*	*No. of members*	*Percentage*
1.	Government	3	3.9
2.	Private	16	20.5
3.	Business	12	15.4
4.	Casual labours	27	34.6
5.	Hotel workers	5	6.4
6.	Transport workers	3	3.9
7.	Construction workers	11	14.1
8.	Military service	1	1.2
	Total	78	100

It is found from the study that only 15 per cent of respondents have non-dependent family members and they were involved in different kinds of occupation in various sectors such as casual labours (34.6 per cent) in unorganized sectors, employee in private sectors (20.5 per cent), construction work (14.1 per cent), business (15.4 per cent), government (3.9 per cent) hotel industry (6.4) and in military service (1.2 per cent) (Table 5.11).

The inference drawn from the analysis is that majority (59 per cent) of respondents family members are engaged in unorganized sectors which gives less and income and least job security.

Table 5.12. Respondents Status in the Family

Sl. No.	*Respondents status in the family*	*No. of Respondents*	*Percentage*
1.	Earner	49	24.5
2.	Earner dependent	67	33.5
3.	Non-earner dependent	84	42.0
	Total	200	100

Table 5.12 shows the status of the respondents in the family. The table has revealed that 42 per cent respondents were non-

earner dependent, 33.5per cent respondents were earner dependent and 24.5per cent were earners for their families.

The conclusion drawn from the table is that the majority (42per cent) of the HIV infected women were non-earner dependents, who are mostly wives.

Table 5.1.13. Place of Residence of Respondents

Sl. No.	*Place of residence*	*No. of Respondents*	*Percentage*
1.	Urban	84	42.0
2.	Urban slums		
	(a) Housewives	95	47.5
	(b) Sex workers	21	10.5
	Total	200	100

The table on the respondents place of residence has identified that majority (42 per cent) of the respondents reside in urban areas and urban slums (58 per cent).

The inference drawn from the analysis is that the urban slum women are highly vulnerable to HIV infection due to promiscuous relationship of their husbands.

Table 5.14. Occupation of the Respondents

Sl. No.	*Nature of Occupation*	*No. of Respondents*	*Percentage*
1.	Commercial sex work	33	16.5
2.	Casual labour	18	9.0
3.	Self Employed	5	1.5
4.	Government services	7	3.5
5.	Others :		
	(a) Private company	16	8.0
	(b) House maids	12	6.0
	(c) N.G.Os	17	8.5
	(d) Support actors	5	2.5
	(e) Construction work	5	2.5
6.	Unemployed	84	42.0
	Total	200	100

The Table 5.14 explains the occupation of the respondents. It is evident from the analysis that significant percentage (42 per cent) of respondents are unemployed and non-earner dependents. The number of respondents employed in various sectors constituted for 58 per cent.

The analysis of the data further shows that a very few percentage of respondents were employed in organized sectors like Government (3.5 per cent) and private companies (8 per cent). But the majority of the respondents were found to be engaged in unorganized sectors such as casual labour (9 per cent) house maids (6 per cent), construction workers (2.5 per cent), cinema artists (2.5 per cent), self employed (1.5 per cent) and field workers in the N.G.Os (8.5 per cent). The respondents who are working in the N.G.Os joined only after their infection. The women involved in commercial sex work constituted for 16.5 per cent.

The conclusion drawn from the analysis is that the majority (30 per cent) of the respondents were employed in unorganized sectors and in commercial sex work (16.5 per cent).

Table 5.15. Ownership of Property of Respondents

	Immovable Assets				*Movable Assets*		
Sl. No.	*Type of Asset*	*No. of Respondents*	*%*	*Sl. No.*	*Type of Asset*	*No. of Respondents*	*%*
1.	Land	2	1.0	1.	TV Radio	83	41.5
2.	House	6	3.0	2.	Fridge	14	7.0
3.	Shop	1	0.5	3.	Motor cycle	4	2.0
4.	No Assets	191	95.5	4.	Jewels	29	14.5
				5.	No Assets	70	35.0
	Total	200	100		Total	200	100

Table 5.15 explains the ownership of property of the respondents. Of the total, very few percentage of respondents own immovable assets like house (3 per cent), land (1 per cent) and shop (0.5 per cent).

As far as movable assets are concerned, a considerable percentage of respondents owned TV/Radio (41.5 per cent), Jewels (14.5 per cent), Fridge (7 per cent) and Motor cycle (2 per cent).

The inference drawn from the table is that many respondents (95.5 per cent) due to gender biased Indian culture do not enjoy the ownership of immovable property and the women who own movable assets (65 per cent) are due to their earning capacity in various occupations.

Table 5.16. Annual Income and Expenditure of Respondent Families

Sl. No.	Amount (in Rupees)	Income		Expenditure	
		No. of respondents	Percentage	No. of respondents	Percentage
1.	Less than 25,000	96	48.0	62	31.0
2.	25,000 – 50,000	43	21.5	66	33.0
3.	50,000 – 75,000	33	16.5	43	21.5
4.	75,000 – 1,00,000	19	9.5	22	11.0
5.	More than 1,00,000	9	4.5	7	3.5
	Total	200	100.0	200	100

Table 5.16 on annual income and expenditure of the respondent families reveal that the majority (69.5 per cent) of the respondent families fall within the income group of Rs. 50,000 followed by the income group of Rs. 50, 000 – 75,000 (16.5 per cent). The respondent families' income of more than Rs.75, 000 constituted around 14 per cent in this study.

The analysis on respondent families expenditure shows that 64 per cent incurred less than Rs.50,000 and the remaining 36 per cent of respondent families annual expenditure was more than Rs. 75,000. The inference drawn from the above table is that the annual expenditure is more than their annual income.

Table 5.17 on indebtedness of the respondent families reveals that 60 per cent of the respondents were indebted to various sources for different purposes. Of the 120 respondents, 59.2 per cent women were indebted for taking treatment for HIV infection for their husband, children and themselves. The other reasons for the indebtedness of the remaining respondents were identified as education of the children (9.2 per cent), business (6.7 per cent), food, and clothes (10.7 per cent), construction of house (1.7 per cent), marriage (5.0 per cent), and other reasons like recreation, celebrating festivals etc (7.5 per cent).

Table 5.17. Indebtedness of Respondent Families

Sl. No.	Purpose of borrowing	*Sources of borrowing, No. of families (in percentage)*					
		Money Lender	Bank	Relatives	Friends	Others	Total
1.	Treatment	47 (66.2%)	-	15 (21.1%)	9 (12.7%)	-	71 (59.2%)
2.	Children education	1 (9.1%)	-	-	6 (54.5%)	4 (36.4%)	11 (9.2%)
3.	Business	3 (37.5%)	3 (37.5%)	-	2 (25.0%)	-	8 (6.7%)
4.	Food and clothes	8 (61.5%)	-	2 (15.4%)	2 (15.4%)	1 (7.7%)	13 (10.7%)
5.	House construction	-	2 (100.0%)	-	-	-	2 (1.7%)
6.	Marriage	4 (66.7%)	-	-	2 (33.3%)	-	6 (5.0%)
7.	Others	2 (22.2%)	2 (22.2%)	1 (11.1%)	4 (44.5%)	-	9 (7.5%)
	Total	*65 (54.2%)*	*7 (5.8%)*	*18 (15.0%)*	*25 (20.8%)*	*5 (4.2%)*	*120 (100%)*

Among the sources of borrowing, moneylender is found to be a dominant source (54.2 per cent) followed by friends (20.8 per cent) and relatives (15.0 per cent).

The inference drawn from the table is that majority (59.2 per cent) of the respondents borrowed for medical reasons to treat HIV infection and the source of their borrower was moneylenders who charged higher interest.

Table 5.18 on amount borrowed by the respondents reveals that the majority (67.5 per cent) of respondents have borrowed amount ranging from 4,000-10,000. The significant percentage (15.0 per cent) borrowed an amount between 2,000-4,000. About 11.7 per cent is borrowed above 10,000 where as 5.8 per cent borrowed upto 2,000 from various sources.

The inference drawn from the analysis is that the majority (67.5 per cent) have borrowed amount from rupees 4000-10000 due to various reasons which lead to heavy burden for them to repay it in time.

Table 5.18. Amount Borrowed by the Respondents

Sl. No.	*Amount (in Rupees)*	*No. of Respondents*	*Percentage*
1.	Less than 2000	7	5.8
2.	2000-4000	18	15.0
3.	4000- 6000	31	25.8
4.	6000-8000	27	22.5
5.	8000-10000	23	19.2
6.	Above 10000	14	11.7
	Total	120	100

Marital Status of the Respondents

Table 5.19 on marital status of the respondents indicates that out of 200 respondents, 82.5 per cent were married and 17.5 per cent were unmarried. Among the married respondents, 38 per cent were living with their husband, 25.5 per cent were found to be widows, 16.5 per cent are separated from their husbands and 2.5 per cent were identified as divorced.

The inference drawn from the table is that the housewives were at higher risk of getting infection in the study area.

Table 5.19. Marital Status of the Respondents

Sl. No.	*Marital Status*	*No. of Respondents*	*Percentage*
1.	Married	76	38.0
2.	Separated	33	16.5
3.	Divorced	5	2.5
4.	Widow	51	25.5
5.	Unmarried	35	17.5
	Total	200	100

Table 5.20 explains the age at marriage of the respondents and their husbands. Of the total 200 respondents 82.5 per cent were married and remaining 17.5 per cent were unmarried. Among the married respondents, the majority (58.2 per cent) of the respondents have got married in between the age of 19—22 years. Child marriage, i.e. marriage age less than 18 years is found among 32.1 per cent of respondents. The respondents who have married at the age of 23 and above are identified as

9.7 per cent. As far as age at marriage of the respondent's husband is concerned, 92.7 per cent got married at the age above 23 years.

Table 5.20. Age at Marriage of Respondents and their Husbands

Sl. No.	*Age at Marriage, years*	*No. of Respondents*	*No. of Respondents Husband*
1.	Less than 18	53 (32.1 per cent)	0 (0 .0 per cent)
2.	19-22	96 (58.2 per cent)	12 (7.3 per cent)
3.	23-27	15 (9.1 per cent)	54 (32.7 per cent)
4.	28-32	1 (0.6 per cent)	61 (37.0 per cent)
5.	Above 33	0 (0.0 per cent)	38 (23.0 per cent)
	Total	165 (100 per cent)	165 (100 per cent)

The inference drawn from the analysis is that 90.1 per cent of women's' age at marriage is below 22 years. These respondents got married the men who are older than them. Due to the younger age, the women can't either negotiate or suggest reproductive health issues and safe sex to their husbands. Moreover, these young women are highly ignorant about sex and its implication of her body and men have all power to with regard to sex and reproductive health. Therefore, younger the age at marriage, higher the chance for getting sexually transmitted diseases including HIV/AIDS.

Table 5.21. Nature of Kins Relationship between Respondents and their Husbands

Sl. No.	*Nature of relationship*	*No. of Respondents*	*Percentage*
1.	Blood relatives	26	15.8
2.	Distant relatives	46	27.9
3.	Not related	93	56.3
	Total	165	100

Table 5.21 shows the nature of kins relationship between the respondents and their husbands before marriage. The analysis reveals that 56.3 per cent of respondent's husbands were not related to their family before marriage. For 27.9 per

cent of respondents, their husbands were distant relatives and 15.8 per cent of respondents got married within the blood relatives.

The inference drawn from the analysis is that the majority (84.2 per cent) of the marriage taken place outside close kin family relationships. According to the respondents, such kind of marriage would not facilitate them to either to collect or to discuss about the health status of the partners. They also revealed that if the partners are within their close family circle, they can know each other behaviour and characters and if the behaviour of the partner is suspeciable and if they have any doubts on their behaviour on pre marital sex they can avoid the marriage with them.

Therefore, the marriage with unknown person may be resulted in the selection of mate whose character may not be well understood before marriage and if the men have pre marital sex before marriage with multiplex sexual partners, it will increases the chance for HIV infection among the married women with single sexual partners.

Table 5.22 projects the type of marriage of the respondents. It explains that 77.6 per cent of respondent's marriage was arranged by their family members. The marriage that is not arranged by their family members is constituted about 22.4 per cent.

Table 5.22. Type of Marriage of Respondents

Sl. No.	*Type of Marriage*	*No. of Respondents*	*Percentage*
1	Arranged	109	66.1
2.	Love with arranged	19	11.5
3.	Love and married by themselves	34	20.6
4.	Living together without marriage	3	1.8
	Total	165	100

The understanding from the table is that the infection rate is found to be high (66.1 per cent) in arranged marriages and it is comparatively low (32.1 per cent) in the marriage based on love. In the Indian context the marriages are arranged by the elders of the family with the good faith that they have selected a good life partner for their daughters. The elders are very keen to collect information with regard to the matching of horoscope rather than health status and other information related to pre marital sexual behaviour of the bridegroom. In the case of love marriage, the loving girl and boy knows each others behaviour and they always have a chance to discuss about their health condition prior to their marriage.

Therefore, HIV infection is found to be high in arranged marriage and low in love marriage.

Table 5.23. Causes for Respondents Widowhood

Sl.No.	*Causes*	*No. of Respondents*	*Percentage*
1.	Husband died due to AIDS	47	92.1
2.	Other causes	4	7.9
	Total	51	100

Among the 200 respondents selected for study, 25.5 per cent were identified as widows. It is observed from the analysis that HIV/AIDS related diseases is the major cause for the death of 92.1 per cent respondents husbands and among them 9 (17.6 per cent) have committed suicide due to the fear of AIDS related stigma. The remaining 7.9 per cent have become widow even before they are infected by HIV (Table 5.23).

The inference drawn from the table is that the AIDS is the major cause for the majority (92.1 per cent) of the women to become widow at younger age.

All the 51 (100 per cent) women became widow within the age of 30 years. The predominant age at widowhood for 88.2 per cent of respondents is identified as 20-25 year and the remaining became widow between the age of 26-30 years. The table also shows that the majority (72.5) of respondents lived with their husband for 1-5 years and the remaining 27.5 per cent respondents life with their husbands ranges between 6-10 years (Table 5.24).

The inference drawn from the table is that AIDS is the major cause for the majority (88.2 per cent) of women to become widow at the younger age of 20-25 years and many (72.5 per cent) have acquired infection within the 5 years of their marital life. Sexual

Table 5.24 Age at Widowhood and Duration of Life with Husband

Sl. No.	*Age at widowhood (in years) No. of Respondents*			*Duration of life with husband (in years) No. of respondents*		
	20-25	*26-30*		*1-5*	*6-10*	
1.	45 (88.2%)	6 (11.8%)	51 (100%)	37 (72.5%)	14 (27.5%)	51 (100%)

encounter or sexual activity is high among the spouses in the early period of their marital life. The aspirations towards giving birth to child force the young couples to avoid condom and other contraception. Unsafe sex in the early period of marital life increases the chances of infection for the women within the less duration of marital life.

The findings of younger age at widowhood also suggest that the pre marital sex with multiple sexual partners is high among the young men and they might have got infection long before their marriage. The men may or may not be aware of their HIV sero status before marriage and they are the sources of transmitting the virus to their young wives.

Table 5.28. Causes for Separation from Husbands.

Sl. No.	*Causes*	*No. of Respondents*	*Percen-tage*
1.	Refused to live with the HIV infected husbands	14	36.8
2.	Deserted by infected husbands	11	28.9
3.	Childlessness	1	2.6
4.	Extra marital affairs of husbands	2	5.3
5.	Extra marital affairs of respondents	8	21.1
6.	Family problems	2	5.3
	Total	38	100

In this study, 18.0 per cent women were identified as either separated 33 (86.8 per cent) or divorced 5 (13.2 per cent)) from their husbands. AIDS is identified as major cause for 65.7 per cent women for the separation from their marital life. Among them 36.8 per cent women refused to live with their infected husbands where as 28.9 per cent were deserted by their infected husbands due to avoid the further spread of infection to the child.. Extra marital affair is the cause for 21.1 per cent respondents' separation from their husbands. Family problem accounted for the separation of 5.3 per cent of women. Husband's extra marital affairs made 5.3 per cent women to break their matrimonial bonds and childlessness is the primary cause for the separation of 2.6 per cent women from their husbands (Table 5.5).

The conclusion drawn from the table is that HIV/AIDS of husbands disturbs family life and forces the spouses either to separate or to get divorce (65.7 per cent) from the infected persons. The findings also reveal that the urban life facilitated many young women to develop extra marital affairs (21.1 per cent) not only for satisfying their sexual urge but also to earn money to meet their personal as well as family requirements.

Table 5.26 on the employment status of the respondents' husbands reveals that the majority (35.8 per cent) are casual labourers and industrial workers (25.4 per cent). The transport workers are identified as 16.4 per cent followed by self employment (12.7 per cent). The remaining are engaged in government service (9.7 per cent) and business (5.4 per cent).

Table 5.26. Employment Status of Husband

Sl. No.	*Employment status*	*No. of Respondents*	*Percentage*
1.	Casual labourers	59	35.8
2.	Transport workers	27	16.4
3.	Government service	16	9.7
4.	Self employed	21	12.7
5.	Industrial worker	42	25.4
	Total	165	100

The inference drawn from the analysis is that the casual labourers, industrial workers, transport workers are more prone to HIV/AIDS.

The above table explains the reasons for the unmarried status of 35 respondents. It shows that involvement in sex work prevented 25.7 per cent of respondents to get marriage followed by dowry problem (229 per cent), HIV infection (20 per cent) and lack of interest by the parents (17.1 per cent). The respondents who are not found suitable alliance for marriage accounted for 8.6 per cent. The 5.7 per cent of respondents have no interest in marriage.

Table 5.27 inference drawn from the analysis is that involvement in sex work and dowry prevented majority (48.6 per cent) of respondents to get marriage.

Table 5.27. Reasons for Unmarried Status of Respondents

Sl.No.	*Reasons*	*No. of Respondents*	*Percentage*
1.	Dowry problem	8	22.9
2.	Not found suitable alliance	3	8.6
3.	Not interested	2	5.7
4.	Parents not shown interest	6	17.1
5.	Involvement in sex workers	9	25.7
6.	HIV infection	7	20.0
	Total	35	100

Circumstances Leading to HIV Infection and Related Behaviours

Table 5.28 explains how long the respondents were suffering from HIV infection. The analysis shows that, of the total, 31.5 per cent respondents were living with HIV infection for less than 5 years followed by 25.5 per cent respondents who were suffering with HIV for 5-6 years. The respondents who carry HIV about 6-7 years constituted 24.5 per cent and the women living with HIV for more than 7 years identified as 19 per cent.

The inference drawn from the analysis is that the majority (81.0 per cent) of the respondents tested HIV within seven years and it shows that they are infected within the sexually hyper active younger age.

Table 5.28. Duration of HIV Infection.

Sl. No.	*Duration (in No. of years)*	*No. of Respondents*	*Percentage*
1	Less than 5	62	31.0
2.	5 - 6	51	25.5
3.	6 - 7	49	24.5
4.	7 - 8	32	16.0
5.	Above 8	6	3.0
	Total	200	100

Table 5.29 observed the sources of HIV infection of the respondents. It is evident from the table that 65.0 per cent respondents got HIV through their husband's promiscuous act. For 31.0 per cent respondents, their heterosexual contact is the major cause for their infection. It is also identified from the study that 3.5 per cent respondents have infection through their pre marital sexual contact with their boy friends. The respondents who have infection through an unsterilized needle while injecting drug accounted for 0.5 per cent.

Table 5.29. Sources of Infection for Respondents.

Sl.No.	*Sources of Infection*	*No. of Respondents*	*Percentage*
1.	Husband	130	65.0
2.	Respondents heterosexual conduct	62	31.0
3.	Injected drug use	1	0.5
4.	Pre marital sex	7	3.5
	Total	200	100

The conclusion drawn from the table is that though the majority (66 per cent) of infected women is innocent victims of HIV infection through their husband, significant percentage (31 per cent) of women got infection through their heterosexual contact. It contradicts the general view that most of the women get infection in the marital life through their husbands.

Among the 62 sex workers, 27 (43.5 per cent) sex workers and one (0.5 per cent) injecting drug user are married and they are living with their husbands. These 27 sex workers and injecting drug user have not revealed their infection status to their husbands and they know that their husbands may also infected by HIV (Table 5.30).

Table 5.30. Husbands Infected by Respondents.

Sl.No.	*Wives behaviour*	*No. of husbands infected*	*Percentage*
1.	Sex work	27	96.4
2.	Injecting drug use	1	3.6
	Total	28	100

Of the 158 married respondents living with their husbands, 130 (65.0 per cent) got infection through their husbands where as the remaining 28 (35 per cent) got infection through their behaviours of sex work and injecting drug use. These 35 per cent of respondents' husbands are highly vulnerable to infection.

The inference drawn from the analysis that sex workers husbands are highly vulnerable to HIV infection.

Table 5.31. Sexual Behaviour of Respondents and their Husbands

Sl. No.	*Sexual Behaviour*	*Respondents*		*Respondent's Husbands*	
		Yes	*Percentage*	*Yes*	*Percentage*
1.	Pre-marital sex	35	17.5	79	47.9
2.	Extra marital sex	30	15.0	26	15.7
3.	Both	4	20.0	31	18. 8
4.	No immoral sex	131	65.5	29	17.6
	Total	200	100	165	100

While analyzing the respondents' sexual experiences, it is identified that significant number of respondents were involved in pre marital and extra marital sex. The analysis revealed that 17.5 per cent have experienced pre marital sex including 7 students. Pre marital and extra marital sex is found among 15.5 per cent women in this study. Among the women who have experienced extra marital sex, 6 are housewives with the social status of either widow or deserted and they have sex with their regular partners and 24 are married commercial sex workers. Besides, the women who experienced both pre and extra marital sex accounted for 4 (2.0 per cent). All these four women were commercial sex workers.

The study also explored the respondents' husbands pre and extra marital sex. It is found from the study that 47.9 per cent respondents' husbands experienced pre marital sex, 15.7 per cent respondents' husbands have an experience of extra marital sex. The men who experienced both pre and extra marital sex accounted for 18.8 per cent (Table 5.31).

Among the 165 married couples, 131 (65.5 per cent) women experienced sex only with their husbands whereas only 29 (17.6 per cent) men experienced sex after their marriage only with their wives.

The inference drawn from the analysis is that the pre and extra marital sex is predominant among the men than the women. However, significant number of women involved in such unapproved sexual activities due to the influence of city oriented life and urban culture. The men experience with pre marital sex increases their vulnerability to sexually transmitted diseases including HIV/AIDS. He may or may not be aware of his infection before marriage. The lack of knowledge on the HIV status of men before marriage increases the vulnerability of their spouse infection after marriage.

It is also clear from the analysis that not only the men are responsible for women infection. But also significant number of women themselves is responsible for their own HIV status through their pre and extra marital sex. These women also increase the vulnerability of their spouse infection.

Table 5.32. Pre and Extra Marital Sexual Partners of Respondents and their Husbands.

Sl. No.	*Sexual partners*	*Pre marital*		*Extra marital*	
		No. Respondents	*No. of Husband*	*No. Respondents*	*No. of Husband*
1.	Relatives	5(12.8%)	8 (7.3%)	1(2.9%)	1(1.8%)
2.	Neighbour	8(20.5%)	13(11.8%)	0(0.0%)	2(3.5%)
3.	Friends	11(28.2%)	17(15.4%)	1(2.9%)	0(0.0%)
4.	Co-worker	3(7.7%)	11(10.0%)	0(0.0%)	0(0.0%)
5.	Customers	9(23.1%)	—	32(94.2%)	—
6.	Family Friend	3(7.7%)	7(6.4%)	0(0.0%)	1(1.8%)
7.	Sex worker	—	54(49.1%)	—	53(92.9%)
	Total	39(100%)	110(100%)	34(100%)	57(100%)

Table 5.32 explains the pre and extra marital sexual partners of respondents and their husbands. Among the respondents who have pre marital sexual experiences, the majority (76.9 per cent) have experienced pre marital sex with the people who are known to her which include friends (28.2 per cent), neighbours (20.5 per cent), relatives (12.8 per cent), co-workers (7.7 per cent) and family friends (7.7 per cent) etc. The 23.1 per cent of women experienced their pre marital sex with their sexual customers.

The majority of the respondents' husbands involved in pre marital (49.1 per cent) and extra marital sex (92.9 per cent) with the sex workers.

The inference drawn from the analysis is that the women are sexually abused and induced to have pre marital sex by the men from the close circle of the women and their families. Sex workers are the major sources for majority of the respondents' husbands pre (49.1 per cent) and extra marital sex (92.9 per cent). It shows that the respondents' husbands sexual behaviour with multiple partners are the primary factors for respondents infection.

Table 5.33. Reasons Behind Respondents Pre and Extra Marital Sexual Behaviour.

Sl.No.	*Reasons*	*Pre marital sex*	*Extra marital sex*
1.	Influence of friends	14(36.0%)	8(23.5%)
2.	Love affairs	17(43.5%)	6(17.7%)
3.	Exposure to mass media	8(20.5%)	3(8.8%)
5.	Difference of opinion	—	17(50.0%)
	Total	39(100%)	34(100%)

The major reasons identified for respondents' pre marital sex are love affairs (43.5 per cent), influence of friends (36.0 per cent) and wider exposure to mass media (20.5 per cent).

Table 5.33 also reveals that difference of opinion between the spouses (50.0 per cent) is the major cause for the extra marital affairs of respondents followed by influence of friends

(23.5 per cent) and love affairs (17.7 per cent). The exposure to mass media influenced 8.8 per cent of respondents to experience with extra marital sex.

The inference drawn from the analysis is that love affairs is the major (43.5 per cent) cause for pre marital sex and difference of opinion between the spouses are the significant (50.0 per cent) reason for extra marital sex of the respondents.

Table 5.34. Methods Adopted for Safe Sex

Sl. No.	*Method adopted for safe sex*	*Pre marital sex (No. of respondents)*	*Extra marital sex (No. of respondents*
1.	Condom	6(15.4%)	3(8.8%)
2.	IUDs	(0.0%)	6(17.6%)
3.	Oral pills	21(53.8%)	3(8.8%)
4.	Sterilization.	0(0.0%)	14(41.2%)
5.	Not practiced any methods	12(30.8%)	8(23.6%)
	Total	39(100%)	34(100%)

The analysis on safe sex practices among the women involved in pre marital (19.5 per cent) and extra marital sex (17.0 per cent) has given a new insight to study. It is found that the condom usage is quite less among the women of pre marital (15.4 per cent) and extra marital sex (8.8 per cent). These women were very much bothered about pregnancy rather than contracting sexually transmitted diseases. Therefore, the lack or insufficient awareness on condom forces women to use other safer method that could avoid pregnancy (Table 5.34).

The major percentage (53.8 per cent) of women who experienced pre marital sex revealed that they have prepared oral pills than any other method to prevent pregnancy. It is also identified that 30.7 per cent of pre marital sexual women have not used any method to safeguard themselves from sexually transmitted diseases and pregnancy.

Among the women who have experienced extra marital sex, 41.2 per cent have undergone sterilization to prevent childbirth. Therefore, they were least bothered and not showed any seriousness to use condom to protect them from all sexually transmitted infections. Besides, 26.4 per cent of women were using temporary birth control measures such as copper T (Intra uterus devices) and oral pills. The respondents who have not at all used any safe sex method when they were in extra marital sex are identified as 23.5 per cent.

The conclusion drawn from the analysis is that the respondents who have pre and extra marital sexual contact are more particular about prevention of birth rather than prevention of sexually transmitted diseases, especially HIV/AIDS. In the Indian culture, giving birth out of promiscuous relationship is considered as taboo and women have to face a lot consequence if such birth is taken place. Culture is acting as a stumbling block to use condom for safe sex since the women are very much hesitant to buy condom from the market. Therefore, majority (53.8 per cent) of respondents used oral pills as safer method which prevents child birth. It is also identified that the majority (41.2 per cent) of the respondents who involved in extra marital sex have undergone sterilization. The practices of sterilization prevented the use of condom because the sterilized women have an attitude that they are free from pregnancy.

Table 5.35. Reasons for Respondents' Husbands Extra Marital Sexual Behaviour.

Sl.No.	*Reasons*	*No. of respondents*	*Percentage*
1.	Frequent migration	16	30.2
2.	Alcoholic behaviour	16	22.6
3.	Difference of opinion between spouse	7	13.2
5.	Lack of sexual satisfaction with wife	5	9.5
6.	Poor health condition of wife	4	7.5
7.	Pregnancy of wife	9	17.0
	Total	57	100

Of the total 165 married respondents, 34.6 per cent have extra marital affairs. Among them majority of the respondents' husbands 30.2 per cent are involved in frequent migration due to their occupation. Alcoholic behaviour is the major causes for the extra marital relationship of 22.6 per cent respondent's husbands. Pregnancy of wife is the major factor for 17.0 per cent of respondents' husbands to seek sex with sex workers.

The other important causes are found to be difference of opinion and lack of understanding between the spouses (13.2 per cent), lack of sexual satisfaction with the wife (9.5 per cent), poor health condition of wife (7.5 per cent).

The inference drawn from the analysis is that the migration and alcoholic behaviour has strong influence on the extra marital affairs of the respondents' husbands.

Table 5.36. Reproductive Behaviour of Housewives Lead to Infection.

SL.No.	*Reproductive behaviour*	*No of Respondents*	*Percentage*
1.	Condom	2	1.5
2.	IUDs	21	16.0
3.	Oral pills	14	10.7
4.	Sterilization.	47	35.9
5.	Not practiced any methods	47	35.9
	Total	131	100

Table 5.36 on reproductive health behaviour of housewives reveals that the majority (35.9 per cent) of the respondents have not adopted any safe sex methods either to avoid pregnancy or to avoid sexually transmitted infections. Adoption of sterilization is found to be high (35.9 per cent) among the respondents to avoid pregnancy. The significant percentage (26.7 per cent) of respondents have adopted non-terminal method of birth control, namely IUDs and oral pills. The adoption of condom for safe sex is very meager (1.5 per cent) among the wives.

Table 5.36 shows that the housewives give more importance to avoid pregnancy rather than sexually transmitted infections. Adoption of sterilization, oral pills and IUDs prevented majority (62.6 per cent) of wives to think about condom as safe sex method to safeguard themselves from sexually transmitted infections.

The above table highlights the marital status of sex workers. It is found from the table that out of 200 respondents, 31.0 per cent were commercial sex workers. Of the 62 sex workers, 45.2 per cent were unmarried women, 43.5 per cent were married and have family with husband and children, 6.5 per cent were widows and 4.8 per cent of them were deserted women.

Circumstances Leading to Commercial Sex Work

It is concluded from Table 5.37 that not only the unmarried but also the married women (54.8 per cent) involved in commercial sex work. Socio-economic responsibility of women to take care of the family led them into sex work which resulted in HIV infection.

Table 5.37. Marital Status of Sex Workers.

Sl. No.	*Marital Status*	*No. of Respondents*	*Percentage*
1.	Unmarried	28	45.2
2.	Married	27	43.5
3.	Deserted	3	4.8
4.	Widow	4	6.5
	Total	62	100

Table 5.38. Circumstances Leading to Commercial Sex Work.

Sl.No.	*Circumstances*	*No. of Respondents*	*Percentage*
1.	Poverty	25	40.4
2.	Lavish spending	16	25.7
3.	Sexual harassments	2	3.2
4.	Influence of pimps	3	4.8
5.	Abandoned by lover	4	6.6
6.	Desertion and widowhood	7	11.2
7.	Influence of friends	5	8.1
	Total	62	100

Table 5.38 on circumstances leading to commercial sex works reveals that poverty is the major cause for the women to choose sex work as a means of their livelihood. The financial strain raised out of poverty forced 32.3 per cent of women to involve in commercial sex works. The analysis also revealed that the poverty is the consequences of lack of employment opportunity

in their native place due to lack of skills (6.6 per cent), unemployment of husband (3.2 per cent), crop failure due to failure of rain (11.3 per cent), indebtedness (9.6 per cent) and insufficient income of the husband (9.7 per cent).

Women's attitude towards luxurious life influenced 25.7 per cent of respondents to involve in commercial sex work to earn more money without much effort. These respondents were influenced by the lavish life of other women who are already in commercial sex work.

The absence of male earning members in the family also identified as another motivating factor for 11.3 per cent respondents to take up commercial sex work as their profession to take care of their family. It included desertion (3.2 per cent) and widowhood (8.1 per cent).

Problems in the family are an influencing factor for 8.1 per cent of commercial sex workers. They involved in this work not only to divert their mind from their problems but also to earn for their livelihood. The problems related to the family include lack of care (3.2 per cent), and parents (1.7 per cent) and husbands (3.2 per cent) force to push the women into sex work.

The influence of peer groups including friends brought 8.1 per cent women into commercial sex works. Besides, 6.6 per cent women were abandoned by their lover in the city that forced them to choose commercial sex work to live in the city. Influence of the pimp is the cause for 4.8 per cent women to enter into this work.

Various sexual harassment pushed 3.2 per cent of women into sex work. This sexual harassment includes harassment in the work place 1.6 per cent and the pressure by the owner of the company to have sex with him to retain job 1.6 per cent.

The inference drawn from Table 5.38 is that the poverty is the major (40.4 per cent) factor to forces women into commercial sex work. The problems which are confined to the family are the primary factor for many women to choose commercial sex as an alternative means to earn and solve the problems of the family. The family conditions make them to become innocent victims for the dreaded disease called HIV/AIDS. The deserted and the widows are deprived of income due to lose of their husbands. The lack of economical resources led these deserted and widows to promiscuous sexual behaviour resulting in HIV/ AIDS.

Table 5.39. Age at Induction in Commercial Sex Work

Sl.No.	*Age at sex work (in years)*	*No. of Respondents*	*Percentage*
1.	Less than 18	18	29.0
2.	19 – 23	14	22.6
3.	24 – 28	21	33.9
4.	29 – 33	5	8.1
5.	34 and above	4	6.4
	Total	62	100

Table 5.39 illustrates the age of the respondents when they initiated into commercial sex work. Of the 62 respondents, 33.9 per cent entered into this work between the age of 24—28 years followed by the 29.0 per cent respondents who were initiated into commercial sex work at the age of less than 18 years. The 22.6 per cent respondents were started this profession at the age between 19—23 years and the remaining 14.5 have chosen this work at 29 and above 29 years.

The conclusion drawn from Table 5.39 is that the majority (51.6 per cent) of the women are initiated into commercial sex work at the younger age of within 23 years. Due to younger age, the women receive more number of customers and involve in frequent sexual activity. The young age also facilitate them to be submissive in sexual encounters. The less or lack of power over the sexual act of their customers strongly influenced the risk of contracting HIV/AIDS.

A. Details of Clients

The statistical analysis of the study explored that the sex workers are not restricted their service with particular categories of clients. They used to engage all kinds of clients irrespective of their age, profession etc. Money is the only criteria for them.

Labourers (38.7 per cent), business people (37.1 per cent), tourist (33.9 per cent), transport workers, including drivers and cleaners (27.4 per cent), students (21 per cent) and men who are away from home for longer duration (17.7 per cent) are identified as dominant categories of clients who visit commercial sex workers quite often.

The analysis of the study also found that the people who are in business (29.0 per cent) and tourist (25.8 per cent) used to pay more for commercial sex workers. The clients from film industry (12.9 per cent) and the transport workers like drivers (9.7 per cent) are paying considerable amount for paid sex. The labourers (6.5 per cent) and the students (4.8 per cent) are not paying much when compared to others for seeking sex from the sex workers.

As far as the safe sex practices are concerned, significant per cent of business people (30.6 per cent), drivers (25.6 per cent), tourist (14.5 per cent) and students (11.3 per cent) are using condom for safe sex. The safe sex practice is found to be low among labourers (3.2 per cent), man away from home (8.1 per cent) etc.

The analysis on the response (97.3 per cent) of the commercial sex workers reveals that the men who seek sex out side the matrimonial relationship have the character of consuming alcohol or using drugs. Therefore, the addicted behaviour of men towards alcohol and drug increases the chances of unsafe sex with commercial sex workers and to acquire HIV infection.

Table 5.40. Number of Clients Engaged Per Day

Sl. No.	*No. of clients engaged per day*	*No. of Respondents*		
		Part Time Sex worker	*Full Time Sex workers*	*Total*
1.	1 - 2	17 (63.0%)	6 (17.2%)	23 (37.1%)
2.	3 - 4	6 (22.2%)	16 (45.7%)	22 (35.5%)
3.	5 - 6	4 (14.8%)	9 (25.7%)	13 (20.9%)
4.	Above 6	0 (0.0%)	4 (11.4%)	4 (6.5%)
	Total	27 (100%)	35 (100%)	62 (100%)

Table 5.40 explains the number of clients engaged by the sex workers per day. Among the 62 sex workers, 37.1 per cent engaged 1-2 clients per day, 35.5 per cent engaged an on average of 3-4 clients and the remaining 27.4 have more than five clients per day. Most (63 per cent) of the part time sex workers were used to engage less than 3 clients per day whereas most (82.8 per cent) of the full time sex workers have more than 3 clients per day. The inference drawn from the table is that the part time sex workers engage less number of clients (1-2) than the full time sex workers (3-6). Due to frequent sexual encounter, the full time sex workers more prone to HIV/AIDS.

Table 5.41. Earning Per Day by Sex Workers

Sl. No.	*Earning per day (In Rupees)*	*No. of Respondents* Part Time Sex worker	Full Time Sex workers	*Total*
1.	Less than 200	13 (48.2%)	7 (20.0%)	20 (32.3%)
2.	200 - 300	11 (40.7%)	9 (25.7%)	20 (32.3%)
3.	300 - 400	3 (11.1%)	13 (37.1%)	16 (25.8%)
4.	Above 400	0 (0.0%)	6 (17.2%)	6 (9.6%)
	Total	27 (100%)	35 (100%)	62 (100%)

Table 5.41 reveals the earnings of the commercial sex workers per day. It shows that the majority (48.2 per cent) of the family based sex workers earn less than Rs. 200 per day. Among the part time sex workers, 51.8 per cent earns Rs. 200-400 per day. Among full time sex workers, majority (54.3 per cent) of women earns more than Rs. 300 per day and the remaining 45.7 per cent of full time sex workers per day earning is found to be less than Rs.300 per day.

The conclusion drawn from the table is that the sex workers are taking risk of contracting HIV/AIDS by exchanging their sex service to the customers for meager amount.

B. Sources of Contact with the Clients

The analysis of the data on various sources used by the sex workers to have a contact with the clients reveals that the majority (33.9 per cent) of the sex workers are picking up men by themselves from the crowded place like bus stand, railway station, market, beach, cinema theater, busy areas of city, tourist attractive places etc. The brokers are the important source for 17.7 per cent of sex workers to meet customers. The modern communication media - phone (12.9 per cent) and cell phone (6.5 per cent) are used to contact the customers. The other sources are found to be the contact person (6.5 per cent), regular clients (6.5 per cent), family members including mother (9.2 per cent), friends including boy friends (4.8 per cent) and the sex workers who are already in services (1.6 per cent).

C. Place of Resident of Sex Workers

The majority (37.1 per cent) of the sex workers in Chennai are found in the slums and urban centers of the city. The significant percentage (27.4 per cent) is coming from near by rural areas of Chennai for their business.

D. Nature of Sex Work

The study also reveals that 50 per cent of the sex workers under the study are involved in sex work individually. The 27.5 per cent of sex workers are doing this sex trade along with the brokers, the 12.9 per cent are engaged in sex work with their friends, and the 9.6 per cent have support from their other family members to meet and catch men who need sex with commercial sex workers. The sex workers who are under the control of brokers are getting their wage either daily or on contract basis.

The sex workers under this study have reported that they have a strong network, which is invisible to the public and police. Their network will help them to develop contact with the brokers, experienced sex workers, clients etc. However, they have no commercial sex workers organisation to protect their interests.

Number of Sex Workers not Asking their Clients to use Condom

The analysis of the study revealed that after knowing HIV infection only 25 (40.3 per cent) sex workers started insisting their clients to use condom and the remaining 37 (59.7 per cent) have not showed any interest to ask their clients to use condom to prevent them from HIV infection. Among them, lack of awareness (45.9 per cent) among sex workers on HIV/AIDS is the major cause for neglecting condom use. The other causes identified in this study for not insisting condom use to the clients by the sex workers are fear of loosing clients (24.3 per cent), lack of faith on the impact of HIV/AIDS (8.1 per cent), restriction imposed by the brokers (16.2 per cent) and stigma attached to the diseases (5.5 per cent). This study also explored that none of the infected sex workers under this study have revealed their HIV status to their clients due to fear of rejection (35.5 per cent), lack of awareness on AIDS (43.5 per cent), vengeance on men (9.7 per cent) and stigma associated with HIV/AIDS (11.3 per cent).

Table 5.42. Reasons for not using Condoms by Clients

Sl. No.	*Causes*	*No. of Sex workers*	*Percentage*
1.	No sexual satisfaction	18	29.0
2.	Fear of asking condoms	8	12.9
3.	Alcoholism hinter usage of condom	24	38.7
4.	Lack of awareness on safe sex	15	19.4
	Total	62	100

Table 5.42 indicates responses of the sex workers with regard to the various causes for not using condom by the clients. It is found from the table that the behaviour of taking alcohol (38.7 per cent) and its associated intoxicated mood prevent the clients to think and use condom while they have sex with the sex workers. The inherent faith on lack of sexual satisfaction owing to condom use prevents 29 per cent of clients to use condoms. The clients also reported that the fears of asking condom (12.9 per cent) from the shops and lack of awareness on safe sex (19.4 per cent) as important causes for not using condom. The finding from the table is that the behaviour of taking alcohol before sex prevents men to take rational decision to use condom whenever they have paid sex. The above table represents the present status of the infected commercial sex workers under this study. The Non-governmental organisations with the sex workers have taken efforts to influence the sex workers to withdraw their

involvement in sex industry. As a consequences many have came out of their profession and started looking for alternative jobs for their survival. Therefore, it is found from the table that after knowing HIV infection, 46.7 per cent has withdrawn their involvement in sex work. Among them (12.9 per cent) were staying in short stay home run by the non-governmental organisations, 11.3 per cent were working as a causal labourers, each 6.5 per cent were employed in non-governmental organisations and as casual labour and 4.8 per cent were found to be housemaid.

Table 5.43. Present Status of the Sex Workers after Knowing HIV Infection

Sl.No.	*Present Status*	*No. of Respondents*	*Percentage*
1.	Unemployed	3	4.8
2.	Employed in N.G.O.	4	6.5
3.	Staying in short stay home	8	12.9
4.	House maid	3	4.8
5.	Self employed	4	6.5
6.	Causal labour	7	11.3
7.	Sex worker	33	53.2
	Total	62	100

The inference drawn from the analysis (Table 5.43) is that the sex workers who came out of sex work engaged in various occupations for their survival.

Table 5.44. Causes for Remaining in Sex Work After Knowing HIV Infection

Sl.No.	*Causes*	*No. of sex workers*	*Percentage*
1.	No alternative jobs	2	6.1
2.	Lack of skill to change the job	5	15.2
3.	Less income in other jobs	17	51.5
4.	People are not willing to give job	9	27.2
	Total	33	100

Table 5.44 explains the number of sex workers who continue the sex work even after knowing their HIV infection. The major causes mentioned by these sex workers are identified as less income in other jobs (51.5 per cent), difficulties in getting alternative jobs (27.2 per cent), lack of skill to change jobs (15.2 per cent) and non availability of alternative jobs (6.1 per cent). The conclusion drawn from the table is that the less income in other jobs prevent majority of the sex workers to find alternative job to come out of the sex work.

F. Sex Workers Awareness on their Role in Spreading HIV/Aids andtheir Willingness to be Lodged in Special Home

The analysis of the data revealed that all the infected sex workers were aware of their role in transmitting the virus to the clients.

Among the 62 infected sex workers, 61.3 per cent have opposed the idea of accommodating infected sex workers in the special home and only 38.7 per cent extended their willingness to be lodged in special home.

It is evident from the analysis, though the sex workers are aware of their role in transmitting the virus, they were not willing to stay in the special home if it is run for the infected people.

HIV Testing

Table 5.45. Places of HIV Testing

Sl.No.	*No. Place of HIV testing*	*No. of Respondents*	*Percentage*
1.	Private labs	41	20.5
2.	Government Hospitals	123	61.5
3.	Voluntary organisations	1	0.5
4.	Private Hospitals	35	17.5
	Total	200	100

Table 5.45 indicates the places where the respondents have undergone HIV positive test. Of the total 200 respondents, 61.5 per cent have undergone HIV positive test in Government hospitals, the 20.5 per cent have tested in private labs, the 17.5 per cent were tested their HIV positive status in private hospital and 0.5 per cent has known her HIV status by testing it in voluntary organisations. It is also evident from the table that the government hospitals played a vital role in providing facilities for HIV test. Therefore, the majority (61.5 per cent) of the respondents under this study have undergone HIV positive test in Government hospitals.

Table 5.46. Factors Influenced for HIV Test.

Sl. No.	*Factors*	*No. of Respondents*	*Percentage*
1.	S.T.D. infections	29	14.5
2.	Continuous illness	21	10.5
3.	Pregnancy	14	7.0
4.	Husband's HIV infection	117	58.5
5.	Others	19	9.5
	Total	200	100

Table 5.46 reflects the factors which influence to take HIV positive test by the respondents. It shows that 58.5 per cent have undergone HIV test after knowing their husband's HIV status. The infection of sexually transmitted diseases (S.T.D.) influenced 14.5 per cent of respondents to take up HIV test. Continuous illness made 10.5 per cent of respondents to undergo HIV test. HIV test is compulsory for the pregnant women in Tamil Nadu. Therefore, the pregnancy forced 7.0 per cent women to go for HIV test. The 9.5 per cent respondents have under went HIV test for various reasons including awareness created by the media (2.0 per cent), influence of N.G.Os. (1.5 per cent), heterosexual contact of the respondents (1.5 per cent), blood donation by the respondents (1.0 per cent), regular health check up (1.0 per cent), blood donated by the husband (1.0 per cent), illness of the child (0.5 per cent), brother in law HIV status (0.5 per cent), partner's HIV status (0.5 per cent).

The inference drawn from the table is that the HIV status of the respondent's husband is the important factor for majority of the women to take up HIV test in Tamil Nadu.

Table 5.47. Sources of Pre and Post Test Counseling to Respondents and their Family Members.

Sl. No.	*Sources of counseling*	*Respondents*		*Respondent's Parents*	
		Pre Test	*Post Test*	*Pre Test*	*Post Test*
1.	Doctors	17 (8.5%)	24 (12.0%)	6 (3.0%)	18 (9.0%)
2.	Counselors	20 (10.0%)	12 (6.0%)	11 (5.5%)	20 (10.0%)
3.	N.G.Os	13 (6.5%)	14 (7.0%)	18 (9.0%)	9 (4.5%)
4.	Others	1 (0.5%)	6 (3.0%)	4 (2.0%)	3 (1.5%)
5.	Counseling not given	149 (74.5%)	144 (72.0%)	161 (80.5%)	150 (75.0%)
	Total	200 (100%)	200 (100%)	200 (100%)	200 (100%)

Table 5.47 explains the pre test and post test counseling given to the respondents and their family members to cope up and living with HIV. The analysis shows that on an average of 75 per cent of respondents and their family members have not given both pre and post test counseling to know and live with HIV.

It is identified that only 25.5 per cent have got pre test counseling from doctors (8.5 per cent), counselors (10.0 per cent), Non Governmental Organisations (N.G.Os) (6.5 per cent) and others including friends (0.5 per cent). The respondents who have post test counseling accounted for 28 per cent. The sources of post test counseling are identified as doctors (12.0 per cent), counselors (6.0 per cent), N.G.Os (7.0 per cent) and others such as friends etc (3.0 per cent).

As far as respondent's parents are concerned, only 19.5 per cent are given pre test counseling and 25 per cent are exposed to post test counseling through the doctors, counselors, N.G.Os and others.

The conclusion derived from the table is that the majority of the respondents and their family members were not exposed to pre and post test counseling to under stand fully about the HIV, its social impact and living with HIV peacefully by coping with social stigma.

Table 5.48. Respondents Knowledge on HIV/Aids At the Time of Testing

Sl. No.	*Knowledge on HIV/AIDS*	*No. of Respondents*	*Percentage*
1.	Killer disease	31	15.5
2.	No Medicine	14	7.0
3.	Spread through sex and blood	7	3.5
4.	No Knowledge	148	74.0
	Total	200	100

The analysis indicates in Table 5.48 that the respondent's knowledge on HIV/AIDS at the time of testing. It shows that out of 200 respondents, 74 per cent have no knowledge on HIV/ AIDS and its implication in their socio-economic life. The respondents who have little knowledge on HIV/AIDS accounted for 26 per cent. Among them 15.5 per cent were aware that the HIV/AIDS is a killer disease, the 7.0 per cent were known that the HIV/AIDS have no medicine and no cure and only 3.5 per cent respondents were well aware that the HIV spread through sex and blood.

The inference drawn from the table is that the majority (74 per cent) of respondents were unaware of HIV/AIDS when they have undergone HIV testing in various centers.

Sexual Behaviour of Respondents After Infection

Table 5.49 on the sexual behaviour of the sex workers after knowing their HIV status shows that 53.3 per cent of sex workers were still remaining in prostitution and only 46.8 per cent have withdrawn their involvement in sex work after knowing their HIV status

Among the women who are continuing prostitution, 19.5 per cent were practicing safe sex, 12.9 per cent have not adopted any changes in their sexual behaviour, 11.2 per cent have avoided students, 6.5 per cent have avoided youth and 3.2 per cent have avoided unmarried men.

Table 5.49. Changes in Sexual Behaviour of Sex Workers After Knowing HIV Infection

Sl. No.	*Nature of changes*	*No. of sex workers*	*Percentage*
1.	Avoided youth	4	6.5
2.	Avoided students	7	11.2
3.	Avoided unmarried men	2	3.2
4.	Withdrawn from sex work	29	46.7
5.	Practicing safe sex	12	19.5
6.	No change	8	12.9
	Total	62	100

It is clear from the table that majority (53.2 per cent) of the women continues sex work even after knowing their HIV status but significant change in the sexual behaviour of the sex workers is observed after HIV infection.

Table 5.50 reveals the changes in the sexual behaviour of housewives after knowing their HIV infection. In this study 130 respondents are identified as innocent housewives and the remaining are sex workers, students and drug user. Among the wives, the majority (80.9 per cent) have not changed their sexual behaviour after their infection. The respondents who are practicing safe sex to avoid pregnancy are accounted for 14.5 per cent. The practice of abstinence is found to be only 4.6 per cent.

The conclusion drawn from the analysis is that there is no significant change in the sexual behaviour of majority (80.9 per cent) of respondents.

Table 5.50 on the revelation of HIV by the respondents shows that 55.5 per cent of respondents revealed their HIV status to their family members where as 44.5 per cent have not revealed their HIV status to their family members. It also reveals that the majority (68.6 per cent) of the full time sex workers (which include 28 unmarried women, 4 widows and 3 deserted) and housewives (66.9 per cent) revealed their HIV status to their family members and the remaining respondents including students. Part time sex workers and injecting drug user deliberately hided their HIV status from their family members.

Table 5.50. Changes in Sexual Behaviour of Housewives After Knowing HIV Infection.

Sl. No.	*Nature of changes*	*No. of sex workers*	*Percentage*
1.	No change	106	80.9
2.	Practicing safe sex	19	14.5
3.	Practicing abstinence	6	4.6
	Total	131	100

Impact of HIV/Aids on the Social Relationship of Respondents

Social Relationship in the Familiy

Table 5.5.1. Revelation of HIV/Aids By Respondents

Sl.No.	*Revelation*	*Revealed (No. of Respondents)*	*Not revealed (No. of Respondents)*	*Total*
1.	Students	0 (0.0%)	7 (100%)	7 (3.5%)
2.	Housewives	87 (66.9%)	43 (33.1%)	130 (65.0%)
3.	Sex workers –Part time	0 (0.0%)	27 (100.0%)	27 (13.5%)
4.	Sex workers-Full time	24 (68.6%)	11 (31.4%)	35 (17.5%)
5.	Injecting drug us	0 (0.0%)	1 (100.0%)	1 (0.5%)
	Total	111 (55.5%)	89 (44.5%)	200 (100%)

The inference drawn from Table 5.51 is that the revelation of HIV infection is high (66.9 per cent) among the housewives and high secrecy is maintained among the women who got HIV through their heterosexual contact and injecting drug use.

Table 5.51 reveal that the majority (90.8 per cent) of the respondents HIV status was known to their family members through their hospital staff where they undergone HIV test.

For respondents' husbands, 64.4 per cent respondents involved in the revelation of HIV status followed by the hospital staff 25.3 per cent and respondents' husbands 10.3 per cent. The inference drawn from the table is that the hospital staff are the major sources of revelation of respondents HIV status where as the respondents are the primary sources of revelation of her husbands HIV status to their family members.

Table 5.51. Person Involved in the Revelation of HIV Status

Sl. No.	*Revelation on*	*Respon-dent*	*Husband*	*In-laws*	*Friends*	*Hospital Staff*	*Total*
1.	Husband	56 (64.4%)	9 (10.3%)	0	0	22 25.3%)	87 (100%)
2.	Housewife	6 (6.9%)	2 (2.3%)	0	0	79 (90.8%)	87 (100%)

Table 5.52. Respondents' Husbands Awareness About HIV Infection Before Marriage

Sl.	*Nature of*	*No. of Husbands*		*Total*
No.	*Knowledge*	*Yes*	*No*	
1.	Aware before marriage	12 (9.2%)	118 (90.8%)	130 (100%)
2.	Disclosed to his parents	0(0.0%)	12 (100%)	12 (100%)
3.	Disclosed to respondents	0(0.0%)	12 (100%)	12 (100%)

Table 5.52 on the respondents' husbands knowledge on his HIV infection reveals that only 9.2 per cent were aware of their infection before marriage. All these 12 also not revealed their HIV status either to his parents or to the bride proposed for him.

The analysis highlighted that the majority (90.8 per cent) of the men were undergoing HIV test only after their marriage. This is mainly because of absence of compulsory blood test for couples before marriage. As a result, even if the men have infection before their marriage, they can easily blame their innocent wife and escape from the social criticism.

Table 5.53 on husband reaction towards his wife after knowing his HIV infection highlights the husbands reaction towards his wife after knowing his HIV infection. Of the 130 couples, 39.2 per cent men showed sympathetic attitude towards their wives due to their guilty over sex outside the marriage. The 35.4 per cent involved in harassing their wives in various forms including physical harassment, 8.5 per cent forcibly deserted their wives and the remaining 16.9 per cent involved in isolating their wives in the home. It is clear from the table that the infected husbands harassed majority (60.6 per cent) the respondents though they are aware their wives are not responsible for their infection.

Table 5.53. Husbands Reaction Towards his Wife After Knowing his Infection

Sl.No.	*Husband's Reaction*	*No. of Respondents*	*Percentage*
1.	Sympathetic	51	39.2
2.	Physical Harassment	46	35.4
3.	Divorced/deserted	11	8.5
4.	Others	22	16.9
	Total	130	100

Table 5.54 on housewife's reaction towards her husband after knowing her husband infection shows that except 42.3 per cent the other 57.7 per cent showed indifferent attitude towards her infected husband by way of not providing care (46.9 per cent) and leaving him (10.8 per cent) with out any considerations. The inference drawn from the table is that the infected men get least support and care from their wives. Generally, the wives neglect most (57.7 per cent) of their infected husbands.

Table 5.54. Housewifes' Reaction Towards Infected Husband

Sl. No.	*Reaction*	*No. of Respondents*	*Percentage*
1.	Supporting	55	42.3
2.	Not provided care	61	46.9
3.	Left the husband	14	10.8
	Total	130	100

The analysis on the relationship between respondents and their husbands reveals that out of 130 couples, except 17.7 per cent the majority samples (82.3 per cent) have indifferent relationships with their husbands like frequent quarrel (43.8 per cent), neglecting each other (33.1 per cent) and other problems like blaming each other (5.4 per cent) etc.

Table 5.55. The Relationship Between Respondents and their Husbands After Knowing HIV Infection

Sl.No.	*Nature of relationship*	*No. of Respondents*	*Percentage*
1.	Compassionate	23	17.7
2.	Frequent quarrel	57	43.8
3.	Neglecting each other	43	33.1
4.	Others	7	5.4
	Total	130	100

It is evident from the analysis (Table 5.55) that the relationship between husband and wife after knowing HIV infection is not compassionate in many cases.

Table 5.56. Reaction of In-laws on Respondents and their Husbands before and After Knowing HIV Infection

Sl. No.	*Nature of Reaction*	*Before Infection*		*After Infection*	
		Husband	*wife*	*Husband*	*wife*
1.	Supporting	118 (90.8%)	110 (84.6%)	45 (51.7%)	12 (13.7%)
2.	Verbal abuse	12 (9.2%)	16 (12.3%)	17 (19.5%)	28 (32.2%)
3.	Physical abuse	0 (0.0%)	4 (3.1%)	5 (5.8%)	19 (21.9%)
4.	Social Isolation	0 (0.0%)	0 (0.0%)	20 (23.0%)	28 (32.2%)
	Total	130 (100%)	130 (100%)	87 (100%)	87 (100%)

The study has identified the responses of the in-laws towards the respondents and their husbands before and after knowing HIV infection. The analysis reveals that among the 130 couples the greater percentage of respondents (84.6 per cent) and her husbands (90.8 per cent) got support from their in-laws before knowing their infection. Among the 130 couple, 87 couple infection is known to their in-laws (Tabnle 5.56).

But after knowing HIV infection, the infected spouses have received verbal abuse, physical abuse, and social isolation from their in-laws in different magnitudes. The data explored that the women get less support (13.7 per cent) from their in-laws than her husband (51.7 per cent). Social isolation by the in-laws is also comparatively high among the respondents (32.2 per cent) than their husbands (23.0 per cent). The verbal (32.1 per cent) and physical abuses (21.8 per cent) are high towards the women by the in-laws whereas men receive less verbal (19.5 per cent) and physical abuses (5.8 per cent) from their parents.

We can infer from the analysis that the discrimination towards the infected women by the in-laws is comparatively high than their husbands.

Table 5.57. Reaction of Parents Towards Respondents and their Husbands

Sl. No.	*Nature of Reaction*	*Before Infection (for 130 couples)*		*After Infection (for 87 couples)*	
		Husband	*wife*	*Husband*	*wife*
1.	Supporting	124 (95.4%)	127 (97.7%)	18 (20.7%)	61 (70.1%)
2.	Verbal abuse	6 (4.6%)	3 (2.3%)	53 (60.9%)	13 (14.9%)
3.	Physical abuse	0 (0.0%)	0 (0.0%)	4 (4.6%)	5 (5.8%)
4.	Social Isolation	0 (0.0%)	0 (0.0%)	12 (13.8%)	8 (9.2%)
	Total	130 (100%)	130 (100%)	87 (100%)	87 (100%)

Table 5.57 on the reaction of parents towards respondents and their husband shows that the significant percentage of respondents (97.7 per cent) and their husbands (95.4 per cent) got all social and economic support from the parents of the respondents before knowing their HIV status.

After disclosing the infection, generally the respondents and their husbands lost importance among their parents and family circles. While compare to the respondents husbands, the majority (70.1 per cent) of respondents got support from their parents than their husbands (20.7 per cent). The respondents husbands are comparatively more abused verbally (60.9 per cent) than their wives. The social isolation by the respondents' parents is also found to be high among respondents' husbands (13.8 per cent) than respondents (9.2 per cent).

The inference drawn from the analysis is that the respondents get more support from their parents rather than their husbands. This is mainly because all the respondents are the innocent victims of HIV and they acquired HIV through their husbands. Therefore, the respondents' parents are against their son in-laws sexual behaviour and they ill-treated them in various forms including verbal and physical abuse and social isolation.

A. Treatment of Parents Towards their Infected Daughters Who are Deserted and Widows Even Before Infection

Furthermore, the study also reveals that 4 women were widow and 3 were deserted even before infection. All these 7 women got full support from their parents before infection. However, after infection all these 7 (100 per cent) lost support and totally isolated by their parents.

B. Treatment of Parents Towards their Unmarried Infected Daughters

Among the 35 unmarried women which include 28 sex workers and 7 students, 88.6 per cent got full support from their parents and 11.4 per cent were socially isolated by their parents before infection due to their unapproved social behaviour. The analysis found that 48.5 per cent sex workers have disclosed their HIV status to their parents whereas 51.4 per cent including 7 students concealed their HIV status from their parents. After disclosing the HIV status to their parents, the majority (64.7 per cent) got support form their parents and the remaining (35.3 per cent) verbally abused and socially isolated from their parents.

The above table represents the nature of restriction imposed by the family members on respondents and their husbands whose infection is revealed to them. It is already stated that among the 130 couple, 33.1 per cent have not revealed their HIV status to their family members. As a result they have not experienced any discrimination from their family members. Like that among 62 sex workers, only 38.7 per cent have revealed their HIV status to their family members where as 61.3 per cent have not revealed their HIV status to their family members. The respondents who hided their HIV status from their family members have no problem with regard to socio-cultural restriction.

Table 5.5.1.9. Nature of Restriction Imposed on People Infected With HIV by their Family Members

Sl. No.	*Nature of Restirction*	*No. of Respondents* Husband	Housewife	Sex worker	Children
1.	No restrictions	18 (20.7%)	13 (14.9%)	11 (45.8%)	6 (42.8%)
2.	Separate place is given	4 (4.6%)	5 (5.8%)	—	0
3.	Restriction on inter dining	9 (10.3%)	2 (2.3%)	—	0
4.	Participation on socio cultural functions	5 (5.8%)	9 (10.3%)	—	0
5.	On sharing articles	16 (18.4%)	7 (8.1%)	—	2 (14.3%)
6.	On touching	23 (26.4%)	17 (19.5%)	—	4 (28.6%)
7.	All above restrictions	12 (13.8%)	34 (39.1%)	13 (54.2%)	2 (14.3%)
	Total	87 (100%)	87 (100%)	24 (100%)	14 (100%)

Among the 87 (66.9 per cent) couple who revealed their HIV status to their family members, only 20.7 per cent men and 14.9 per cent women have not experienced any discrimination from the family. The remaining couple (79.3 per cent men and 85.1 per cent women) (Table 5.58) have experienced various forms of discrimination in the form of separate place in the home, restriction on inter dining, participation on socio-cultural functions, sharing articles and touching.

Majority of the sex workers (54.2 per cent) and children (57.2 per cent), whose infection is revealed out also experienced same discrimination from the family members.

It is found from the analysis (Table 5.58) that the difference in gender discrimination is not significant between men and women. Irrespective of sex, the people living with HIV are generally restricted in socio and cultural activities of the family in day today life.

Table 5.59. Decision taken in the Family Before and After Infection

Sl. No.	*Person involved in taking decisions*	*Before infection*	*After infection*
1.	Husband	81(40.5%)	43(21.5%)
2.	Respondent	19(9.5%)	8(4.0%)
3.	Both	49(24.5%)	16(8.0%)
4.	Others	51(25.5%)	133(66.5%)
	Total	200(100%)	200(100%)

The analysis (table 5.55) on the decision-making process in the family before infection shows that the respondent's husbands (40.5 per cent), respondents (9.5 per cent) and both by consultations (24.5 per cent) are involved more in taking decision in the family. The involvement of parents (16.5 per cent) and in-laws (9.0 per cent) in taking decision is seems to be less before knowing the infection of the samples under the study.

But after infection, the participation of the infected people [respondent's husbands (21.5 per cent), respondents (4.0 per cent) and both (8.0 per cent)] in making decision to their own family have gone down to the per cent of (33.5 per cent) while compare to before infection (74.5 per cent). The parents (29.0 per cent) and in-laws (27.5) became a dominant figure in taking decision for respondents and their families. Considerable percentage of respondents family members like brothers (6.0 per cent), son (2.0 per cent) and uncles (2.0 per cent) also entered into the decision making process of the families of people living with HIV positive.

As far as gender role in decision-making process is concerned, men dominated more in taking decision related to family affairs before (40.5 per cent) and after (21.5 per cent) knowing infection. Women role in decision making process is considerably reduced after their infection.

Therefore, it is evident from the study the role of people living with HIV positive in decision-making process has affected due to their infection.

Table 5.60. Participation in the Socio-cultural Activities in the Family

Sl.No.	*Participants*	*Before infection*	*After infection*
1	Husband	27 (13.5%)	9 (4.5%)
2.	Respondent	12 (6.0%)	7 (3.5%)
3.	Both	102 (51.0%)	36 (18.0%)
4.	In-laws	15 (7.5%)	62 (31.0%)
5.	Parents	41 (20.5%)	53 (26.5%)
6.	Others	3 (1.5%)	33 (16.5%)
	Total	200 (100%)	200 (100%)

The analysis (Table 5.60) also explored the participation of the respondents in socio-cultural activities of the family before and after infection.

It is found from the study that the majority (51.0 per cent) of the married couples have participated in all socio-cultural functions of the family before knowing their HIV infection. In 20.5 per cent of cases including 17.5 per cent unmarried women, the respondent's parents were taken part followed by respondents' husbands (13.5 per cent) and in-laws (7.5 per cent). The respondents who participated in socio-cultural activities are accounted for 6.0 per cent. In few cases, (1.5 per cent) respondent's siblings are participated in the family functions.

However, after knowing HIV infection, 157 (78.5 per cent) respondents have withdrawn their participation in all functions of their families. The participation of the infected people has gone down to 18 per cent from 51 per cent before infection. In-laws (31.0 per cent), parents (26.5 per cent) and other members in the family (16.5 per cent) are taking part in socio-cultural activities of the families. The respondents (3.5 per cent) and their husbands (4.5 per cent) have reduced their participation due to infection.

The inference drawn from the analysis is that the participation of respondents in social and cultural ceremonies of their family have adversely affected due infection.

Table 5.61. Reasons for Non-participation in Socio-cultural Ceremonies

Sl.No.	*Reasons*	*No. of respondents*	*Percentage*
1.	Not getting invitation	33	21.0
2.	Reluctant to participate in ceremonies	88	56.1
3.	Fear on discrimination	36	22.9
	Total	157	100

Majority (56.1 per cent) of the respondents are reluctant to participate in ceremonies and functions. They imposed self restriction in the participation of social and cultural ceremonies of families. The significant percentage (22.9 per cent) avoided their participation due to the fear of facing discrimination followed by not getting invitation (21.0 per cent) from their family members to take part in the family functions (Table 5.61).

The analysis highlighted that the majority of the respondents have self imposed restriction in participating socio-cultural activities due to shame and guilty though most of their HIV status is not known to others.

It can be understood from the analysis that the infected people are not participating much in the family functions in general and women in particular due to guilt and shame.

Table 5.62. Maintenance and Property Given to Deserted and Widows

Sl. No.	*Maintenance and property*	*No. of respondents*		*Total*
		Yes	*No*	
1.	Deserted	2 (8.0%)	23 (92.0%)	25 (100%)
2.	Widows	12 (25. 5%)	35 (74.5%)	47 (100%)

It is already stated that four women became widow and three became deserted even before infection. However, it is observed from the study that 25 women became deserted and 47 became widows due to AIDS. Among the 25 deserted women only 8.0 per cent have given maintenance from their husbands and the others (92.0 per cent) have denied maintenance from their husbands. With regard to property for the widows, only 25.5 per cent got property of their husbands share and the remaining 74.5 per cent have not got share from the property of their husbands from their in-laws (Table 5.62).

The analysis reflected that the infected women were deprived of either getting property or maintenance from their husband's side due to the perception that the infected people will have short life.

Table 5.63. Place of Present Stay of Respondents

Sl. No.	*Places of present stay*	*No. of Respondents*	*Percentage*
1.	Parents	39	19.5
2.	In-laws	16	8.0
3.	Husband	69	34.5
4.	Children	48	24.0
5.	Alone	4	2.0
6.	N.G.Os	24	12.0
	Total	200	100

Table 5.63 on the present stay of the respondents reveals that 34.5 per cent of respondents live with their husbands. The 24.0 per cent found to be along with their children followed by parents (19.5 per cent). The 12.0 per cent respondents stayed in the short stay home run by the N.G.Os. The 8.0 per cent of respondents are under the care of their in-laws and the remaining 2.0 per cent staying alone without their family members support.

The analysis indicates that the majority of the infected women living either with their husbands (34.5 per cent) or with their children (24.0 per cent). The abundant sex workers are staying with the N.G.O. in the short stay home at Chennai.

Social Relationship in Neighbourhood

Neighbourhood relationship is indispensable for any individual to sustain in the society. The study has attempted to bring out the social relationship of infected women with their neighbours.

Table 5.61. Infection Known to the Neighbours

Sl. No.	*Infection known to neighbours*	*No of Respondents*		
		Yes	*No*	*Total*
1	Wives	3 (2.3%)	127 (97.7%)	130 (100%)
2	Sex workers	0 (0.0%)	62 (100%)	62 (100%)
3	Students	0 (0.0%)	7 (100%)	7 (100%)
4.	Drug user	0 (0.0%)	1 (100%)	1 (100%)
5.	Children	0 (0.0%)	14 (100%)	14 (100%)
6.	Respondents' Husbands	3 (2.3%)	127 (97.7%)	130 (100%)

Table 5.64 has identified that the infected men and women have adopted the strict principles of hiding the infection from their neighbours. Therefore, the neighbours were not aware of the majority of the respondents (97.7 per cent) and respondent's husbands (97.7 per cent) infection.

Table 5.65. Social Relationship of Respondents and their Husbands with Neighbours Before Infection

Sl. No.	*Nature of Interaction*	*No. of Respondents*	*Percentage*
1.	No Interaction	4	2
2.	Discuss and participate in all activities	184	92
3.	Just based on needs	12	6
	Total	200	100

The inference drawn from the table is that the people living with HIV positive are maintaining secrecy of their infection from their neighbours due to the problem of stigma and discrimination.

The respondents have very good social relationships (92.0 per cent) with neighbours before knowing their infections. They have participated in the social functions of marriage, childbirth, death, community festivals and other rituals and ceremonies organized by the neighbours. Majority of the married respondents (86.7 per cent) have participated in these functions along with their husbands and children.

It is found from the analysis that the respondents have established very good social relationship with their neighbours before infection.

Table 5.66. Social Relationship of Respondents and their Husbands with Neighbours After Infection

Sl. No.	*Nature of relationship*	*No. of Respondents*	*Percentage*
1.	Withdrawn relationship	144	72.0
2.	Discuss and participate in all activities	23	11.5
3.	Just based on needs	33	16.5
	Total	200	100

However, after knowing infection many respondents have felt guilt and shame to interact with the neighbour as like before infection. It is found from the analysis that the majority (72 per cent) of the respondents have themselves withdrawn their relationship from their neighbours and they hesitated to participate in the social functions freely due to the fear of facing social stigma attached to the HIV/AIDS though their infection in not known to their neighbours. The responses of the married respondents revealed that their husbands were more reluctant to participate in the functions outside the family because of shame and guilt. It is found from the analysis that only 11.5 per cent of respondents maintained good relationship with their neighbours and 16.5 per cent respondents relationship with their neighbour is just based on needs.

The conclusion drawn from Table 5.66 is that the people living with HIV positive withdrawn themselves from the socio-cultural activities with their neighbours due to the impact of stigma and discrimination.

A. Neighbour's Interaction Towards People Living with HIV Positive whose Infection is Known to Them

Of the 200 respondents, the 3 (1.5 per cent) of respondents infection was known to their neighbours. All the three respondents are not getting support from their neighbours. They are all socially distanced from their neighbours.

It is clear from the analysis that social distance is the common response from the neighbour towards the people living with HIV positive.

Table 5.67. Reasons for Discrimination by the Neighbours

Sl. No.	*Reasons for discrimination*	*No. of Respondents*	*Percentage*
1.	Lack of knowledge on HIV/AIDS	47	23.5
2.	Fear of infection	134	67.0
3.	Fear about other's comments	11	5.5
4.	Respondent's deviant behaviour	5	2.5
5.	Husband's deviant behaviour	3	1.5
	Total	200	100

It is evident from the above said analysis that the misconception about the spread of HIV is the major cause for discrimination as the fear of infection was reported by 67 per cent of respondents.

The understanding from the table is that the fear of contracting infection is the major cause for stigmatizing and discriminating the infected people.

B. Person Blamed for Respondents Infection by the Neighbours

Among the 200 respondents, only three respondents infection was known to their neighbours. All the three are blamed for their infection by the neighours for their ignorance and inability to control their husband from having extra marital affairs.

C. Effects of Discrimination on the Respondents

The discrimination by the neighbour produced certain negative impact on the socio-economic life of the people living with HIV positive. Because of discrimination, the 3 respondents have changed their residence and moved to the place where no one is aware of their infection. All the 200 (100 per cent) respondents have developed fear towards social isolation, and complex of inferiority and guilt and they restricted their social mobility.

Social Relationship with Friends

Every individual life is in one or other way linked with friendship settings. The friends are called as peer groups or reference groups. Many individual have close tie-up with the friends than their family members and relatives. They share all their happiness and sorrows with them. Each and every event of individual life is closely associated with their friends. If the individual is affected by any chronic illness, the friends are the first person in providing courage, moral, psychological and financial support, care and other needs expected by the sick persons. But in the case of HIV/AIDS, stigma makes certain difference between the infected persons and their friends. The study also made an attempt to find out the discrimination in friendship settings.

The above table reflects the respondents and the husbands of married respondent's involvement with their friendship circle before and after infection. It shows that the majority of both the respondents (53 per cent) and their husbands (59.5 per cent) were often with their friends before knowing their HIV-status.

Their associations with their friends have drastically changed after knowing their infection. The infected men and women were themselves reluctant to meet their friends and share their feeling. When compared to infected men, the majority (42.5 per cent) of infected respondents were completely out of their friendship circle and many (41.5 per cent) have developed the attitude of rarely meeting their friends instead of often (13.5 per cent) or very often (2.5 per cent) meeting them.

Table 5.68. Frequency of Respondents and their Husbands with their Friends before and after Infection

Sl. No.	Frequency of involvement with friends	Before Infection Respondents	Before Infection Husbands	After Infection Respondents	After Infection Husbands
1.	Not at all	9 (4.5%)	1 (0.6%)	85 (42.5%)	17 (10.7%)
2.	Rarely	56 (28.0%)	35 (22.2%)	83 (41.5%)	53 (33.5%)
3.	Often	106 (53.0%)	94 (59.5%)	27 (13.5%)	79 (50.0%)
4.	Very Often	29 (14.5%)	28 (17.7%)	5 (2.5%)	9 (5.8%)
	Total	200 (100%)	158 (100%)	200 (100%)	158 (100%)

As in the case of infected men, though they are gradually coming out of their friendship circle, more than 50 per cent have still maintaining their close relationship with their friends.

The analysis of data given in Table 5.68 also identified that the unmarried women, sex workers and separated/divorced are more particular in hiding themselves from their friends as a result of their guilt and fear on stigma with their behaviour and infections.

Out of 35 unmarried women, 28 (80.0 per cent) are sex workers and 7 (20.0 per cent) are students. All the 7 (20.0 per cent) students are completely out of their friendship circle after knowing their infection. As far as the unmarried sex worker is concerned, they have developed the attitude of meeting their friends very rarely after infection. Among the 27 family based sex workers, majority (77.8 per cent) have rarely meeting their friends after infection.

It is evident from Table 5.68 that the infection has brought significant changes in the respondents' relationship with their friends than the infected men. The infected women were more reluctant to meet their friends as before their infection.

Table 5.69. Revelation of HIV Status to the Friends

Sl. No.	*Revelation of HIV status*	*No. of Respondents*		*Total*
		Yes	*No*	
1.	Housewives	4 (3.1%)	126 (96.9%)	130 (100%)
2.	Part time sex workers	19 (70.4%)	8 (29.6%)	27 (100%)
3.	Full time sex workers	13 (46.4%)	15 (53.6%)	28 (100%)
4.	Students	0 (0.0%)	7 (100%)	7 (100%)
5.	Drug user	0 (0.0%)	1 (100%)	1 (100%)
6.	Respondents' Husbands	23 (17.6%)	107 (82.3%)	130 (100%)

The analysis explored that only 3.1 per cent respondents and 17.6 per cent husbands of respondents were disclosed their HIV status to their friends. Among the 200 respondents, majority (82.3 per cent) have not revealed their HIV status to their friends. Among the 158 husbands of married respondents, 27 part time sex workers husbands and 1 injecting drug user husbands are ignorant about their of their infection which they got through their wives. These husbands were not undergone HIV test. Among the remaining 130 husbands, majority (82.3 per cent) not revealed their HIV status with their friends. The hiding of infection is mainly due to the negative impact of HIV on the affected people (Table 5.69).

Part-time sex workers (70.4 per cent) followed by full time sex workers (46.4 per cent) are predominant among the respondents who have revealed their HIV status to their friends. Majority of the housewives (96.9 per cent), students (100 per cent) and drug user (100 per cent) are deliberately hiding their HIV status from their friends.

The finding drawn from the table is that the majority of the respondents (82.0 per cent) and their husbands (82.3 per cent) have not disclosed their HIV status to their friends. The revelation of HIV status is found high among the sex workers (51.6 per cent) than the housewives, students and drug users.

Table 5.70. Reaction of Friends Towards Respondents and their Husbands After Infection

Sl. No.	*Reaction of the friends*	*No. of Respondents Respondents'*	*No. of Husbands*
1.	Sympathetic	4 (11.1%)	3 (13.0%)
2.	Withdrawn friendship	3 (8.3%)	0 (0.0%)
3.	Disclosed HIV status to others	8 (22.2)	3 (13.0%)
4.	Supporting – moral/financial	21 (58.4%)	17 (74.0%)
	Total	36 (100%)	23 (100%)

Table 5.70 on the reaction of the friends towards the respondents shows that among the 36 (18 per cent) respondents whose infection is revealed to their friends, 58.4 per cent got moral and financial support from their friends. All these 21 respondents are sex workers. The friends have disclosed 22.2 per cent respondents HIV status to others including their family members and relatives. The 11.1 per cent respondents got sympathy from their friends. All these four respondents are housewives and innocent victims of HIV. The 8.3 per cent respondents' friends have withdrawn their friendship from the infected respondents.

Except eight friends, others have not disclosed the infection of the respondents to their family members.

Out of 23 men who have disclosed their HIV status to their friends, 74 per cent have got moral and financial support and 13 per cent have got sympathy from their friends. The remaining 13 per cent respondents were discriminated from their friends by disclosing their HIV status to others.

The inference drawn from the analysis is that majority (58.4 per cent) of the respondents and their husbands (74.0 per cent) are getting moral and financial support from their friends. But when compared to men, less number of infected women is getting support from their friends.

Social Relationship with Relatives

Relatives are part and parcel of every individual's life. Individual is not only very close to their family members, but also with their relatives and they used to take part in all social events of their relatives. Sharing of emotional feelings with the close kin and kith used to bring psychological support for the individual. Everyone normally *get al.*l supports including moral, financial, physical etc. during crisis. This part of the analysis will highlight the discrimination and support experienced by the women living with HIV positive from their relatives.

Table 5.71. Respondents and their Husbands Infection Known to the Relatives

Sl. No.	*The person's infection known to relatives*	*No. of respondents*	*Percentage*
1.	Respondents	27	37.0
2.	Respondent's Husband	6	8.2
3.	Both	40	54.8
	Total	73	100

Table 5.71 shows that 127 (63.5 per cent) respondents have not revealed their HIV status to their relatives and only 73 (36.5 per cent) respondent's infection was known to their relatives. Among them, 37.0 per cent respondent's infection alone known to their relatives of whom 70.4 per cent are housewives and 29.6 per cent are sex workers. In the cases of respondents living with husbands, 54.8 per cent couples infection is known to their relatives and only 8.2 per cent respondent's husband's infection alone revealed to their relatives.

The inference drawn from the analysis is that the majority of the infected housewives and their husbands' infection is known to their relatives. The infection of sex workers and students infection is not known to their relatives.

Table 5.72. Reaction of Relatives Towards People Infected with HIV

Sl. No.	*Nature of Reaction*	*No. of Respondents*	*No. of Respondents' Husbands*
1	Isolated	24 (32.9%)	13 (28.3%)
2	Verbal abuse	13 (17.8%)	6 (13.0%)
3.	Physical abuse	1 (1.4%)	0 (0.0%)
4.	Withdraw their visit of coming	16 (21.9%)	3 (6.5%)
5.	Supporting-moral, financial	12 (16.4%)	23 (50.0%)
6.	Others.	7 (9.6%)	1 (2.2%)
	Total	73 (100%)	46 (100%)

Tanle 5.7 reveals that among the respondent's infection known to their relatives, only 16.4 per cent of respondents have got financial and moral support from their relatives. All these 12 respondents are housewives who got infection through their husbands. The remaining respondents are discriminated by their relatives in the form of social isolation (32.9 per cent), withdraw their visit to respondents house (21.9 per cent), verbal abuse (17.8 per cent), other form of discriminations like not inviting the respondents to take part in the social events of relatives house (9.6 per cent) and physical isolation (1.4 per cent).

Among the respondents HIV status known to relatives, eight are sex workers and the remaining are housewives. All these eight sex workers are socially isolated by their relatives.

Of the 46 men's infection known to their relatives, 23 (50.0 per cent) have got both moral and financial support from their relatives and the remaining 50.0 per cent are discriminated by their relatives.

The inference drawn from the table is, irrespective of sex if the infection is known to relatives, they are discriminated by them as a result of fear of contagious and stigma associated with the mode of infection. While comparing the discrimination experienced by infected respondents and their husbands, the infected women are subjected to severe discrimination and criticism by the relatives.

Table No. 5.73. Frequency of Visit to Relatives House Before and after Infection by Respondents

Sl.No.	*Frequency of visit*	*Before Infection*	*After Infection*
1	Not al all	6 (3.0%)	107 (53.5%)
2	Rarely	15 (7.5%)	72 (36.0%)
3.	Often	74 (37.0%)	19 (9.5%)
4.	Very often	105 (52.5%)	2 (1.0%)
	Total	200 (100%)	200 (100%)

The analysis of the data on the social participation of respondents before knowing their infection status showed that the majority of the respondents visited their relatives house for various social functions either very often (52.5 per cent) or often (37.0 per cent). Very few respondents rarely visited their relative's house (7.5 per cent). Only 3.0 per cent of women have not at all participated in any social events of their relative's house due to certain dispute and misunderstanding between them.

After knowing the infection, the analysis observed drastic changes in the social participation of respondents with their relatives. It is identified that 54.5 per cent of respondents have stopped their social participation in their relatives house due to guilty and fear about stigma and discrimination. Among them the 16.5 per cent unmarried girls are more reluctant to take part in the social events of their relatives house. The 36.0 per cent respondents have rarely taking part in the social gathering of their relative house. Very few respondents either often (9.5 per cent) or very often (1.5 per cent) participated in the social events of their relatives house.

The inference drawn from the analysis is that the majority (53.5 per cent) of respondents are not visiting their relatives' house after knowing their infection.

Table 5.74. Reason for not Visiting Relatives House After Infection by Respondents

Sl.No.	*Reasons*	*No. of Respondents*	*Percentage*
1.	Self imposed restriction	127	63.5
2.	Fear on discrimination	56	28.0
3.	Due to guilt and shame	17	8.5
	Total	200	100

The analysis identified that, though the majority of the infected women not disclosed their HIV status to their relatives, they themselves developed self imposed restriction (63.5 per cent) to visit their relatives house. Fear on discrimination restricted 28.0 per cent of respondents to restrict their visit to relatives house followed by guilty and shame (8.5 per cent).

Table 5.75. Participation in Socio-cultural Activities of Relatives House Before and After Infection

Sl.No.	*Participants*	*Before infection*	*After infection*
1.	Parents	35 (17.5%)	78 (39.0%)
2.	In-laws	24 (12.0%)	59 (29.5%)
3.	Respondents	44 (22.0%)	16 (8.0%)
4.	Respondent's husbands	41 (20.5%)	13 (6.5%)
5.	Respondents and her husbands	56 (28.0%)	7 (3.5%)
6.	Others : Brothers	0	21(10.5%)
	Son	(0.0%)	6(3.0%)
	Total	200 (100%)	200 (100%)

Fear owing to stigma associated with AIDS majority (63.5 per cent) of the respondents developed self imposed restriction to visit their relatives house.

Table 5.75 reveals the people who have participated in the socio-cultural activities of relative's house before and after the infection of respondents.

Before infection the majority of the respondents were participated along with their husbands (28 per cent) in the socio cultural activities of relatives. Majority of the respondents, especially married respondents (22.0 per cent) were empowered to take part with their relative's social events followed by their husbands (20.5 per cent). In the case of unmarried 35 (17.5 per cent) girls the parents are participated where as in the case of widows and deserted/divorced majority of the in-laws (12.0 per cent) are participated in the socio-cultural activities of relatives.

After infection, significant changes have taken place in the participation of respondents in the socio-cultural activities of relatives house. The table showed that only 36 (18 per cent) of respondents including their husbands were willingly participated after infection as against 70.5 per cent in before infection. The respondents participation is replaced by their parents (39.0 per cent) followed by their in-laws (29.5 per cent), brothers (10.5 per cent) and son (3.0 per cent).

The inference drawn from the table is that the respondents have themselves isolated from the socio-cultural activities of relative's house after infection due to various reasons.

Table 5.76. Person Blamed for Respondents and their Husbands Infection by Relatives

Sl. No.	*Person Blamed for Infection*	*No. of Respondents*	*Percentage*
1.	Respondents	49	67.1
2.	Respondents' Husbands	24	32.9
	Total	73	100

The analysis revealed that only 36.5 per cent respondent's infection was known to their relatives. Among them except eight respondents (sex workers), the remaining were housewives.

In majority of the cases (67.1 per cent) the women were blamed for her as well as her husband's infection. In the remaining cases (32.9 per cent) the respondent's husbands are blamed for respondent's infection.

Table 5.77. Reasons for Blaming the Respondents By Relatives

Sl. No.	*Reasons*	*No. of Respondents*	*Percentage*
1.	Promiscuous behaviour	8	16.3
2.	Ignorance and inability to control husbands promiscuous behaviour	16	32.7
3.	Frequent stay with parents	11	22.4
4.	Fidelity is suspected	14	28.6
	Total	49	100

In the case of majority (32.7 per cent) of respondents are blamed due to their inability and ignorance to control their husbands promiscuous behaviour. Fidelity and morality is suspected for 28.6 per cent of respondents by their relatives. Besides, 22.4 per cent of respondents blamed for their frequent stay with their parents and 16.3 per cent of respondents blamed due to their promiscuous behaviour.

The inference drawn from the analysis is that the majority (32.7 per cent) of respondents are blamed for their infection by the relatives due to their ignorance and inability to control their husbands' promiscuous behaviour.

Table 5.78. Impact of Relatives Discrimination on Respondents

Sl. No.	*Impacts*	*No. of Respondents*	*Percentage*
1.	Changed the place of residence	19	26.0
2.	Developed the complex of inferiority	47	64.4
3.	Restricted the activities in the public	7	9.6
	Total	73	100

As a result of discrimination, the majority of the respondents (64.4 per cent) have developed the complex of inferiority followed by changing the place of residence (26.0 per cent) and restriction of activities in and out side home (9.6 per cent) (Table 5.78).

The conclusion drawn from the analysis is that the majority of the respondents were blamed not only for her infection but also for her husband's infection though they got infection through their husbands. The gender biased and baseless discrimination created inferiority complex among the infected women.

Discrimination in Treatment

The study has made an attempt to identify the gender discrimination existed between men and women in taking treatment for opportunistic infections.

Table 5.79 on treatment seeking behaviour of the people living with HIV positive reveals that the infected men are regularly taking treatment than the infected women. Among the housewife the majority (59.3 per cent) takes treatment whenever they fall sick and 31.5 per cent have not taken any treatment for their infection.

As far as sex worker is concerned, the full time sex workers are non family based sex workers which includes unmarried girls, deserted and widows are taking treatment either whenever they fall sick (77.1 per cent) or in monthly once (22.9 per cent) than the family based sex workers Table 5.79. The 27 part time sex workers are family based sex workers and have husbands and children. The part time sex workers infection was not known to their husbands. These men might also get infected by HIV by their infected wives. To hide their HIV status these part time sex workers are not taking treatment for their illness.

The seven students and one injecting drug user are not taking treatment for their infection.

The inference drawn from the table is that the treatment seeing behaviour for the infection is found to be high among the full time sex workers and housewives. While comparing the treatment seeking behaviour with infected husband, the women give less priority than men.

Table 5.79. Treatment Seeking Behaviour of Infected People

Sl. No.	*Frequency of Treatment*	*No. of Respondents*					
		House wife	*Part Time Sex worker*	*Full time Sex worker*	*Student*	*Drug user*	*Husbands*
1.	Weekly	0 (0.0%)	0 (0.0%)	0 (0.0%)	0 (0.0%)	0 (0.0%)	12 (9.2%)
2.	Monthly	12 (9.2%)	0 (0.0%)	8 (22.9%)	0 (0.0%)	0 (0.0%)	68 (52.3%)
3.	When ever fall sick	77 (59.3%)	0 (0.0%)	27 (77.1%)	0 (0.0%)	0 (0.0%)	43 (33.1%)
4.	No Treatment	41 (31.5%)	27 (100%)	0 (0.0%)	7 (100%)	1 (100%)	7 (5.4%)
	Total	130 (100%)	27 (100%)	35 (100%)	7 (100%)	1 (100%)	130 (100%)

Table 5.80. Place of Treatment

Sl. No.	Place of Treatment (Hospital)	No. of Respondents					
		House wife	Part Time Sex worker	Full time Sex worker	Student	Drug user	Husbands
1.	Government	29 (22.3%)	0 (0.0%)	9 (25.7%)	0 (0.0%)	0 (0.0%)	19 (14.6%)
2.	Private	6 (4.6%)	0 (0.0%)	0 (0.0%)	0 (0.0%)	0 (0.0%)	87 (66.9%)
3.	N.G.O	54 (41.5%)	0 (0.0%)	26 (74.3%)	0 (0.0%)	0 (0.0%)	17 (13.1%)
4.	No treatment	41 (31.6%)	27 (100%)	0 (0.0%)	7 (100%)	1 (100%)	7 (5.4%)
	Total	130 (100%)	27 (100%)	35 (100%)	7 (100%)	1 (100%)	130 (100%)

Table 5.80 show that the treatment taken by the respondents and their husbands reveals that majority of the housewives (41.5 per cent) take treatment in the N.G.Os followed by government hospitals (22.3 per cent) and very few housewives (4.6 per cent) are taken treatment in the private hospitals.

Majority of the full time (74.3 per cent) of sex workers are taking treatment in the N.G.Os. Significant number of full time sex workers (25.7 per cent) also seeks treatment in Government hospitals.

The students and drug user are not taking treatment for their illness in order to maintain secrecy with regard to their infection.

As far as respondents husbands is concerned, majority (66.9 per cent) are taking treatment in the private hospitals followed by Government hospitals (14.6 per cent) (Table 5.80).

The inference drawn from the table is that the N.G.Os played a vital role in providing treatment to the respondents either at free of cost or by charging very less amount. In the same time men take treatment in the private hospital by paying huge amount for treatment. This is the clear indication of gender discrimination prevailing in the treatment for HIV/AIDS related illness.

Table 5.80 explains the expenditure incurred by the person towards the medical treatment of respondents and their husbands. Of the 130 housewives, 31.6 per cent is not taking treatment for their HIV/AIDS related illness. In the remaining 89 housewives, majority of their medical expenditure is met by their parents (39.2 per cent) followed by respondents' husbands (14.6 per cent).

All the 100 part time sex workers not taking treatment in order to hide their inflectional status from their family members. All the 35 full time sex workers and one injecting drug user incurred their medical expenditure by themselves.

Table 5.80 shows that as far as respondents' husbands are concerned, 32.3 per cent of respondents' husbands met their own medical expenditure. Significant percentage (26.9 per cent) of respondents' husbands' expenditure is incurred by their wives. Respondents' in-laws incurred 20.8 per cent of respondents'

Table 5.81. Expenditure Met by the Person for Respondents' Treatment

Sl. No.	*Expenditure met by*	*No. of Respondents*				
		Housewife	*Drug User*	*Part Time Sexworker*	*Full time Sex worker*	*Respondents Husbands*
1.	In-laws	6 (4.6%)	0 (0.0%)	0 (0.0%)	0 (0.0%)	27 (20.8%)
2.	Parents	51 (39.2%)	0 (0.0%)	0 (0.0%)	0 (0.0%)	19 (14.6%)
3.	Respondents	13 (10.0%)	0 (0.0%)	0 (0.0%)	35 (100%)	35 (26.9%)
4.	Respondents' Husbands	19 (14.6%)	0 (0.0%)	0 (0.0%)	0 (0.0%)	42 (32.3%)
5.	No Treatment	41 (31.6%)	1 (100%)	27 (100%)	0 (0.0%)	7 (5.4%)
	Total	130 (100%)	1 (100)	27 (100%)	35 (100%)	130 (100%)

husbands medical treatment. Respondents' parents met the expenditure of 14.6 per cent of respondents' husbands.

The inference drawn from the analysis is that significant percentage (26.9 per cent) of housewives gives preference to their husbands for treatment and they spent amount for the treatment of their husbands. It is also evident from the analysis that the majority of the housewives medical expenditure is met by their parents rather than their husbands and in-laws. Besides, among the sex workers the full time sex workers are giving importance for their treatment and they themselves incurred the medical expenditure for the treatment. In the same time the full time sex workers, students and injecting drug user are not taking treatment due to the fear of exposure of their infection to others.

Table 5.82. Problems Faced by the Respondents in Hospitals

Sl. No.	*Nature of problems*	*No. of Respondents*	*Percentage*
1.	Hospital admission	42	21.0
2.	Care in the wards	39	19.5
3.	Confidentiality of report	33	16.5
4.	All	78	39.9
5.	No discrimination	8	4.0
	Total	200	100

The analysis on the problems faced by the people living with HIV positive reveals that except few (4.0 per cent) respondents the others (96.0 per cent) have experienced various discriminations in the hospitals with regard to hospital admission, care in the wards, confidentiality of report etc. As far as the magnitude of the problems is concerned, the women were comparatively facing more (96.0 per cent) problems than men (91.1 per cent) (Table 5.82). According to the respondents, the people in the health care sectors are thinking that all the infected women are sex workers and they are responsible for transmitting the virus to the innocent men. Therefore, every infected woman is treated as a sex worker in the hospitals though they got infection through their husbands. The medical personnel, though aware of HIV/AIDS, show reluctance over the affected persons. As like common populace, they also fired them with wounding words. While treating these people, they denied touching them and diagnosing the HIV/AIDS related illness. Majority of the women (58.0 per cent) also reported that they have not find much difference in discrimination between men and women in the hospitals.

The inference drawn from the analysis is that the practice of discrimination on HIV/AIDS is high in health care institutions.

Discriminatiion in the Place of Work

Many studies have revealed that the discrimination experienced by the people living with HIV positive in the place where they are working. Majority of the people living with HIV positive have lost their job and faced various discriminations and humiliations in the work place after revealing their HIV status to their employer and colleagues. The present study also made on attempt to explore the discrimination faced by the respondents in the place of their working.

Table 5.83. Employment Status Of Respondents

Sl.No.	*Employment Status*	*No. of Respondents*
1.	Working from before infection	48(41.4 per cent)
2.	Working after infection	68(58.6 per cent)
	Total	116(100 per cent)

In this study, of the total 200 respondents, 58 per cent were employed in various sectors. Among the employed women, the 58.6 per cent have started working only after knowing their HIV infection.

The inference drawn from the analysis is that the majority (58.6 per cent) of the respondents were taken up job only after knowing their HIV status (Table 5.83).

Table 5.84 shows that the causes for taking up jobs by the respondents after knowing their HIV status is identified as widowhood (26.5 per cent), to meet medical expenses (23.5 per cent), to get free from mental torture and tension (20.6 per cent), separation or desertion from husband (16.2 per cent) and husband's unemployment and his inability to do work (13.2 per cent) due to sickness.

Table 5.84. Reasons for Taking Job after Knowing HIV Status

Sl. No.	*Reasons*	*No. of Respondents*	*Percentage*
1.	Widowhood	18	26.5
2.	To meet medical expenses	16	23.5
3.	To get rid of mental torture and tension	14	20.6
4.	Separation or desertion from husband	11	16.2
5.	Husband's unemployment and his inability to do work due to sickness.	9	13.2
	Total	68	100

The conclusion drawn from Table 5.84 it is that the widowhood due to AIDS and heavy medical expenses to treat opportunistic infection are the major cause for the women to go for employment after knowing their HIV status.

A. Discrimination Experienced by the Respondents and their Husbands in the Place Of Work

As for the analysis, 158 respondents were with their husbands. Among these husbands, 93.0 per cent were employed in various sectors. Their employers known about 6.1 per cent respondent's husband's infection and they discriminated all these men by throwing them out of jobs.

Among the 116 (58.0 per cent) employed respondents, only 20.7 per cent have revealed their HIV status in their working places under the circumstances of getting sympathy and jobs in Tamil Nadu State AIDS Control Society and in voluntary organisations working in AIDS prevention and control. The revelation of HIV status brought employment opportunity for all these 24 respondents in voluntary organisations (17 (70.8

per cent)) and Tamil Nadu State AIDS Control Society (7 (29.2 per cent)). By knowing the HIV status of these respondents, the employer showed sympathy and immediately agreed to observe them for their organisations.

However, these respondents reported that they have experienced different kinds of discrimination both from their employer and colleagues. According to them, whenever visitors come to their organisations, their employers used to introduce them as a HIV infected person to get name and fame. They revealed that such kind of introduction to unknown persons make them to think about their HIV status with fear of guilt and death. Besides, their colleagues are also maintaining social distance in the work due to lack of knowledge and the fear of contracting infection through causal contacts.

The discrimination produced certain psychological impact on their personality development. They felt that their working condition was not favorable for them to forget their infection and get relief from tension and fear. Therefore, in the beginning many have thought of resigning their jobs and find some other organisations where no one is aware of their infection. Nevertheless, the reasonable income and other facilities for their treatment made them to continue their work in the NGOs and Tamil Nadu State AIDS Control society. Now, they are all adjusted with the present circumstances and mould their mind to work for the people living with HIV positive and to create awareness to the general population and high risk groups on HIV/AIDS and its impact.

B. Organisation to Fight for Women Living with HIV Positive Against Stigma and Discrimination

The infected women have an organisation in Chennai under the name of "Positive Women Net Work". It fights against the discrimination of AIDS and involved in providing counseling, support and care to the women living with HIV positive. It is functioning under the financial support of Tamil Nadu AIDS Control Society.

The analysis clearly revealed that the infected women were maintaining secrecy with regard to their HIV infection in the place where they are working. The infected women were very much scared about the impact of stigma associated with AIDS if they revealed their infection with their employer and colleagues. Therefore, stigma and discrimination played a vital role to prevent the infected people to share their infection with others.

Respondents Attitude Towards Pregnancy and Childbirth after Infection

The status of women in India is determined by her fertility status. Motherhood is glorified in all religion and the children are essential to perform all religious rituals and last rites of the parents. The infertility of women is stigmatized and it discriminate women throughout her life and it may end with divorce, separation or desertion. Therefore, the women in particular and family in general give more importance for pregnancy and childbirth.

Pregnancy and child birth is purely personal. But in the context of HIV/AIDS, it is proved that the infected women can transmit the virus to the infant if she is not taking antiretroviral treatment and adopt breast feeding to the infants. Once the child is infected by HIV, its survival is questionable and the child also has to face all discrimination like adult without knowing anything about HIV/AIDS.

The analysis makes an attempt to understand the women's attitude towards pregnancy and child birth, sexual behaviour after infection etc.

Table 5.85. Number of children born before and after infection to respondents

Sl. No.	*No. of Children*	*No. of Respondents*			*Total*
		1-2	*3-4*	*4-5*	
1.	Before infection	74 (46.5%)	82 (51.6%)	3 (1.9)	159 (100%)
2.	After infection	27 (93.1)	2 (6.9%)	0	29 (100%)
3.	Children infected	14	0	0	14 (48.3)
4.	Children died due to infection	2	0	0	2 (14.3%)

Table 5.85 shows that among 165 married respondents 96.4 per cent have children even before knowing infection and 14.5 per cent of respondents delivered babies after infection. Among the babies born to infected mother, 48.3 per cent were infected with HIV and among 14.3 per cent children have died due to HIV/AIDS. All these children living with HIV are under the age group of 1-5 years.

The conclusion drawn from Table 5.85 is that the majority of the children (48.3 per cent) born to the respondents after infection are infected by HIV.

Table 5.86. Causes for Pregnancy after Infection

Sl.No.	*Causes for Pregnancy*	*No. of Respondents*	*Percentage*
1.	Not practiced birth control	13	44.8
2.	To fulfil the role as mother	6	20.7
3.	Not aware of infecting the child	10	34.5
	Total	29	100

Of the 29 respondents who have given birth to child after infection, 44.8 per cent have not practiced any birth control measures to prevent child birth, 20.7 per cent have decided to have children to fulfill the role as motherhood and the remaining 34.5 per cent aware not aware that the infection of mother will infect the child.

Lack of awareness on mother to child transmission (34.5 per cent) and lack of practices of birth control measures (44.8 per cent) are the major causative factor for the pregnancy of women after infection.

A. Reaction of Respondents and her Husbands about Pregnancy after Infection

Of the 29 respondents who have conceived after infection, the majority of the respondents 89.7 per cent were decided to terminate the pregnancy, but it couldn't possible for them due to their advanced stage of pregnancy and the remaining 10.3 per cent prepared to have children with the support of their husbands (Table 5.87).

Of the 29 respondents who have given birth to child after HIV infection were stated that they are all consulted the doctors by knowing their HIV status. Among them 48.3 per cent of respondents (Table 5.87) are asked by the doctors to terminate the pregnancy and 41.4 per cent have reported that they were discriminated and denied treatment in the hospital. Only 10.3 per cent respondents have been advised by the doctors to take antiretroviral treatment.

Table 5.87. Reaction of Doctors Towards Infected Pregnant Respondents

Sl.No.	*Reaction of Doctors*	*No. of Respondents*	*Percentage*
1.	Asked to take treatment regularly	3	10.3
2.	Asked to terminate the pregnancy	14	48.3
3.	Refused to give treatment	12	41.4
	Total	29	100

The inference drawn from the table is that the HIV infected women are highly discriminated in the hospitals by doctors.

B. Preventive Method Adopted by the Respondents to Avoid Mother to Child Infection

The high cost of antiretroviral drugs prevented all the respondents from taking antiretroviral treatment to prevent mother to child transmission.

Table 5.88. Strategy Adopted by the Respondents for Delivery

Sl. No.	*Strategy adopted for delivery*	*No. of Respondents*	*Percentage*
1.	Getting admission in the hospital at the time of labour pain without informing HIV status	17	58.6
2.	Delivered at home with the support of local midwives without informing HIV status	12	41.4
	Total	29	100

The discrimination experienced by the respondents in the hospital made 58.6 per cent respondents to get admission in the hospital only at the time of labour pain without informing their HIV status. The remaining 41.4 per cent were scared to face the discrimination in the hospital and therefore they have delivered baby in the home with the support of local midwives.

The findings suggested that the discrimination in the healthcare settings made many infected pregnant women either to get admitted into the hospital at the time of emergency by hiding their HIV status or to prepare to deliver at home with the help of midwives by hiding their HIV status. The tendency of hiding the infection status further facilitates the spread of infection among the innocent people who have attended delivery.

Table 5.89. Reproductive Sexual Behaviour After Infection to Avoid Pregnancy

Sl.No.	*Reproductive sexual behaviour*	*No. of Respondents*	*Percentage*
1.	Sterilization	34	17.0
2.	Oral pills	21	10.5
3	Condom	28	14.0
4.	IUD (Intra Uterine Device)	32	16.0
5.	Abstinence	3	1.5
6.	Avoided Marriage	35	17.5
7.	Sterilized before infection	47	23.5
	Total	200	100.0

Table 5.89 represents the reproductive behaviour of the respondents to avoid pregnancy in order to prevent mother to child transmission.

The table shows that 23.5 per cent respondents have undergone female sterilization even before knowing infection. These respondents have reported that there is no need of using any other preventive method to avoid pregnancy as well as transmission.

All 35 (17.5 per cent) of unmarried respondents have decided to avoid marriage due to the fear of infecting their husbands as well as the child. Among the married women 17.0 per cent have undergone sterilization 16.0 per cent have adopted the temporary method of contraception or non-terminal measures called IUDs (Intra Uterus Devices). The 14.0 per cent were using condom to avoid pregnancy and among them majority (25 respondents) were female sex workers who were motivated by the non-governmental organisations to use condom to prevent transmission to their male sexual partners. Oral pills is used by 10.5 per cent of respondents to avoid pregnancy and only 1.5 per cent of respondents were adopted the concept of abstinence to prevent their child from infection.

The conclusion drawn from the table is that the unmarried women were well aware of the passing of infection to their husbands if they get married. So they have all avoided marriage. Among the married respondents, the majority have prepared terminal method followed by non terminal method called IUDs. Condom usage is not popular among the married women rather than the women in sex work.

Table 5.90. Attitude of Respondents Towards Pregnancy and Child Birth

Sl.No.	*Respondents Attitude*	*Yes*	*No*	*Total*
1.	Infected women must have pregnancy	48 (24.0%)	152 (76.0%	200 (100%)
2.	Pregnancy of infected women is unadvisable	128 (64.0%)	72 (36.0%)	200 (100%)
3.	Infected women can have pregnancy to experience motherhood	56 (28.0%)	144 (72.0%)	200 (100%)
4.	Pregnancy right should not be denied to infected women	45 (22.5%)	155 (77.5%)	200 (100%)
5.	Child will get infection from infected mother	105 (52.5%)	95 (47.5%)	200 (100%)
6.	Infected child will have less survival	100 (50.0%)	100 (50.0%)	200 (100%)
7.	Regular Antiretroviral treatment prevent child from infection	57 (28.5%)	143 (71.5%)	200 (100%)
8.	Government can ban the pregnancy of HIV positive women	156 (78.0%)	44 (22.0%)	200 (100%)

Table 5.90 reveals the respondent's attitude towards pregnancy and child birth by the women living with HIV positive.

The table reflects that though the majority of the women were against the pregnancy of HIV infected women, they were not supported the denial of pregnancy right to the HIV infected women either by the public or by the Government. At the same time almost 50 per cent of the respondents were unaware of mother to child transmission and the less survival chance for the infected child. The table also shows that the majority (71.5 per cent) of the respondents were unaware of the antiretroviral treatment and its administration to prevent child from infection.

The inference drawn from the table is that the infected women were against the denial of pregnancy right to the infected women and most of them were ignorant about mother to child transmission and the antiretroviral treatment to safeguard the child from infection.

Table 5.91. Facilities Expceted by the Respondents to Take Care of Infected Child and Positive Parents

Sl.No.	*Facilities Expected by the Respondents*	*No. of Respondents*	*Percentage*
1.	Treatment along with other patients	193	96.5
2.	Free antiretroviral drugs	200	100.0
3.	Financial assistance to take up self employment	164	82.0
4.	Insurance for people with HIV positive	157	78.5
5.	Admission in the school for the infected children	200	100.0
6.	Special care home for the abundant people	189	94.5
7.	Reservation in the employment	83	41.5
8.	Alternative avenue to the infected sex workers	163	81.5

Table 5.91 represents the facilities expected by the respondents to take care of infected child and positive parents. All the respondents (100.0 per cent) were expected free

antiretroviral drugs for both the child and infected parents and all the respondents (100.0 per cent) were demanded admission for the infected child in the schools. Besides, majority (96.5 per cent) of the respondents were expected the facilities of treatment which is free from stigma along with other patients instead of treatment in special isolated ward and the larger proportion of respondents were suggested special care home for the abundant people with HIV positive. Greater percentage (82.0 per cent) of respondents were in need of financial assistance from the government to take self-employment to compensate the loss of income due to unemployment as result of their infection status.

The 81.5 per cent of respondents were in favour of creating alternative employment avenue for the sex workers to prevent them to continue their sex work after infection. The facilities of insurance for the people living with HIV positive are suggested by 78.5 per cent of people followed by reservation in the employment (41.5 per cent).

It is found from the table that all the infected people were expected the facilities of antiretroviral treatment, treatment along with other patients and financial assistance to cope up with the loss of employment due to HIV/AIDS.

CASE STUDIES

Case : 1

Vennila (name changed) is aged 31, studied upto 12th standard and working as a clerk in garment industry in Chennai. She got married at the age of 21 and her husband is a taxi driver working in a travel agency in Chennai. His frequent tour to various parts of the country influenced him to enjoy sex with various sex workers of different states and got infection even before his marriage. He confirmed his HIV positive status by blood test before getting marriage but he has not revealed it to any one including his parents. When his parents arranged marriage for him, he happily agreed without any guilt and he has not disclosed his HIV status to his wife and her family members not only before marriage but also after marriage. When Vennila became pregnant, her doctor suggested her to take HIV test which is mandatory test for pregnant women in

Tamil Nadu. The blood test confirmed that she is HIV positive. By knowing her HIV status she was shocked and made a lot of quarrel with her husband, her mother in-law and parents. She blamed her husband for passing HIV virus to her and refused to continue living with him. But her parents and in-laws forced her to live with him due to the fear of social criticism on the family as a result her desertion from her husband. She delivered a male baby with HIV negative status and now she is living with her husband and continue her work in garment industries in Chennai.

It is clear from this case that the women are the victims of HIV infection in the male dominated society. It is a social crime committed by men for transmitting the virus to his loyal and innocent wife

Case : 2

Gangammal (name changed) is aged 24, studied upto 10th standard and belong to poor agricultural family in Thirupathi, Andra Pradesh. She has aged parents and 3 adolescent sisters and 2 brothers. Her family is perennially marked by poverty, unemployment and inadequate income as a result of large family size and crop failure. Since her old parents are unable to involve in any productive activity, the family commitment has fallen on her shoulder. In view of her family's economic distress, taking advantage of possibility of getting employment in Tamil Nadu she moved out of her native place and entered into Chennai city with a view to seek decent gainful employment to take care of her family. Her hopes shattered when she understood that Chennai is not providing decent opportunity for her livelihood as against her previous understanding about Chennai.

Due to family compulsion and her disinterest to get back home forced her to come under the influence of women pimps in Chennai. Her involvement in prostitution is not informed to her family members. She visits to her family once in a month and provides money and gifts to parents and sisters and brothers. Her sexual engagement with a number of clients brought sexually transmitted diseases. She went for treatment in the sexually transmitted diseases clinics and she tested HIV positive. When she was told about her HIV/AIDS, she was unable to understand the infection. Later she understood that the infection carries severe stigma and discrimination and it affects not only her but also her family. Therefore, she has decided to keep it secretly unto herself. She continued her commercial sex work even after knowing her infection as there is no option left for her.

The inference is that there are a number of Gangammas living in our society. The social health of society would be affected severely if more number of Gangammas continue to involve in commercial sex even after knowing their infection status. Hence the social implication is severe. The strong taboo and stigma prevented Gangamma to reveal her HIV status and the economic necessity forced her to continue her sex work. She is infecting her clients every day, as she is young. Her clients may be young and unmarried; their future life is uncertain and dangerous

It is evident from this case that social and economic problems forced women to take to prostitution as an option for their survival without recognizing their social responsibility to prevent others from infection. Social taboo and stigma compelled sex workers to hide HIV status, if they are infected

Case : 3

Savithiri (name changed) is aged 23, illiterate and belong to a poor agricultural labour family in the remote village of Villupuram in Tamil Nadu. She has lost her parents during her childhood (at the age of 6) and was brought up under the care of her maternal grandmother. Being the agricultural labour family, her grand parents also lived under the condition of poverty and they harassed her and forced her to go for any work which generates income. Therefore, she ran way from her grand parents and went to Villupuram as a stranger. She was helped by a woman-a hotel owner. While she is working in the hotel she met another woman and believing her words she went along with her at the age of 8 with a view to get better job and income. Actually, the woman is the pimp and she has close contact with the brokers of child trafficking. The woman pimp sold Savithiri to the brokers at Villupuram. Then she is taken to Bangalore and from there to Mumbai.

The 8 year old Savithiri was harassed and severally beaten up and raped by the gang in the Bombay red light area. At this tender age she was forced to have sex with the older men with superstitious belief that sex with a child will cure all sexually transmitted infections. With no other option to escape, she started living with similar girls. During her routine check up for sexually transmitted diseases she was identified as HIV positive at the age of 17. She was not given any counselling. She knew nothing about AIDS except that it is a killer disease. The brothel keeper took her to Thambaram Thoracic Sanatorium, at Chennai and disappeared without informing her. The World Vision of India – an N.G.O. working for care and support for the people living with HIV positive helped her and shifted her to the short stay home.

In this case, it is clear that child racketing took place and violated the rights of the child and abused her, which is an incident of violence against childhood. The myth associated with sex with child and the cure of sexually transmitted disease increases child rape and child prostitution. Here also the girl child succumbs to innocent victim.

Case : 4

Nirmala (name changed) is a 21-year old woman, studied upto 10th standard and belong to an agricultural family in Ottanchatram in Dindigul District, Tamil Nadu. She got married at the age of 19 to her maternal uncle who is a lorry driver aged 27. From the third month of her marriage her husband fell sick frequently and took treatment in a private hospital at Coimbatore where he tested HIV positive. The medical advice forced Nirmala to take HIV test and her positive status was confirmed and revealed to her and family members. She was shocked to know her HIV status because she knew some thing related to AIDS, its route of transmission and its implication through various media. Since then she vehemently neglected her husband and refused to provide care and support to him. Her husband was given treatment by her parents and he died eight months after the marriage. She lived with him only for three months and got infected as a result of her marriage and she became widow at the younger age for none of her fault. She is now under the care and support of her parents and in-laws.

It is evident from this case that the innocent women are getting infected mostly through their marital partner.

Case : 5

Rathakrishnan (name changed) is a casual labour, aged 39, and studied upto higher secondary. He has two wives and 2 children aged 3 and 1. His nature of work necessitated him to move frequently to many places. During his mobility he had a contact with the sex worker and got infected and it was transmitted to his wives. When he tested HIV positive as a result of his continuous illness in the private hospital at Palani he was mentally shocked and fearful of his immature death. His mental shock made him to behave like an insane person and he unconsciously revealed his HIV status publicly in the village. He died within 6 months of his HIV test and none participated in his funeral except his family members. As a result of this revelation, the whole family is subjected to social boycott and social sanctions by the community. Their uninfected children are also facing the same discrimination and stigma. They are also not allowed to play with the children in the neighborhood. The widowed women are denied cooly work and all economic avenues outside their family are closed to them.

In this case the women again became the innocent victim of HIV infection in marital life. It is also evident that the stigma and discrimination are very strong in HIV/AIDS.

6

Summary of Major Findings, Suggestions and Conclusion

The study has been undertaken among the women living with HIV positive in Chennai City, Tamil Nadu. The major findings derived from the analysis and interpretations of primary data are summarized in this chapter.

MAJOR FINDINGS

The Social and Economic Status of Women Living with HIV Positive

Age of Respondents

The study revealed that a large number of respondents living with HIV positive fall in the age group of 20-29 years (66.5 per cent). The women in this age group are hyper active in reproduction as well as in social and economic activities. The increasing infection among women in sexually active age group will lead to great damage to human resources, national economy and social fabric of the society.

Community of Respondents

HIV/AIDS epidemic is not restricted to particular community. Though the infection is found among all the communities, women from the backward (46.6 per cent) and schedule caste (26 per cent) communities are worst affected by this dreaded disease. Limited or lack of access to information, lower social and economic status always force women to be sexually submissive to their sexual partner which prevent them to adopt safe sex mechanism.

Religion of Respondents

HIV/AIDS is not confined to particular religion. The people from all religions including Hindu, Muslim and Christian are vulnerable to HIV/AIDS. In this study, an overwhelming majority of respondents (85 per cent) belong to Hindu religion which is well known for its high moral and social values. The rapid spread of HIV among Hindus might be due to the changes occurring in the religious attitude of the youth in the contemporary society.

Education ofRespondents

A vast majority of the women (81.6 per cent) in the study are literate. Therefore, it is a myth that illiterate women are more vulnerable to HIV infection.

Social status of Respondents

Social status of the respondents is concerned, the majority (65.5 per cent) are housewives. The sex workers (31.0 per cent.) and students (3.5) are considerably less in this study. Housewives are more vulnerable to HIV/AIDS due to their husbands promiscuous behaviour.

Family Structure

As far as the structure of the family is concerned, the nuclear family (77 per cent) is predominant among the respondents. The joint family system can act as informal social control agent to check and control the behaviour of the individual. But in the contemporary society the elders have less control over the youth which led to the rapid spread of HIV infection in the nuclear families.

Dependent Family Members

Majority (63 per cent) of the respondents have dependent family members that increased the burden of the HIV infected women.

Educational Status of the Family Members

Literacy rate is high (81 per cent) among the members of respondents family.

Employment Status of Family Members

Overwhelming majority (59 per cent) of respondents family

members are engaged in unorganized sectors which give less income. The transport workers are found to be less (3.9 per cent) in the families of respondents.

Causes for Migration of Respondents to Chennai

Majority (62.5 per cent) of the respondents migrated to Chennai due to two major reasons namely marriage, and HIV infection. Marriage necessitated 27 per cent of women to migrate to Chennai whereas 13.5 per cent of respondents migrated to Chennai in order to hide their HIV status from their family members, relatives and friends as well as for treatment in the Tambaram Sanitarium nearby Chennai.

Economic Status of Respondents

Non-earner dependent (42.3) and earner dependents (33.5 per cent) are predominant in this study. The dependent women have either less or no power over their reproductive health which led to the contract of HIV/AIDS through their husbands.

Place of Residence

The study has identified that majority (42 per cent) of the respondents reside in urban areas and urban slums (58 per cent).

Occupation

The overwhelming majority (42 per cent) of respondents are unemployed. At the same time 30 per cent of women are engaged in unorganized sectors. The women in commercial sex work are also found in significant per centage (16.5 per cent). The power of negotiation about safe sex is strongly influenced by the economic empowerment of women. The unemployed and the women in unorganized sectors are economically deprived and they have less control over their reproductive health. The less or lack of power on reproductive health makes women more vulnerable to HIV/AIDS.

Ownership of Property

The majority (95.5 per cent) of women do not own any immovable assets. Women property right is not encouraged in the Indian society. In the patriarchal society, men dominate in all resources and the women are subordinate to men and hence lack ownership.

Annual Income and Expenditure

More than 65.5 per cent of respondents family incurred annual expenditure more than their annual income. The significant per centage (60 per cent) of respondents have borrowed amount ranging from Rs. 2,000-10,000 from various sources. Majority (59.2 per cent) of respondents borrowed money for medical treatment for HIV related illness of their husbands and children. Money lender is found to be the dominant sources of (54.2 per cent) lending money to the respondents. The medical treatment for HIV/AIDS made respondents to become indebted.

Marital Status of the Respondents

Marital Status

Married women are predominant (82.5 per cent) in this study. The unmarried women account for only 17.5 per cent. It is revealed that the married women are at the higher risk of contracting HIV infection.

Age at Marriage

The overwhelming majority (90.1 per cent) of the respondents got married when they were below 22 years. All the respondents married men who are 3-8 years older than them. The women have either no or less negotiation power with regard to their reproductive health choice due to their younger age. The age at marriage is an important factor for women in the Indian context to accept the male domination over their reproductive health. Therefore younger the age at marriage, higher the chance for getting infection through their husbands who experienced pre marital sex with multiple sexual partners.

Nature of Relationship between Respondents and their Husbands

Majority (84.2 per cent) of the respondents' marriage have taken place out side the close kin family relationship. Marriage with unfamiliar persons has high risk of contracting HIV. In this study, majority of husbands are not familiar with the respondents at the time of marriage. The sexual behaviour of the bride or bridegroom can be observed among the known person rather than the unknown person. Marriage among the familiar person has least chance for contracting HIV.

Type of Marriage

The infection rate is found to be high (66.1) in arranged marriages than the marriage based on mutual love (32.1 per cent). Arranged marriage with unknown persons has the high risk of contracting HIV rather than the marriage based on mutual love. In arranged marriages consideration is given only for horoscope and related matters of match making instead of personal background of individual proposed for marriage.

Causes for Respondents Widowhood

One-fourth (25.5 per cent) of the respondents are widows. Majority (92.1 per cent) of the respondents became widows due to the death of their HIV infected husbands. It revealed that their husbands got infected long back and even before marriage. Therefore, mortality rate is high among the infected men.

Age at Widowhood and Duration of Married Life

The majority (88.2 per cent) of the women age at widowhood is identified as 20-25 years and majority (72.5 per cent) of respondents lived with their husbands only for 1-5 years. Therefore, younger the age at marriage higher the chance for becoming widow at younger age due to HIV/AIDS.

Causes for Separation

Nearly one-fifth of the respondents (19.0 per cent) are separated women. HIV/AIDS is identified as major cause for the separation of majority (65.8 per cent) of respondents. The infection of HIV among any one of the spouse disturb the family life and it challenge the sacramental nature of marital bonds.

Employment Status of the Husbands

Of the 165 married respondents, the majority (35.8 per cent) of their husbands are casual labourers and industrial workers (20.0 per cent). The transport workers are comparatively less (16.4 per cent). Due to the migratory nature work the casual labourers are more prone to HIV infection

Reasons for Unmarried Status of Respondents

Involvement in sex work and dowry prevented majority (48.6 per cent) of respondents to get marriage.

Circumstances Leading to HIV Infection and Related Behaviours

Duration of HIV Infection

Majority (81.0 per cent) of the respondents understood their HIV status since seven years during their young and sexually hyper active age.

Sources of Infection

The overwhelming majority (65.0 per cent) of the women were infected through their husbands. At the same time significant per centage (34.5 per cent) of women got infection through their multi sexual behaviour which includes married women (31.0 per cent) and students (3.5 per cent). It revealed that the promiscuous sexual behaviour of women not only led her to acquire HIV/AIDS but it also increases the vulnerability of infection to their husbands and it is identified that 17.6 per cent of respondents husbands might be infected with HIV/AIDS due to the promiscuous behaviour of women.

Husbands Infected by Respondents

Of the 158 married respondents, 130 (65.0 per cent) got infection through their husbands whereas the remaining 35 per cent got infection through their behaviours of sex work and injecting drug use. Their husbands are highly prone to HIV infection. These 35 per cent of respondents' husbands are highly ignorant about their infection and they are also not aware of their wives HIV infection.

Pre and Extra Marital Sexual Behaviour

The majority (76.9 per cent) of women experienced pre marital sex with the men who are known to her, for example, relatives, family friend, friends, neighbour and co-workers. It revealed that the women pre marital sex is confined with the people who are close to them. Significant per centage (15.0 per cent) of respondents experienced extra marital sex with those who are regularly patronising them. It increases not only their vulnerability towards HIV but also their innocent husbands.

Majority (82.4 per cent) respondents husbands are promiscuous and among them the significant per centage (66.7 per cent) have experienced pre marital sex mostly (49.1 per cent) with sex workers. Pre marital sex of the men increases the vulnerability of infection of innocent wives.

Reasons for Respondents Husbands Extra Marital Sexual Behaviour

Majority (51.8 per cent) of the respondents husbands also involved in extra marital sex with sex workers (92.9 per cent). Their sexual involvement with commercial sex workers resulted in HIV/AIDS. Migration (30.2 per cent) and alcoholic behaviour (22.6 per cent) appears to be important factors for the development of extra marital affairs of the respondents husbands. Since they satisfy their sexual urge with sex workers they have increased chance of contracting infection and spreading it to their wives.

Reasons for Respondents Pre and Extra Marital Relationships

Love affair is the major (43.5 per cent) cause for pre marital sex and difference of opinion between the spouses are the significant (50.0 per cent) reason for extra marital sex of the respondents.

Safe Sex Practices in the Pre and Extra Marital Relationship

Condom usage is found to be low among the respondents who have experienced pre (15.4 per cent) and extra marital (8.8 per cent) sex. The practice of oral pills is higher among the women experienced pre marital sex (53.8 per cent) and adoption of sterilization is high among the respondents experienced extra marital sex (41.2 per cent). These respondents are very much bothered about avoiding pregnancy due to cultural implications of giving birth out side wedlock. The culture surrounding around the notion of pregnancy increases the vulnerability of women towards HIV/AIDS.

Significant per centage of respondents engaged in pre (30.8) and extra marital (23.6 per cent) sex are not practicing any method of safe sex to prevent sexually transmitted infection as well as child birth. The culture of silence around sex and the fear to ask or to buy condom increases the vulnerability of women's HIV infection. The sterilization also led women not to use condom since they are already safe in avoiding pregnancy.

Reproductive Behaviour among Housewives

Housewives give more importance to avoid pregnancy rather than sexually transmitted infections. Adoption of sterilization, oral pills and IUDs prevented majority (62.6 per cent) of housewives to think about condom as safe sex method to safeguard themselves from sexually transmitted infections.

Circumstances Leading to Commercial Sex Work

Marital Status of Sex Workers

The majority (54.8 per cent) of sex workers are married women and among them 43.5 per cent have husbands and children. The unmarried respondents in sex work are accounted for 45.2 per cent. The responsibilities on catering the needs of the family members force the women, especially the married women to involve in exchanging sex for money. Their engagement in multiple sex is considered as potential sources of contracting HIV/AIDS. The husbands of these sex workers also have greater possibility of contracting HIV/AIDS through them.

Reasons for the Involvement in Commercial Sex Work

Poverty and related economic deprivation of the family is the central factor for the involvement of 77.3 per cent respondents in commercial sex. The economical necessities force the commercial sex workers to be less empowered with regard to demanding condom use with their customers. Unsafe sex is the major contributing factor for contracting HIV.

Age at Induction in Commercial Sex Work

The significant per centage (51.6 per cent) of sex workers inducted in sex at the young age of within 23 years. It indicate that early involvement in sex involve longer duration of sexual participation which has strong influence on the risk of contracting HIV/AIDS. Due to younger age the sex workers have less negotiation power with regard to safe sex which has strong influence both for contracting and spread of HIV/AIDS.

Clients of Commercial Sex Workers

Labourers (38.7 per cent), business people (37.1 per cent), tourist (33.9 per cent), transport workers, including drivers and cleaners (27.4 per cent), students (21 per cent) and men who are away from home for longer duration (17.7 per cent) are identified as dominant categories of clients who visit commercial sex workers quite often.

Safe Sex Practices of Clients

Safe sex practice is significant among business (30.6 per cent) people and transport workers (25.6 per cent). The safe sex practice is found to be less among labourers (3.2 per cent). Unsafe sex practice and use of alcohol is closely related HIV/AIDS. The overwhelming majority (97.3 per cent) of respondents customers have the habit of drinking alcohol and due to the influence of alcohol the customers are not in a mental state to use condom as safe sex. The unsafe sex between the sex workers and their customers increases the vulnerability of infection for sex workers and their customers.

Number of Clients Engaged Per Day

All the 27 part time sex workers are married and they have husband and children. The part time sex workers engage less number of clients (1-2) per day rather than the full time sex workers (3-6). The full time sex workers include 28 unmarried girls, four widows and three deserted. As a result of frequent sexual encounter with multiple partners the full time sex workers are more prone to HIV/AIDS.

Earning Per Day

The majority (88.9 per cent) of part time sex workers earn less Rs. 300 per day where as the majority (62.8 per cent) of the full time sex workers earn upto Rs. 400 per day. The sex workers are taking risk of contracting HIV/AIDS by involving in multiple sex for earning considerable amount for their survival.

Sources of Contact with the Clients

Most of the full time sex workers (33.9 per cent) contact and pick their clients directly from the crowded places like bus stand, railway station, market, beach, tourist centres etc. The majority (19.4 per cent) of the part time sex workers use modern communication technology including mobile phone, e-mail to contact the customers who are regular to them. The 17.7 per cent of part time sex workers also have a close link with the brokers to meet their customers. The part time sex workers choose particular place for their sex work and they returned home like other employed women.

Network and Place of Residence

The sex workers have strong invisible net work to contact fellow sex workers as well as customers in Chennai and most (37.1 per cent) of the sex workers are residing in slums which is known for many illegal activities. The poor social and economic background of the sex workers residing in slum will not acquire power of negation of safe sex with their customers.

Nature of Sex Work

The majority (50 per cent) of the respondents involved in sex work independently and 27.5 per cent are under the influence of brokers. The economic necessity resulted many impoverished women to choose prostitution as a means for their survival.

Reason for not Insisting the Clients to use Condom

Lack of awareness on the implication of HIV/AIDS is the major factor for 59.7 per cent of sex workers who do not insist their clients to use condom. The lack of safe sex practices has spread effect for both the sex workers and their customers.

Reason for not Using Condoms by the Clients

Drinking of alcohol prevents majority (38.7 per cent) of customers to use condom during paid sex. The intoxicative mental state has direct influence on unsafe sex and behavioural change with regard to sex and sexuality.

Changes in the Sexual Behaviour of the Sex Workers after Knowing their HIV Infection

Majority (53.2 per cent) of women continues sex work even after knowing their HIV status but significant change in the sexual behaviour of the sex workers with regard to safe sex is observed after HIV infection. At the same time significant per centage (46.7 per cent) of sex workers are withdrawn their involvement from sex work after knowing their HIV infection. It revealed that these sex workers have realized their role in transmitting the virus to the innocent clients.

Present Status of the Sex Workers after Knowing their HIV Infection

After the withdrawal from the sex work due to infection, the 42 per cent of sex workers found alternative avenues for their survival with the support of non-governmental and governmental organisations.

Causes for Remaining in Sex Work after Knowing HIV Infection

Lack of alternative job and less income in other job made 53.2 per cent of sex workers to remain in the same work even after knowing their HIV status. The spread effect of HIV is higher due to the involvement of women in sex work with HIV status.

Awareness on HIV/AIDS and Willingness to be in Special Home

After knowing the infection all the sex workers are aware of their role in transmitting the virus to their clients. At the same time they are not willing to stay in the special home if it is run for the infected people. The stigma and discrimination prevent the infected sex workers to be lodged in special home since it has the label which carries HIV positive.

HIV Test

Places of HIV Test

Majority (61.5 per cent) of the respondents tested their HIV status in government hospitals. The government hospitals have the facilities for HIV test at free of cost. It facilitated the respondents to take HIV test in government hospitals.

Factors Influencing HIV Test

HIV status of the respondents husband influenced more than 50 per cent of respondents to take HIV test. The Sexually

Transmitted Diseases (STD) and its related illness in other important factors which forced the women to take HIV test.

Pre and Post Test Counseling to the Respondents and their Family Members

More than 75 per cent of the respondents and their family members are not exposed to pre and post test counseling to understand fully about the HIV, its social impact, care and support and living with HIV peacefully by coping with social stigma. The absence of pre and post test counseling for the respondents and their family members led to discrimination, personality disorder and lack of confidence to live with HIV status.

Knowledge on HIV/AIDS at the Time of Testing

The majority (74 per cent) of respondents have no knowledge on HIV/AIDS when they have undergone HIV test in various hospitals. Lack of awareness on HIV/AIDS at the time of testing created fear and lost confidence and courage to share their infection with their family members.

Impact of HIV Status in the Social Relationship in Family

Revelation of HIV/AIDS of the Respondents

The revelation of HIV infection is high (66.9 per cent) among the housewives and high secrecy is maintained among the women who got HIV through their heterosexual contact and injecting drug use. The cultural taboo on promiscuous relationship not allowed the multisexual women to share their infection with their family members.

Sources of Revelation of HIV

Majority (90.8 per cent) of respondents HIV status is revealed to their family members through the hospital where they underwent HIV test. Respondents husbands HIV status revealed to the family members mostly (64.4 per cent) through the respondents. HIV revelation to any individual is insisted only after proper guidance and counseling. More than 90 per cent of the respondents HIV status is revealed without counseling.

Guidance and counseling have direct influence on the social relationship of infected persons.

Respondents Husbands Awareness about his HIV Infection before Marriage

The vast majority (90.8 per cent) of respondents husbands are not aware of their infection before their marriage. They married with the ignorance of their HIV status and they infected their innocent wives unknowingly. The absence of mandatory HIV test before marriage increases the vulnerability of infection for the women after their marriage.

Husbands' Reaction Towards Wives after Knowing Infection

Majority (60.6 per cent) of respondents infected husbands harassed their wives after knowing their HIV status. Though the men fully aware that their wives got infection through them and they are the innocent victims of infection, they involved in harassing their wives due to guilt and shame.

Respondents Reaction Towards Husbands Infection

Majority (57.7 per cent) of respondents have not provided care and support for their infected husbands. At the same time 42.3 per cent of respondents supported their husbands due to the cultural bound existed between husband and wife in the Indian Society. The culture of marriage and family made majority (42.3 per cent) women to remain with their infected husbands.

The Relationship between Respondents and Husbands after Knowing HIV Infection

The relationship between husband and wife after knowing HIV infection is not compassionate and majority (49.2 per cent) have involved in frequent quarrel with each other. The stigma associated with promiscuous relationship and HIV/AIDS led to family dispute resulting in family disintegration.

Reaction of in-laws

Discrimination towards the infected women by the in-laws is comparatively higher (86.3 per cent) than their husbands (48.3

per cent). The significant per centage (32.2 per cent) of respondents are socially isolated by their in-laws. The Indian culture is always favourable to men and his promiscuous relationship is tolerated by their family members. Due to the tolerance based on cultural influence the infected men is comparatively experience less discrimination than infected women.

Reaction of Parents

The majority (70.1 per cent) of respondents parents give support to the respondents rather than the respondents husbands (20.7 per cent). Very less number of respondents and their husbands are socially isolated by the parents of respondents. In view of the fact that the housewives get infection through their husbands they get more support from their parents. At the same time the widowed and deserted (3.5 per cent) women have not got support from their parents due to the infection as a result of promiscuous relationship. The majority (64.7 per cent) of the unmarried sex workers got support from their parents after sharing their HIV status with them. It revealed that they are involved in sex work with the knowledge of their parents.

Nature of Restriction Imposed by Family Members on HIV Infected Persons

Majority of the housewives (85.1 per cent), their husbands (79.3 per cent), sex workers (57.2 per cent) and infected children (57.2 per cent) are restricted to casual contact, for example, touching and sharing articles and to take part in the socio cultural ceremonies of the family. The stigma associated with HIV/AIDS is the primary factor for such restriction imposed on people living with HIV positive.

Decision taken in the Family before and after Infection

The role of people living with HIV positive in decision-making process has affected due to their infection. Before knowing HIV status, the respondents husbands (40.5 per cent) played a dominant role in taking decision with regard to their family affairs. At the same time significant per centage (24.5 per cent) of respondents are consulted by their husbands while taking decision. The parents and in-laws played insignificant role in taking decision related to respondents families. But after infection majority (33.5 per cent) of the respondents and their husbands have not participated in decision making and it indicated a way to their parents and in-laws to take decision with regard to their family affairs.

Participation in the Socio-cultural Ceremonies in the Family

More than 70 per cent of the respondents are not participating in the socio cultural ceremonies of the family due to the fear of discrimination. They voluntarily restricted their participation in such functions. The status of HIV resulted in self imposed restriction and lack of courage to associate with the family members.

Maintenance and Property given to the Deserted and Widows

The majority of the widows (74.5 per cent) and separated women (92 per cent) have not been given property or maintenance support for their survival. The infected women are deprived of getting property or maintenance from their husbands side due to the perception that the infected people will have short life.

The Place of Present Stay of the Respondents

The significant per centage (58.5 per cent) of infected women are living along with husband or children. The abundant infected sex workers (12 per cent) got accommodation in short stay home run by the NGOs.

Social Relationship with Neighbourhood

Infection Known to the Neighbours

The people living with HIV positive are maintaining secrecy of their infection from their neighbours due to the problem of stigma and discrimination. The overwhelming majority (97.7 per cent) of respondents and their husbands infection is not known to their neighbours.

Social Relationship of Respondents and their Husbands with Neighbourhood

The majority (92.0 per cent) of respondents and their husbands have good relationship with their neighbours before they know their HIV positive status. They participated in all socio cultural functions of their neighbours. But after knowing their infection, 72 per cent have voluntarily withdrawn their participation in socio cultural ceremonies of their neighbours due to guilt and shame. The fear of stigma associated with the diseases resulted in self imposed restriction among the people living with HIV positive.

Neighbours Interaction Towards People with HIV Status

Very least per centage (1.5 per cent) of respondents infection is known to their neighbours. All these respondents were socially distanced by their neighbours. Therefore, social distance is the common response from the neighbours towards the people living with HIV positive.

Reasons for the Discrimination by the Neighbours

Fear of contracting infection is the major (67.0 per cent) cause for stigmatizing and discriminating the infected people. The general population still has a belief that they get infected if they have a causal relationship with the infected persons. The poor awareness on the mode of spread of infection created such kind of fear among the general population

Person Blamed for Respondents Infection by the Neighbours

Only three (1.5 per cent) respondents infection was known to their neighbours. All the three are blamed for their infection by the neighbours for their ignorance and inability to control their husband from extra-marital affairs.

Effects of Discrimination on theEespondents

The three respondents migrated to other areas as they were fear of facing the isolation by the neighbours. The discrimination by the neighbours led to migration of infected people.

Social Relationship with Friends

Frequency of Respondents, their Husbands with their Friends before and After Infection

The majority (64.5 per cent) of the respondents and their husbands (77.2 per cent) have frequent contact with their friends before knowing their HIV status. Their relationship with the friends has drastically changed after knowing their HIV status. The majority (42.5 per cent) of infected respondents were completely out of their friendship circle and at the same time 50 per cent of their husbands have frequent contact with their friends. The infected women were more reluctant to meet their friends than their husbands. The myth that the immoral people or the multisexual alone get HIV made women to restrict their contact with their friends.

Disclosure of HIV Status by Respondents to the Friends

The majority of the respondents (82.0 per cent) and their husbands (82.3 per cent) have not disclosed their HIV status to their friends. The revelation of HIV status is found to be high among the sex workers (51.6 per cent) than the housewives (3.1 per cent), students (0.0 per cent) and drug users (0.0 per cent). The stigma and discrimination associated with AIDS made the respondents to maintain high confidentiality about their infection.

Reaction of the Friends Towards the Respondents Infection

Majority (58.4 per cent) of the respondents and their husbands (74.0 per cent) are getting moral and financial support from their friends. But when compared to men less number of infected women are getting support from their friends.

Social Relationship with Relatives

Respondents, Husbands Infection Status known to the Relatives

Very few (36.5 per cent) respondents and their husbands have revealed their HIV status to their relatives. The revelation is high among the housewives (70.4 per cent) than the sex workers (29.6 per cent). The housewives innocent victims and they got infection through their husbands. Therefore, they are comparatively comfortable to share their infection to their relatives. The cultural restriction towards promiscuous contact prevents sex workers in sharing their infection with their relatives.

Reaction of the Relatives Towards Respondents and their Husbands

One-third of the respondents are isolated by their relatives after revelation of their HIV status. Social isolation by the relatives is high among the sex workers than the housewives. One fifth of the relatives have restricted their visit to the respondents house. Very few (16.4 per cent) respondents got moral and financial support from their relatives. While comparing the discrimination experienced by infected respondents and their husbands, the infected women are subjected to severe discrimination and criticism by the relatives than their husbands. The 50 per cent Of respondents husbands got moral and financial support from their relatives. It revealed that due to the influence of culture, men's extra marital sex is tolerated by the society.

Frequency of Visit by Respondents and their Husbands to the Relatives House

Before knowing their infection status more than 50 per cent of the respondents and their husbands visited their relatives house regularly for various social functions. After knowing the infection status around 55 per cent of respondents and their husbands have stopped their visit to their relatives house due to the fear of criticism and discrimination. Though the majority of the infected women and men were not disclosed their HIV status to their relatives, they themselves felt guilty and developed fear owing to stigma associated with AIDS and withdrawn their social participation with their relatives.

Participation in the Socio-cultural Ceremonies by Respondents

Before infection, 70.5 per cent of married respondents participated in the socio-cultural ceremonies of relatives house along with their husbands. In the case of unmarried respondents, deserted and widows their parents have participated in the socio cultural ceremonies of their relatives house. After infection, significant changes have taken place in the participation of respondents in the socio-cultural ceremonies of relatives house. As against 70.5 per cent of participation, only 18 per cent have taken part in the socio-cultural ceremonies after infection. The fear of discrimination resulted in self imposed restriction by the respondents in participating all functions in the relatives house.

Persons Blamed for Respondents and their Husbands Infection

The majority (83.7 per cent) of the respondents are blamed not only for their infection but also for their husbands infection though they got infection through their husbands. The gender biased and baseless discrimination created inferiority complex among the infected women resulting in self imposed isolation from the society.

Discrimintion in Medical Treatment

Medical Treatment Seeking Behaviour of the Infected People

Treatment seeing behaviour for the infection is found to be high (100 per cent) among the full time sex workers and housewives (68.5 per cent), part time sex workers (0.0 per cent), students (0.0 per cent) and drug user (0.0 per cent). The respondents who maintain high confidentiality with regard to their infection is not taking treatment for their HIV related illness. While comparing the treatment seeking behaviour with infected husband, the women get less priority than men. The majority (94.6 per cent) of respondents husbands avail treatment for their illness. The gender discrimination in medical treatment prevents many women from availing treatment for their illness.

Place of Treatment

The N.G.Os played a vital role in providing treatment to the respondents either at free of cost or by charging very less amount. Majority of the housewives (41.5 per cent) and sex workers (74.3 per cent) availed treatment in the N.G.Os which is working in AIDS intervention programmes. While comparing the place of treatment by the respondents and their husbands, 66.9 per cent of respondents' husbands got treatment in the private hospital by paying considerable amount. The economic power vested with the men facilitated them to avail treatment in private hospitals. Taking treatment in the private hospitals also helped them to hide their infection status from others. Lack of control over economic resources increased gender discrimination in treatment.

Person Met the Expenditure of Medical Treatment

Significant per centage (26.9 per cent) of housewives gave preference for their husbands treatment rather than their treatment. They are also involved in incurring the expenditure of their husbands treatment. The sex workers spent amount by themselves for their treatment. Besides, 39.2 per cent of housewives medical expenses had been met by their parents rather than their in-laws and husbands.

Problem Faced by the Respondents in the Hospitals

The overwhelming majority (96 per cent) of women faced discrimination in the hospitals. The health care personnel have an opinion that the women get infection through their promiscuous contact. Though the health care personnel are aware of the means of the spread of HIV, they are more reluctant to treat the infected patients and they discriminated them by denying admission in the hospitals, maintaining confidentiality of infection, calling them with the label of AIDS patient etc. The discrimination in the health care sector is mainly due to irresponsibility of medical personnel.

Discrimination in the Place of Work

Employment Status of the Respondents

The majority (58.6 per cent) of the respondents have taken up job only after knowing their HIV status. The widowhood and separation due to AIDS and heavy medical expenses to treat opportunistic infection are the major causes for the women to go for employment after knowing their HIV status.

Discrimination Experienced by the Respondents and their Husbands

The 20.7 per cent of respondents employed in Tamil Nadu State AIDS Control Society and N.G.Os working in AIDS intervention and Control Project have revealed their HIV status to their employer and colleagues. Though the revelation of HIV status brought them certain monetary benefit, they faced discrimination in different forms. Whenever the visitors come to these organisations, the employee with HIV status is introduced by them as HIV infected people. Such kind of introduction resulted in certain psychological problem which always made them to think about early death due to AIDS.

Attitude Towards Pregnancy and Childbirth after Infection

Number of Children Born before and after Infection of Respondents

The majority (96.4 per cent) of respondents gave birth to children before infection. The respondents who gave birth after infection account for14.5 per cent and the majority of the children (48.3 per cent) born to the respondents after infection are infected by HIV.

Causes for Pregnancy after Infection

The respondents who have given birth after infection is accounted for 17.5 per cent from the 165 married respondents. Lack of awareness on mother to child transmission (34.5 per cent) and lack of practices of birth control measures (44.8 per cent) are the major causative factor for the pregnancy of women after infection.

Reaction of Respondents and her Husbands about Pregnancy after Infection

The majority (89.7 per cent) of respondents and their husbands have decided to terminate the pregnancy after knowing the impact of infection on their children. The high cost in antiretroviral treatment to prevent mother to child transmission force the respondents and their husbands to think about the termination of pregnancy.

Reaction of the Doctors Towards the Infected Pregnant Respondents

The majority (82.8 per cent) of respondents have asked to terminate the pregnancy by the doctors and they denied admission and treatment in the hospitals. Due to the fear of facing discrimination, 41.4 per cent of respondents delivered their baby in the home with the support of local midwives without informing their HIV status. At the same time 58.6 per cent of pregnant respondents went to the hospital only at the time of labour pain and got admission without revealing their

HIV status. The existing discrimination towards people living with HIV positive increased the possibility of taking treatment by the infected people by hiding their infection status. It may increase the risk of infection for the people working in the health care sectors.

Reproductive Sexual Behaviour of Respondents

The majority (40.5 per cent) of respondents have adopted non-terminal method of contraception including oral pills (10.5 per cent), IUDs (14.0 per cent) and condom (16.0 per cent) to avoid pregnancy. Significant per centage (17 per cent) has undergone sterilization to avoid pregnancy after knowing their infection. Condom usage is not popular among married women rather than the women in sex work. The unmarried women have taken the decision to avoid marriage in order to further spread of infection to others.

Attitude of Respondents towards Pregnancy and Child birth

The infected women are in favour of pregnancy right and many (47.5 per cent) respondents are unaware of mother to child transmission and the availability of antiretroviral treatment (50.0 per cent) to prevent child from getting infection from mothers.

Respondents Expectation for Child Care and Positive Parenthood

Majority of respondents expected the facilities of antiretroviral treatment (100 per cent), treatment along with other patients (96.5 per cent), financial assistance (82.0 per cent) to cope up with lose of employment due to HIV/AIDS and life insurance (78.5 per cent) for the people living with HIV positive. They also expected the provision of admission of children in schools (100 per cent), special care home for the abundant women and children with HIV/AIDS (94.5 per cent) and rehabilitation of sex workers by providing alternative employment opportunities (81.5 per cent). They have all suggested that the Government should ensure these facilities for the people living with HIV positive.

SUGGESTIONS

1. Since most of the women are getting infection only after their marriage from their infected husband. Therefore, both the women and men should be motivated to voluntary testing of HIV before marriage for both bride and groom. In order to ensure HIV test, all marriage should be registered under the Marriage Act and a certificate of HIV positive test should be produced at the time of registration.
2. Poverty plays a vital role in the existence of prostitution. The women who are in sex work should be rehabilitated or they should be provided alternative avenues for their survival. This can be possible by associating the sex workers with the women self help group for micro credit. The Department of Social Welfare and Corporation for Women's Development could play a significant role in this regard.
3. Defective socialization is the primary cause for sex outside the marriage. Family and schools are the primary agencies to socialize the individual in accordance with the expectation of the societal norm. Counseling centres should be established in all schools and colleges with the involvement of Sociologist. Community counseling centres should also be established in all villages and towns in co-ordination with local N.G.Os to provide counseling and education to the parents and youths.
4. Exposure to multi media due to the implication of globalization, peer group pressure, modern communication facilities and easy availability of paid sex directly influence the youth to experience pre marital sex. The youth should be advocated the implication of pre marital sex and the importance of having sex after marriage. The youth forum should be formulated in all schools, colleges, villages, towns and cities with the support of N.G.Os , academicians and local government leaders to sensitize the implication of pre marital sex in the context of HIV/AIDS.

5. HIV/AIDS information, its implication and preventive mechanism should reach to the door step of each and every house. This is only possible through mass media, especially through television. The information related to AIDS should be telecasted in all channels frequently between the serials or programmes like other advertisements. The same may also help to overcome stigma and discrimination associated with HIV/AIDS.
6. HIV/AIDS Care Centre should be established in every district with financial support of Government to provide shelter to the abandoned people living with HIV positive.
7. Migration, especially rural to urban migration has direct influence on contracting HIV by youth and transmitting the virus to the housewives. Rural migration owing to economic necessity should be controlled by creating employment opportunities by using locally available resources in the villages and extending financial support to the youth to establish their own enterprises in the village.
8. Gender inequalities should be addressed in all possible ways to empower the women to control over their reproductive health. Women should be educated to negotiate safe sex with their husbands without any hesitation. Gender Sensitization through mass media is a step in the right direction.
9. Culture and tradition of Indian society acting as stumbling block for the implementation of AIDS intervention programmes. The culture prevents people to negotiate issues on reproductive health. Therefore, the culture and tradition of each and every society should be taken into consideration while planning AIDS intervention programmes.
10. Sex education should be incorporated in school and college curriculum in order to influence the students to share their feelings and doubts with regard to their general health and reproductive health without any inhibitions.

11. Government should enact strict law to prevent cross border and internal trafficking of women and girls for sexual exploitation.
12. The reproductive health programme should be incorporated with the programmes of family planning in order to educate the women not only on the methods of fertility control but also the AIDS, route of spread, its implication, safe sex and prevention and control.
13. People living with HIV positive are experiencing various kinds of discrimination in the hospitals. The health care personnel should have the commitment to treat all the patients equally irrespective of their diseases. The discrimination in the hospitals resulted in strengthening the discrimination in the society. Therefore, the health care personnel should be given regular orientation with regard to the treatment of people living with HIV positive.
14. Every Government hospital should have exclusive ward for HIV/AIDS patients with specialized doctors and other medical personnel. It will promote treatment seeking behaviour among the people living with HIV positive.
15. All red light areas in India should be abolished in order to arrest sale of illegal sex, trafficking of girls and the spread of HIV to the general population.
16. Under existing law the sex workers are punished rather than the men who seek sex from them. Therefore, effective law should be enacted to give severe punishment to the women who involve in prostitution as well as to the men who seek sex from prostitutes.
17. The Members of Parliament and Legislative Assemblies should be given target to ensure AIDS free status to their respective constituency.
18. In India, especially in Tamil Nadu, women self help groups are emerging as powerful agents in the social transformation of villages as well as empowering the women in family and community. Therefore, women

self help group should be encouraged to participate in implementing AIDS intervention programmes in their respective areas. Their participation in AIDS intervention programmes will help to eliminate stigma and discrimination associated with AIDS and to bring family and community care to the people living with HIV positive.

19. The local panchayat members should be trained to take up AIDS intervention programmes in their panchayat. The participation of panchayat members in the AIDS intervention programmes will help to prevent and control HIV/AIDS in rural areas.

20. Financial support should be strengthened to the N.G.Os by the Government to ensure regular intervention programmes in all sections of the community.

CONCLUSION

In the span of just two decade, AIDS has turned into an epidemic affecting millions of men, women and children in all countries. It becomes a serious public health problem and expresses the intensity of seriousness the popular term 'Pandemic' is associated with AIDS. The continued spread of HIV is not only threatening millions of lives, but is also either slowing or reversing the progress made in the social and economic development of the countries. The epidemic continues to develop in the atmosphere of fear, prejudice, stigma, silence and discrimination. In spite of serious AIDS intervention programmes to create awareness and advocacy, denial still exists in all sections of society. India is rapidly becoming the epicenter of the AIDS epidemic. Its mobile population and their families, women and children living under hazardous or exploitative conditions and women and children under trafficking are highly vulnerable to HIV/AIDS. Effective law is the urgent requirement to create internal employment opportunities and to check migration, criminal net work of prostitution and trafficking.

Social inequalities, gender discrimination and cultural prejudice made women and children to become the worst victims of HIV/AIDS. The low social and economic status of women and dependence on men limit their control over their sexual and reproductive lives. The power imbalance, violence, and abuse in the family and society increase the chances for women to get exposure to HIV and other sexually transmitted diseases.

Women in sex work are most defenseless and they have no power to insist their customers to use condom. They have not taken this profession on their own choice. Abject poverty, domestic abuse and violence, destitution and abduction and trafficking have pushed these women into this profession. Appalling living condition, entertaining many clients in a day, lack of power to negotiate condom use make them most vulnerable to HIV infection.

Economic uncertainty and growing rural unemployment and underemployment resulted in rural migration. Separation from the family and the hazardous nature of work forces the migrant to seek pleasure with sex workers. The poor access to reproductive health information and AIDS increased not only their vulnerability to HIV but also to their wives. In the context of HIV/AIDS, housewives are adversely affected and they are prone to get infection through their husbands in the marital life which is described as sacrament. Gender insensitivity, discrimination, lack of social and economic status and basic rights reduce the access of women to gain knowledge on HIV/AIDS and its prevention. Economic dependence, social expectations of wives and fear of disrupting family life are powerful disincentives for wives to insist on the use of condoms, especially in environments in which sexual issues are not an acceptable topic for discussion even between husbands and wives. Marriage has given right to men to have unprotected sex with their wives and it also expected wives that accepting unprotected sex of their husband is their responsibility. Moreover, where conception is the desired outcome of marital sexual relations, the use of a condom for protection is unavailable and it is considered as taboo in India. Advocating condom usage in the marital life will not help to promote safe sex and preventing HIV among the innocent wives. Alternative strategy is needed with the consideration of cultural implication and traditional attitude towards sex and sexuality in the marital life.

As consequences of HIV/AIDS, women has to shoulder triple burden – facing stigma and discrimination and caring sick and bearing loss of income in the family. The study has revealed that women experienced more discrimination in the society rather than men. The discrimination is higher in the family due to lack of counseling to the family members and poor knowledge and misconception of HIV/AIDS.

The study further highlighted that the care and support system to the people living with HIV positive in the society is non-existent. Family and community care is essential not only to provide moral support to the infected people but also to control further spread of HIV to the innocent women and to the larger society.

The awareness and knowledge in the practice of safe sex is not correlated in the marital life due to certain cultural importance given to sex and procreation. The notion of sex and sexuality in the Indian context is acting as an obstacle to create safe ground for women to protect themselves from the dreaded infection HIV/AIDS. The power imbalance in interpersonal relationships and in society which create women's subordination must change if women are to be able to protect themselves from HIV/AIDS infection and its consequences. This can be possible through empowerment of women with regard to their reproductive health and it should be given high priority in all matters related to HIV/AIDS. The empowerment of women alone help to realize the dream of AIDS free society.

Commitment from all sections – political, religion, academic, family, health care sector, Government, Non-governmental organisation, public, mass media – is essential to mobilize the people to join together to fight against AIDS to create AIDS free India. Social transformation through Millennium Development Goals in Indian context involves this coordination to realize the vision of HIV/AIDS free world with a missionary zeal. The success depends through value education, morality and social ethics based life among people. The task in this regard is voluminous, l*et al.*l people living in the 21st century take a collective pledge to root out this Global killer as a challenge. IF THERE IS WILL DEFINIELY THERE IS A WAY.

7

Implication of the Research

Based upon the issues highlighted in this study, an attempt is made here to suggest a suitable plan of action towards prevention and control of HIV/AIDS. The major aspects considered under the plan are stated below along with relevant details.

AIDS is not only a medical problem but it is also a social problem. Social responsibility or collective responsibility is the prerequisite for tackling any social problems. With this perspective the model suggested for action is an Integrated Model. This model integrates social and medical aspects with due consideration of cultural values in the society.

Integrated Approach to Provide Care and Support to Women Infected with HIV Positive

Integrated approach is needed to ensure commitment from all sections of population in India to provide care and support to women infected with HIV positive and to establish AIDS free society. The social institution of family, community, hospitals, N.G.Os, women self-help groups and government can be integrated to fight against AIDS and to provide care and support and relief and rehabilitation to the infected and affected people.

Creation of Mechanism for Collection of DATA

Collection of relevant primary data with regard to number of women infected by HIV and circumstances leading to HIV is highly important to formulate policy and plan appropriate intervention programmes for the care and support and relief and rehabilitation of women infected with HIV positive. At present, the Government of India is estimating the number of women with HIV positive based on the sentinel surveillance cases from different government hospitals. The present method provides no accurate information about the number of women infected with HIV and causes and consequences of HIV on women. Therefore, alternative mechanism can be evolved to get the reliable data and information about women infected with HIV positive.

The data on women infected with HIV can be collected not only from Government hospitals and its voluntary testing and counselling centres butlllllll also from private hospitals and private labs. It will help to know the actual rate of infection among women and to plan policy and programmes for prevention and control of HIV among women, care and support and relief and rehabilitation of infected women.

Sensitization of Women with HIV Positive to Take Self Care

Women with HIV positive are either ignorant or lack of knowledge about HIV/AIDS and positive living. The insufficient knowledge on HIV/AIDS made many women to get more depression and lack of hope in life soon after they were told that they are HIV positive. It leads to family disintegration and separation of spouses. Therefore, the infected women must be sensitized with correct information. It will help them to accept the infection and lead a positive life without infecting others. The infected women can also be sensitized on safe sex to protect themselves from reproductive tract infection, safe pregnancy and delivery, breast feeding and non-transmission of infection to their babies.

Family and Community Sensitization

To promote family and community care and support, the basic social institution of family and community can be sensitized in all possible ways with the support of mass media. The integration of infected women into social life is only possible when the family and community accept the reality of HIV/AIDS infected people. The social health of the infected women can be protected by integrating them into family and community life in the society.

Review of Law

The law can be reviewed to protect the civil and human rights of women infected with HIV positive. The review of law is highly essential due to following reasons :

(*a*) **Monitoring of atrocities** : The infected women are subjected to various abuse and violence both in the family and in the society. The HIV infection is feminized in India and all infected women are looked down as immoral women. As a consequence of this notion the infected women are experiencing trauma which affects their total personality. Therefore, law can be reviewed to monitor the atrocities against women infected with HIV positive in order to guarantee a decent and dignified life for them.

(*b*) **Inheritance of property right** : The infected women finds very difficult to inherit the property of her husband after his death. Therefore, the newly formulated property inheritance right of the women can be strengthened to help the infected women get their share like any other women in India.

(*c*) **Job of deceased husband** : The infected women are subjected to severe economic hardships after the death of their husbands. To ensure economic security, law can be enacted to support the infected women to get the job from their husbands' employers.

(*d*) **Life Insurance** : At present the people with HIV positive are denied life insurance scheme by the insurance companies of India. Therefore, law can be formulated to cover the people infected with HIV positive in insurance schemes to enable them to ensure for the benefit of their children and family.

(*e*) **Legalisation of marriage between infected man and woman** : To get mutual care and support, the marriage between infected people can be encouraged by enacting appropriate legalisation. This will also help to control the spread of infection to the larger society. There is no provision in the existing marriage Act of India for legalising the marriage between the HIV infected people. Therefore, the Marriage Act should be reviewed to give provision for legalising the marriage between people living with HIV positives.

(*f*) **Law against HIV/AIDS discrimination** : At present severe stigma is associated with HIV/AIDS. The stigma resulted in social discrimination in which the infected people are subjected to social boycott and social distancing. The elimination of discrimination is only possible by taking the issue under the influence of law. The person or any organisation which involved in discriminating the infected people in general and women in particular can be punished as per legal provisions. The formulation of law against HIV/AIDS discrimination will ensure a decent and dignified life for the people infected with HIV positive.

Formulation of Social Policy and Planning

Social policy and its related planning and implementation are important to secure the right to life of women infected with HIV positive. Formulation of social policy for the welfare of people infected with HIV positive will help to build movements for social justice, economic equality, and participation of infected people in AIDS prevention and control programmes. Social policy can be formulated to ensure the following activities for the care and support and relief and rehabilitation of women infected with HIV positive :

(*a*) **Involving women infected with HIV positive in formulation of policy** : Women infected with HIV can be given representation in the formulation of policy. By involving the infected women in the formulation of policy, the policy-makers will receive first hand information about the urgent needs of the infected women to survive in the society in a dignified manner.

(*b*) **Benefits to infected women under poverty alleviation programme** *:* The women infected by HIV positive are suffering due to economic deprivations. Economic support from government is essential to empower them and motivation towards self care and participation in AIDS prevention and control activities. The government can consider the women infected with HIV positive as economically deprived and marginalized segments and they are to be included in poverty alleviation programmes so as to avail the benefits to sustain their livelihood.

(*c*) **Integration of positive women net work with Women Development Corporation :** The State AIDS Control Societies are encouraging emergence of positive women net work in all districts to provide platform for the infected women to get peer support to share their feelings and problems, information and counseling, and to get economic and medical support in coordination with State AIDS Control Societies and various national and international funding agencies. Women Development Corporation is functioning in Tamil Nadu for the empowerment of women through the concept of women self-help groups. The positive women net work can be integrated with Women Development Corporation to get the status of self help groups and avail financial assistance with subsidy from banks to generate assets and employments. Support for generation of assets and employment will empower the infected women to control their reproductive health as well as to improve their socio-economic status in the society.

(*d*) **Integration of positive women with Women Self-Help Groups :** Women self-help groups in Tamil Nadu are emerging as movement for the empowerment of women. They must be sensitized to participate in AIDS intervention activities as well as in providing care and support to women infected with HIV positive in their respective areas. The integration of positive women with women self-help groups will promote de-stigmatization of diseases, empowerment of infected women and social support system for the women infected with HIV positive.

(*e*) **Integration of Panchayat Raj Institution with State AIDS Control Societies in AIDS prevention and control and care and support programmes for infected people :** Panchayat Raj Institution play an important role in various aspects of Indian social life. It has contributed a lot for the socio-economic transformation in India. Evolving people's participation from identification of problems to evaluation of development programmes implemented for them are the principal areas of Panchayat Raj Institutions. Panchayat Raj Institution can easily mobilize public commitment towards AIDS intervention programmes. Therefore, they can be integrated with State AIDS Control Societies to mobilize public commitment towards AIDS prevention and control, care and support and relief and rehabilitation. It will help for creation of awareness, de-stigmatization of disease and promotion of community care and support for the people infected with HIV positive in general and women in particular.

(*f*) **Creation of free legal cell** : Free legal cell can be created in all State AIDS Control Societies in order to provide legal support to the infected women to fight against atrocities, to avail social security measures and inherit property from their parents and in-laws. Creation of free legal cell also help to protect the women infected with HIV positive from social discrimination and boycott.

(*g*) **Creation of HIV/AIDS information Cell in all hospitals** : HIV/AIDS information cell can be created in all hospitals of rural and urban areas. The HIV/AIDS information cell can have all updated information with regard to medicine, availability of treatment, counselling, availability of provision and benefits and the mechanism of availing these benefits etc. It will help the infected women to sensitize themselves to lead a life with HIV positive without fear and confusion.

(*h*) **Creation of short stay home for women with HIV positive :** Short stay home can be established in all district head quarters in co-ordination with N.G.Os to provide care and support to infected women who are abandoned by their family members. These homes can be provided financial and technical assistance to built infrastructure for the capacity building of inmates. Relief and rehabilitation of infected women can be ensured through these short stay homes.

(*i*) **Integration of media in mobilizing public commitment to create awareness on HIV/AIDS** : Public commitment is essential both for creating awareness on HIV/AIDS without myth and promoting care and support and relief and rehabilitation of people infected with HIV positive. The media can play a vital role as change agents in the society. The regular dissemination of message of HIV/AIDS and the problems experienced by the infected people can bring attitudinal change among the public. The positive attitudinal change among the public will help to build social support system and community care and support for the women infected with HIV positive.

(*j*) **Capacity building** : Capacity building means to equip the people to do things by their own based on 'what they know', 'what they have', 'what they are capable of', and 'what they can do'. The women infected with HIV positive can be helped to identify their innate capacities and accordingly the capacity building programmes are formulated to improve their knowledge, competencies, and vocational, managerial and marketing skills.

Holistic and Non-judgemental Medical Care

Comprehensive medical care and support is the immediate need of women infected with HIV positive. The widespread discrimination in the health-care system created guilt and fear in the minds of infected women to take treatment in the hospitals. In general, treatment seeking behaviour is less among the Indian women. The stigma and discrimination associated with AIDS prevents women to take early treatment for their ailment in the hospital. When compared to other diseases, the cost for the treatment of HIV/AIDS related illness is high and most of the Indian women are not in a position to spend large amounts for availing treatment. The infected women can be given care and support without considering the root cause of infection. There is no need of separate ward for HIV/AIDS patients. They can be given equal treatment like any other patient. The infected women can have easy access to Anti-Retro Viral (ARV) drugs. Therefore, the Government can plan to distribute ARV to the AIDS patients in all Government hospitals including Primary Health Centre. All Primary Health Centre can be equipped with all necessary medical equipments and it can be upgraded to provide treatment for HIV related illness. The upgrading of Primary Health Centre will help to promote treatment seeking behaviour among infected women in India.

Operation of Action Plan

The plan can be operated with the strategy of integration of the social institution of family, community, hospitals, organisations such as N.G.Os, women self help groups and the Government. The role of N.G.Os is very important to sensitize family, community and women self help group to extend their support to the infected women to lead a normal life in the society. Government is the powerful institution to mobilize political commitment towards AIDS intervention by formulating appropriate policy, programmes and reviewing the laws for the welfare of people infected with HIV positive in India.

Institutional Approach for Creating AIDS Free Society

The network of invisible rules and institutional arrangements which guide the behaviour of individual are the base for Indian social structure. By interacting with each other, people are governed by cultural patterns of norms, values, beliefs and symbols. It defines the behaviour of individual towards the fulfillment of social goals. All social institutions are interrelated and interdependent to accomplish basic social tasks. Institutions provide established answers to recurring problems of living. Each institution is a sort of societal master plan – a kind of "grand design" – whereby essential activities are organised, directed, and executed. Because of institutions, every one in the society feels that there is some measure of regularity, efficiency and certainty in daily activities. In the context of HIV/ AIDS, every institution can contribute by taking up certain specific social function to realise the goal of AIDS free society.

The institutions of family, marriage, community, religion, social organisations, government, academic institution, hospitals, industries, media, N.G.Os and women self help groups can be motivated and mobilized towards the activities of AIDS prevention and control, care and support and relief and rehabilitation of people infected by HIV/AIDS.

Family

Family is the primary agent of socialization of individual. If there is any defect in socialization it will lead to the unapproved social behaviour of individual resulting in pre or extra marital sex and using drugs for enjoyment. Therefore, the family can be made aware of its important role in socializing the individual according to the expectation of the society with regard to moral values and ethics. Throughout the world, the family has been assigned the responsibility for shielding, protecting, sustaining and otherwise maintaining children, the infirm and other dependent members of the community. Healthy family relationships afford companionship, love, security, a sense of worth and a general feeling of well being.

Each and every family can be integrated in the AIDS intervention programmes to sensitize the family members to take active part in prevention and control of HIV/AIDS in the family and providing care and support to the infected and affected members of the family. By sensitizing the family with regard to care and support of people infected with HIV positive and destigmatization of disease, it is possible to mobilize the family to take the role of advocacy to provide the community care and support to the infected people.

To prevent and control the spread of HIV in the society, the family can be motivated to socialize the individual on the line of values of society to avoid sex out side marriage and to integrate the infected people within the family. Family harmony is important to prevent extra marital sex which leads to acquiring

HIV infection. Gender equality with regard to reproductive health and women empowerment can be promoted in the family to prevent HIV infection. The family can be motivated to create friendly atmosphere to the adolescents to share their doubts on sex and sexuality with their parents. Sharing and getting information related to sex and sexuality from the parents will prevent the adolescents from sexually transmitted infections including HIV/AIDS. The family can also be made aware of taking early treatment for their sexually transmitted diseases to avoid the possibility of acquiring HIV infection.

To promote care and support in the family, the HIV infected people can be advocated to stay within the family instead of absconding from the family. All family members can be advocated to take care of infected people like any other sick persons and to provide financial and moral support for treatment. Destigmatization of disease can start from the family by considering HIV/AIDS like any other disease. The infected people, especially the women can get their property share of husbands and parents to lead a decent life and they can be encouraged self employment by the parents to sustain in the society.

The N.G.Os and mass media can take a leading role to sensitize the family about HIV/AIDS and integration of infected people within the family.

Marriage

The rate of HIV infection is high among married women who are in monogamous relationship. In many cases the men who experienced pre marital sex with multisexual partners and got infected by HIV are not aware of their infection before marriage. They are married with out being aware of their HIV status. The women are also socialized to be a passive partner in sexual life with their husband. Woman's assertive role in sexual life is condemned by the society in general and husband in particular. This rigid notion on sex and sexuality in marital life is the major cause for the rapid spread of HIV among married women in India. Therefore, changes can be made in the Institution of marriage with regard to sex and sexuality of women in order to empower women over their reproductive health.

Voluntary HIV testing can be advocated among youth before marriage to prevent HIV infection through marriage. Pre-marriage counseling on sex related issues, mutual trust and marital harmony and creation of awareness on sex and reproductive health can be imparted to prevent HIV infection in marital life. Awareness on safe sex, early treatment for STD and parent to child transmission can be imparted to infected couples to control HIV infection in society. Mutual care giving can be promoted among the infected couples in order to prevent separation of spouses due to HIV/AIDS. Marriage between infected male and female can be encouraged as a part of providing relief and rehabilitation for the people infected with HIV positive.

Community

Community sensitization is the urgent need today to control the spread of HIV/AIDS and to provide care and support and relief and rehabilitation of people infected with HIV positive. Since HIV/AIDS is considered as social problem, it is the responsibility of the community to provide care, support, relief and rehabilitation to the infected and affected people. If the community is sensitized, people can be easily mobilized to achieve AIDS free society and to promote care and support and relief and rehabilitation to the people infected with HIV positive.

The HIV/AIDS sensitized community can prevent and control the spread of HIV infection through social mobilization with community participation to promote gender equality in reproductive health and empowerment of women to control over their reproductive health. The community has to take a key role to ensure availability and accessibility of condom for needy people and access to health care to all to control the spread of infection. The community can exercise control over the sale and use of injecting drugs to control infection through contaminated needles. Destigmatization of HIV infection is essential to promote community care and support for the infected people. Community can encourage the marriage between infected male and female in order to promote mutual care and support as well as to mobilize community care and support to people infected with HIV positive. For relief and rehabilitation of infected people, the community can involve in generation of funds to infected people in order to help them to establish self employment.

Sensitization of community on HIV/AIDS can be done with the support of N.G.Os, State AIDS Control Societies, Academic Institutions, local panchayats, mass media and women self help groups.

Religion

Norms, beliefs and rituals provide the cultural fabric of religion. It act as an informal means of social control agent to regulate and shape the behaviour of individual in the society. Each religion has its own structural organisation to mobilize people to impart religious values in their life. These religious organisations or missionaries can be mobilized to take part in creating AIDS free society as well as to provide care and support and relief and rehabilitation to the people infected with HIV positive. The religious missionaries can bring changes in the attitude and behaviour of people by disseminating message on morality, ethics and values of behaviour. Attitudinal change in the minds of people will help to control the spread of HIV infection by promoting gender equality and empowerment of women. Religious institutions can influence people to provide care and support to the infected people. These institutions can also establish care home and funding support to N.G.Os for the welfare of people infected with HIV positive. The religious institution can also mobilize to start employment programmes for the deprived people in general and infected people in particular. The religious missionaries can be sensitized on HIV/AIDS with the support of government and religious leaders.

Social Organisations

Social organisations, especially the Panchayat Raj Institutions are working for the welfare of the people with the principal with people's participation in all its activities. People participation is the core essence for the stability of Panchayat Raj Institutions in India. Panchayat Raj Institutions can be integrated with AIDS intervention mission along with government organisations to prevent and control the spread of infection in India. The local panchayat can be mobilized to work with N.G.Os to promote women empowerment, impart value education to public and to create awareness on safe sex practices and condom use to prevent and control HIV infection in society. It can also destigmatize the disease by involving in AIDS intervention programmes, creating information cell on HIV/ AIDS and its related issues and extending funding support to infected people to take treatment. The panchayat raj institution can provide relief and rehabilitation by providing financial support to infected people for the generation of self employment for their dignified survival in the society.

The members of the Panchayat Raj Institution can be given training and motivation by the State AIDS Control Society to take part in AIDS intervention activities.

Government

Government has the power to give direction to human affairs and to mobilize people's actions towards collective goals towards realizing welfare state ideals. It also has power to bring about changes in people's attitude and behaviour. Therefore, government has to play a vital role in prevention and control of HIV/AIDS, care and support and relief and rehabilitation of people infected with HIV positive by formulating policy, reviewing law and planning and implementing programmes.

To prevent and control HIV/AIDS in India, the Government can make policy for creating AIDS free society with the support of all social institutions. It has to involve in planning, implementing, monitoring and evaluating AIDS intervention programmes in order to find the success and to frame alternative measures to reach the goal of AIDS free society. The government can frame policy to include infected people in all intervention programmes in order to enhance the effectiveness of the programmes. It has to organise regular campaigns against HIV/ AIDS in all districts to create awareness on HIV/AIDS in the society. To control the spread of infection poverty alleviation programmes can be strengthened to generate employment opportunities for women to prevent their involvement in sex work. It has to create treatment facilities for STD in all public health centres to control the possibility of infection through STD.

To promote care and support, the government can influence the health care sectors to give treatment to HIV infected people along with other patients. It will help to destigmaitize the disease in the society. The Government can ensure the availability of ARV drug in all districts hospitals to promote the access of ARV drug to all infected people. Legislation can be enacted to include HIV infected people under Life Insurance Scheme. It will help not only the infected people but also their family members. To provide relief and rehabilitation to the infected people the Government can establish care home in all district headquarters. It has to rehabilitate the sex workers by creating alternative employment opportunities.

Academic Institutions

Academic institutions are considered as an important agent of socialization of individual in the society. The academic institutions - schools and colleges - not only provide formal, and systematic training to the students but it also teach more than the skills and information specified in the curriculum. Students learn values, morality, responsibility, conscientiousness, reliability, thoroughness, self-control, efficiency and emotional stability from their schools and colleges. The healthy future of the nation is vested with younger generation, especially with the students. Therefore, the students can be made aware of HIV/AIDS and their role in creating AIDS free society.

Value-based education, reproductive health education, education on gender sensitization and HIV/AIDS is important to prevent and control HIV/AIDS. This type of education can be imparted to the students through schools and college curriculum. All academic institution can have tutorial system to have close interaction with students. The tutorial system will help to understand the problems of the students in all aspects. The academic institutions can be insisted to establish counseling cell to counsel the students, especially the girl students on reproductive health and HIV/AIDS. The academic institutions can be motivated to organise meetings, workshops and seminars to create awareness on HIV/AIDS and reproductive health among students. It can also be encouraged to develop curriculum on extension activities in coordination with N.G.Os to generate awareness on HIV/AIDS and family and community care for people infected with HIV positive which leads to prevention and control of HIV infection in India. As a part of providing care and support, the academic institution can promote the involvement of parents-teacher association in its AIDS intervention activities. It will help to destigmatize the disease among the parents. Enrolment of infected children in schools and colleges is important to ensure care and support for people infected with HIV positive. It can be made possible by sensitizing parents and students through parent-teacher associations. The academic institutions can organise campaign for the promotion of relief and rehabilitation to people infected with HIV positive through their extension activities with the support of N.G.Os.

Teachers may be trained to take up AIDS intervention activities with the support of N.G.Os and State AIDS Control Society.

Hospitals

Society's well-being depends upon a healthy labor force for carrying out vital tasks. Consequently, disease and illness must be socially controlled and the people under sick can ensure holistic and non-judgemental medical care and support for proper societal functioning. Physicians, nurses and other practitioners have vital role in ensuring equal and client friendly treatment to all patients. It is the duty of the hospitals to destigmatize the diseases and to provide healthy service to care seekers to promote treatment seeking behaviour among the infected people.

The hospitals can play a vital role in prevention and control of HIV/AIDS by promoting client friendly treatment, syndromic management for STD/RTI (Reproductive Tract Infection) and counselling to sterilized couples about safe sex to prevent HIV and other sexually transmitted infection. Counselling must be made compulsory in the hospital for both the patients and parents about HIV/AIDS before and after HIV test. Destigmatization of HIV/AIDS, non-judgemental and equal treatment to HIV/AIDS patients and creating the access to ARV drugs to HIV infected people will ensure care and support in the hospitals. The health care institutions can also involve in providing relief and rehabilitation to the infected people by way of supporting infected inmates of short stay home run by the government and N.G.Os.

The health care providers can be sensitized on HIV/AIDS to treat HIV/AIDS patients like any other patients without any discrimination.

Industries

Migrant labourers are more prone to HIV infection due to their multisexual contacts with sex workers. These labourers are ignorant about HIV/AIDS and its prevention and implications. Therefore, they can be given correct information about HIV/AIDS in their workplace by the management of industries as part of Workers Education. The involvement of industries in AIDS intervention activities can help to prevent and control the spread of HIV infection among the labour community.

Involvements of industries in HIV/AIDS intervention programmes are very essential to control and prevent HIV/AIDS among migrant labourers. The management of industries can be sensitized to frame work place policy to take work place intervention programmes and influence the trade unions to take part in HIV/AIDS intervention programmes to control and prevent the infection among labourers. The industries can also involve in providing care and support to the HIV infected workers by way of retaining them in work and giving equal opportunities in recruitment for infected people. The human resource management of industries can take up advocacy role to eliminate stigma and discrimination against HIV infected people in workplace. The Employees State Insurance (ESI) hospitals can be linked with AIDS intervention mission to provide treatment to the HIV infected labourers. The industries can also involve in relief and rehabilitation of HIV infected people by opening employment opportunities for the infected people and by providing medical leave and financial assistance to infected labourers to take treatment for their HIV related illness.

The State AIDS Control Societies and N.G.Os can take responsibilities to mobilize and sensitize industries towards creating AIDS free society.

Mass Media

Media is an important agent to disseminate the message to larger society. In all societies people are very keen to know day to day events of the world through various media. Television plays a vital role in attracting all categories of people and it disseminates the information at the doorstep of the people. The print and visual media can be sensitized and mobilized to give regular coverage on HIV/AIDS news and to mobilize the public opinion towards AIDS intervention mission to control and prevent the spread of HIV infection. It can also develop networking with N.G.Os to collect case studies of infected people for their projection. The media can have social responsibility to protect the people from the dreaded diseases. Therefore, it can give correct information about HIV/AIDS to public. It will help to destigmatize the disease in the society. As a part of providing care and support and relief and rehabilitation to the infected people, the media have to cover the violation of human rights experienced by the infected people in the society and disseminating message on family and community care. The projection of HIV/AIDS related issues in media will help to mobilize community support to the people infected with HIV positive.

Non Government Organisations (N.G.Os)

N.G.Os are really interested to provide care to the uncared sections and the people at the bottom of the social stratum. Their work is people centered and hence they reach the unreached rural poor and live and work with them. They strive to promote the lives of the oppressed, deprived, marginalized, impoverished, downtrodden, hopelost, helpless, powerless, deserted and poverty stricken in the society. Therefore, the N.G.Os involvement is essential to provide care and support and relief and rehabilitation of women infected by HIV/AIDS.

There are two kinds of N.G.Os working in AIDS intervention activities. One is funding agencies which provide funds to the N.G.Os working in the field and the second is field agencies which implement the programmes for the benefit of larger society.

The funding agencies are expected to involve in :

1. Conducting research on women infected with HIV/AIDS among different cross sections.
2. Extending funds to the N.G.Os which focuses on care and support and relief and rehabilitation of women infected with HIV positive.

3. Establishment of Relief and Rehabilitation Cells in all States with partnership of Government. It can have common phone number in order to facilitate the infected and affected people to get immediate relief and rehabilitation for survival.
4. Co-ordination and networking of N.G.Os to know the success and difficulties faced in the implementation of care and support and relief and rehabilitation programmes to the infected women. It will help to find out alternative strategy for the sustainability of care and support services in the society for the people infected with HIV positive.

The N.G.Os working in the field can take up the following action for care and support and relief and rehabilitation of women infected with HIV positive :

1. Family and community sensitization to integrate the HIV infected women into the family and community.
2. Awareness building – (health and gender awareness) creation of awareness on HIV, STD, RTI, safe sex.
3. Promotion of treatment seeking behaviour among women infected with HIV positive and creation of awareness on the access to treatment.
4. Creation of positive women network to motivate the infected women to involve in positive prevention programmes.
5. Capacity building – promotion of vocational training to the infected women to generate self employment to sustain in the society.
6. Building hopes – promotion of self care and self support among the women infected with HIV to develop confidence in their life.
7. Networking with Human Right Organisations to represent the problems and humiliation experienced by the infected people.

N.G.Os can bring attitudinal change in the minds and behaviour of people related to their sexual behaviour in order to prevent and control HIV/AIDS in the society through its effective involvement in AIDS intervention activities in coordination with Government and other funding agencies.

N.G.Os are capable of mobilizing grassroot leaders and SHG members towards advocating the family and community care and support for the people infected with HIV positive. It can also conduct research on various issues of HIV/AIDS in order to help policy makers and programmes planners to prevent and control HIV/AIDS in India. The N.G.Os can influence HIV infected people to bring their co-ordination in disseminating information on HIV/AIDS to the public in general and target groups in particular. The taboo and rigidity on the usage of condom among Indian women can be removed with the support of N.G.Os working with the people.

Women Self-help Groups

Women self-help groups are emerging as a movement in Tamil Nadu in women's empowerment. The women self-help groups are more powerful in mobilizing the people towards common cause. The Integration of the women self-help group in AIDS intervention activities will help to sensitize the larger women folk within short period.

The women self-help groups can be motivated to involve in mobilizing the women to take part in AIDS intervention activities. It will help in awareness creation on safe sex as well as to sensitize the women on reproductive health and their rights. The women's awareness and their empowerment on reproductive health will prevent and control HIV infection among women of different categories. The stigma and discrimination can be removed from the society if the infected women are accepted and assisted by the members of women self-help groups. The women self help group can be motivated to provide care and support and relief and rehabilitation by accommodating sex workers and infected women in their groups and assist them through micro credit facilities in the promotion of income generation activities. Family and community care and support can be realized with the active participation of women self help groups in AIDS intervention programmes.

The N.G.Os and State AIDS Control Societies can take up the responsibility of providing training and other technical support to women self help groups in AIDS intervention activities.

Criteria to Implement Action Plan

Joint effort is an urgent need to prevent and control HIV/AIDS in the society. The institution of Government, N.G.Os,

Academic Institution and Mass Media can take a lead role to sensitize other social institutions of family, marriage, community, religion, social organisations, hospitals, industries and self help groups. Sensitization of social institutions definitely helps to sensitize the public and mobilize public commitment towards the mission of creating AIDS free society.

Scope for Further Research

The present study has been conducted with specific objectives in Chennai City, Tamil Nadu. As there are certain issues remaining unexplored in this research, the researcher presents the following suggestion for further research.

1. A similar study can be conducted throughout Tamil Nadu to obtain comprehensive view on impact of HIV/AIDS on women's social and economic life and the nature of discrimination experienced by them.
2. A study can also be conducted to find out whether the practices of reproductive health choice have a link with unsafe sexual practices in marital life.
3. A study can be conducted to find out the psychological problems of people living with HIV positive.

Integrated Approach to Provide Care and Support to Women Infected with HIV Positive

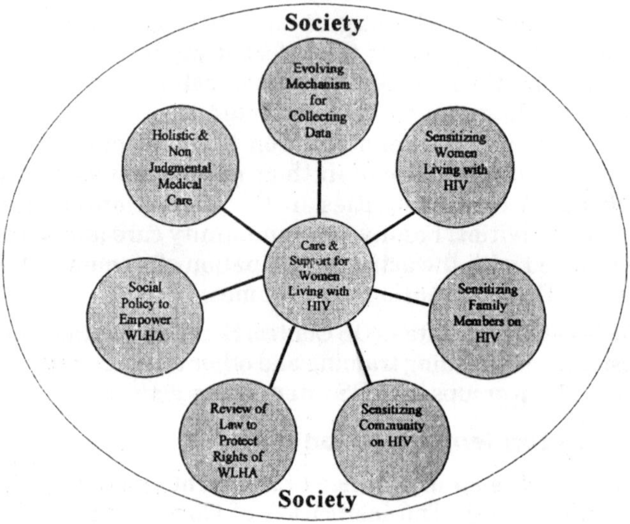

Institutionalized Approach for AIDs Free Society-Action Plan

INSTI-TUTIONS	ACTIVITIES PREVENTION AND CONTROL	CARE AND SUPPORT	RELIEF & REHABILITATION
FAMILY	❖ Socialization of individual based on morality, values and ethic ❖ Perception, motivation and learning about sex ❖ Gender equality and women empowerment ❖ Integration of HIV infected people ❖ Sharing of information on safe sex and early treatment for STD	❖ Support to treatment for infected ❖ Caring of sick and orphaned children ❖ Moral & psychological support ❖ Property sharing	❖ Financial support to the infected to establish self employment ❖ Marriage between infected can be encouraged
MARRIAGE	❖ Pre-marriage counseling ❖ Motivation to voluntary HIV test ❖ Awareness on sex and reproductive health ❖ Mutual trust and marital harmony ❖ Knowledge on the prevention of parent to child transmission	❖ Living together ❖ Facilitating treatment to the infected people and children ❖ Mutual care giving	❖ Marriage between infected male and female
COMMUNITY	❖ Community participation to create knowledgeable community ❖ Gender equality and empowerment of women ❖ Creation of awareness on safe sex ❖ Social mobilization to generate social responsibility	❖ De-stigmatization of disease ❖ Social interaction with the infected ❖ Acceptance of marriage between infected	❖ Generation of funds to self employment for sex workers and to the networks of positive people.
RELIGION	❖ Involvement of religious missionaries in AIDS prevention programmes and advocacy ❖ Networking with NGOs ❖ Imparting morality, ethics and values of individual behavior	❖ Establishing care homes with treatment ❖ Funding support to NGOs ❖ Advocating the public with regard to care and support of the infected people	❖ Providing employment to the infected people

A I D S F R E E S O C I E T Y

(Contd.)

INSTI-TUTIONS	ACTIVITIES PREVENTION AND CONTROL	CARE AND SUPPORT	RELIEF & REHABILITATION	
SOCIAL ORGANI-SATION	❖ Involving caste panchayat and local panchayat in intervention ❖ Empowerment of women ❖ Value education	❖ De-stigmatization of disease ❖ Non -discriminatory approach towards infected people ❖ Funding support to infected to take treatment	❖ Support to infected and sex workers for self employment	A I D S F R E E S O C I E T Y
GOVERNMENT	❖ Legislation, funding support to NGOs, policy, planning, programme, monitoring & evaluation ❖ Formulation of policy on non-discrimination in work place ❖ Regular campaign against HIV / AIDS in all districts ❖ Generation of local self employment ❖ Treatment facilities in all PHCs	❖ Orientation to health staff ❖ Distribution of ARV through all district hospitals ❖ Insurance to HIV positive ❖ Infected people can be included in poverty alleviation programmes ❖ Allotment of fund to care and support programmes	❖ Care homes in all district headquarters ❖ Nutritious food to infected people ❖ Contact phone no. for needy for help (Help line)	
ACADEMIC INSTI-TUTIONS	❖ Value based education ❖ Reproductive health education ❖ School and College intervention on HIV/AIDS ❖ Creation of guidance counseling cell ❖ Sensitization of Parents-Teachers Association	❖ De-stigmatization of disease ❖ Enrolment of infected children	❖ Design vocational training programmes	
HOSPITALS	❖ Syndromic management ❖ Counseling before and after HIV test to patients and family members ❖ Client friendly treatment and ❖ Counseling to the sterilized couples about safe sex ❖ Integration of AIDS intervention with family planning ❖ Sensitization of health care personnel ❖ Breast feeding counseling		❖ Counseling cell ❖ Networking with NGOs for better treatment	

(Contd.)

INSTI-TUTIONS	ACTIVITIES PREVENTION AND CONTROL	CARE AND SUPPORT	RELIEF & REHABILITATION
INDUSTRIES	❖ Workplace intervention ❖ Creation of awareness through workers education programme ❖ Counseling cell ❖ Involvement of trade unions in intervention	❖ Employment to infected people ❖ Equal treatment ❖ Advocacy ❖ Linking ESI hospitals with AIDS intervention	❖ Employment to infected people ❖ Medical leave and financial assistance / loan for treatment
MASS MEDIA	❖ Compulsory coverage on HIV / AIDS ❖ Mobilize people participation ❖ Documentary on HIV/AIDS to educate the mass ❖ Dissemination of information and education	❖ Information for de-stigmatization of disease ❖ Projection of the violation of human rights	❖ Dissemination of message on family care ❖ Projecting the issues of abandoned
NGOs	❖ Intervention for prevention and control ❖ Mobilization of grass root leaders ❖ Advocacy to family, community ❖ Coordination with NGOs & Govt. ❖ Involving infected people in intervention	❖ ARV distribution ❖ Counseling ❖ Liaison with hospitals ❖ Advocacy to family members	❖ Care homes ❖ Capacity building through income generation activities ❖ Integration of infected in the society
WOMEN SELF HELP GROUPS (SHG)	❖ Involvement in intervention programmes ❖ Mobilization of people ❖ Creation of awareness on safe sex	❖ Integration of infected in SHGs	❖ Support to creation of income generation activities

A I D S F R E E S O C I E T Y

Bibliography

BOOKS

Abraham, Francis, 1982. *Modern Sociological Theory : An Introduction*. Oxford University Press, New Delhi.

Ahuja, Ram. 1999. *Social Problems in India*. Jaipur and New Delhi: Rawat Publications.

Benedict, B.B. Naanen. 1999. *Itinerant Gold Mines : Prostitution in the Cross River Basin of Nigeria, 1930-1950*. In Women in Prostitution by Mary A. Yeager, Cheltenham. U.K., Edward Elgar Publishing Limited.

Bongaarts.1988. *Approach to Prevention*. New York. Elsevier Science Publishing Co.

Digumarti Bhaskara Rao. 2000. *An Introduction to HIV/AIDS*. New Delhi: Discovery Publishing House.

Digumarti Bhaskara Rao. 2000. *HIV/AIDS AND NGOs*. International Encyclopedia of AIDS. New Delhi. Discovery Publishing House.

Digumarti Bhaskara Rao. 2000. *Issues and Challenges*. International Encyclopaedia of AIDS. Discovery Publishing House. New Delhi.

Doshi, S.L. 2003. *Modernity, Post modernity and Neo-Sociological Theories*. Jaipur and New Delhi. Rawat Publiations).

Dube, Siddharth. 2000. *Sex lies and AIDS*. New Delhi. HarperCollins.

Dutta, P.K. 1998. *Public Health and Social Aspects : Some Selected Essay*. Atlantic Publishers and Distributors. New Delhi.

Ellison, Bryan J. and Peter H. Duesberg. 1994. *Why we will Never Win the War on AIDS*. California. Inside Story Communication. El Cerrito.

Erving, Goffman 1963. *Stigma : Notes on the Management of Spoiled Identity*. New Jersey : Prentice-Hall.

Francois-Xavier Bagnoud Center for Health and Human Rights. 1995. *"AIDS, Health and Human Rights – An explanatory manual"*. International Federation of Red Cross and Red Crescent Societies. Harvard School of Public Health.

Harry, W. Kestler, Ronald Medley and Tim Horn. 1998. *HIV, Description of*. In Encyclopedia of AIDS : A Social, Political, Cultural and Scientific Record of HIV Epidemic, by Raymond A. Smith, Fitzroy Dearborn Publishers, Chicago, London.

Horton, Paul B. and Leslie, Gerald R.. 1970. *The Sociology and Social Problems*. (4th Ed.), Appleton Century Crofts, New York.

Hospedales, 1988. *Approach to Prevention*. New York: Elsevier Science Publishing Co.

James, W. Vander Zanden. 1990. *The Social Experience – An Introduction to Sociology*. New York: McGraw-Hill Publishing Company.

Jon, Tinker. 1988. *Extract from Ranee Sabatier's Blaming others – Prejudice, Race, and World wide AIDS*. London, Panos Institute.

Jonathan, H Turner. 2002. *The structure of Sociological Theory*. Jaipur: Rawat Publications.

Jones, Pip. 2005. *Introducing Social Theory*. Cambridge: Polity Press.

Kapadia, K.M. 1966. *Marriage and Family In India*. Calcutta: Oxford University Press.

Khorshed, M. Pavri. 1992. *Challenge of AIDS*. National Book Trust.

Khurana, Pushpa. 1998. *The Awesome Challenge AIDS*. New Delhi: Diamond Pocket Books (P) Ltd.

Kimberly, B. Sessions and Richard Loftus. 1998. *Immune System*. In Encyclopedia of AIDS : A Social, Political, Cultural and Scientific Record of HIV Epidemic, by Raymond A. Smith, Fitzroy Dearborn Publishers, Chicago, London, 1998.

Mark, Preston. 1998. *HIV, Origin of*. In: *Encyclopedia of AIDS : A Social, Political, Cultural and Scientific Record of HIV Epidemic, Raymond A. Smith,* Fitzroy Dearborn Publishers, Chicago, London.

Marx, Karl 1964. *Early Writings*. (Transulated and editated by T.B. Bottomore). New York: McGraw-Hill.

Merton and Nisbet. 1971. *Contemporary Social Problems*. Harcourt Brace. New York.

Merton, R.K. Social Structure and Anomie. *American Sociological Review*. October 1938.

Merton, R.K. *Social Theory and Social Structure*. Free Press, Glencoe, New York, 1957.

Prakasa Rao, V.V. and Nandini Rao V. 1982. *Marriage, the family and Women in India*. New Delhi: Heritage Publicity.

Ramamurthy, V. 2000. *AIDS and the Human Survival*. Authors Press, India Health Foundation.

Ramamurthy, V. 2000. *Global Patterns of HIV/AIDS Transmission*. Delhi: Authors Press.

Ramamurthy, V. 2003. *HIV/AIDS Vulnerability in South Asia*. Delhi: Authors Press.

Randy and Shills. 1987. *And the Band Played on*. New York: St. Martin's Press.

Reid., Elizabeth 2000. *Young Women and the HIV Epidemic*. In Internatioanl Encyclopaedia of AIDS – Intrduction to HIV/AIDS edited by Digumarti Bhaskara Rao. New Delhi: Discovery Publishing House.

Sabatier, Renee. 1988. *Blaming Others : Prejudice, Race and Worldwide AIDS*. London: The Panos Institute.

Sahmi, Ashok, 1993. *HIV and AIDS in India – An Update for Action*. Indian Society of Health Administrators. YES YES Prenters. Bangalore.

Sethi, Praveen. 2000. *Hand Book of Modern Tourism*. New Delhi: Anmol Publication Pvt Ltd.

Sinha, S.P. 1999. *India Sits on AIDS Bomb*. B.R. Publishing Corportation, Delhi.

Thai, Myo. 2000. *The Economic Implications of AIDS in Southeast*

Asia : Equity Considerations. In: *Economic Implication of AIDS in Asia,* David E. Bloom and Joyce V. Lyons (Eds.). United Nations Development Programme Division. Regional Bureau for Asia and the Pacific. New Delhi.

Theresa, McGovern and Raymond A. Smith. 1998. *AIDS, Case Definition of*. In: *Encyclopedia of AIDS : A Social, Political, Cultural and Scientific Record of HIV Epidemic,* Raymond A. Smith (Eds.). Fitzroy Dearborn Publishers. Chicago, London.

Thomas, Gracious. N.P. Sinha, Johnson Thomas K. 1997. *AIDS, Social Work and Law*. Rawat Puplications, New Delhi.

JOURNALS

Ainsworth, Martha and Mead Over. 1994. "AIDS and African Development". *The World Bank Research Observer*. 9(2).

Alessandro, Cozzi Lepri. Patrizio Pezzotti Maria Dorrucci. 1995. "HIV Disease Progression in 854 women and men infected through injecting drug use and heterosexual sex and followed for up to nine years from seroconversion". *British Medical Journal*. Vol. 10. No. 12. February.

Amanda, Kolburn Kawal and Lynn Blinn Pike. 2004. "Role of older siblings in protectying adolescents from engaging in unsafe sexual practices". *Family Relations. Inter disciplinary Journal of Applied Family Studies.* 53(4) July.

Anastasia, J. Gage. 1998. "Sexual Activity and Contraceptive Use : The Components of the Decisionmaking Process". 29(2).

Anjum, Suresh K. 1998. "Indian women and AIDS". *Social Welfare.* 45(1).

Ann, E. Biddlecom, Beth Fredrick and Susheela Singh. 2004. "Women, Gender and HIV/AIDS – Women bear the heaviest HIV/AIDS burden, but they can't prevent its spread by themselves". *In Countdown 2015 (Special Issues)* – Sexual & Reproductive Health & Rights for all. Special Report, ICPD At Ten where are we now? Published by Population Action International, Washington D.C.

Ann, E. Biddlecom. John B. Casterline and Aurora E. Ferez. 1997. "Spouses Views of Contraception in the Pilippines". International Family *Planning Perspectives.* 23(3) September.

Ann, K. Blanc and Ann A. Way. 1998. "Sexual Behavior and Contraceptive knowledge and use among Adolescents in Developing Countractives". *Studies in Family Planning.* 29(2) June.

Any, Coen, Geeta Rao Gupta and Dina Bogecho. 2004. "Are We there yet?". *In Countdown 2015 (Special Issues)* – Sexual & Reproductive Health & Rights for all. Special Report, ICPD At Ten where are we now? *Published by Population Action International, Washington D.C.*

ARROW FOR CHANGE. 2000. "Research on Sex, Contraception and Reproduction among young Filipinas in Australia". 6(2).

Bai, Lakshmi Krishna Murthy. Bima P. Charles. 1999. "Communication Approaches to Sex workers in a Highway Project". *Health Education in South East Asia.* 13(4).

Baingana, Gladys. Kyung-Hee Choi, Donald C. Barrett Ronald Byansi and Norman Hearst. 1995 "Female partners of AIDS patients in Uganda : reported knowledge, perceptions and plans". *AIDS.*

9 (suppl 1). July.

Banatuvala, J.E. 1995. "Unlinked anonymous HIV screening Programme in England and Wales". *British Medical Journal (BMJ).* 11(12) April.

Barbara, S. Mensch, Deniel Bagah, Wesle H. Clark, and Fred Binka. 1999. "The Changing Nature of Adolescence in thssena-Nankana District of Northern Ghana". *Studies in Family Planning.* 30(2) June.

Basia, Zaba and Simon Gregson. 1998. "Measuring the impact of HIV on fertility in Africa". *AIDS.* 12(i).

Baylay, A.C. 1984. "Aggressive Kaposis' Sarcroma in Zambia, 1983". *Lancet.* 23 April.

Berkley, S. Naamara W. Okware S. 1990. "AIDS and HIV infection in Uganda : are more women infected than men? *AIDS.* No. 4.

Bhave, G. Wagle U. Desai S. 1992. "HIV surveillance and prevention". *II International Congress on AIDS in Asia and the Pacific.* New Delhi. November.

Bhave, Geeta. Christina P. Lindan. Esther S. Hudes. Seema Desai. Usha Wagle. Shrivam P. Tripathi and Feffrey S. Mandel. 1995. "Impact of an intervention of HIV, sexually transmitted diseases, and condom use among sex workers in Bombay, India". *AIDS* Vol. 9. (suppl 1).

Biggar, R.J. 1984. "Epidemiology of AIDS in Europe". *European Journal of Cancer and clinical Oncology.* 20(2).

Carael, Michel. Bernhard Schwartlander. 1998. "Demographic impact of AIDS". *AIDS*. 12. (Supp. 1)

Carovano, K. 1992. "More than mothers and whores : Redefining the AIDS prevention needs of women". *International Journal of Health Services.* Vol . 21(1).

Celentano, David C. 2000. Preventive intervention to reduce sexually transmitted infections : A field trial in the Royal Thai Army. *Achieves of Internal Medicine.* No. 160.

Chuttani, 1991. "Awareness and knowledge about AIDS among rural population in India". *CARC CALLING.* 3(4).

Dalla, Rochelle 2004. "I Fell off (The Mothering) Track : Barriers to effective Mothering among Prostituted women". *Family Relations. Inter disciplinary Journal of Applied Family Studies*. 53(2).

Deneberg, Risa. 1997. "Childhood Sexual Abuse as an HIV Risk Factor in Women". GMHC Treatment Issues. *A Publication of the Gay Men's Health Crisis.* VI(7/8).

Dev, Vasu 2005. "Ore Eravu –Highways Alahiyaha Namathu Nirubar. *Kumutham*. May 23.

Elfkord, J. Dwyer J. 1993. "HIV and AIDS in Asia and the Pacific". *AIDS Care.* Vol 5.

Evasius, K. Bauni and Ben Obonyo Jarabi. 2000. "Family Planning and Sexual Behaviour in the Era of HIV/AIDS : The Case of Nakuru District, Kenya". *International Family Planning Perspectives.* 31(1) March.

Feffrey, O'Malley. 2004. "SAHR with HIV – Can This Marriage work? Linking the response to AIDS with sexual and reproductive health and rights". In *Countdown 2015* (Special Issues) – Sexual & Reproductive Health & Rights for all. Special Report, ICPD At Ten where are we now? Published by Population Action International, Washington D.C.

Fleming, P.L. Ciesielski, C.A. Byers, R.H. Castro K.G. Berkelman R.L. 1993. "Gender Differences in reported AIDS-indicative diagnoses". *Journal of infectious Diseases*. No. 168.

Foley, M, Skurmic. 1994. "Family Support for hetrosexual partner in HIV – Serodiscordant Couples". *AIDS*. October. 8(10).

Frances, A. Althaus. 1997. "Female Circumcision : Rite of Passage or Violation of Rights". *International Family Planning Perspectivesl*. 23(3), September.

Friedlan, G.H., Saltzman, B. Vileno, J. 1991. "Survival difference in Patients with AIDS". *Journal of Acquired Immune Deficiency Syndrome*. 4.

Gangakhedkar, 1997. "Spread of HIV infection in married monogamous women in India". *Journal of the American Medical Association*. 20(2). *In International Family Planning Perspectives*. 278(23).

Gangakhedkar, R.R. 1999. " Chemoprophylaxis to Reduce Mother-to-Child Transmission of HIV-1 Infection". *AIDS Research & Review*. 2(3).

Garenne, Michel Stephen Tollman and Kathleen Kahn. 2000. "Premarital Fertility in Rural South Africa : A Challenge to Existing Population Policy. *Studies in Family Planning*. 13(1).

Golmare, 2002. 'Adopting strategic approach for reaching out to inaccessible population viz'. Abstract WePeF6707F abstract, *The XIV International AIDS Conference.*

Grosskurth, H. 2000. "Link between control of STD and HIV prevention: Mwanza and Rakai Studies". *Lancet*. No. 355. *In AIDS update*. 2000. 5(3).

Halperin, D.R. Bailey. R.C. 1999. "Male Circumcision and HIV infections : 10 years and counting. *Lancet*. 35A(192).

Hardman, K. 1997. "A Social work group for prostituted women with children". *Journal of Social Work with groups*. No. 20.

Here, GM. 1999. " AIDS and stigma". *Am Behav Scientist*.42(7) :1106-16. Available at : http :// psychology.ucdavis.edu/rainbow/html/bibabs.html.

Herek, GM, Gillis JR, Cogan J. 1999. "Psychological sequelae of hate crime victimization among lesbian, gay, and bisexual adults". *Journal of Consultation Clinical Psychology*.67(6).

Hirve.S.S. and Sathe. P.V. 1997 "AIDS awareness among Married Women in Reproductive Age group from Rural Areas of Three Coastal Districts". *AIDS Research and Review*. Vol. 2. No. 4. Oct-Dec.

Inn Mackinnon and Adam Piore .2001. "The Quiet AIDS crisis". *SPAN*. Vol. XLII. Number. 5. September/October.

Isabelle de Zoysa. Michael D. Sweat and Julie A. Denison. 1996. "Faithful but fearful : reducing HIV transmission in stable relationships". *AIDS*. Vol 10, (Suppl A)

Jacob K. John. 2000. "Do most individual with HIV/AIDS consider suicide?". *Abstract in First International Conference of AIDS*. India.

Jacob K.S. Eapen V. 1987. "AIDS Phobia". *British Journal of Psychiatry*. No.150.

Jagatheeswary. P.A.T. Shameem Banu and Rosy Vennila. 2000. "HIV/AIDS and STD – A Five year study at Chennai Medical College". *First International Conference of AIDS*. India.

Jeanette J. Rodrigues. Snjay M. Mehendala. Mary E. Shepherd. Anand D. Divekar. Raman R. Gangakhedkar. 1995. "Risk factors for HIV infection in people attending clinics for sexually transmitted diseases in India". *British Medical Journal*. Vo. 11. No. 8. Oct.

Jeff Goodwin. 1978. "The Libidinal Constitution of a High Risk Social Movement : Affected ties and solidarity in the Huk Rebellion 1946-1954. In *American Sociological Review*. Vol. 62. No. 1. 1997.

John C. Caldwell, Pat Caldwell, Bruce K. Cald ell, and Indrani. 1998. "The Construction of Adolescence in Changing World : Implications for Sexuality, Reproduction, and Marriage". *Studies in Family Planning*.Vol. 29. No. 2. June.

John Stover and Peter Way. 1998. "Projecting the impact of AIDS on mortality". *AIDS*. Vol. 12. Supplement. 1

John T. Babu P. Jayakumari H. Simoes E. 1987. "Prevalence of HIV infection in risk groups in Tamilnadu, India". *Lancet*.

Jones, Heidi. Nafissatau Diop. Ian Askew and Inoussa Kabore. 1999. "Female Genetal Cutting practices in Burkina Fasa and Mali and Their Negative Health Outcomes". *Studies in Family Planning*. 30(3).

Karen Hardee, Kokila Agarwal, Nancy Luke, Ellen Wilson, Margaret Pendzich, Marguerite Farrell and Harry Cross. 1999. "Reproductive Health Policies and Programs in Eight Countries : Progress Since Cairo". *International Family Planning Perspectives*. Vol. 25. Supplement. January.

Kelly. R.J. and Gray. R.H. 2003. "Age Differences in Sexual Partners and Risk of HIV-1 Infection in Rural Uganda". *Journal of Acquired Immune Deficiency Syndrome*. No. 32.

Kim, Best. 2001. " Removing Specialized Cells may Explain Protection Effect. *Net Work. Family Health International*. 20(4).

Kim, Best. 2001. "HIV Infected women less fertile". *Net Work*. Vol. 20. No. 4.

Kim, Best. 2001. "HIV Positive Women have Different Needs". *Net Work*. Vol.10. No. 9.

Kim, Best. 2001. Does Circumcision Reduce HIV Risks?. *Net Work. Family Health International*. 20(4).

Korber, Bette. Muldoon. M. Theiler J. Gao F. Gupta R. Lapedes A. Hahn B.H. Wolinsky S and Bhattacharya T. 2000. "Timing the ancestor of the HIV-1 pandemic strains". *Science*. No. 288. 9 June.

Krishnamurthy, Vijaya Srinivasan. Charles B. Lakshmim Bai. 1999 "HIV/AIDS and safe sex practices among female sex workers in India – Risk perception". *Health Education in South East Asia*. 13(4).

Lamey, B and Malemeka. N. 1982. "Aspects cliniques at pidemiologiques de la cryptococcose a Kinshasa" *Medecine Tropicale*. Sep-Oct. 42(5).

Limsuwan, Y., Kanapa S., Siristonapun Y. 1986. "Acquired immune deficiency syndrome in Thailand, a report of two cases". *Journal of Medical Association Thai*. 69

Lobo, Francis. 1999. "HIV/AIDS and the meaning of life : Lessons for community services". *Leisure Issues*. 2(4).

Maclure, Malcolm. 1998. "Inventing the AIDS virus hypothesis : An example of scientific versus unscientific induction". *Epidemiology*. No. 9.

Martin, S.L. 1999. "Domestic Violence in northern India", *Amercian Journal of Epidemiology*, 150 (4).

Martin, S.L. 1999. "Sexual Behaviour and Reproductive Health Out comes : associations with wife abuse in India". *Journal of the American Medical Associations*. 282(20).

McEwan, R.T. 1992. "Sex and the risk of HIV infection : the role of alcohol". *British Journal of Addict*. 87(4).

McGrath, J.W. Ankrah M. Schumann D.A. Nkumbi S. Lubega M. 1993. "AIDS and the Urban family : its impact in Kampala, Uganda". *AIDS Care*. No.5.

Melkote, Srinivas R. Sundeep R. Muppidi and Goswami, D. 2000. "Social and economic factors in an integrated behavioral and societal approach to communications in HIV/AIDS". *Journal of Health Communication.* No. 5.

Michal, C., Latham and Elizabeth A Preble. 2000. "Appropriate feeding methods for infants of HIV infected mothers in sub-Saharan Africa". *British Medical Journal.* 16.

Morbidity. and Mortality Weekly Report. 1982. *"Opportunistic Infection and Kaposis' Sarcoma among Haitians in the United States"*. 13(2).

Moses, Stephen, Francis A. Plummer, Elizabeth N. Nagugi. Nico J.D. Nagelkerke, Aggrey O. Anzala and Jackonaiah O. Ndinya-Achola. 1991. "Controlling HIV in Africa : Effectiveness and cot of an intervention in a high-frequency STD transmitter core group". *AIDS.* No. 5.

Nair, B.K.K. Viswan. M.P. Venugopal. B.S. Nair. P.S. 1973. "An Epidemiological study of Veneral Diseases". Vol. 6.

Nancy, L. Sloan, Beverly Winikoff, Nicole Haberland, Christa Coggins, and Christopher Elias. 2000. "Screening and Syndromic Approaches to Identity Gonorrhea and Chlamydial Infection among Women". *Studies in Family Planning.* 31(1).

Nataraj, Hyamala, 2002. "Women in Prostitution – Need for Informed Intervention" *Manushi.* No. 124.

Naveed, Syed V. 1998. "Interpersonal Relationships of Relatives and Friends of HIV/AIDS Patients". *Layola Journal of Social Science.* 12(2).

Offenstadt, G. 1983. "Multiple Opportunistic Infection Due to AIDS in a Previously Healthy Black Woman from Zaire". *New Englnd Journal of Medicine.* 308.

Osinubi., Tokunbo Simbowale 2003. "Perception Change is Crucial". *Health Action.* January.

Panda, S. 2000. " Transmission of HIV from injecting drug users to their wives in India". *International Journal of STD and AIDS.* 11(7).

Panda, S. 2000. "Indian Council of Medical Research Project on HIV/AIDS and Substance Abuse, Calcutta". *Indian Journals of STD and AIDS.* 11(7).

Pape, J.W. 1983. "Characteristics of the Acquired Immuno Deficiency Syndrome (AIDS) in Haiti". *New Englnd Journal of Medicine.* 309(16).

Phanuphak, P, Locharernkul C, Panmuong W., Wilde H. 1985. "A report of three cases of AIDS in Thailand". *Asian Pacific Journal Allergy Immunol*. No. 3

Potterat, J.J. Phillips. L. Rothenberg. R.B. and Drrow w.w.w. 1985. "On becoming a Prostitute : An exploratory case-comparison study". *Journal of Sex Researh*. No.20/21.

Pottert, J.J. Rothenberg R.B. Muth. S.Q. Darrow W.W.W and Phillips Plummer L. 1998. "Pathways to prostitution : The Chronology of sexual and drug abuse milestones". *The Journal of Sex Research*. No. 35.

Punia, Deepa, Punia, P.K. and Kaur, S.1996. "Sexual Victimization of female Children in Haryanvi Folk Songs". *Social Defence*. 38(125). July.

Rajkumar, R. Chellam Balasundaram and Ravi Chandran M. 1996. "AIDS Control-Awareness and Action Needed". *Social Welfare*. 42(12).

Ramasamy, P, Sabhesan S. 1988. "Promiscuity and family pathology". *Indian Journal of Social Work*. 44(2).

Richard, W Goodgame. 1990. "AIDS in Uganda". *The New England Journal of Medicine*. 323(6).

Rutenberg, Naomi Carol E. Kaufman. Kate Macintyre. Lisanne Brown. AliKarim. 2002. "Pregnant or Positive : Adolescent Child bearing and HIV risk in South Africa". *Working-Policy Research Division. Population Council*. No. 162.

Ryder, R. 1989. "Deprivations caused by Poverty increases AIDS among women". *New England Journal of Medicine*. 320(25).

Sandala, Luciano, Peter Lurie. M. Rosemary Sunkutu. Edgar M. Chani. Esther S. Hudes and Norman Hearst. 1995. "Dry Sex and HIV infection among women attending a sexually transmitted diseases clinic in Lusaka, Zambia". *AIDS*. 9 (suppl 1).

Singh, Richa. 2001. "Masculine Identity Workers and HIV/AIDS". *Economic and Political Weekly*. 36(2).

Singh, Susheela, Deirdre Wulf, Renee Samara and Yvette P. Cuca. 2000. "Gender Differences in the Timing of First Intercourse : Data from 14 Countries". *International Family Planning Perspectives*. 26(1).

Srinivasan, Vijaya Prasanthi R. and Yayanthi. V. 1999. "Evolving an Innovative Strategy for Control of Sexuallyn Transmitted Diseases in a Developing Country". *The Gandhigram Institute of Rural Health & Family Welfare Trust Bulletin*. 34(1).

Szabo, Robert Roger V Short. 2000. "Does male circumcision protect against HIV infection?". British Medical Journal. No. 320. In *AIDS update*. 2000. 5(3).

The United Nations Documents. 1998. "On the Impact of HIV/AIDS on Adult Mortality in sub-Saharan Africa". *Population and Development Review*. 24(3).

Thomas, William A, Christoper, A.J. and Saravanan. 1996. "Awareness is shield Education is the Sword". *Social Welfare*. 43(9).

Ties Boerma J. Andrew J. Nunn and James A.G. Whiteworth. 1998. "Mortality impact of the AIDS epidemic : evidence from community studies in less developed countries'. *AIDS*. 12 (supp. 1).

Tobia, Nahid Amany Abouzied and Eimn Sharief. 2004. "Health Risk Vs Defending Rights". *In Countdown 2015 (Special Issues) – Sexual & Reproductive Health & Rights for all*. Special Report, ICPD At Ten where are we now? Published by Population Action International, Washington D.C.

Usha, M.S. 2001. "Women and AIDS in India". *Women'Link*. 7(2).

Vandepitte, J. 1983. "AIDS and Cryptococosis Zaire 1997. *Lancet*. 23 April.

Weiss, Helen A. Maria A. Quigley and Richard J. Hayes. 2000. "Male circumcision and risk of HIV infection in Sub-Saharan Africa : A systematic review and meta-analysis". *AIDS*. No. 14.

Weniger, B.G. 1991. 'The epidemiology of HIV infection and AIDS in Thailand'. *AIDS*. No. 5 (suppl 2)

William, R. Finger, 2001. "Reaching Youth, Men May Improve Services". *Net work*. Vol. 20. No. 4.

WISE Words. 2000. "Power and Prevention". *Am Publication of Project Information*. No. 6. October.

Young, Ellie Wright. 1991. "The effects of Family structure on sexual behaviour of adolescents". *Adolescence*. 26(104).

Zabin, Laurie Schwab and Karungari Kiragu. 1998. "The Health Consequences of Adolescent Sexual and Fertility Behavior in Sub-Saharan Africa". *Studies in Family Planning*. 29(2).

Zhu, Twofu. Bette T. Korber. Andre J. Nabmias. Edward Hooper. Paul M. Sharp. and David D. Ho. 1998. "An African HIV-1 sequences from 1959 and implications for the origin of the epidemic". *Nature*. No. 391. Supplement. 5 February.

REPORTS

AIDS Update, 2000

Ainsworth, Martha, Chris Beyrer and Agnes Soucat. 2000. *"Thailand's response to AIDS : Building on success, confronting the future"*. Bangkok. World Bank.

APAC. *"HIV Risk Behavior Surveillance Survey in Tamil Nadu and Pondichery". Report on Sixth Wave.* AIDS Prevention and Control Project. Voluntary Health Services. Chennai.

APAC. *"HIV Risk Behavior Surveillance Survey in Tamil Nadu" Report on Fourth Wav".* AIDS Prevention and Control Project. Voluntary Health Services. Chennai.

APAC. *"HIV Risk Behavior Surveillance Survey in Tamil Nadu". Report on Fifth Wave.* AIDS Prevention and Control Project. Voluntary Health Services. Chennai.

APAC. 1998. *"Community Prevalence of Sexually Transmitted Diseases in Tamil Nadu. A Report on Third Wave".* AIDS Prevention and Control Project. Voluntary Health Services. Chennai.

APAC. 1998. *"HIV Risk Behaviour Surveillance Survey in Tamil Nadu". AIDS Prevention and Control Project.* Voluntary Health Services. Chennai.

Asian Red Cross and Red Crescent Regional AIDS Task Force. 1997. *"Regional workshop on Home and Community Care for People living with HIV/AIDS (PLWHA)".* Chiang Mai, Thailand, 3-7 June.

Bharat, Shalini 2000. *"India : HIV and AIDS-related Discrimination, Stigmatization and Denial".* Geneva : UNAIDS

Ekstrand M. 2003. *"HIV/AIDS in India".* AIDS Policy Research Centre. University of California. August.

Joyce, V. Lyons. 2000. *"Economic Implication of AIDS in Asia".* United Nations Development Programme Division. Regional Bureau for Asia and the Pacific. New Delhi.

Karuppaih. 2000. *"A Study of Socio-cultural and Economic correlates of HIV/AIDS in Madras City".* Report of the Research Project Sponsored by University Grant Commission. University of Madras. Chennai.

Mennonite Central Committee. 2005. *"Report on HIV/AIDS in Nepal".* June. 18. http ://www.mec.org/getinv.html

NACO. 1998. *Country Scenario 1997-1998.* National AIDS Control Organization, Ministry of Health and Family Welfare, Government of India.

NACO. 2003. *Facts & Figures – HIV Estimate (2003) : A note on HIV estimate*

NACO. 2004. *Annual Report 2002-2003 and 2003-2004*

NACO. 2004. *Facts and Figure*

National Family Health Survey. 1993. *"Tripura Summary Report"*. International Institute for population Science. Bombay.

Parliamentary Forum on HIV/AIDS (PFA). 2004. *"Young Ambassadors' Fight against HIV/AIDS – National Students & Youth Parliament Special Session on HIV/AIDS". New Delhi. November 6-7.* Supported by UNAIDS, NACO, Delhi Govt., NYKS, AIU & Students Organization.

Peter, Piot. 2000. *"Gender Is Crucial Issue In Fight Against Aids, Says Head of UNAIDS"*. Press Release. UNAIDS. 5 June.

Reid, G. and Costigan G. 2002. *"Revising the Hidden Epidemic : a situation assessment of drug use in Asia in the context of HIV/IDS"*. The Centre for Harm reduction, The Burnet Institute, Australia January.)

Sathiamoorthy and Suniti Solomon. 1997. *"Socio-economic Realities of Living with HIV"*. In Socio-economic Implications of the Epidemic, ed. Peter Godwin .New Delhi : United Nations Development Program. Asia-Pacific Office. May.

Status of Women in India. 1975. *"A Synopsis of the Report, National Committee on the Status of Women, (1971-74)"*. New Delhi: The ICSSR. Allied Publications.

Tamil Nadu State AIDS Control Society. 1998. *"Meeting the challenge – Annual Report 1997-98"*. Tamil Nadu AIDS Control Society, Chennai.

Thomas, Cox and Bal K. Suvedi. 1994. *Sexual Networking in Five Urban Areas in the Nepal Terai - An Assessment* AIDS and STD Prevention Network, Valley Research Group, Kathmandu, Nepal, March.

UNAIDS. 1997. *Briefing paper.*

UNAIDS. 1998. *Report on gender related vulnerability and obstacles to prevention and coping.*

UNAIDS. 1999. *Report on the global HIV/AIDS epidemic.*

UNAIDS. 2000. Report on the Global HIV/AIDS epidemic.

UNAIDS. 2001. *Children and young people in a world of AID"S.* August.

UNAIDS. 2002. *Mother to Child Transmission.*

UNAIDS. 2002. *Report on the global HIV/AIDS epidemic.*

UNAIDS. 2002. *Report on the global HIV/AIDS epidemic.*

UNAIDS. 2002. *Report on the global HIV/AIDS epidemic.* July

UNAIDS. 2003. *A Joint Response to HIV/AIDS*

UNAIDS. 2004. *Questions & Answers : Basic facts about the HIV epidemic and its impact.* 1/10, July.

UNAIDS. 2004. *Report on the Global Epidemic.*

UNAIDS/WHO. 2004. *AIDS epidemic update. December*

UNDP (undated). *AIDS in South and Southwest Asia : A development Challenge.* New Delhi.

UNDP. 1999. *AIDS in South and Southwest Asia – A Development Challenge.* HIV and Development Project. South and Southwest Asia.

UNDP. 2004. *Migration and HIV in South Asia.* New Delhi.

United Nations Development Fund for Women (UNIFEM). 2002. *Reducing Vulnerabilities of Young Women to STI / HIV / AIDS.* New York.

United Nations/Commission on the Status of Women. *Effects of the Acquired Immunodeficiency Syndrome (AIDS) on the advancement of women.* E/CN.6/1989/6/Add.1. in Expert Group Meeting on Women and HIV/AIDS and the Role of National Machinery for the Advancement of Women. Vienna. 24-28 September 1990. In Interrelationships between the status of women and HIV-Epidemic : a Review of published Literature. EGM/AIDS/1990/ bp 2. 21 July.

US. Centre for Disease Control. 1981. "Pneumocystic pneumonia – Los Angeles". *Morbidity and Mortality Weekly Report.* 30(21).

WHO. 1988. *Social Aspects of AIDS, Prevention and Control.* AIDS ACTION, Issue 2 March.

WHO. 2001. *HIV/AIDS in Asia and the Pacific Region.*

WHO. 2003. *AIDS Epidemic Update.*

WHO. 2003. *HIV/AIDS in Asia and the Pacific Region. Western Pacific-South-East Asia.*

World Bank (2000) *'Thailand's Response to AIDS : Building on Success, Confronting the Future* Thailand Social Monitor.

ABSTRACT

Reid, Jeanette Brown. 1998. "*HIV/AIDS : The Emotional Impact on Two Young Women Whose Mothers are HIV-infected (Immune Deficiency*). DAI—A 59/03, University of South Florida.

Riedel, Marion C. 1998. "Women Living with AIDS : How do family role tasks affect the custody plans and mental health of their adolescent children? (Immune Deficiency). DAI—58/12. Columbia University.

Rwabukwali, Charles Barwogeza. 1998. "*Gender, Poverty, and AIDS in Kabarole, Western Uganda : The socio-cultural context of risk and prevention behaviors (Immune Deficiency).* DAI—A 58/10. Case Western Reserve University.

Schneider. 1989 "*AIDS in women in the Federal on Federal Republic of Germany*" by Bunikowski, J. Estermann, M.A. Koch, abstract presented at International Conference on the Implications of AIDS on Mothers and Children, Paris. November.)

Schoultz, Kristasn Kay. 1998. "*Understanding Social Vulnerability : Gender and sexually Transmitted Infection in Niamey, Niger (Hausa, Prevention).* DAI—A 59/04, Brown University.)

Shankaran. S.S. 2002. "*Intervention for women and children in the red light area*". Abstract WePeF6910. The XIV International AIDS Conference.)

Singh and Malavia. 1990. "*HIV prevention interventions among prostitutes in India : Delhi experience*". Abstract published in VI international Conference on AIDS. San Francisco. Vol. 3.)

Sivaramamurthy. V. 2000. "*Sexuality, Sexual behaviour and Awareness about HIV/AIDS among rural men near Salem*". Abstrct in First International Conference of AIDS. India.

NEWS LETTER

AIDS IN INDIA. 1995. "*Women and AIDS : Issues and Concern*". Newsletter of the National AIDS Control Organization. March.

Lawyers Collective HIV/AIDS Unit Positive Dialogue. 2000. "Criminalisation of Livies". *Newsletter*. 7. November.

Machika TANNO. 1997. "The Agony of a family of AIDS patients : A case study about 42 year old single man died of AIDS". Proceedings of the 11th Congress of the Japanese Society for AIDS Research. *AIDS Research Newsletter*. Dec. 4-5. Kumadmoto.

Meena Gopal. 2000. "Gender and Disease : A Research Note". *Social Sciences and Health News Letter*. 1(1)

National Institute of Social Defence 2004. "Tackling the Challenge of HIV/AIDS". A Newsletter of National Institute of Social Defence. 5(11).

National Institute of Social Defence. 2004. *"Condom use declines drastically in urban India : Survey". A Newsletter of National Institute of Social Defence.* 5(11)

National Institute of Social Defence. 2004. *"HIV among married Indian women likely to increase : report". A Newsletter of National Institute of Social Defence.* 5(11).

NEWS PAPERS

Aarthi Dhar. 2005. "AIDS vaccine may be available in eight years". *The Hindu*. 8 February.

Aarti Dhar. 2005. "Sharp fall in number of new HIV cases – India continues to have most number of cases after South Africa". *The Hindu*. 26 May.

Anandhi Subramanian. 2004. "Pushing at the barriers". *The Hindu*. Magazine. 12 December.

Biswas, Ranjita. 2005. "Of human bondage". *The Hindu*. 3 April.

Break Through Organization. 2005." Married women are increasingly affected by HIV". *Thinamalar (Tamil Daily)*. 23 April.

Deenabandu. K. 2003. "Policy shift in Battle against AIDS – Health department to offer district specific, micro-solutions". *The Hindu*. 27 August.

Dinesh Varma. 2004. "AIDS awareness high, but access to information inadequate". The Hindu. 3 May. http :// www.thehindu.in

Gayathiri Devi, R. 2004. "Measures sought to stop violence against women". *The Hindu*. 30 November.

Kannan, Ramaya. 2005. "They live under the shadow of HIV/AIDS – Over 10 per cent of street children had STD". *The Hindu*. 25 August.

Kannan, Ramya. 2003. *The Hindu*. 1 November.

Kannan, Ramya. 2004. "Treatment in Government Hospitals/ Discrimination – HIV-affected women will be on advisory panels". *The Hindu*. 5 March.

Krishnamurthy. 2005. "Need to check sexually transmitted infections – Study among two high-risk groups". *The Hindu*. 6 May.

Ledger, Wendy. 1997. "It's a delicate issue for business sector-Special issue". *East African Standard*. 21 July.

Menon, Meena. 2005. "Suicides by HIV positive patients in Mumbai – People feel there is a feeling of neglect". *The Hindu*. 3 May.

News Today. 2002. "Police, prostitutes nexus cannot be denied – Southern belles in brothels up North". 10 February.

Olson, Elizabeth. 2000. "Red Cross say three diseases kill many more than disasters". *The New York Times*. 29 June.

Paul, George. 2005. "HIV/AIDS patients and doctors". *The Hindu*. 4 September

Prasad. R. 2005. "HIV : trial shows male circumcision cuts risk". *The Hindu*. 25 August.

Quraishi. 2005. "India seized of AIDS problem". *The Hindu*. 21 April.

Samgaeswaran K.T. 2004. "Is it yet another crime against women?". *The Hindu*. 22 September.

Sharma, K. 2005. " Blaming women". *The Hindu*. 12 June.

Sharma, Kalpana. 2005. "Is this what we call progress? – What is happening to women in U.P. makes for a relentless horror story". *The Hindu*. Magazine. 17 April.

The Hindu 2004. "AIDS Study/Violation of Rights – Women face stigma, discrimination". 6 December.

The Hindu. 1991. "To Err Is Human, But At What Cost?". 5 January.

The Hindu. 1996. "Dissemination of information to combat AIDS mooted". 13 December

The Hindu. 2002. "Open Page – Crime in Chennai". 19 March.

The Hindu. 2003. "AIDS patients in 6 States to get free drugs". 1 December.

The Hindu. 2003. "Slum women show the way to fight HIV stigma". 1 December.

The Hindu. 2004. "$9 billion needed to fight HIV/AIDS". 22 April.

The Hindu. 2004. "A ticking time bomb", 5 December.

The Hindu. 2004. "AIDS Meet/Asia Facing Grave Threat - Leaders not doing enough : Annan". 12 July.

The Hindu. 2004. "AIDS spreading fast in areas near highways". 30 November.

The Hindu. 2004. "Hospitals lacking in positive attitude to HIV patients" 21 April.

The Hindu. 2004. "ILO'S ominous estimates". 11 July.

The Hindu. 2004. "India reaffirmed political commitment to the spread of AIDS" 12 July.

The Hindu. 2004. "Innocent Victims". 30 November.

The Hindu. 2004. "Make HIV test before marriage mandatory : victims". 30 November.

The Hindu. 2004. "Partner in the anti—AIDS battle". 2 December.

The Hindu. 2004. "Project for home-based care for AIDS patients". 1 December.

The Hindu. 2004. "Women at Risk". 1 December.

The Hindu. 2004. "Women near mines suffer untold misery". 26 April.

The Hindu. 2005. "AIDS vaccine may be available in eight years". 8 February.

The Hindu. 2005. "Caring for children orphaned by HIV/AIDS". 29 March.

The Hindu. 2005. "Editorial- Death in a booming economy". 17 April.

The Hindu. 2005. "HIV Cardinal supports condom use". 10 February.

The Hindu. 2005. "India rebuts U.N. Claim on HIV prevalence – Number of infections less than 1 per cent". 26 May.

The Hindu. 2005. "India seized of AIDS problem". 21 April.

The Hindu. 2005. "Life insurance for the HIV positive". 10 March.

The Hindu. 2005. "Supporting HIV/AIDS – affected children". 31 March.

The Indian Express. 1990. "The Plight of AIDS Patients". 8 July.

The Indian Express. 1999. "Homosexuals educated on safe sex". 14 October.

The Indian Express. 2001. "HIV patients can do all the work that others are doing as long as they feel physically comfortable". 29 May.

The New Indian Express. 2004. "The Positive side of life". 1 December

The New Indian Express. 2004. "World AIDS Day 2004- "Care, support, treatment" 1 December.

The Week. 2001. "What you must know about AIDS". 19 August

Thinamalar. 2005. "AIDS infected husband, wife approached District Collector along with three female children for care and support. 29 June.

Thinamalar. 2005. "AIDS Noie pathippil Manilathil muthalidathai nokki Theni Mavattam". 15 February.

Thinamalar. 2005. "Paathikkapadum Appavi Pengal". 1 January.

Thinamalar. 2005. "Salaththai kalakkum teem sex : Padukuliel vilum manaviyar". 14 June.

Thinathanthi. 2003. "Kanavan-Manaiveyaga Enaintha AIDS Jodi" 17 January.

Venkatarangam, Lily. 2002. *The Hindu*. 24 November.

WEB SITES

Amnesty International. http ://web.amnesty.org/library/index/ ENGACT770012004

and sexually transmitted Inductions, 2004 Update, India.

Avert Organization. 2004. *HIV / AIDS in Eastern Europe and Central Asia*. http ://www.avert.org/ecstatea.htm.

Avert Organization. *People living with HIV*. www.avert.org. Last updated December 10, 2004.

Avert Organization. www.avert.org. Last updated Jan.5, 2005

http ://www.avert.org/indiaaids.htm.

http ://www.eurasianet.org/htm

http ://www.unaids.org/bangkok 2004/report.html

http ://www.walnet.org/csis/groups/nswp/

Jawahar, K.R. 2004. *Central Asian Republic – A Demographic Profile*. http ://www.asthabharathi.org/oia Aproz/Central/20 asian.htm.

Jo Bindman, Jo Doezema. 1997. *Net work of sex work Project.*

Monthly updates on AIDS, NACO, 31 March 2005. http :// www.avert.org/indiaaids.htm

NACO. 2003. *Facts and Figures*. http ://www.nacoonline.org/ facts.hitestimates.htm.

NACO. 2003. *State wise HIV Prevalence (1998-2003)*. http :// www.avert.org/indiaaids.htm

NACO. 2004. *Monthly update on AIDS. 31 August*. http :// www.avert.org/indiaaids.htm.

NACO. 2004. State wise HIV Prevalence (1998-2003). http :// www.nacoonlinc.org/facts.hitestimates.htm

Naz Naza. 2004. *Central Asia : What is being done about AIDS?*

Noble, Rob. 2004. *Caribbean Statistics Summery*. Avert Org. September 2004. www.avert.orgn/aidstarget/htm

Noble, Rob. 2004. *South and Central American Statistics Summery*. Avert Org. September 2004. www.avert.orgn/aidstarget/htm

Population Reference Bureau. 2005. *Without My Consent—Women and HIV related Stigma in India*. www.prb.org

Ramya Kannan. 2003. *Study to address gender bias against AIDS victims*. The Hindu. March 7, 2003. http ://www. Thehindu.com/ 2003/03/07/stories/2003030705529 0500.htm

Tamil Nadu State AIDS Control Society. 2005 – *Home page*. http :// tnsaacs.tn.nic.in

The Hindu. Debate, dithering and deadly AIDS – Opinion News Analysis. November 17. www.thehindu.in

The World Bank Group. 2005. *World Bank Assist Central Asia in Combating AIDS*. www.worldbank.org/eca/aids.

UNAIDS. 2004.*HIV/AIDS statistics on Myanmar*.

UNAIDS/WHO. 2004. *Epidemiological facts sheets on HIV/AIDS*

WHO HIV/AIDS programme : http ://www.who.int/hiv/en/

NEWS

Sun News. 2005. 1.30 pm on 17 March.

HIV/AIDS and Law
Ethics and Human Rights

INTERNATIONAL ENCYCLOPAEDIA OF AIDS - 4

HIV/AIDS AND LAW, ETHICS AND HUMAN RIGHTS

PART - I

Editor

Dr. Digumarti Bhaskara Rao
M.Sc., M.A., M.A., M.Ed., Ph.D.
Dean, Faculty of Education
Member, Academic Senate
Ex-Chairman, Board of Studies in Education
Member, Research Advisory Committee
Acharya Nagarjuna University
D-43, S.V.N. Colony
Guntur - 522 006 (India)

DPH

DISCOVERY PUBLISHING HOUSE PVT. LTD.
NEW DELHI-110 002

HIV/AIDS AND LAW, ETHICS AND HUMAN RIGHTS

First Published - 2000

Reprinted - 2015

ISBN: 978-81-7141-526-7 (Set)

HIV/AIDS and Law, Ethics and Human Rights

Published by:

DISCOVERY PUBLISHING HOUSE PVT. LTD

4383/4B, Ansari Road, Darya Ganj

New Delhi-110 002 (India)

Phone: +91-11-23279245, 43596064-65

Fax: +91-11-23253475

E-mail: discoverypublishinghouse@gmail.com

sales@discoverypublishinggroup.com

web: www.discoverypublishinggroup.com

Printed at:

Infinity Imaging Systems

Delhi

Preface

The HIV/AIDS is a new phenomenon in the human society. HIV destroys the immune system of human individuals, producing a defenselessness fatal state known as AIDS. The World Health Organisation has estimated that already one in every two hundred and fifty adults in the world is infected with Human Immunodeficiency Virus and according to WHO's projections a total of forty million men women and children worldwide will have been infected with HIV by the turn of this twentieth century. Visualising the devastating effects of the HIV/AIDS epidemic within our life times and beyond is difficult. Probably, no other disease in recent times has had the impact on human society generated by HIV/AIDS.

The HIV/AIDS epidemic has brought into focus many health related ethical, legal and human rights issues. This epidemic requires immediate and effective responses in new programming areas: attitudinal and behavioural changes, community-based care and support initiatives, and the maintenance of human development in the face of increasing rates of illness and deaths. At this point, education enters the scene as it can alter the HIV/AIDS situation since it brings change in the behaviour of the people.

This *'International Encyclopaedia of AIDS'* presents the worldwide information about HIV/AIDS, issues and challenges, reports and reviews, ethics laws and human rights, and educational activities and programmes to keep the policy makers, planners, professionals, activists, researchers, educationists, teachers and students well informed of the epidemic.

Dr. Digumarti Bhaskara Rao,
26 January 1999
The Republic Day of India

Acknowledgement

I am thankful to the World Health Organisation and its associated offices for using their material namely School Health Education to prevent AIDS and STD: A Resource Package for Curriculum Planners-Handbook for Curriculum Planners. Student's Activities, Teachers' Guide, Global Programme on AIDS-HIV Prevention and Care: Teaching Modules for Nurses and Midwives, Global Programme on AIDS–Community HIV Prevention Handbook; STD care Management-workbooks 1-7, Facing the Challenge of HIV/AIDS STDs: A Gender-based Response; HIV/AIDS and STD surveillance Data Management and Use-Report, Bangkok, 1995; Carrying out HIV Sentinal Surveillance–A Guide for Programme Managers, AIDS Prevention and Care in the workplace: Enhancing the Role of Private Sector; HIV Testing Policies and Guidelines; Carrying out HIV Sentinel surveillance; AIDS Prevention; Understanding and Living with AIDS; AIDS: A Modern Epidemic; HIV/AIDS in South-East Asia: IXth meeting of the National Programme Managers, New Delhi, 1993; Information, Education and Communication: A Guide for AIDS Programme Managers, Handbook on AIDS Home Care; HIV/AIDS in South-East Asia: A Pictorial Summary; etc.

I am thankful to the United Nations Development Programme, UNDP's HIV and Development Programme, and UNDP's Regional Projects on HIV and Development for using their material namely Economic Implications of AIDS in Asia; Socio Economic Implications of the Epidemic; NGOs Working with Sex workers; NGO Responses to HIV/AIDS in Asia-Case Studies; HIV in the Workplace: Dealing with the Issues-Role Plays, Development and the HIV Epidemic, Law Ethics and HIV; HIV Law and Law Reform; Issue Papers; Study Papers; Working Papers; etc.

I am thankful to the Health and Nutrition Centre, Republic of

Philippines for using its material namely sourcebook on HIV/AIDS Prevention Education for Tertiary Educational Institutions.

I am thankful to the Curriculum Development Programme, Ministry of Education, Government of Thailand for using its material namely Institutional Modules for AIDS Education.

I am thankful to US Department of Health and Human Services; Whitman-Walker Clinic, Inc., USA; East-West Centre, USA; National AIDS Control Organisation, Government of India; Academy of Culture Communication Education Science and Service, Guntur, United Nations and its agencies for using their material.

I am grateful to Bhaskar Bhattacharji; V. Alexeev, Geeta Sethi, Elizabeth Reid, Mina Mauerstein-Bail, A. A. Trinidad, Palomi Cuchi, D. Pushpa Latha for their kind co-operation.

Dr. Digumarti Bhaskara Rao,
Secretary
ACCESS
D-43, S.V. N. Colony,
Guntur-522 006

Contents

1

The Role of Judiciary and HIV Law

Michael Kirby
President
International Commission of Jurists
Special Representative of UN Secretary General for Human Rights in Combodia

Consciousness

Judges, by definition, are leaders of their communities. They are invariably educated above the average. They ordinarily enjoy a privileged lifestyle. Typically, they are respected because of their office. Their special position in society imposes upon them a responsibility of leadership. Nowhere more is that responsibility tested than when a completely new and unexpected problem presents itself to society. All the judges' instincts for legality, fairness and reasonableness must then be summoned up, to help lead society towards an informed, intelligent and just solution to the problem.

It is dangerous to generalize about the judiciary. In the region of the world in which this book is likely to be used (Asia and the Pacific) several legal systems may be found. In each of them, the role of judiciary will be different. As the Special Representative of the Secretary-General for Human Rights in Cambodia I have observed quite different traditions and conventions than does a judge in Australia, Fiji or India. Typically, in common law countries which derive their legal systems from England, the judge enjoys a specially important place in the place exposition, development and application of the law. The judge's creative role in developing the common law gives him or her opportunities and responsibilities of lawmaking, which are probably greater than in most countries of the civil law tradition.

But even within common law countries, the opportunities of legal development will differ at different levels of the judicial hierarchy. Thus, a judge of the final appellate court will have an enormously important role in applying the Constitution, in expounding basic human rights, in sometimes striking down legislation as unconstitutional, and in keeping the other branches of government in check. A judicial officer at the other end of the spectrum, a magistrate, will have much less opportunity to develop and expound new legal principles. He or she will generally be bound simply to apply statute law or common law as elaborated by the higher courts. Yet a magistrate will see many more citizens than higher court judges do. Typically, the magistrate's court processes about ninety per cent of criminal and small debt proceedings. This is where most people see the judiciary. It is a mistake to conceive of the role of the judiciary as limited to judges of the highest courts.

As a judge of twenty-one years in a common law country (Australia), now serving also in another common law country of the region (Solomon Islands), I am much more familiar with the role of the judiciary in common law countries. Although I am now quite familiar with the legal system of another country of the region (Cambodia) whose traditions are those of the civil law, I hope the readers will understand my concentration upon the case work of judges in common law countries. Yet in the face of HIV/AIDS, judicial officers everywhere must marshal their talents to give leadership. The epidemic presents many problems of a legal character; but still more problems of prejudice, ignorance and discriminatory attitudes. This is why discrimination against people living with HIV/AIDS, or thought to be in that position, is sometimes described as the "second epidemic".

This chapter is organized in terms of the "5 C's". These are Consciousness; Courts; Cases; Colleagues and Community. I will also offer some conclusions. In each context, the judiciary has personal and collective responsibilities. They are universal, and not limited to any particular legal system. But necessarily, my treatment of cases will be confined to the system which I know best—that of the common law. Doubtless similar cases could be presented in civil law systems.

Inevitably, in a brief contribution, I cannot do justice to all of the aspects of the judiciary's response to the HIV/AIDS epidemic. But that response is not confined to interpreting, developing and applying HIV/AIDS law. The judiciary must do more than this, for the epidemic is fundamentally about human beings, fellow citizens. It is not about statistics. It is not about law, as such. Jurists, as educated leaders of the community, must understand this.

The first responsibility of the judiciary is consciousness about HIV/AIDS, and about the relevant legal principles which affect the performance of their professional tasks.

Long ago, at the outset of this epidemic, I was taught by Dean June Osborn, of the Michigan School of Public Health, that the first rule in HIV/AIDS law and policy was to base all action and responses upon sound data. That data will require those involved in relevant decisions and the exercise of governmental power (including the judiciary) to know what they are dealing with, and what they are talking about.

This is why it is important that all judicial officers today, in every country, should have more than a layman's understanding of HIV/AIDS. The epidemic is coming to affect millions of people. It will have enormous implications for the running of courts, the decision-making in cases, relationships with colleagues, and the judiciary's role in the community.

In Australia, the Judicial Commission in 1992 published an *HIV Outline—Source Material for Judicial Officers in New South Wales.*[1] This is an excellent work. It starts with basic facts about AIDS and HIV infection with rudimentary information on what AIDS is; when it first appeared; how HIV is transmitted; how many people in Australia have been infected; which groups of people have been particularly infected; what the life expectancy of a person with HIV or AIDS is; how it is diagnosed; what are its symptoms; whether health care workers and other professionals are at risk of HIV infection; and what risk still exists in donated blood, blood products of human tissue.

The booklet continues with basic information on public health legislation in New South Wales applicable to people with HIV/ AIDS, and with chapters on relevant statutory and common law principles applicable to such topics as liability for HIV transmission; application of anti-discrimination laws; the rules on confidentiality; the relevance of HIV/AIDS to sentencing; and the impact of HIV/AIDS on family law.

Doubtless, with the passage of time, some of the data

concerning the epidemic has been overtaken. Certainly, much of the treatment of particular legal issues would now have to be elaborated by reference to recent developments. But the beginning of wisdom is a knowledge of the features of the epidemic. Judicial officers, by their privileged position, and responsibilities to make decisions relevant to people with HIV/ AIDS, owe it to their communities to inform themselves about the basic facts. They should not rely solely upon the general media, for it is often guilty of misinformation and extravagant reporting on this topic. That is why the first step in the role of the judiciary in this area is consciousness about HIV/ AIDS. That consciousness should extend globally, but should be supplemented by a detailed knowledge of the best data available on the spread of the epidemic in the judge's own jurisdiction, as well as the most relevant statutory and common law principles, that a judge, suddenly facing a problem involving HIV/ AIDS, will need to be aware of.

It is the responsibility of the Executive Government in every jurisdiction to provide to judicial officers the basic information contained in the HIV outline mentioned above. It does not, the judges must inform themselves.

Courts

The professional judicial function is typically performed in courts, and sometimes in chambers. It is here that the judge, as jurist, meets citizens involved in legal cases, and their representatives. Some of those citizens will have problems relevant to HIV/AIDS. These will call for sensitive application of statute law and general legal principles. But before the judge gets to this, he or she will have to know how to conduct a case which concerns an infection which is not just an ordinary medical condition. Around various medical conditions there can gather elements of prejudice and stigma. It is found in community attitudes to various venereal conditions, and even to cancer. But HIV/AIDS in the courtroom is specially sensitive. In part, this is because of its association with death. In part it is also because the modes of transmission are frequently by sexual intercourse and injecting drug use. The association of HIV/AIDS with drugs, sex, and in particular, groups which have often been (and sometimes still are) the subject of stigma and even criminalization (homosexuals, drug-addicted persons, sex workers etc.), makes community responses to the epidemic highly sensitive, and sometimes over-reactive. The judiciary are members of their communities. They cannot be entirely free from the attitudes, fears and prejudices of the societies they live in. But it behaves the judiciary to be better informed, and especially to so perform their functions as to reduce unnecessary burdens upon those who come before them who are living with HIV/AIDS.

When AIDS first came along, there was often gross over reaction to its presence in the courtroom. Prisoners, actually infected or suspected of being infected with HIV/AIDS, were brought into court by guards wearing space suit protection, completely unnecessary and highly prejudicial to the fair trail rights of the accused. There is no need for special courtroom procedures, such as the wearing of surgical masks or gowns or protective gloves, still less for the exclusion of the defendant from the courtment. In the United States it has been suggested that such courtroom precautions, without any scientific basis, would be a violation of constitutional rights to due process of law.[2] Requests by court staff for the testing of prisoners, or for the provision of special gloves to sheriff and bailiff officers, should ordinarily be rejected. It is a duty of the presiding judicial officer to make sure that his or her court staff are protected from risks of infection, or exposure to such risks. But it is now well known that casual social contact will not transmit HIV. The judiciary should not permit court process to be distorted, invariably to the disadvantage of the accused, by generally unnecessary isolation, or disadvantageous treatment:

> "We are employers, of sorts, with large personal and official staffs, whose safety and security are our utmost concern. Judges are independent and are paid a salary which is not based on whether they win or lose... Our job is to do the right and just thing, without fear or favour. Ensuring the right to an attorney, the right to have one's case heard, the fundamental rights of fairness and due process are the cornerstones of the halls of justice".[3]

Because of the nature of the sensitive questions that can arise in cases involving HIV/AIDS, it will often be the duty of the judge to afford a measure of confidentiality to the persons involved. This is because it is usually permissible and proper to report court proceedings which are open. It would be wrong to close every court proceeding which involved some issue concerning HIV/AIDS, or concerned a person living with the virus. The principle of open justice is fundamental to the role of the judiciary. On the other hand, the need to protect confidentiality can be secured by judicial orders in appropriate cases, forbidding the naming of those who are infected. In such cases, the courts try to balance the public interest in protecting confidential information against the public interest which favours disclosure.[4] In X v Y[5], the English Court of Appeal considered the public interest exception in relation to the disclosure of information about a person's HIV status. An injunction was sought to prevent a newspaper from publishing the names of two doctors infected with HIV who were working in a particular hospital. The newspaper had obtained the information from confidential hospital records. The newspaper argued that there was an overriding public interest in disclosing the information, because the public was entitled to know that the doctors had HIV. However, the court held that the public interest in preserving the confidentiality of hospital records outweighed the public interest in the freedom of the press to publish the information, because people with HIV must not be deterred from seeking appropriate testing and treatment. This decision is important because the judges recognize that confidentiality in relation to a person's HIV status, could be important, not only to protect the interests of the infected person, but also for public health strategies generally against the spread of the epidemic.

In Australia, there have been similar orders by the superior courts protecting the confidentiality of people infected with HIV.[6] Sometimes these have proved controversial. Occasionally, the media attack the confidentiality orders of the judge. But the judiciary will know, and give value to, the competing interests at stake. So it was in the Bombay High Court where an interim order was issued suppressing the information of the identity of a person infected with HIV. Both were allowed to sue by pseudonyms (Mr. M X and Ms. Z Y). The applicants challenged a public corporation's dismissal of Mr. M X because he had tested HIV positive. The corporation's policy permitted discrimination on that basis. Mr. M X had been a casual labourer for a public sector corporation. He was due for promotion, subject to medical clearance. The medical examination declared him to be fit. He was then required to undergo a further examination for permanency. He was found to be physically fit. But the HIV test revealed that he was sero-positive. The corporation sought to justify its discriminatory policy— although it is hard to see how, before any onset of disability, such a policy could be justified especially in the case of a labourer. Mr. M X challenged it as contrary to law and a violation of the non-discriminatory clauses (ss 14, 15 and 16 of the Constitution of India). The Bombay High Court showed considerable sensitivity in its name suppression order. Some people, denied confidentiality, would simply abandon their rights at law and never come to court.7

Another consideration in such cases is the need for urgency. Particularly at an advanced stage of AIDS, unless judges become pro-active, and take control of litigation involving people suffering from HIV/AIDS, the litigant may be improperly denied a right or remedy, and such loss may prove irreparable:

> "If attorneys will not vigorously represent or refuse to represent HIV defendants, or if a defendant is denied access to the courtroom, time is critical. Similarly if an AIDS litigant does not receive a fair trial because of bias or hostility, given the pace of the appellate process, the probability is that he or she won't be around for a retrial. Finally, if a defendant is sentenced to prison merely because of his or her HIV condition, the person usually receives sub-standard medical care and other deprivations before an appeals court can rectify the situation.[8]

It is the duty of a judge, as the exemplar of due process, to insist upon fairness in the court, and to prevent discrimination from showing its ugly face.

A recent article in the *Victorian Law Institute Journal* described the kind of problem that can arise in the context of a litigant's sexual orientation. The same problem might arise in the context of HIV/AIDS status:

> "Often it is simply a matter of homosexuality being unnecessarily dragged into a case. The criminal lawyer ... whose gay clientele is ten per cent of his practice and growing, says that a lot of his work is in making sure the courts don't dwell on who his clients prefer to spend their lives with. 'Sexuality is rarely an issue in criminal matters and it should certainly not impinge on a person's equality in the eyes of the law. Having a client's gay status thrown about in court doesn't always help get a fair judgment".[9]

I was once greatly affected by a Canadian judge (Justice Louise Arbor) when she told a conference of judicial colleagues in Quebec that she never tolerated sexism in her court —whether it came from a litigant, the lawyer or a colleague. She always intervened to correct the perpetrator and the record, and to insist upon manifestly equal justice under the law. The judiciary must do so in the courtroom upon every ground of irrational discrimination, including the HIV/AIDS status of litigants, witnesses or others in front of the court.

Cases

The cases involving aspects of HIV/AIDS are now legion. Whole texts are written about AIDS and the law[10]. From something which began rather modestly[11], this is now a very large enterprise. In many countries, including my own, special series are now published on aspects of HIV/AIDS and the law. Thus, in Australia, there is a quarterly newsletter on HIV/AIDS law and policy called *HIV/AIDS Legal Link*. There is a similar journal in Canada called *Canadian HIV/AIDS Policy and Law Newsletter*. There are many similar publications in the United States. I cannot attempt in this brief essay to analyze the role of the judiciary in responding to the many issues which HIV/AIDS has presented to the law.

A number of examples may, however, illustrate the way in which informed judges, and other quasiudicial decision makers, can render a service by the sensitive application of the law to novel problems presenting as a result of HIV infection.

Let me start in the criminal law area. In common law countries, bail before trial is quite normal. It is not a feature of most civil law traditions. In the United States, it has sometimes been argued that the defendant's HIV status is relevant to whether or not he or she should be released pending trial. This is because of the shortened lifespan of most people found HIV positive. Typically, constitutional and statutory standards refer to the central question of whether the defendant will return to court to face the charges. Few, if any, refer specifically to HIV status. According to one analysis, it is no so much the category in which the person belongs, as the behaviour in which he or she engage, which is relevant. The stereotyping views about dangers to the public should be expelled by the judge, who should confine his or her decision to the actual known conduct of the applicant. An appellate court in New York held that it was an abuse of discretion to impose a condition of a negative HIV/AIDS test prior to release on bail, insofar as this was not mentioned in the statutes, and could involve an injustice to the particular applicant.[12]

Increasingly, judges are being faced by applications of the general criminal law, with special HIV/AIDS statutes designed to penalize persons who know that they are infected, but proceed to have unprotected sex and spread the virus. A Kenyan visitor was recently convicted in New Zealand under the general law.[13] But in Victoria, Australia, a judge directed a jury to acquit a person accused, following consensual, unprotected intercourse, because he considered the risks of infection unreasonably slight.[14]

In the criminal area, the main questions which have come before judges involve issues such as sentencing persons who are known to be infected with HIV, and ordering parole release of such person. In Australia, the principle that has been applied was stated by King C.J. in the South Australian Court of Criminal Appeal in R v. Smith:[15]

> "The state of health of an offender is always relevant to the consideration of the appropriate sentence for the offender. The courts, however, must be cautious as to the influence which they allow this factor to have upon the sentencing process. Ill health cannot be allowed to become a licence to commit crime, nor can offenders generally expect to escape punishment because of the condition of their health. It is the responsibility of the correctional services authorities to provide appropriate care and treatment for sick prisoners. Generally speaking, ill health will be a factor tending to mitigate punishment only where it happens that imprisonment will be a greater burdenon the offender by reason of his state of health, or where there is a serious risk of imprisonment having a gravely adverse effect on the offender's health".

In R v. McDonald,[16] the accused had been aware at the time of his original sentencing that he had HIV, but did not disclose the fact to the court. Evidence as to his HIV status was brought out in an appeal. There was also evidence that the appellant, by reason of his HIV infection, had been transferred to a special wing of the prison, where conditions were more restricted than in any other part of the prison system. The New South Wales Court of Criminal Appeal said:

> "The very nature of the confinement in the assessment unit imposes hardships, including the lack of opportunity that would exist in other sections of the prison for the appellant to determine who his associates would be. He is necessarily confined with other AIDS sufferers ... While so confined, the appellant would have reduced opportunities for courses of education ... A further consequence of confinement .. is the loss of opportunity for remissions".

The Queensland Supreme Court ordered that an HIV positive prisoner should have his application to parole reconsidered. It over ruled the Parole Board's original determination that special circumstances had not been shown by reason of HIV status.[17]

Other areas where judges are called upon to make sensitive decisions include family law;[18] immigration decisions on permanent residence or refugee status;[19] adoption;[20] disturbance of a will which fails to make provision for a life partner and is contested by the family;[21] discrimination cases involving employment, including in the military;[22] superannuation rights;[23] insurance benefits;[24] and industrial cases concerned with family leave entitlements.[25] All of those, and doubtless many other, cases call forth sensitive understanding by the judge of the high passions which tend to be engendered by the element of HIV/AIDS. In such cases especially judges need to ground all decisions upon sound data resting on the evidence—not on prejudice, stereotypes, myths or pre-judgment.

Many cases are now coming before the courts concerning claims for negligence. The cases may involve an accusation that a medical practitioner did not test the patient for his or her HIV status; did not inform the patient's partner of a positive HIV test of a patient, so as to warn him of the risk of infection;[26] and the failure to advise against the risks of exposure to accidental infection.[27] The cases are virtually infinite in their variety. Whilst it is unlikely that some of the more esoteric cases will come before courts in many countries of the Asia/Pacific region, claims in negligence provide the vehicle for assertions that medical practitioners, other health workers, public authorities, and the like, have not acted with due care. Where a person has become HIV-infected, it is natural that he or she should look to others to provide financial protection during life, and protection for dependants thereafter. Some of the most difficult decisions arise in the area of family law. Cases have been decided whereby access to a child was denied to a father found to be HIV-positive.[28] The basis of the decision, however, was not any real risk to the child, but that it was "not unreasonable" for the child's mother to have concerns without the risk of infection from fatherly social contact. This was an irrational fear, and the judge should not have given effect to it. A better approach was suggested in another case, where a wise judge held that it was a more appropriate response to the risk of stigmatization to bring the child up in a way that assists him or her in coping with it, and not to shield the child from it altogether.[29]

The call to the proper judicial function in all of the cases which I have mentioned, and doubtless many other, is to rest the decision, as all good judges do, upon sound evidence. Insofar as the judge may take judicial notice, he or she must inform the decision about the real nature of HIV/AIDS, so that prejudice is replaced by knowledge; and stereotyping by the judicial commitment to equal justice in the courts.

Colleagues

It is inevitable that as HIV/AIDS penetrates more societies and every branch of society, the judiciary will become aware of colleagues who are living with HIV/AIDS, either in the judiciary, or in the legal profession. Because the judiciary is still generally made up, in most countries, by elderly males, the modes of transmission of the virus may be less likely to have consequences affecting judges, than other groups in society. But this is not necessarily so. These suppositions sometimes collapse in the face of reality.

I myself have known a number of legal practitioners who have been infected with HIV. I have sat at the bedside of one, a fine attorney, born in New Zealand, who acquired the virus in a time that he worked in New York in the early days of the epidemic. He was an outstanding lawyer. He told me how he was determined to "beat the virus". He did not. But it is important that jurists should reach out to their colleagues facing this predicament. They should ensure that they are received without discrimination, but with support, where that is appropriate, and accommodation where it is necessary. Bar Associations, in Australia, and doubtless elsewhere, have provided special assistance to members of the legal profession who cannot continue in their professional work because of HIV/ AIDS. Judges, as leaders of the profession, must not forget their duties of professional comradeship and support where colleagues are affected. This means not just other judges, but court staff, police and bailiffs, their families and friends.

Community

Finally, judges are members of their communities. They must give a lead to community discussion of HIV/AIDS, its causes, and the behavioural modifications that are necessary to arrest the spread of the epidemic.

Judges cannot be interested in everything. But many of the features of HIV/AIDS are relevant to the professional duties of judges. Typically, laws stigmatize, and often criminalize conduct which is relevant, e.g., the sexual activities outside marriage; prostitution; homosexual activities; and injecting drug use. It is therefore the duty of judicial officers to reflect upon the effectiveness of current laws, insofar as they are relevant to the epidemic. Where law has become part of the problem, judicial officers (being better informed and usually more powerful) have a responsibility to add their voices to the discussion of reform. In default of a cure for, or vaccine against HIV/AIDS, the only weapon in society's armoury is behaviour modification. Alas, it is the lesson which judges can tell society that strong criminal sanctions are of limited use only in securing and reinforcing behaviour modification in such basic activities as sex and drug use.

That is why, in many countries, the advent of HIV/AIDS has led to a rare, and long delayed, re-examination of rules of law long established. Although the law in most countries no longer punishes (as once it did) adultery, as a criminal offence, legal vestiges from the same time intrude upon other consensual adult conduct of citizens. Because judges are the instruments of enforcing such laws, their moral sense is bound to be enlivened by what they are forced by the law to do. That given them both the motivation and the legitimacy to add their opinions to the suggestion of reform.

It is surely no coincidence that, since the advent of HIV/ AIDS, very significant pressures have built up, particularly in developed countries, for re-examination of laws concerning sex and drug use. In several parts of Australia, including New South Wales, prostitution (paid sex work) and the running of brothels have been decriminalized so far as they affect adult consensual conduct.[30] Similar moves have occurred in other states of Australia.[31] But the reforms are uneven. In many countries, people are asking what business it is of the law to intervene in such matters, save to prevent oppression, and to protect minors. The AIDS paradox teaches that criminalization and stigmatization make it more difficult to reach the minds of those affected. The first step on the path to effective behaviour modification will often be decriminalization, and the provision of educational messages. It is in this sense that informed judges can contribute to AIDS prevention by participating in discussion of legal reform.

The same message is relevant to the re-evaluation of laws on homosexual conduct and drug use.[32] In Australia, leading judges have begun to contribute to public discussion about the problems of homophobia, and the causes of injustice to fellow citizens by reason of their sexual orientation. Although HIV/AIDS is a human virus, and not limited to any sub-group, its early unequal impact upon gays has directed a lot of attention, particularly in developed countries, to the alienation of this group of the community, and the need to redress the unequal laws and policies which drive its members into a dangerous ghetto.[33]

In a number of parts of Australia, the advent of the AIDS epidemic has also promoted a debate on euthanasia. In two jurisdictions (the Australian Capital Territory and the Northern Territory)[34] the criminal law has been modified to permit assistance to aid peaceful death under given conditions. A significant part of the momentum towards law reform in this area has been the predicament of young people dying prematurely by reason of HIV/AIDS. In this connection, the judicial function remains: of protecting the vulnerable and defending their human dignity against well-meaning, or avaricious, family and friends.

Conclusion

The judiciary has an important role to play in the response to the HIV/AIDS epidemic. It should be aware of the causes of HIV/AIDS, and familiar with the body of law that is growing up as a consequence of its unexpected advent. It should ensure justice and equality in every courtroom, and be alert to the differential way general laws fall upon those who are living with HIV/AIDS, their families and dependants. Because judges have choices in deciding cases, where their decisions are relevant to HIV/AIDS, they should rest them upon sound data. They should expel from their minds the stereotypes, the myths and the prejudice. The judiciary should be alert to colleagues in the court process who suffer because of the epidemic. To the best of their ability, they should reach out with help and understanding. And as leaders of the community, they should contribute to the discussion of law reform which the HIV/AIDS epidemic demonstrates to be needed.

We are only at the beginning of this unpredicted challenge to our species. The Asia/Pacific region, which is promised enormous economic growth in the decades ahead, faces both economic and personal challenges unless behaviour can be modified and the spread of HIV contained. Harsh laws will not achieve these objectives, as any judge san tell. Instead, sensible policies, redress to discrimination and suitable law reform—as well as unyielding honesty—will be the chief weapons against the spread of HIV/AIDS.

Judges, as leaders and teachers, must play their part in responding to AIDS.[35]

REFERENCES

1. Judicial Commission of New South Wales, *HIV Outline—Source Material for Judicial Officers in New South Wales, Sydney, 1992.*

2. *Wiggins v. Maryland* 315 MD 232; 554 A 2d 356 (1989) (Maryland CA). See Judges' Journal, No .2, 25 (1990).
3. R. T. Andrias, "Shed Your Robes—Three Reasons for Aggressive Judicial Leadership in Coping with the HIV Epidemic." *29 Judges Journal*. No. 2,7,(1990).
4. *See Woodward* v *Hutchins* [1977] 1 WLR 760 (CA); *W. v Edgell* [1990] 1 All ER 835.
5. *X* v *Y* [1988] 2 All ER 648. See also R. Sarre, "HIV/AIDS and Suppression Orders", (1995) 17 (3) *Bulletin of Law Society of South Australia*, 11.
6. See *Loker* v *St. Vincents Hospital (Darlinghurst) and Anor,* unreported, Supreme *Court of New South Wales, Australia*, 11 October 1985 (Allen, M.). See also *Australian Red Cross Society* v B. C., Supreme Court of Victoria (Appellate division), unreported, 7 March 1991. Noted in Judicial Commission, above No.1,29.
7. A. Grover, "Names Suppressed in Indian Discrimination Case", (1995) 6 *HIV/ AIDS Legal Link*, No. 3, 26.
8. R. T. Andrias, "Shed Your Robes—Three Reasons for Aggressive Judicial leadership in Coping with the HIV Epidemic," 29 *Judges Journal*, No.3,7,(1990).
9. K. Derkley, "The Hard Earned Pink Dollar", *Law Institute of Victoria Journal*, August 1995, 742, 743.
10. See, for example, J. Godwin *et al., Australian HIV/AIDS Legal Guide*, 2 ed., The Federation Press, Sydney, (1993).
11. See e.g., M. D. Kirby, "AIDS Legislation—Turning Up the Heat?" (1985) 60 ALJ 324.
12. See *People* v *McGreevy* 514 NYS 2d 622 (1987) (NYCA).
13. MC Morgan. "The Problems of Testing for HIV in the Criminal Courts" 29 Judges Law Journal No. 2, 25 (1990).
14. Two charges were brought under the *Crimes (HIV) Act of Victoria*. The accused was acquitted on the direction of Teague J. of the Supreme Court of Victoria.
15. (1987) 44 SASR 587:27 A Crim R 315 (CCA SA).
16. (1988) 38 A Crim R 470 (CCA NSW).
17. Decision of Fryberg J. in the Supreme Court of Queensland, noted (1995) 6 *HIV/AIDS Legal Link*, No. 2,13.
18. K. B. Glen, "Parents with AIDS, Children with AIDS", 29 *Judges Journal* No. 2 14 at 17 (1990). See also Judicial Commission, above, No.1,33.
19. Decision of Refugee Review Tribunal (Aust.) N 94/04178, noted in (1994) 5 *HIV/AIDS Legal Link*, No. 4,3. See also M. Alexander, "HIV and Permanent Residence" (1995) 6 *HIV/AIDS Legal Link,* No. 2,8.
20. K. B. Glen, "Parents with AIDS, Children With AIDS", 29 *Judges Journal* No.2 14 at 17 (1990). See also Judicial Commission, above, No.1, 18.
21. K. Derkley, "The Hard Earned Pink Dollar", *Law Institute of Victoria Journal*, August 1995, 743.
22. *Canadian HIV/AIDS Policy and Law Newsletter*, April 1995, 14.
23. K Derkley, "The Hard Earned Pink Dollar", *Law Institute of Victoria Journal*, August 1995, 742.
24. A. Anderson, "Landmark Discrimination Case—Gay Family Wins Right to Family Health Insurance", (1995) 6 *HIV/AIDS Legal Link,* No. 3,18.
25. M. Alexander, "Success in the Family Test Case" (1995) 6 *HIV/AIDS Legal Link*, No. 4,12; *ibid*, Family Leave Test Case (1995) HIV/AIDS Legal Link, No.1,3. The case referred to is a decision of the Australian Industrial Relations Commission in the *Family Leave* Test case. The principle has been accepted in State Industrial Commissions. See note (1995) 6 *HIV/AIDS Legal Link,* No. 2,4 (NSW Industrial Relations Commission).

26. See reference (1995) 6 *HIV/AIDS Legal Link,* No. 3,5.
27. See e.g. *Johnson v West Virginia University Hospitals Inc.* 6 ALR 5th (1991) (CAW Va).
28. *In the marriage of B & C* (1989) FLC 92. 043 (Family Ct. of Aust.).
29. *Jarmen v Lloyd* (1982) 8 Fam LR 878 (Family Ct. of Aust.).
30. *Disorderly Houses (Amendment) Act* 1985 (NSW).
31. M. Fahey, "Prostitution Law Reform in South Australia", (1995) 6 *HIV/AIDS* Legal Link, No. 2, 16; See Ryan, "Prostitution Law Reform In WA" (1995) 6 *HIV/AIDS Legal Link,* No.3, 13.
32. As to Canada, see Canadian HIV/AIDS Policy and Law Newsletter, January 1995, 12.
33. See e.g. the comments of Nicholson CJ. Family Court of Australia (1994) 5 *HIV/AIDS Legal Link*, No. 4, 13 about same sex relationships.
34. See B. Delahunty, "ACT Approved Passive Euthanasia", (1994) 5 *HIV/AIDS Legal Link*, No. 4, 10 (Medical Treatment Act 1994 ACT); P. Leach and S. McLean, "Euthanasia Law Passed in the Northern Territory", (1995) 6 *HIV/AIDS Legal Link*, No. 2,1.
35. See generally D. C. Jayasuriya (ed.) *HIV Law and Law Reform. Asia and the Pacific*, UNDP, New Delhi, 1995.

2

The Nature and Scope of HIV Law

Dr. D. C. Jayasuria
UNDP
New Delhi, India

Within a short period of the first cases of an unusual breakdown in the human immune system were first reported in the United States, there were indications that this was not going to be merely a medical or scientific problem. As more HIV cases came to be reported, there were manifestations of 'homophobia' and of 'xenophobia'—the former because men who have sex with men were disproportionately represented among those infected, and the latter because individuals from certain countries or parts of the world were implicated as having spread a deadly virus to the rest of the world.

The medical or public health model of disease management had to compete with another–a model based on prejudice, discrimination, value judgments and religious and moral sanctions. Even after a decade of having lived with the virus, the spirit of the "stigma model" still lingers on.

The HIV epidemic has brought into sharp focus some fundamental and basic issues such as

- permissible limits on state interventions to regulate human conduct;
- the linkages between poverty and human behaviour; and
- the nature of the multisectoral and community responses needed to address the problems brought in its wake.

Among the many responses to the HIV epidemic have been those of a legislative, ethical and human rights nature. While early legislative interventions focused on case detection and compulsory notification, some countries have introduced measures of a more restrictive nature, including compulsory detention of infected persons and restrictions on international travel, to name only two of the many restrictions in place.

Since 1983, when the first AIDS-related legislative measure was introduced by Sweden, over 100 countries or some 150 sub-national jurisdictions have enacted such measures. In some countries, existing laws, such as those dealing with communicable or sexually transmitted diseases have been extended to the new HIV/AIDS context; in others legislative measures of a more comprehensive nature have been introduced.

'HIV-Law' or 'AIDS-Law' serves several functional roles such as the following:

1. Monitoring, Case Detection, Reporting and Surveil-Lance

This has taken different forms, ranging from the collection of statistics of cases to the identity of infected cases being recorded without concern for privacy or confidentiality.

2. Regulating Conduct/Behaviour

Regulations are in place based on

- Activities (prohibiting blood donations or commercial sex)
- Classification/Labelling (such as high risk groups)
- Status: Occupational (licences for commercial sex workers) or Marital (classification of partners of persons having multiple partners); and
- Sexual Orientation (such as men having sex with men).

3. Establishing Policy Framework/Infrastructure; Institutional Mechanisms; Resource Allocation; NGO Recognition

In the policy evolution process, beginning with the Short-Term Plan, Medium-Term Plan I and Medium-Term Plan II, legal, ethical and human rights issues have come to be reflected more often only during the latter stages.

4. Standard-Setting, Licensing and Quality Control

These have been done with respect to

– Blood and Blood Products

- Organs, Tissue, Semen, and Breast-Milk
- HIV Test Kits
- Sex Establishments
- Drugs, Vaccines

Legislative measures in. these areas are in place mainly in developed countries. Very few developing countries have accorded attention to matters such as mandatory standards–a situation compounded by the lack of enforcement machinery.

5. Mandating Interventions and Programmes

In some countries interventions such as free needle and syringe exchange schemes were introduced after a consultative process, involving, among others, AIDS service organizations, while in others the absence of a human rights environment helped the introduction of restrictive measures with little opposition or concern for the rights of infected persons.

Interventions have included coercive measures such as

- Compulsory Testing, and
- Traditional Public Health Strategies as well as those that have had a positive impact such as
- Public Information and AIDS Education;
- Needle and Syringe Exchange Schemes;
- Condom Distribution; and
- Counselling/Testing.

6. Mandating the Establishment of Services

Among the services the establishment of which have been mandated by law are:

- Counseling and Testing, Particularly of a Vol-untary and Anonymous Nature;
- Treatment;
- Community-Based Interventions; and
- Training and Research

Legislative provisions mandating services are found more frequently in the HIV-related laws of developed countries. Developing countries, on the other hand, tend to provide for such services more on an ad-hoc basis, often resulting in lack of continuity.

7. Creating A Supportive and Enabling Environment

It has taken time to develop a package of legislative and related measures that help to create and sustain an environment within which practical, humane and reasonably balanced HIV-related legislative, ethical and human rights approaches can be best formulated. Examples exist, particularly in the laws of developed countries, of measures dealing with:

— Recognition of Rights;
— Guarantees of Non-Discrimination;
— Empowerment;
— Qualitative Improvements;
— Harm Reduction Choices;
— Legal Aid;
— Liability Recognition; and
— Representation of Interest Groups.

While HIV-related laws have many functional roles, we should have no illusions that the record with HIV laws is that of an unqualified success story. Some legal provisions have been counter productive, a classic example being travel-related laws in more than 50 countries around the world. Moreover, only the laws of a few countries have addressed the broader HIV and development agendathe agenda that poses a challenge to the way in which we tend to approach issues such as confidentiality, privacy, liberty, gender equality, economic and social equity, and fundamental social obligations. This agenda can be properly addressed only if there is a supportive legal, ethical and human rights environment, the elements of which include the following:

— Capacity building;
— Policy/legal practice reforms;
— Existence of legal structures to determine complaints;
— Facilitating access to legal/administrative reforms; and
— Current awareness/information sharing/strategic questioning.

The UNDP HIV and Development Project is conducting a series of regional training workshops on HIV law and law reform. These workshops seek to create a better understanding of the nature, roles and functions of HIV law and the legal, ethical and human rights considerations that must permeate the law review and law reform process. They also seek to strengthen national capabilities to establish and sustain national networks on HIV law, ethics and human rights. As so long as the virus remains a part of human society, we will need such networks to maintain a dialogue to develop and sharpen the responses that could make a difference between a high quality of life and that which is subordinate to the elements of the 'stigma model'.

3

The Role of the Law in HIV/AIDS Policy

Julie Hamblin
Partner
Ebsworth and Ebsworth Solicitors
Sydney, Australia

INTRODUCTION

Much has been written about legal rights and duties in the AIDS epidemic and the importance of an appropriate legal response. With many policy responses being shaped by the all too familiar and often misconceived debate about public health versus individual rights, the delineation of legal rights and duties has heen a necessary part of the policy debate. Moreover, the ongoing reports of serious and unjustified encroachments on the civil liberties of people with HIV have established beyond doubt that the law has a central role to play in HIV/AIDS policy.

The precise definition of this role, however, has not always been given such careful attention. We know that the legal response to HIV/AIDS is important, but what should the legal response actually be? Can legislation, HIV/AIDS specific or otherwise, assist in strategies for the care and treatment of people with HIV and help to reduce the spread of HIV? What has been the experience, a decade into the epidemic, in seeking legal remedies for HIV/AIDS-related discrimination? Are legal sanctions ever helpful in bringing about the changes that will be necessary to respond effectively and appropriately to HIV/AIDS?

Underpinning these questions is a central theme that will be explored in this article. This theme relates to the need to recognise and distinguish between the different levels on which the law can operate, and which are seen with all their nuances in the context of HIV/AIDS policy. At one end of the spectrum is the role of the law which follows an essentially proscriptive model, whereby certain forms of conduct are prohibited and made subject to criminal sanctions. The complex social and ethical dimensions of HIV/AIDS, however, have called for more creative approaches to how the law can contribute to HIV/AIDS policy. This requires an exploration of not only the proscriptive function of the law but also the ways in which the law can be used—or on occasions, not used—in a constructive way to promote and reinforce the goals of HIV/AIDS strategies.

At this point in the epidemic; with the experience of a decade of different legal responses to HIV/AIDS to reflect upon, it is constructive to analyse the various models by which the law can be incorporated into HIV/ AIDS policy. Three main models will be analysed here. The first is the traditional proscriptive model that penalises certain forms of conduct. The second model focuses on the protective function of the law and the need to uphold the rights and interests of particular classes of people, notably those infected with HIV or at risk of infection. Both these models have been widely used in responses to HIV/AIDS to date. The third model, however, has been explored less fully. This model seeks to use the law actively to promote the changes in values and patterns of social interaction that lead to susceptibility to HIV infection.

The distinction between these different models is not always clear-cut and a particular legal intervention may display elements of more than one model. However, an understanding of the distinctions is important in order to identify clearly what is sought to be achieved by a proposed legal intervention. This analysis can guide any decisions about when we should intervene using the force of law and when, in the interests of certain policy objectives, we should refrain. Unless these different roles are recognised, there is a risk that the full potential of the law to assist HIV/AIDS policy will be overlooked or, worse, that the law may actively obstruct an appropriate response to HIV/AIDS.

The Proscriptive Role of the Law

The impact of the law in its proscriptive mode on HIV/AIDS policy became apparent very early in the epidemic because of the particular epidemiology of HIV infection in developed countries. The two groups most affected by HIV in the West—homosexual men and injecting drug users—were people whose sexual or drug-using activities constituted (and in some cases still constitute) a criminal offence in many jurisdictions. The existence of these criminal sanctions meant that legal concerns were drawn into the policy debate right from the outset. Our response to the activities that were placing people at risk of HIV infection had to be formulated in the context of legal prohibitions on these activities.

The involvement of the law in HIV/AIDS policy in this way can be seen to have often obstructed rather than facilitated effective policy implementation. These are the laws, for example, that have imposed criminal sanctions on the sale of condoms in Ireland.[1] and have led workers in needle exchange programmes to fear they may be prosecuted for aiding and abetting an illegal activity or for possessing the traces of illegal drugs that remain in used needles and syringes[2]. They have caused those people who are most at risk of HIV infection to be reluctant to identify themselves as being at risk for fear of adverse legal consequences. In short, the law has presented yet another obstacle to effective strategies to minimise the spread of HIV and meet the needs of people already infected.

Similarly, it can he argued that the enactment of proscriptive laws directed specifically at HIV/AIDS has been counterproductive in the context of broader HIV/AIDS strategies. Examples of this type of proscriptive law are laws for the compulsory reporting of HIV seropositivity*, laws which require HIV testing of certain population groups, such as prisoners[3], and immigrants[5], and laws that compel the disclosure of an individuals HIV status in certain circumstances** The coercive nature of these laws, which often impose criminal sanctions for non-compliance, far from encouraging

* Provisions requiring reporting of cases of AIDS and HIV infection are now common in many jurisdictions; for Australia see [2] the United States [3] and Canada [4].

** This most commonly occurs as the result of a compulsory contact tracing policy, such as that which is currently in place in Ontario, Canada and which in some circumstances requires physicians to disclose the identity of HIV-infected patients to public health authorities for contact tracing purposes. This programme is carried out pursuant to 960 which permits the identity of HIV-infected persons to be disclosed where the disclosure is made for purposes of health administration.

conduct that will reduce the spread of HIV, may actively impede prevention efforts by alienating those people who are at risk of HIV and making it less likely that they will cooperate in prevention measures. For those working in the field of HIV/AIDS, this is a familiar debate, and I do not propose to canvass it in detail here. For the purposes of the present analysis, the significant point is that lawmakers must be sensitive to not only the direct but also the indirect impact of legal sanctions.

In the case of proscriptive and punitive laws, therefore, an appropriate legal response to HIV/AIDS will most often have as its desired outcome the absence rather than the presence of applicahle law. This may not be as easy to achieve as it might seem. Where criminal offences exist in relation to certain HIV risk activities, for example, a policy of decriminalization may be politically unpalatahle because of public controversy surrounding homosexuality or drug use which may be unrelated to HIV/AIDS. Where absence of law is already the *status quo*, a policy that proposes essentially no legal reforms may fly in the face of the political imperative that policy makes be seen to take wift and decisive action to the threat of HIV. It requires us to resist the appeal of the 'quick fix' in favour of a less tangible response that recognises the complexities and subtleties involved in effecting changes in behaviour.

The particular dynamics of AIDS and HIV infection suggest that proscriptive laws will rarely be an appropriate policy response if they seek merely to target the conduct of people with HIV or activities that give rise to HIV infection risks*. In this guise, the role of the lasv is a negativc rather than a positive one, and the challenges of HIV/AIDS are such that an effective policy requires more than negative prohibition. Of all the different models the law can follow, the proscriptive model has the least scope for a creative application to policy formulation.

The Protective Role of Law

A second model for the role of law in HIV/AIDS policy focuses upon how the law can protect individuals or classes of individuals from harmful and undesirable occurrences. This model has been of central importance in the context of the legal response to HIV/

* Whether, in exceptional circumstances, proscriptive laws may have a role to play is a question not canvassed in detail here. It could be argued for example that criminal sanctions may still be appropriate in cases of deliberate or wilful HIV transmission. The critical issue however is whether the overall thrust of the legal response to HIV/AIDS is essentially proscrintive in nature or whether it conveys a different message.

AIDS because of the proliferation of discrimination against people with HIV[7-9] and because of the increasing recognition, both nationally and internationally, of the interplay between AIDS and human rights[10,11]. Accordingly, legal instruments such as human rights and anti-discrimination legislation that embody the protective role of the law have heen proposed as practical and effective svays in which the lavv can assist HIV/AIDS policy.

Laws that protect individual rights and interests must, to be effective incorporate a proscriptive element that imposes certain penalties for non-compliance, but they are not essentially proscriptive in their thrust. Equal opportunity legislation, for example, may prohibit certain conduct on the part of employers, landlords and others that is held to amount to unlawful discrimination, hut the philosophy underpinning the legislation is that of protecting individuals against discrimination. The oblective of the legislation is positive rather than negative: to engender respect for individuals and to promote human rights rather than merely to impose a prohibition on, for example, homosexual activity. It could be conceded that the distinction is one of emphasis rather than degree, but there is nonetheless an important conceptual shift hetween, on the one hand, regarding the role of the law as that of enforcing legal prohibitions and, on the other hand, viewing it as a mechanism for promoting and protecting individual rights.

The legal response to HIV/AIDS has drawn on the protective role of the law in many ways, but two protective functions of the law have been dominant, namely protection against discrimination and the protection of confidentiality for people with HIV or suspected HIV infection. In the area of protection against discrimination, human rights instruments have been invoked in the interests of people with HIV and, in some jurisdictions, new legislation has been passed strengthening human rights protection in this context[12,13]. Judges have heen called upon to decide whether pre-existing human rights legislation can or should be given a sufficiently broad interpretation to cover new circumstances presented by HIV/AIDS-related discrimination[3]. Consideration has been given to drawing upon international human rights conventions and declarations embodied in international law to strengthen human rights protection within domestic legal frameworks[14].

In relation to protection of confidentiality, the law has heen invoked in a range of different ways. It has been used, for example, to uphold obligations of confidentiality relating to information about HIV status obtained by a hospital[15], to provide a remedy for defamation in a case of threatened disclosure of HIV status[16], and in some cases to justify with holding the identify of an HIV-infected blood donor*. In some cases, where existing confidentiality protection has been considered inadequate, legislation has been passed strengthening confidentiality safeguards[19].

These examples are not intended to suggest that the law has necessarily been exemplary in this context, for indeed many would argue that the law has fallen far short of what is required to protect the interests of people with HIV. Moveover, legal protection in theory may not translate into legal protection in practice if the legal process is too cumbersome, time-consuming or costly to enable people with HIV to exercise their legal rights. Legal remedies that apply in the event of unjustified discrimination or breaches of confidentiality must also be recognised as dealing only with the symptoms of the problem and not with the cause which lies with community prejudice and lack of sensitivity to the rights and needs of people with HIV. Even bearing these limitations in mind, however, the examples described above nevertheless demonstrate the extent to which the model of the law as a protective instrument has been incorporated into the response to HIV/ AIDS.

It must he recognised that both the proscriptive and the protective model for legal intervention involve fundamental value judgments and, often, value conflicts in relation to what should be protected and what prohibited. As a result, each model operates on two levels, first by defining specific legal rights and obligations and second by creating or reflecting certain values and rejecting others. These statements of values which are inherent in the law can influence and shape other policy responses.

The distinction between the proscriptive and the protective roles of the law is important because it assists in determining whether active legal intervention is an appropriate policy response. While proscriptive and coercive laws may be counterproductive if they discourage the voluntary participation hy people at risk of HIV in measures to reduce HIV transmission, protective laws may help to enlist the support and co-operation of these people in prevention strategies. Thus, although decriminalization or the absence of law may be what is sought within the context of the proscriptive legal model, decisive and firm legal intervention may be what is required

* The decided cases are divided on the question of whether the identity of an HIV-infected blood donor should remain confidential in relation to the position in the United States [3]. See [17] for the United Kingdom and [18] for Australia.

in the context of measures to protect the rights of people with HIV. The identification of what is primarily sought to be achieved by a particular legal intervention therefore provides insight into its likely impact on broader HIV/AIDS strategies.

The Instrumental Role of Law

The third model for legal intervention is the most controversial and its application is arguably the most problematic. Whereas the proscriptive and the protective models of legal intervention focus on the conduct of individuals or on the adjustment of rights and obligations as between individuals, the third model envisages a legal response to HIV/AIDS that will operate on a broader and more far-reaching level. This is the model which suggests that the law can play a proactive role not merely in mediating rights and obligations as between individuals but also in seeking to change underlying values and patterns of social interaction that create vulnerability to the threat of HIV infection.

An appreciation of the potential role of the law in this context requires an appreciation of the emerging socio-economic patterns of HIV infection during the 1990s. In April 1991, the World Health Organisation estimated that the cumulative total of people infected with HIV worldwide was in the order of 8-10 million[20]. Of this total, more than 7 million infections were estimated to have occurred in the developing countries of suh-Saharan Africa, the Caribbean and South and South East Asia[20]. Increasingly, it has heen said, the disease is one that affects poor women of colour[21], as race and gender patterns emerge in the demography of HIV infection. In the United States, for example, the incidence of new cases of HIV infection is affecting blacks and Hispanics disproportionately, while in some areas of Sub-Saharan Africa the rate of new infections is estimated to be almost three times higher among women than among men[22].

These patterns suggest that one of the most significant risk factors for HIV infection during the 1990s relates not to sexual or drug-use activities as such but rather to socio-economic dependency. Because HIV infection is preventable, people who have access to information and appropriate preventive measures and have the means to implement these will he able to protect themselves against infection. At this point in the epidemic, therefore, the people who remain most vulnerable are those who are denied the means of protecting themselves against the risks of HIV because of economic need or powerlessness to control the basis upon which their sexual relationships take place. This may occur, for example, because a person's sexual activity is directed by his or her need for economic support, because preventive measures, such as condoms, are not accessible and affordable, or because poor health care (in particular, inadequate treatment of sexually transmitted diseases) increases transmission risks. For women, it may occur because their sexual relationships with men are determined by cultural values which are beyond their control and which are often compounded by lack of economic independence[22], or because of the absence of HIV prevention measures, such as virucides, that are exclusively within the control of women[23].

The challenge for HIV/AIDS policy during the 1990s is to recognise the need to address not only what might he called the 'HIV/AIDS-specific' issues, such as HIV education programmes and research into new harrier methods to prevent HIV transmission, hut also the underlying social and economic factors that deprive individuals of the power to protect themselves against HIV infection. Put in this context, the task is an enormous one and extends far beyond what is most commonly perceived as the scope of HIV/AIDS policy. Nonetheless, efforts to address the socio-economic risk factors for HIV infection are a critical part of an effective strategy to reduce the spread of HIV in the years to come.

The changes required are dramatic and clearly far transcend the law and the legal system. But can the law he used as an instrument to provoke or reinforce these changes? One could coin a well-known legal metaphor (albeit one with somewhat aggressive connotations) by suggesting that in this context, there is the potential to use the law as a sword rather than a mere shield.

One must he careful about making grandiose claims as to the extent to which the law can be used to bring about social and economic change. By the same token however, the potential of the law to complement and reinforce other policy initiatives in this regard should not be overlooked, because legal interventions can address some of the social and economic factors that render particular groups of individuals susceptible to HIV infection*. In many developing countries, for example, there exist legal regimes that

---

* Many of the ideas in this section grew out of my discussions and collabourative work with Elizabeth Reid, Policy Adviser on HIV/AIDS for the United Nations Development Programme, and I am grateful to her for her contribution. The ideas are elabourated in [24].

entrench the economic dependence of women through land ownership and marital property laws which deny women independent ownership of property or through laws which deny women access to certain forms of paid employment[25]. Law reform in this area could have an immediate impact on patterns of economic support in these countries, which in turn could assist in permitting access to health care and in reducing reliance upon sexual activity as a source of income. Similarly, laws can be enacted which require minimum levels of participation and representation of socially disadvantaged groups in the policy process, either in relation to HIV/AIDS specifically or to more general matters, such as economic assistance and health care. Such laws can help to ensure access to relevant information about HIV and, by the mere fact of participation, help to redress the social imbalance.

One of the primary reasons why law reform has the potential to he effective in this way is that law in any form is an important expression of social and cultural values and can therefore be used to change these values. Where laws uphold certain customs or behaviours that give rise to HIV transmission risks, such as traditional marriage patterns in some cultures[25], the abolition of these laws can provoke a questioning of the customs and values that underpin them. The active prohibition of certain conduct which may hitherto have been considered acceptable but which places individuals at risk of HIV can also be a powerful force for change. There is, therefore, a need to harness the symbolism of the law in all its manifestations - proscriptive, protective, instrumental or otherwise—and to use it to promote rather than impede the changes necessary to reduce the spread of HIV.

With most policy initiatives for HIV/AIDS, it is possible to envisage a legal intervention that could complement and reinforce the desired objective. These interventions will require a creative approach to the law which recognises that the law can play more than just a direct proscriptive or protective role. They will also require a recognition of all the implications of a particular legal intervention on the direct, indirect and symbolic levels. With such an approach, there is a real potential to use the law proactively and constructively in the response to HIV/AIDS.

CONCLUSIONS

The three models of legal intervention that have been described illustrate the range of different ways in which the law can play a role in the response to HIV/AIDS. All three models are potentially relevant, but it is important to distinguish between them in order to direct policy appropriately.

The proscriptive and the protective roles of the law have already been widely utilised in legal responses to HIV/AIDS. With the epidemic continuing to spread at alarming rates in many parts of the world, however, it is important that HIV/AIDS policy in the 1990s explores new and creative measures for dealing with the challenges facing it. We must fully exploit the potential of the law to promote and buttress other HIV/AIDS strategies and, where necessary, to change the traditions and values that place people at risk of HIV infection. This is the most pressing and critical role for the law in HIV/ AIDS policy in the 1990s.

REFERENCES

1. Anonymous St. Valentine's Revenge. *Lancet* 1991. 337.548
2. Godwin J., Hamblin J., Patterson D., *Australian HIV/ALDS Legal Cuisle* Sydney. The Federation Press, 1991. P. 182
3. Gostin Lo the AIDS Litigation Project: A national review of court and human rights commission decision Part I. The social impact of AIDS: *Jama* 1990. 265.1961-1970.
4. Hamblin J., Somerville Ma. Surveillance and reporting of HIV infection and AIDS in Canad: ethics and law. *Univ Toronto Law of* 1991 41. 224-246.
5. Duckett M., Ornin AJ., AIDS-related migration and travel policies and restrictions a global survey. *AIDS* 1989. 3 (suppl 1)S231-S242.
6. *Health Protection Antl Promotion Act 1983 (ontario)* S O 1983 C10 S38.
7. Tindall B., Tillett G., HIV-related discrimination. AIDS 1990 4 (Suppl.) S251-S256.
8. Gostin Lo The AIDS Litigation Project: A national review of court and human rights commission decisions. Part II Discrimination *Jama* 1990. 263.2086-2093
9. Somerville Ma. Ornin AJ., Human rights, discrimination and *AIDS* concepts and issues AIDS 1989, 3 (suppl 1) S283-S2S7.
10. United Nations Centre for Human Rights *Ȓeport of an International Consultation on AIDS and Human Rights* New York United Nations. 1991.
11. World Health Assembly *Resolution of the Avoidance of Discrimination in Relation to HIV Infected People and the People with AIDs.* Geneva World Health Assembly, May 1988.
12. *Theamericasis uvith disahilitiesact(i990)* pl 101 33c. 104 stat 327 (1990)
13. *Equal Opportullity Act* (*Victoria*) 1984. S4(1).
14. Hodge D. Smith A., Patterson D., HIV status, sexuality and discrimination in Australia whose turn to (en) act? *Nati AIDS Bull.* 1990. 4.48-51
15. *X v Y & Ors* (1988)2 All ER 648 (Queen's Bench Divisionx UK).
16. *X v Sattler and Western Broad casting Services Pty Limited (unreported).* Supreme Court of Western Australia. Mr. Justice Kennedy, 31 may 1989.
17. *AB v Glasgou and West Scotland blood Transfusion Service (unreported)* cited in Centre of Medical Law and Ethics Despatches 1990, 1(1), at 5.
18. *Australian Ped Cross Society & Anor v 'BC' (By ber Litigation Guardian J* (unreported). Supreme Court of Victoria (Appeal Division). March 1991.

19. Public Health Act 1991 *(New South Wales)*. S-17.
20. World Health Organisation Global Programme on ALDS Current *and future Dimensions of the HIV/AIDS Panaemic A Capsale Summary*, Geneva, WHO. April 1991.
21. Carovano K. More than mothers and whores: redefining the AIDS prevention needs for women. *Int J Health Ser* 1991. 21:131-142.
22. United Nations Division for The Advancement of Women *Interrelationships between the status of women and HIV epidemic. A review of Published Literature report Prepared for the Expert group meeting on women and HIV/ aids and the role of national machinery for the Advancement of* Women, Vienna, September 1990 (EGM/AIDS/ 1990/BP.2, 31 July. 1990.
23. Stein Z. HIV Prevention: the need for methods women can use. *Am. J. Public Health* 1990. 460-462.
24. Hamblin J., Reid E. *Women, the HIV Epidemic and Human Rights. A Tragic Imperative PREPARED for the International Workshop on AIDS. A Question of Rights and Humanity.* the HAGUE, may 1991.
25. Longwe Sh., Clarke R. *Proposed Methodlology for Combating Women's Suborblination as a Means Towards Improved AIDS Prevention and Control Report prepared for the Expert Group Meeting on Women and HIV/AIDS and the Role of National Machinery for the Advancemtn of Women* Vienna, September 1990 (EGM/AIDS 1990 W5 5. 24 September*).

4

HIV Law: The Expanding Frontiers

Dr. D.C. Jayasuriya
Regional HIV & Development Advisor,
UNDP, New Delhi, India

Background

When the first AIDS cases came to be reported in the early 1980s, most countries had on their statute book laws dealing with communicable diseases. These represent some of the earliest health-related laws to be enacted.[1] In most developing countries in Asia,[2] Africa and the Pacific[3] these laws have continued to remain in force without being updated to address current infection control and disease management systems or the rights and duties of affected individuals and communities. In Sri Lanka, for instance, the Contagious Diseases Ordinance and the Quarantine and Prevention of Diseases Ordinance are both 19th century enactments that have remained in force without undergoing any significant or far reaching changes.[4]

During the early years of the epidemic, the most common legislative approach was to require the notification of persons with AIDS and/or HIV to the authorities.[5] While case reporting contributed to the efforts to monitor the evolving epidemic, the reporting systems in place in some countries were not structured around the concept of confidentiality, with the result that in such countries the identity of infected persons was very much a matter in the public domain. With growing pressures to protect the identity of infected persons, some countries have updated their notifications laws, but quite a large number still continue to have in place laws providing for systems that do not provide any assurance of protection.

In some countries, the communicable disease laws apply to Sexually Transmitted Diseases (STDs) as well, while in others there are separate or special laws for the purpose. Pressures to respond to the growing epidemic resulted in a few countries[6] classifying HIV and AIDS even as a STD. This resulted in persons with haemophilia and other recipients of blood transfusions who contracted the virus through non-sexual means being legally classified into the same group along with those who had contracted STDs through sexual means.

Comprehensive HIV/AIDS prevention and control laws have been enacted only by a few countries. In the Asian region,[7] countries such as China, Indonesia, Japan, Mongolia and Vietnam have enacted special laws that address several dimensions of the epidemic that are not generally covered in traditional communicable disease or sexually transmitted disease statutes.

While these special laws help redress some of the problems brought in the wake of the application of the older laws, the effectiveness of the former depend on as much on the lawmaking process as on the content of the legal provisions. The HIV epidemic has a number of stakeholders, including most importantly affected individuals and communities. Where the enactment of legislation had involved consultations with representatives of groups or communities affected by the epidemic, the final text is likely to reflect some or all of their needs and concerns. Where the law (or the legislative policy) reflects such needs and concerns, concerned individuals and communities will more readily assume the responsibility for taking the initiative to ensure due compliance by mobilizing existing networks and support systems. In some countries, such as Australia, for instance, the consultative process thus spawned by the HIV epidemic is being extended to other areas of law reform.

This chapter provides an overview of legislative responses from different parts of the world. It seeks to exemplify the diversity in the scope and content of HIV-related laws and regulations. It is, by no means, a comprehensive survey; the examples cited are primarily intended to serve as a backdrop to the discussions contained in the other chapters in this publication.

2. Definition of "HIV-related Law"

Since 1983 when a number of countries began to turn their attention to the role of law, more than 115 countries around the world have enacted HIV-related laws, regulations, decrees, orders and related instruments. If sub-national jurisdictions such as states, provinces and territories are also taken into account, HIV-related laws or legal provisions can be found in more than 150 legal jurisdictions.

"HIV-related Law" can be defined as that branch of the law that specifically addresses the problems, issues and challenges posed by the HIV epidemic by (i) supporting and channelling resources for epidemiological surveillance, policy initiatives and interventions; (ii) mandating interventions for healthier life styles and other preventive measures such as education, counselling, treatment and disease management; (iii) establishing the rights and duties of persons with HIV/AIDS as well as of others; (iv) regulating human behaviour and laying down norms for conduct; (v) specifying the quality and use of products such as blood, semen, organs, tissue, HIV test kits and condoms; and (vi) creating a supportive and an enabling environment in which affected individuals and communities as well as others can mutually co-exist to enhance their quality of life.

The above definition includes within its scope most of the key elements thus far addressed by HIV-related laws. It also covers the functional roles served by HIV-related legislation.

3. Evolution of HIV-related Legislative Measures

Two years after the first AIDS cases came to be reported, several countries began to have recourse,to legislative measures to deal with the impending crisis. By 1983 little was known about the virus itself and how it affects the immune system; far less was known about effective preventive measures .

The first generation of HIV-related laws enacted in 1983 essentially focused on notification of cases, blood safety, institutional mechanisms, education, funding and research and safety precautions but not in great detail. Table 4.1 lists the scope of the laws enacted by some 12 countries in 1983:

TABLE 4.1
SCOPE OF HIV/AIDS LEGISLATION ENACTED IN 1983
(31 JANUARY-22 DECEMBER, 1983)

- **REPORTING**
  Canada (British Columbia, Alberta, Ontario) United States (California) Sweden, Denmark, Italy, Norway, Greece, Israel, Austria, New Zealand
- **BLOOD SAFETY**
  France, Greece
- **INSTITUTIONAL MECHANISMS**
  (e.g., Research Institute (R); Advisory Council (A)) United States (New York (R); California (A))
- **PRECAUTIONS: HEALTH WORKERS**
  Austria, Greece
- **EDUCATION/INFORMATION United States (New York; California) Italy**
- **FUNDING**
  United States (New Jersey; California)
- **RESEARCH**
  Germany (ex-Federal Republic of)

What is significant about the above list is that, in 1983, apart from the United States, Canada and a few European countries, only New Zealand had enacted an HIV-related legal provision. What is also significant about this list is that it does not include even a single developing country. It was, in fact, in 1984, that three developing countries—Chile, Uruguay and Venezuela—enacted HIV-related legislation. But, as can be seen from Table 4.2, most developing countries introduced legislation only in 1987, the year in which the World Health Organization created the Special Programme on AIDS.

TABLE 4.2
INITIAL INTRODUCTION OF HIV/AIDS LEGISLATION

Year	*Developed Countries*	*Developing Countries*
1983	11	-
1984	4	3
1985	9	11
1986	7	8
1987	2	21
1988	2	7
1889	-	7
1990	-	6
1991	1	3
1992	2	1
1993	-	1
1994	-	2
Total	**38**	**70**

Source: Information extracted from International Digest of Health Legislation.

During the first decade of HIV-related law-making, most countries with ten or more reported AIDS cases had enacted HIV–related laws, compared with those with no cases[8] or only a few cases. Countries in Africa are, however, an exception to this trend. Even countries such as Cote d'Ivoire, Ghana, Malawi, Zaire and Zambia that had reported more than 10,000 cases by the end of 1992 had not enacted any legislation specifically related to HIV. With few exceptions, the health legislation framework in most African countries is relatively rudimentary, and it is not surprising, therefore, that the enactment and enforcement of HIV-related legislation did not receive priority.

Table 4.3 lists the year of initial enactment of HIV-related legal provisions or HIV-related laws.

TABLE 4.3
COUNTRIES WITH LEGAL INSTRUMENTS DEALING WITH AIDS AND HIV INFECTION AND RELATED MATTERS AND YEAR OF FIRST ADOPTION

Country	Year	Country	Year
Albania	1993	Chad	1991
Algeria	1989	Chile	1984
Andorra	1994	China	1987
Angola	1987	Colombia	1988
Argentina	1988	Comoros	1988
Australia	1984	Costa Rica	1986
Austria	1983	Croatia	1992
Bahrain	1990	Cuba	1986
Barbados	1985	Czechoslovakia	1984
Belgium	1985	Czech Republic	1987
Belize	1987	Denmark	1985
Bermuda	1985	Dominican Rep	1987
Bolivia	1989	Ecuador	1985
Brazil	1985	Egypt	1986
Brunei Darussalam	1987	El Salvador	1988
Bulgaria	1985	Equatorial Guniea	1988
Burundi	1987	Estonia	1992
Canada	1983	Finland	1985
France	1983	Netherlands	1987
French Polynesia	1985	New Zealand	1983
German, Dem. Rep.	1986	Niger	1987
Germany, Fed.		Norway	1983
Rep. of	1983	Oman	1990
Greece	1983	Panama	1985
Grenada	1986	Paraguay	1985
Guatemala	1986	Peru	1987
Guinea Bissau	1989	Philippines	1986
Guyana	1989	Poland	1986
Haiti	1987	Portugal	1986
Hong Kong	1988	Rep. of Korea	1987
Hungary	1985	Romania	1985

Iceland	1986	Russian Federation	1985
India	1987	Rwanda	1987
Indonesia	1987	Sao Tome & Principe	1989
Iraq	1987	Saudi Arabia	1990
Israel	1983	Senegal	1990
Italy	1983	Singapore	1985
Japan	1988	Slovak Republic	1984
Jordan	1987	South Africa	1987
Kenya	1987	Spain	1985
Kazakhstan	1994	Sri Lanka	1987
Lebanon	1990	St. Lucia	1991
Libyan Arab Jamahiriya	1987	Sweden	1983
Liechtenstein	1987	Switzerland	1986
Luxembourg	1984	Syrian Arab Rep.	1987
Madagascar	1990	Thailand	1985
Malaysia	1985	Togo	1987
Malta	1986	Tunisia	1989
Mauritius	1987	Turkey	1983
Mexico	1985	Uganda	1992
Monaco	1986	Ukraine	1991
Mongolia	1989	USSR	1985
Mozambique	1986	United Kingdom	1985
Myanmar	1995	USA	1983
		Uruguay	1988
		Uzbekistan	1992
Venezuela	1984	Yugoslavia	1986
Viet Nam	1989	Zimbabwe	1991

(*Source*: Information extracted from *International Digest of Health Legislation*).

It should be noted[9] that the above listing is not necessarily exhaustive because some countries that are not listed may nevertheless have had recourse, through administrative measures, for instance, to existing laws and regulations that had been extended to cover HIV/AIDS.

4. Scope and Content

As noted earlier, legislation dealing specifically with AIDS came to be first enacted around 1983.[10] During the early years, laws addressed only AIDS or AIDS patients. Subsequently, legislative provisions were made applicable to HIV infection, ARC, and high-risk groups. Laws which began with blood donors as the target group, now address other groups such as sex workers and intravenous (IV) drug users. As far as homosexuals and bisexuals are concerned, most laws identify only the former as a specific group; references to both groups, however, are to be found most commonly in administrative guidelines, and educational materials. "Persons with many sexual partners" is also a concept that is used in some laws.

There is no uniformity in the descriptive labelling attached to AIDS, ARC or HIV. In most countries these conditions are classified as 'communicable' or 'infectious' or 'notifiable' diseases; in others as a 'sexually transmitted disease' or 'venereal disease'. In some legal instruments, AIDS and HIV are referred to without any descriptive labelling. In most societies a certain degree of social stigma is attached to persons with 'venereal diseases', and the application of this label to persons with HIV infection or AIDS might have resulted in further discrimination.

In the evolution of AIDS-related laws, developments in medical technology have come to be reflected particularly with regard to the identification of persons with HIV. With the availability of the Western blot test as a confirmatory test, some laws now specify that only persons who are seropositive after a 'confirmatory test' should be notified to the authorities.[11] At a time when diagnostic tests were being refined to reduce the incidence of false-positive alid false-negative results, this was a particularly significant legislative development.[12] The high cost of the Western blot test has made it difficult for many developing countries to offer such a confirmatory test as a matter of routine in all cases where a seropositive finding has been initially recorded.

Within the scope of this chapter it is not possible to provide a comprehensive or detailed catalogue of the varied and diverse issues that have been covered in AIDS-related legislation[13]. Hence, some of the key areas that have been the subject matter of legislation are listed below by way of example:

A. Regulation of Blood and Blood Products

The main concern is to protect the supply of blood by requiring screening tests to be undertaken and by actively discouraging AIDS patients or HIV infected persons or those engaging in high-risk activities from donating blood. Concern with blood has led to similar requirements and restrictions being imposed with regard to semen, tissues, organs etc. Some state legislatures in the United State have found it necessary to authorize designated blood donations when the recipient has a foreseen medical need.[14] Denmark[15] and several other countries have made provision for the payment of compensation to persons with haemophilia who have contracted HIV infection. In most US jurisdictions blood is considered as a "service" and not as a "product", and hence there is no strict liability for the transfusion of contaminated blood. Declarations by potential donors that they do not have AIDS or HIV infection are being used to eliminate samples that must not be used. In order to stem the tide of requests for blood donations from persons primarily for the purpose of finding out their HIV status, a network of alternative testing sites to provide confidential test results has been established in the United States and in several other developed countries. In some developing countries, too, results of blood tests can be obtained without necessarily divulging the identity of the person. This is often done administratively, rather than as part of a legislative scheme.

B. Regulation of Sexual Activity

Measures to restrict sexual activity which is likely to spread the virus have concentrated on certain high-risk groups such as commercial sex workers. In Austria, for instance, they must get themselves tested at periodic intervals and the licences of those who are seropositive will be cancelled.[16] However, in many countries in the world, there is no official registration system for commercial sex workers. Nor is compulsory medical examination a legal requirement. Some jurisdictions have ordered the closure of establishments such as bathhouses and massage parlours where high-risk activities occur. Some laws require the distribution of information leaflets to patrons of such establishments. The Dominican Republic requires condoms to be made available at hotels, motels, bars and restaurants.[17]

Under the Penal Code or other criminal laws of some countries it is an offence to intentionally or through negligence to cause or aggravate the danger of the introduction or spread of an infectious human disease.[18] Some laws specifically declare it to be an offence, punishable with imprisonment, to knowingly expose a person to AIDS or to transmit AIDS when the person is aware that he or she is infected.[19] In Las Vegas, a prostitute was sentenced to 20 years' imprisonment for violating a state law which makes it an offence to solicit after testing HIV positive.[20]

C. Screening

The mandatory versus voluntary screening debate still continues to rage in many parts of the world. In some developing countries, the debate has not assumed much importance due to the unavailability of adequate facilities for screening.

In the United States where the issue of screening has been the subject of much heated debate, some states have mandated compulsory screening in a wide variety of special populations, including marriage applicants, pregnant women, newborns, hospital patients, mentally ill or mentally retarded patients, prisoners, commercial sex workers, intravenous drug users, and sex offenders.[21] Outside the United States, several countries have mandated the screening of one or more of such populations and of foreigners. The October 1990 USSR Regulations on medical testing for detection of HIV contained probably the most exhaustive list of categories for testing.22 More than 15 categories were listed:

(a) Donors of blood, blood plasma, and other biological fluids and tissues, on the occasion of each donation;
(b) Soviet citizens returning from service-related, business, and private journeys abroad of more than three months' duration;
(c) Aliens and stateless persons who have come to the USSR for study, work, or other purposes, in the 10 days following their arrival, with the exception of aliens and stateless persons coming from countries whose certificates of testing for antibodies to the virus are recognized by the USSR;
(d) Soviet citizens travelling abroad to countries whose requirements necessitate a certificate of testing for infection by the human immunodeficiency virus;
(e) Soviet citizens and aliens who have had sexual contacts with AIDS patients or carriers of the virus and who are identified during an epidemiological investigation (to be examined once every six months for one year);
(f) Patients with the following clinical symptoms:
(g) Patients with the suspected or confirmed diagnosis of:
(h) Children born to HIV-infected mothers, at birth and at six and 12 months after birth;
(i) Patients systematically receiving transfusions of blood and blood products (for haemophilia, etc.), (to be tested once a year);
(j) Pregnant women, upon being recorded as pregnant and at 30 weeks of pregnancy, where data from an AIDS test are not available, upon admission to the maternity unit;
(k) Pregnant women undergoing examination for artificial termination of pregnancy;
(l) Children admitted to intensive care, cancer, chest, and haematology units:
(m) People suffering from sexual transmitted diseases, on applying for medical care and subsequently as indicated;

(n) Medical personnel working with the virus or providing diagnoses, treatment, and direct services for AIDS patients (to be tested once a year);

(o) People in risk groups: drug abusers, drug addicts, homosexuals and bisexuals, and people engaged in prostitution (to be tested twice a year);

(p) People in risk groups placed in solitary confinement or in corrective labour establishments and preventive therapeutic/labour units, on admission and before release; and,

(q) People of no fixed abode engaged in vagrancy.

Legal provisions on the testing of foreigners are more common than those that apply to nationals. Over 50 countries require one or more of the following categories to be tested on arrival or to submit a certificate of a test done previously:

1. Applicants for work permits.
2. Applicants for residence permits.
3. Applicants for naturalization.
4. Immigrants.
5. Tourists.
6. Nationals returning to country.
7. Refugees.
8. Foreign students
9. Cabaret artists.
10. Foreign defence contractors.
11. Nationals who are pilots or marine crew members.
12. Returning nations who are seamen or entertainers.
13. Truck drivers crossing national frontiers.
14. Visitors coming frequently.
15. Foreigners wishing to marry nationals.
16. Persons who have developed clinical symptoms.

Countries that require the above categories to be tested may not necessarily require all those coming under each category to be tested. Certain criteria have been laid down by some countries to determine the categories to be subjected to testing. Among the criteria are the following:

1. Country of origin (based on a geographical basis or on the incidence of HIV and AIDS)
2. Age limit (minimum and/or maximum)
3. Length of stay
4. Purpose of visit

Some nationalities and categories of professionals are often excluded from the screening requirements—e.g. persons entitled to diplomatic status; officials of United Nations and similar agencies; nationals and servicemen of certain countries; persons accompanied by spouses; official delegations; and, accredited journalists. The rationale underlying such exemptions is not evident.

With regard to the test itself, different countries have different requirements. Some countries require, for instance, the test to be done immediately on arrival or within a specified period thereafter, while others permit the test to be done before arrival. If the test is to be done prior to arrival or prior to the submission of the application, some countries specify the doctor or clinic. A certificate from another doctor or clinic may not necessarily be admissible. Some laws require a repeat test to be performed. Many countries have traditionally applied the requirement of a medical examination for all migrants, students and long-term visitors, and a test for HIV antibodies may or may not be included among the tests to be routinely performed as part of such examination.

Different consequences flow depending on the outcome of the test. If the certificate has been submitted prior to entry and the applicant is seropositive, he or she may not be granted the visa or work permit, or even the scholarship in the case of students, and denied entry. If the test is done after arrival or if the authorities become aware that a person who has entered the country is HIV infected or is having AIDS, a number of options may be available, depending on the applicable laws and regulations. While these vary from country to country, among the measures that may be taken, are the following: deportation or expulsion; observation, surveillance and isolation; termination of visa or permit; and, imposition of a fine. In some countries the law permits consideration on a case by-case approach, while in others the consequences will apply automatically.

D. Reporting and Contact Tracing Systems

In most countries with HIV-related legislation there is a requirement to notify AIDS cases. ARC is reportable only in a few countries.[23] Similarly, only a few countries specifically require cases of *Pneumocystis carinii* pneumonia to be reported.[24] Increasingly, more and more countries require HIV seropositive cases to be notified; in a few countries there is a requirement that seropositive findings must be confirmed by another (such as the Western blot) test.[25]

Contact tracing is a public health strategy traditionally used in the context of sexually transmitted diseases. In the United States, some states have classified HIV infection as a sexually transmitted disease, thus making the provision concerning contact tracing applicable to HIV and AIDS, while others have specifically provided for the tracing of the sexual contacts of HIV- infected persons.[26] Legislation in Hungary requires the sexual partners of AIDS patients and seropositive persons to be placed under epidemiological surveillance.[27]

E. Detention, Isolation and Quarantine

In the absence of a drug or vaccine, issues of individual liberty and functional effectiveness of coercive measures tend to loom large when measures such as detention, isolation and masantine are considered. In some countries where AIDS has been subsumed under existing classifications of communicable, infectious, notifiable or sexually transmitted disease, it is possible to have recourse to measures that curtail individual liberty either by restricting mobility or by requiring submission to tests, examinations and treatment. In some countries these measures extend to the identification of sexual partners. In the United States, some states provide for both quarantine and isolation.[28] Similar legal provisions exist in countries like China.[29] In Cuba HIV seropositive persons have been sent to a sanatorium located in a Havana suburb.[30]

Increasingly, the view that such coercive and restrictive measures are counterproductive is gaining currency, but countries have been slow to repeal existing provisions.

F. Restrictions

Closely related to the requirement of screening is the issue of discrimination. This issue has loomed large ever since the discovery of AIDS. Homosexuals, bisexuals and commercial sex workers, in particular, have been discriminated by linking AIDS to so-called "promiscuous" conduct. Some nationalities and ethnic groups have also been victimized. Despite uncontroverted evidence that HIV or AIDS cannot be transmitted by casual contact, children with HIV/ AIDS have been barred from schools, workers have been summarily dismissed; insurance companies have refused coverage; and tenants have been from houses.[3]

In relation to reporting, screening and discrimination, the issue of confidentiality assumes importance. Some countris that require reporting have devised a means of protecting the identity of the person by the use of a code for reporting purposes. The code may contain, for instance, the initials of tht person wlth the year of birth or another combination of figures with the social security number and some letters from the family name. Ihe failure to guarantee confidentiality of HIV status results in compromising the privacy and many related rights and freedoms of persons with HIV or AIDS.

Legal restrictions placed upon persons with HIV/AIDS that have lead to all forms of discriminatory treatment include the following:

1. Restrictions on the movement of persons across national frontiers;
2. Restrictions on freedom of internal travel due to compulsory hospitalization or other reason such as quarantine or isolation;
3. Restrictions on sexual behaviour;
4. Restrictions on donation of blood, semen, breast-milk or organs;
5. Restrictions on freedom of occupation; and,
6. Other miscellaneous forms of restrictions (e.g. marriage contracts).

Within less than a decade there has emerged a substantial body of restrictions applicable to persons with HIV or AIDS not all of which are entirely new to the field of public health legislation. In many instances, these restrictions have been extended to apply to or to cover HIV or AIDS disregarding the fact that these restrictions were initially formulated to deal with the specific context of contagious or communicable diseases or conditions; neither HIV or AIDS fits this label of a contagious or communicable disease or condition in the strict sense of the term. Even after 10 years of close monitoring HIV is not known to have been transmitted except through one of the three well-documented modes, thus reinforcing the view that it is a virus difficult to 'catch'. To varying degrees, these restrictions limit the rights and freedoms of individuals with HIV and AIDS even in the absence of definitive evidence that such restrictions are necessarily effective in slowing down HIV transmission.

G. The Role of Criminal Law

Several states in Australia and countries like the Republic of Korea and Singapore in the Asian region have made it a criminal offence for a person who is aware of his or her HIV status to have sexual intercourse with another unless that fact had been disclosed and the other person had voluntarily agreed to accept the risk. This is an area of the criminal law where difficulties in obtaining evidence loom large.[32] Courts in some other jurisdictions, such as the United State have, however, entered convictions in cases involving the transmission of infections.[33]

Another area in which criminal sanctions have been provided is in respect of donations of blood, semen or organs when one is aware of his or her HIV seropositive status. While it is obviously safer and more cost-effective to exclude contaminated blood samples from entering the system in the first place, some countries have found that where blood donations to earn money are ubiquitous, there are few options available to blood banks. According to one report, an estimated 20,000 to 30,000 professional blood donors in India sell roughly 15-16 units for a month, for as little as 85 US cents a unit.[34]

The regulation of the sex industry has always attracted the use of criminal sanctions. In several countries in the regio laws exist which, to varying degrees, seek to criminalise certain activities such as soliciting or loitering for purposes of prostitution, maintaining brothels and making a livelihood out of the earnings of sex workers. Discriminalization has been the subject of much discussion in Asian countries like Australia and Thailand. In the State of Victoria in Australia brothels are now legal, provided a town planning permit has been obtained. In terms of the Health (Brothels) Regulations 1990,[35] a proprietor must provide a free supply of condoms and water based lubricants, and take reasonable steps to ensure that prostitutes and their clients use condoms in vaginal, anal and oral sex. Under the regulations it is not permissible to display on the premises any HIV-free certificates. It is the responsibility of proprietors to provide written information concerning sexually transmitted diseases. Due to the presence of many ethnic groups in the country, the regulations require that information be provided in a variety of languages. It is still uncertain as to what impact the Victorian model has had on slowing HIV transmission.

H. Access to Needles and Syringes

Some countries now provide for a system of exchanging new needles and syringes for those that have been used.[36] There has also been a relaxation of prescription requirements applicable to the supply of needles and.syringes from pharmacy outlets. Travellers to high-risk areas are often urged to carry a small consignment of needles and syringes because clean needles and syringes may not always be available, particularly in some developing countries. However, there are several countries around the world where the possession of needles and syringes constitutes a serious offence under the relevant narcotic and dangerous drugs laws. Some countries mandate by law the compulsory treatment of persons dependent on drugs.[37]

I. Education and Counselling

In many countries priority has been accorded to education and counselling programmes. In the United States, some states that mandate AIDS education programmes require schools to stress abstinence until one is ready to form an exclusive relationship within the institution of marriage.[38] Education and information laws may not necessarily have been formulated at a time when health education was expected to play a more pro-active role. Some laws, for instance, still do not allow condoms to be advertised in the public.

Pre-testing and post-testing counselling requirements are important in order to minimize the psychological trauma associated with an HIV seropositive finding. Some countries have made such counselling a mandatory requirement.

J. Treatment, Services and Research

In the USSR new regulations of 1990 addressed the issue of making drugs available to AIDS patients and persons who are HIV infected. A parent can be on leave with pay to look after a child who is HIV infected or who has AIDS.[39] In the United States specific laws are in place that are designed to promote AIDS research and to facilitate treatment and related services. Some states have made medical, mental health, social, housing, testing and financial services available to patients with AIDS and their families.[40]

K. Pharmaceutical Laws and Clinical Trails

Over one hundred drug companies and scientists in research based institutions have embarked on what might well turn out to be a very long voyage of discovering a drug or vaccine.

Clinical trails have brought into sharp focus legal and ethical issues.[41] In the context of developing countries—the setting for many clinical trails—these issues assume critical importance.[42] Few developing countries regulate clinical trails.

In the United States, the Food and Drug Administration has been quick to appreciate the need to adapt the procedures governing the investigational use of new drugs. However, there is as yet no consensus of opinion on how drug regulatory authorities can best respond to the crisis and support the research-based industry.

5. Implementation and Impact of Legal Measures

It is not unusual to have a long gestational period before the real impact of a new law can be measured in relation to stated goals and objectives.

In some areas of intervention, however, the results are quite evident. A clear example is the screening of blood and blood products. Transmission of HIV through this source has been virtually eliminated or greatly minimized since legal and policy measures for screening blood were introduced.

One rationale for legal interventions is the symbolic effect of legislation. Since HIV transmission is largely behaviour-related, behavioural and attitudinal changes play an important role. It is perhaps true of many countries that the debates that have taken place in the public and in the legislatures, and mass media coverage, have sensitized the public to a great extent.

The extent to which a country can contain the HIV/AIDS problem through legal measures is still unknown. What is perhaps clear is that certain legal measures that can be introduced can have a deflnite impact. An example is the development of the health infrastructure, through improved mechanics of colle cting, screening and storing blood. To give another example, mandating the use of good quality condoms might have the effect ot slowing down HIV infection, where one partner is already seropositive or whose I IIV status is unknown.[43]

6. The Unfinished Agenda

The brief overview presented in this chapter illustrates how 'HIV Law' has evolved within just over a decade and the ever widening scope of matters addressed by HIV law. What was once perceived as a simple matter of tracking down infected cases has now turned out to offer a 'window of opportunity' to assess the role of law in regulating human behaviour in a context where individuals—infected or otherwise—demand that their r ights be respected. Had the HIV epidemic manifested itself two or three decades ago, and not in the early '80s, the legislative, ethical and human rights response might have been quite different.

The E IIV epidemic is not simply a matter concerning a virus. It is an epidemic that challenges the ways in which we regulate inter-personal relationships and the ways in which we seek to regulate what others may do or may not do. It is an epidemic that challenges the rationale of many things we have taken for granted in the past. For instance, until recent times in most countries, the very process of reviewing and drafting laws was the prerogative of a few—the individuals and communities who will be affected by these very laws never came into the mainstream of events. The HIV epidemic has sharpened the focus on the role of 'stakeholders'—the affected individuals and communities. Increasingly, the affected individuals and communities assume the responsibility for bringing about changes in perception, behaviour and lifestyles that will enable a more humane and effective response to emerge.

Initially, 'HIV Law' was conceived within the narrow confines of traditional communicable disease statutes that were based on a strict regime of case notification, isolation, quarantine or similar restrictions. As countries began to progressively adopt a broader-based and multi-sectoral approach to HIV prevention and control, the scope and content of 'HIV Law' changed quite rapidly. 'HIV Law' then came to be concerned with the broader social, economic, cultural, ethical, legal and human rights environment that regulates behaviour. Abandoning centuries of thinking based on the coercive role of law in bringing about attitudinal and behavioural changes, it was realized that there must be an enabling and supportive environment within which policy and legislative changes can be best formulated and implemented.

Experience with over a decade of the epidemic has clearly demonstrated the vulnerability of individuals, communities and societies to HIV. Vulnerability is exacerbated by a multiplicity of factors including social prejudices; unequal power relations within families, communities, nations and as well as between nations; and, last, but not least, by ineffective, inequitable or unjust laws. Given that HIV/AIDS will continue to remain a threat to the well-being of individuals and societies for man decades to come, the march towards a better quality of life requires many hurdles being cleared. This calls for 'HIV Law to be concerned more aggressively with those aspects of development that directly or indirectly affect the quality of life of individuals and the ability of individuals to function as fully and effective members of civilized society. While providing the fine tuning that is required of existing laws and policie the new task of those concerned with 'HIV Law' is to address the developmental implications of the HIV epidemic and to help formulate policy. legislative and practice reforms that will make a difference to the impact of the epidemic on the quality of life.

REFERENCES

1. Mills, M., C. B. Wofsy and J. Mills, "The Acquired Immunodeficiency Syndrome: Infection control and Public Health Law", *NEJM,* 261, 1986, 931-6.
2. Jayasuriya, D. C. ed., *HIV Law and Law Reform in Asia and the Pacific,* UNDP, New Delhi, 1995.
3. *Ibid.*
4. Jayasuriya, D. C. and S. Jayasuriya. *The Health Legislation System of Sri Lanka. ICHPL,* Nawala, 1992, 42-9.
5. Fluss S.S. "National AIDS Legislation: An Overview of Some Global Developments" in Gostin, L. and L. Porter eds. *International Law and AIDS. International Responses, Current Issues. and Future Directions,* American Bar Association, Chicago, 1992, 15-7.
6. For example, Iceland (Law No. 7 of 7 April 1986 amending Law No. 16 of 1978 on the prevention of venereal diseases).
7. Jayasuriya, D.C. "A Comparative Review of AIDS Legislation in Asia and the Pacific", *International and Comparative Law Quarterly,* 43 (2), 1994, 391-405.
8. Notable exceptions, however, were Albania, Mongolia and Kyrgyztan.
9. The Table is based on information made available to the Health Legislation Unit of the World Health Organization, in terms of Article 63 of its Constitution. The current legal status of the HIV-related laws of some countries (eg. former USSR) that have undergone geo-political and constitutional changes in recent years is not clear.
10. Regulation No. 6 of 8 March 1983 of the National Board of Health and Welfare [Sweden] concerning: notification of AIDS *(Int. Dig. Hlth. Leg.,* 34, 1983, 748).
11. E.g. Austria, Denmark.
12. Jayasuriya, D.C., "AIDS-related Health Legislation" in Fleming, A.F. *et al. The Global Impact of AIDS,* A.R. Liss, Inc., New York, 1988, 313.
13. For a more comprehensive comparative review of the legislation, see Jayasuriya D.C. *AIDS: Public Health and Legal Dimensions,* Martinus Nijhoff Publishers, Dordrecht, 1988, 11-37 and Jayasuriya D.C. *AIDS: Health, Policy and Legal Aspects,* Commonwealth Secretariat, London, 1993. For US legislation, see further, Lamboi, S.E. et. al. "The Impact of AIDS on State Public Health Legislation in the United States: A Critical Review", *AIDS Education and Prevention,* 1, 1989, 324-339. US judicial and tribunal decisions are analyzed in Gostin, L. "The AIDS Litigation Project", *tAMA.* 263, 1990, 1961-1970 and *JAMA* 263, 1990, 2086-2093.
14. Gostin, L.O. "Public Health Strategies for Confronting AIDS', *JAMA*, 261, 1989, 1624; and Zuck, T.F. "Legal Liability for Transfusion Injury in the Acquired Immunodeficiency Syndrome Era", *Arch. Pathol. Lab. Med.,* 114, 1990, 309-315.
15. Order of 14 June 1988 *(Int. Dig. Hlth. Leg.,* 39, 1989, 824).
16. The AIDS Law of 16 May 1986 *(Int. Dig. Hlth. Leg.,* 37, 1986, 533).
17. Resolution of 13 April 1987 of the Secretary of State for Public Health and Welfare *(Int. Di8. Hlth. Leg.,* 39, 1988, 627).
18. For example, Notice of 2 December 1987 of the Ministry of Justice of the Czech Socialist Republic establishing the list of communicable diseases in man for the purposes of the Penal Code *(Int. Dig. Hlth. Leg.,* 39, 1988, 626).
19. For example, Decree of 25 August 1987 of the Presidium of the USSR Supreme

Soviet on measures for the prevention of infection by the AIDS virus (*Int. Dig. Hlth. Leg.*, 38 1987, 769 and 41, 1990, 433).

20. *State v. Kearns*, New Dist Ct. Clark Cty. No. C86584X.03 September 1989, cited in Gostin, L. "The AIDS Litigation Project", *JAMA* 263, 1990, 1963.
21. Gostin, L. "Public Health Strategies for Confronting AIDS: Legislative and Regulatory Policy in the United States", *JAMA*. 261, 1989, 1621-1630; and Lamboi, S.E. *et. al*. "The Impact of AIDS on State Public Health Legislation in the United States: A Critical Review", *AIDS Education and Prevention, 1*, 1989, 324.339.
22. Regulations of 4 October 1990 on medical testing for detection of the human immunodeficiency virus (AIDS) (*Int. Dig. Hlth. Leg.*, 42, 1991, 21).
23. E.g. Costa Rica.
24. For example; Israel: The Public Health (Communicable Diseases) Regulations, 1983 (*Int. Dig. Hlth. Leg.*, 38, 1987, 767).
25. E.g, Cuba and Hungary.
26. *Op. cit.* note 21.
27. Instructions No. 10 of 1985 of the Mirwister of Health (*Int. Dig. Hlth. Leg.*, 37, 1986, 21).
28. *Op. cit.* note 21.
29. Regulations of 26 December 1987 on surveillance and control measures applicable to AIDS (*Int. Dig. Hlth. Leg.*, 39, 1988, 623).
30. Bayer, R. and C. Healton "Controlling AIDS in Cuba: The Logic of Quarantine", *NEIM*, 320, 1989, 1022-1024.
31. Jayasuriya, D.C. "AIDS-Related Legislation in the Context of the Third AIDS Pandemic", *Law, Medicine and Health Care*, 18, 1990, 41-47.
32. Kirby, Michael "The Ten Commandments for AIDS Law", AIDSED Newsletter 2, 1991, 26-28.
33. Gostin, L. Lane Porter and H. Sandomire, AIDS Litigation Project: A National Survey of Federal, State and Local Cases Before Courts and Human Rights Commissions (Washington, D.C: Public Health Service, Department of Health and Human Services, 1990).
34. Girimaji, P. "Professional Blood Donors Protest", *World AIDS*, 22, 1992, 9-10.
35. The regulations have been made under the Prostitution Regulation Act 1986.
36. Brettle, R.P. "HIV and Harm Reduction for Injection Drug Users", *AIDS*, 5, 1991, 125-136.
37. Curran, W.J., A.E. Arif and D.C. Jayasuriya, Guidelines for Assessing and Revising National Legislation on Treatment of Drug-and Alcohol Dependent Persons, (*Int. Dig. Hlth. Leg.*, 38 (Supplement 1), 1987; and Gostin, L. "An Alternative Public Health Vision for a National Drug Strategy: "Treatment Works", *Houston Law Review*, 28, 1991 285-308.
38. *Op. cit.* note 21.
39. Resolution No. 947 of 18 September 1990 (*Int. Dig. Hlth. Leg.*, 42, 1991, 20).
40. *Op. cit.* note 21.
41. Mariner, W. "The Ethical Conduct of Clinical Trials of HIV Vaccines", *Evautation Review* 14, 1990, 538-564.
42. Jayasuriya, D.C. "Law, Ethics and Biomedical Research Involving Human Subjects in Developing Countries", *Journal of Clinical Research and Drug Development, 33*, 1989, 83-88.
43. Jayasuriya, D.C. *AIDS and Condoms*, ICHPL, Nawala [Sri Lanka], 1989; and Jayasuriya, D.C. "The Formulation and Implementation of a National Policy on Condoms in the Context of HIV/AIDS', *AIDS Care, 3*, 1991, 3-9.

5

HIV and Liability in Tort

Dr. Hemamal Jayawardena
Head, Department of Forensic Medicine & Medical Law
University of Kelaniya, Sri Lanka

INTRODUCTION

A tort[1] is a form of civil injury or wrong. An action in tort arises when the defendant, without just cause or excuse commits an act (or an omission) which results in some form of harm to the plaintiff.

The distinguishing feature between a contract and a tort is that in the former the duties of the parties towards each other are fixed by themselves, whereas in the latter, the duties towards persons in general are laid down by law.

Unlike in a criminal lawsuit, the main aim of a tort action is to compensate the victim for damages. Sometimes, a punitive element may be incorporated into an award of damages. Another aim of tort law is to deter people from harming one another in respect of their property, person or reputation.

An action of tort is a claim for pecuniary compensation in respect of damages suffered because of an invasion of a legally protected interest.[2] As all human interests cannot be legally protected, courts have been vested with the responsibility of deciding which interests should receive legal protection.

Originally, the Anglo-American courts interpreted these interests very narrowly. However, in recent times they have recognized less obvious, yet convincing, interests such as emotional security, disease phobias, or stress trauma. This is an important development in the light of the AIDS pandemic. Credit should be given to judges with foresight such as Sir John Halt C J[3] and Sir Charles Prat C J[4] who, as early as 1702, established that novelty in form is no bar to an action in tort.[5] Torts have evolved to meet new demands of society.

Tort law has its origins in the common law. The corresponding term used in Roman Law is "delict". The subsequent developments in various parts of the world have been varied. They have been influenced by economic, cultural, constitutional and social factors. For example, a review of English cases on medical malpractice suggests that the English judges have taken a pro-doctor approach. But in the United States the approach has been more pro-patient. This may be attributed to Britain[6] primarily having a government-based National Health Service, while the American health service is mainly private insurance-based.

This chapter discusses the long established common law causes of action in tort as well as the newly emerging ones related to HIV/AIDS. It is not implied that all courts throughout the world will abide by the same guidelines referred to in this chapter. For example, the courts in Sri Lanka, guided by a tort system based mainly on the Roman Dutch Law of Delict, may not recognize non-pecuniary damages such as 'disease phobias'.

CAUSES OF ACTION IN TORT AND THEIR RELEVANCE TO HIV/AIDS

1. Trespass to the Person

Trespass to the person has long been established as a cause of action in tort. Interference with personal liberty is actionable even without damage.

1.1 Battery

In the United States, the Restatement (second) of Torts sec. 525 defines battery as an intentional, harmful or offensive, and unjustifiable contact with the body of another made without that person's consent. English law simply defines battery as the intentional application of force to the person of another without lawful justification.[7]

1.1.1 Willful Transmission of HIV/AIDS

Transmission of diseases through sexual contact[8] or other means such as wilful needle pricks, or knowingly sharing intravenous (IV) needles would amount to battery. The defendant in such cases may be liable to the person who becomes infected with the virus. In the event of death of a victim, liability may extend to his or her survivors in a wrongful death claim.

It is clear from the wording of the restatement that the intention need not be to cause harm (e.g., spread HIV), but to commit the unjustifiable contact (e.g., have sex). If the defendant can prove that he did not know his HIV-positive status, he would not be held liable, as having sex would then not be unjustifiable.

Battery is not only a civil wrong but a criminal one. In *State v. Lankford*[9] the defendant was convicted for criminal assault and battery for infecting his wife with syphilis.

1.1.2 Compulsory Medical Examination and Informed Consent

Compulsory examination or treatment of a patient without informed consent is tortuous.[10] The words of the English judge, "No man of professional skill can justify the substitution of the will of the surgeon for that of his patient"[11] and his American counterpart, "Every human being of adult years and sound mind has a right to determine what shall be done with his own body"[12] amply exemplify the legal recognition that it is the patient who knows what is best for him or her. The doctor should only give the relevant information to the patient so as to help the latter to make his or her own decision. He should never impose what he thinks is best for the patient against the patient's will since the medical decision-making process is strictly not a clinical one. It is a complicated combination involving moral and cultural values, socio-economic circumstances, and other individual biases which the doctor may be ignorant of.[13]

In an emergency, when immediate therapeutic measures have to be taken without delay or when the patient is unconscious,[14] consent may be considered to be implied. But expressed consent should be taken at the earliest opportunity. As a means of avoiding frivolous lawsuits, it is advisable for doctors to get an attestation from another medical officer, confirming that it is an emergency, before starting therapy in such cases. Implied consent also covers non-invasive examination of a patient who has wilfully come to the doctor for treatment.

Consent to medical examination and treatment is a legal

concept rather than a question in traditional medical ethics. For example, the Hippocratic Oath does not refer to consent, as it does to confidentiality and other ethical norms.

The doctor is required to give detailed information about the procedure before obtaining the signature indicating consent. This includes informing the patient about the adverse effects of the envisaged procedure, its complications, the alternatives available, and their advantages and disadvantages.

There are two principal standards of disclosure described in medico-legal literature. According to the American standard laid down in *Canterbury v. Spence*,[15] all information necessary for the patient to make a therapeutic decision should be divulged. This leaves room for "wisdom after the event". The British standard, laid down in the Sideway case,[16] requires the doctor to inform only details which an ordinary doctor in the community would inform a patient in like circumstances.

The consent of the guardian should be obtained when the person is a minor or of unsound mind.

Before blood transfusions[17] in the United States, the information that should be divulged includes the possibility of the occurrence of a false negative HIV test result in blood used for transfusion. Since paid donors have a higher chance of withholding information, making their transfusions more riskier, information about the type of donor (paid/voluntary) too should be given to the patient. Some states require that such blood be specially labelled. It is yet to be seen whether such standards will be expected by the courts of countries that do not still record or have minimal numbers of transfusion acquired HIV/AIDS.

Medical examinations without consent have been recognized under certain limited circumstances. Examples include mandatory vaccination requirements, statutes requiring quarantine.[18] and court ordered medical examinations. The settings under which actions against compulsory testing have been brought include employment, health, judiciary, insurance and industry.

Although the current World Health Organization (WHO) recommendations are against mandatory testing for HIV, there are countries that provide for such testing at least in a limited way. Except in such jurisdictions under the stipulated circumstances, any person who trespasses the person of a HIV/AIDS suspected individual would be liable in tort, even when no clear damage has occurred.

1.2 Unaurhotized Detention. Isolation and Quarantine

False imprisonment is a well-established tort. It is also a criminal offence in all the common law countries.[19] It refers to the arrest or imprisonment of a person without lawful justification and includes restraining the movement of a person by not allowing the person to leave. Since it is the curtailing of personal liberty and not the actual incarceration[20] that matters, any form of unjustifiable restraint would be covered by this tort.

Mandatory blood testing may be considered as an illegal search, barred under the Fourth Amendment to the US constitution. In *Glover v. Eastern Nebraska Community Office of Retardation,*[21] it was held that forced testing of employees of a mental hospital was a violation of the Fourth Amendment.

However, public health criteria may be considered as a lawful justification[22] for isolation. For example, in England, an AIDS patient may be detained in a hospital when a Justice of the Peace is satisfied that the patient may not take proper precautions to prevent the spread of the disease upon discharge.[23]

As in mandatory testing, WHO does not recommend quarantine in general for HIV/AIDS, as there is no public health rationale. The courts have expressed a similar view.[24] But the AIDS phobia, especially in the initial phase of the epidemic, influenced certain legislators to legalize the quarantining of persons suspected to be infected with HIV.[25] Except in such jurisdictions, a person who has been wrongfully confined or falsely imprisoned by virtue of his or her HIV status may invoke the authority of the court for compensation.

2. Negligence

Negligence is one of the grounds for most tort actions related to HIV/AIDS. It is based on fault liability theory, i.e., that the plaintive must prove fault on the part of the defendant.

A plaintiff who has been injured by the negligent conduct of the defendant should establish the existence of the following elements for compensation:[26]

* A duty of care
* Breach of this duty
* Causation
* Damages

The defendant would not be liable if he or she succeeds in establishing a legally valid excuse for the conduct. Voluntary assumption of risk and contributory negligence are commonly pledged defences in alleged negligence.

2.1 Duty of Care

The law does not impose a legal duty of care in all moral circumstances in which a duty to care seems to exist. "The rule that you are to love your neighbour becomes in law, you must not injure your neighbour."[27] A neighbour, here, refers to any person who is so closely and directly affected by one's act (or omission) that one should have such person in contemplation as being so affected by the act in question.[28]

2.1.1 Sexual Partners

Based on the neighbourhood principle, a person has a legal duty to protect his or her sexual partners from any reasonably foreseeable harm sex can bring about. A person having a sexually transmittable disease (STD) or a communicable disease has a legal duty to take precautions against transmission. In Berner v. Caldwell,[29] the courts held that one who knows or should reasonably know that he has genital herpes is under a duty to abstain from sexual contact or to warn others before engaging in risky behaviour. It is the intimateness of the sexual relationship that casts the duty to care. Whether the persons involved are married or not would not be relevant.

2.1.2 IV Needle Sharers

Under the above doctrine, IV drug addicts who use needles have a legal duty to inform their HIV status to persons who share these with them. Failure to do so gives rise to a cause of action. A prudent person would foresee the risk of sharing IV needles.

Since needle sharing is known to be a high-risk behaviour, it may also be presumed that the persons concerned have assumed the risk of contracting HIV. (see 2.5.2).

2.1.3 Doctors and Hospitals

Health care or health services providers have a duty to care for their patients. This duty arises when the doctor-patient relationship begins. Unless the doctor terminates the relationship, giving the patient adequate notice, or the patient terminates it by getting discharged, it lasts as long as the particular illness (and its direct complications, if any) lasts.[30] Except in an emergency, the doctor is not obliged to accept all patients who come to him or her.[31] The hospitals have a similar responsibility. However, government hospitals in some countries may be obliged to treat all patients who come to these hospitals under all circumstances. In such instances, the doctors employed by the government may have to accept all patients, including non-emergency cases, based on their service agreement.

A doctor who unlawfully terminates a doctor-patient relationship may be liable in malpractice for abandonment.[32] Refusing to treat an AIDS patient is illegal under the anti-discrimination law, where such a law exists, and may also be considered as abandonment. When the doctor is employed by a hospital, the hospital can be held vicariously liable for the actions of the doctor. The hospital may also be held vicariously liable for actions of other hospital employees such as nurses and attendants.

2.1.4 Blood Banks

Blood banks have a duty to avoid reasonably foreseeable harm towards the persons who may be placed at risk through their products or services. It includes not only the person who is directly transfused but also the foetus in the case of a pregnancy.

2.2 Breach of Duty to Care

Negligence[34] may be defined as a failure to exercise a reasonable degree of skill and care. This will include an omission of an act that a reasonable and prudent man would door the commission of an act that a reasonable and prudent man would not do. A reasonable person is expected to take steps to prevent foreseeable harm.

The application of the reasonability test will depend on the circumstances of the case. The standard expected may be that of a reasonable blood donor or a blood bank in a case of negligent blood transfusion. It may be a reasonable doctor in a case of negligent misdiagnosis.

The standard expected from a professional is higher than that of the average individual. A professional is expected to show a fair, reasonable and competent degree of skill in the practice of his or her art. The standard expected from a doctor is that of an average practitioner of that particular field.

Courts have decided that service providers such as blood banks and blood product manufacturers provide a professional service, and that they should be held to a professional and not a general standard of care.[35]

A doctor (or hospital) is required to exercise a reasonable degree of care and skill throughout the management of a patient. This includes diagnosis, treatment, and follow-up of the patient. It applies to therapeutic measures as well as professional advice and counselling. An action might be brought to recover damages as a result of negligent counselling after a positive HIV test result.[36]

2.2.1 Non-Diagnosis and Misdiagnosis

To avoid malpractice liability, the doctor should exercise care and skill throughout the diagnosis process, from history taking, to examination, ordering the relevant investigation,[37] and interpreting the findings to arrive at a diagnosis.[38]

This includes eliciting, in the history, associations such as homosexuality, IV drug addiction and previous blood transfusions; examining the respiratory system for repeated lung infections; examining other organs for opportunistic infections and malignancies; and ordering relevant tests such as HIV antibody and CD4 cell counts. A higher standard would be legally expected from a teaching hospital than from a rural village hospital with minimal facilities. The courts would need the assistance of experts from that locality to establish the expected standard of care.

Since prophylactic and symptomatic treatment is available for AIDS/HIV patients, a delay in diagnosis can cause damage through a premature death. It can also cause damage by the spread of infection through unprotected sex or needle sharing which would not have occurred had a diagnosis of HIV been made in time.

2.2.2 HIV-infected Blood and Blood Products.

The majority of AIDS-related tort cases in United States in the early period of the epidemic involved the receipt of HIV-infected blood or blood products.[39]

Since the duty of care owed to a patient is judged based on the standard applicable at the time of the transfusion, it is not a basis of liability for transfusions that occurred before the discovery of the syndrome. Before the Centers for Disease Control reported cases of *Pneumocystis carinii* pneumonia in persons with haemophilia and blood transfusion recipients in 1982,[40] blood banks would not have had a reason to foresee a risk of HIV.

For transmission after the discovery of AIDS, but before the availability of screening tests, plaints based on negligence may be filed.[41] However, arguments such as that blood donors should have been subjected to surrogate testing[42] have been rejected by most courts.[43]

Although an HIV antibody screening test became available in 1985, the existence of a window period and the possibility of false negativity have not made the whole scenario foolproof. Therefore, it is the duty of the doctor to inform patients of the option of autologous[44] blood donations, especially prior to elective surgery. The next best option is a direct blood donation.[45]

Prescreening test guidelines drafted with the aim of excluding high-risk persons from donating blood are now available in the medical literature. Therefore, non-adherence to these recommendations may lead to suits for damages.

A negligent HIV-infected blood transfusion may not only lead to an action for personal claim of damages, but also to a wrongful death tort action in the United States. Action may be brought by a survivor for damages caused by the death of his or her relative, such as in the case of death of a child due to antenatal injury caused by HIV. However, in most common law countries, death as such is not actionable in tort, but loss to the estate and certain dependants may be compensated.

In addition to negligence, a breach of implied warranty, strict liability, and lack of informed consent are other bases for recovery in blood-related HIV transmissions.

Products liability law generally establishes contractual warranties for the sale of products but not for services. Therefore, if blood is interpreted to be a product, a seller who breaches the implied warranty that the blood is fit for transfusion may be liable to the injured party.

Most American courts have held that transfusion is a service rather than the sale of a product, thereby making blood banks not liable to pay damages.[46] Most jurisdictions in the United States have enacted legislation along the same lines.[47]

Although courts have been reluctant to hold hospitals[48] under strict liability in tort for HIV-infected blood transfusions, they have been more liberal in holding blood banks for same.[49]

2.2.3 Spread of HIV through Personnel and Equipment

Needles and scalpel blades and other equipment used in medical and surgical procedures which are contaminated with HIV-infected blood can transmit HIV through injury. It may be accidental, negligent[50] or wilfully caused. Action has been brought against hospitals that have failed to dispose hazardous waste such as HIV-contaminated needles. Plaints have been made even of reusing disposable swabs on mucous membranes, causing anxiety in the plaintiff. Although the statistical risk of transmission through these means is minimal, the phobia it causes may be substantial.

The Centers for Disease Control (CDC) published in 1991 a case of a dentist transmitting HIV to five patients.[51] Thereafter, the American Medical Association (AMA), through its news release dated 17 January 1991, informed its membership that "physicians who are HIV positive have an ethical obligation, not to engage in any professional activity which has an identifiable risk of transmission of infection to the patient." The courts have held a similar view[52] and allowed hospitals to regulate the types of procedures HIV seropositive doctors can engage in.

The risk of spreading the infection through an infected health care provider to a patient is minimal and in most cases only a theoretical possibility. But due to ignorance, even in developed countries such as the USA, people have been anxious after learning that their doctor had died of AIDS. However, the courts have refused to consider mere fear of a disease transmittable by a doctor as one deserving compensation.[51]

Although when, in fact, such a transmission occurs due to negligence, the plaintiff deserves substantial compensation, an unjustified phobia or anxiety need not be compensated. Condoning such phobias through court sanction can be adverse to public health.

2.2.4 False Communication/Non-Communication

The shock and emotional pain brought about by a negligent false communication that a person is HIV positive may be actionable. In *Beadling* v. *sirotta,*[54] the plaintiff succeeded in a malpractice action against the doctor who conducted his pre-employment medical examination, for negligently diagnosing him as having active tuberculosis.

The patient's righf to know is well-established in the West.[55] But there may be doctors, especially in Third World countries, who consider that it is only ethical to keep the patient uninformed of his or her HIV status, provided that there is no risk to others. Their reasons may be that AIDS is a condition with no cure or resources for prophylaxis or meaningful counselling. It will be up to the courts of the respective countries to decide this matter. However, it should be noted that the patient's right to know should not be compromised without a logical and scientific basis.

2.2.5 Failure to Warn at-risk Partners

Courts have not hesitated to hold physicians liable for foreseeable injury that has resulted from their patient's spread of infection to third parties.[56]

The doctor's legal duty to protect an individual from harm caused by a patient was discussed in *Tarasoff v. Reagents of the University of California.*[57] Action was brought against the doctor for not adequately warning and taking steps to prevent a murder by his psychiatric patient who had confided in the doctor his intentions.

It was held that although common law does not hold a person responsible for controlling the risky conduct of another or imposes a duty to warn a person endangered by such conduct, an exception arises when there is a special fiduciary relationship. When there is such a relationship, the doctor has a duty that extends to care to all persons who are foreseeably endangered by the patient's conduct. Both the American Medical Association[58] and the American Psychiatric Association[59] have recommended warning partners who are known to be at risk after all other efforts to persuade an HIV-positive patient to inform his or her at-risk partners have failed.

2.3 Causation

The prosecution must establish the *cause in fact* and the *proximate cause* for damages. A plaintiff may establish the former using expert testimony, i.e., that a particular type of activity transmits HIV.

The latter would have to be established by showing that the injury could not have occurred but for the negligence of the defendant. This is one of the main problems in HIV-related tort litigation, as it is difficult to say whether the person already had the virus at the time of the alleged negligent conduct (by doctor, sexual partner, needle sharer, etc.). The window period, and the fact that not all persons who come in contact with the virus become infected, compound the problems in proving causation.

The plaintiff would have to prove that he or she did not have the virus until the alleged negligent conduct, and that he or she has not engaged in any behaviour or procedure known to transmit the disease subsequently.

Wrongful Birth and Wrongful Life

The probability of maternal transmission of HIV to foetus is high (about 65 per cent). A congenitally-infected child would usually have a painful and short life span, needing expensive medical care.

Parents may claim damages for wrongful birth if they can prove that they would have avoided giving birth to a child with congenital defects, had they been advised of the potential risk. Usually the plaintiff can recover only special damages[60] in such cases (e.g. expenses for lifetime medical care).

An impaired child can claim damages for wrongful life if such child can establish that the impairment was a result of the health care provider's negligence. Therefore, a doctor who does not offer HIV testing to a mother risks being sued in jurisdictions that recognize these causes of action.

2.4 Damages

A plaintiff is usually not compensated for mere negligence of the defendant unless the person has suffered damages. There are different forms of damages:

Nominal damages - a small sum of money, that is awarded to the plaintiff as an expression of the recognition of a right, rather than for actual compensation - e.g. one pound.

Exemplary damages - a form of exaggerated damages, awarded for outrageous conduct of the defendant. Such awards have been criticized by some jurists as bringing a criminal element into civil law. At least in the UK, the scope for such awards is now quite narrow.61

Real damages - awarded with the aim of putting the person whose right has been invaded in the same posit on as if it has been respected[62] Consideration is given to the loss of the plaintiff rather than to the ability of the defendant to pay.

General damages[63] - what the law presumes to follow the wrong complained of. Therefore, they need not be expressly mentioned in the pleadings.

Special damages - damages that do not generally follow the alleged wrong. Therefore, the plaintiff should expressly mention them in the plaint. The defendant will thus have the opportunity for negating such allegations.

Calculation of damages may be a problem in HIV/AIDSrelated litigation as the effects of HIV will vary depending on the individual. It would be difficult to predict at the time of litigation the actual damages that might follow. Sometimes a positive result for the HIV antibody may be due to a "false positive"[64] test. In such cases the defendant may not have caused any damage to the plaintiff.

In HIV/AIDS-related litigation, awards may be made to compensate losses such as loss of earning capacity, loss of occupation, and medical expenses. Although the Roman Law of Delict does not compensate non-pecuniary loss, under current tort law even emotional damage may be compensated. For example, in *MacMahon v. Nelson,*[65] it was held that the emotional distress caused by an eight-month delay in the diagnosis of the plaintiff's cancer was actionable.

AIDS Phobia

Courts have generally been reluctant to recognize emotional distress, loosely referred to as "AIDS phobia," as a form of damage in the absence of proof that the plaintiff, in fact, came into contact not just with blood but infected blood.[66] A much publicized exception to the rule is the case of *Christian v. Sheft.*[67]

2.5 Defences[68]

2.5.1 Contributory Negligence and Comparative Negligence

Application of universal precautions is one of the effective methods of preventing the spread of HIV. The courts should encourage universal precautions by attributing some degree of responsibility to the plaintiff in cases of transmission that have been within his or her control. This would include the practice of unsafe sex and sharing needles. However, it should be born in mind that in certain societies, women are not in a position to insist that a man should use a condom or practice safe sex.

A defendant's liability may be proportionally reduced or totally exempted through the applications of the principles of contributory negligence and comparative negligence. The plaintiff is judged by the reasonable and prudent man's standard in proportioning his or her contribution.

2.5.2 Assumption of Risk (Volenti Non Fit Injuria)

This is a common defence against negligence. No person can enforce a right which has been voluntarily abandoned.[69] This would be a defence for doctors who have obtained informed consent for damages in the course of proper and standard treatment. An HIV person voluntarily having 'safe' sex after informing the partner of his or her HIV status would also be covered under this defence.

However, it is questionable whether the same would apply for IV needle sharers as consent does not cover an act that is likely to result in death, except when it is meant to save the life of the person consenting. Another factor that has to be considered is whether the plaintiff was of sufficient age, experience, intelligence and maturity to know that needle sharing is a high-risk activity.

2.5.3 Interspousal Immunity

A husband who has allegedly transmitted HIV to his wife may claim interspousal immunity as a defence. However, most progressive jurisdictions have rejected this doctrine. Jurisdictions that have not totally rejected this defence may still entertain such cases after divorce of the respective parties. However, whether it would cover torts committed before divorce would be a question for courts to decide.

2.5.4 Parent—Child Immunity

This common law exception to liability has also been rejected in many jurisdictions in recent years. A parent who transmits HIV to a child during pregnancy may be held liable for damages. Courts have recognized the liability of a mother who injects drugs during pregnancy, causing defects in the newborn. However, the illegality of the latter makes it a more convincing case than the former. Arguments based on women's autonomy do not favour such an approach.[70]

2.5.5 Illegality[71]

Certain high-risk behaviours that help spread HIV are illegal in many parts of the world, e.g., sodomy, adultery, commercial sex, IV drug use. In case where HIV has been transmitted through the plaintiff's participation in such behaviour, the defendant may claim illegality as a defence as 'no one should be rewarded for his or her own wrong.'

The defence of illegality has lost its recognition in relation to sexually transmittable diseases. However, in cases of transmission through illegal IV drug use, the plaintiff's voluntary participation would affect the defendant's liability.

2.5.6 Right to Privacy

In jurisdictions that recognize a right to privacy, the plaintiff may first have to overcome the concept that the state has no business to oversee domestic relationships. This has not been a problem as all concepts have their limits.[72] If the defendant's act is a threat to others, his near and dear ones, it is no more a private matter and becomes a matter of public concern.

English law does not recognize a general right to privacy,[73] but in the United States it is considered an unwritten constitutional provision.[74]

2.6 Procedural Problems

2.6.1 Statutes of Limitation

Most statutes of limitations bar the filing of tort plaints after two to three years of the onset of the cause of action.[75]

If the limitation is considered to start running from the moment the defendant breached his or her duty, most victims may nqt be compensated as the development of AIDS generally takes a few years.

However, in cases of latent diseases, the statutes of limitations are usually considered to run upon the manifestations of injury or the date the plaintiff discovered (or should reasonably have discovered) the breach of duty.[76] This should be borne in mind when fixing statutory time limits to file HIV-related cases.

2.6.2 Burden of Proof

Usually, the burden of proving negligence is on the plaintiff. He should prove by a "preponderance of evidence" the existence of a duty to care, negligence, causation and damages. But in some instances the occurrence may speak for itself *(res ipsa loquitur)*. In such cases, the plaintiff has only to prove the occurrence of the damage, and negligence is presumed. Then, the burden will shift to the defence to prove otherwise.

3. Defamation

Defamation refers to the unlawful publication of a false statement concerning another person, making him subject to ridicule and contempt. In *McCune v. Neitzel,*[77] the defendant was held liable for spreading a false rumour that the plaintiff had AIDS.

Since the legal personality is an essential criteria sought by English courts, a statement regarding a deceased or unborn person is not generally actionable.[78] It will be up to the courts to decide in the future whether this principle should continue in light of the HIV/

AIDS pandemic. It should be emphasized that a trend of defaming persons using HIV-related statements, even after the death of that person, can have catastrophic public health consequences.[79]

4. Breach of Confidentiality

4.1 Breach of Pofessional Secrecy[80]

Once a doctor accepts to care for a patient and a doctor patient relationship begins, there is an ethical duty to keep all information acquired through the professional relationship confidential.[81]

However, a breach of an ethical duty is not necessarily actionable in tort. In *Coralluzzo v. Fass,*[32] it was held that common law does not prohibit disclosure of information without consent, although it may violate ethical standards. It was not covered by defamation either, since defamation essentially refers to a false statement.

Subsequently, the American courts evolved a new course of action in tort against breach of confidentiality,[83] based on theories such as invasion of privacy,[84] breach of an implied contract, and negligence.[85] A doctor who violates this duty may now be liable in tort[86] and may also be guilty of professional misconduct.

An HIV-infected person can sue the doctor, hospital or other persons for unauthorized release of information when as a consequence he or she suffers damages, e.g., loss of job or housing.[87] In *Doe v. Borough of Barrington,*[88] the court held that a municipality which did not train its employees in the need for confidentiality of AIDS-related information would be liable for improper release of that information.

A doctor's ethical and legal duty to keep medical information confidential is not absolute. There may be an overriding duty towards society when the benefits of disclosure outweigh its harm, such as when an HIV-infected patient is acting irresponsibly—engaging in risky behaviour without warning the partner. But it would not be reasonable to divulge the identity of a blood donor for 'discovery' before litigation as it would discourage voluntary blood donations.

4.2 Invasion of Privacy

Damages may be claimed for a public disclosure of private facts, which are highly offensive to the plaintiff, in jurisdictions that specifically recognize a right to privacy. Under this principle liability may arise for publication in the media of unauthorized HIV/AIDS-related information of an individual. A valid defence in such cases would be that the information published was of lngitimate public or general interest. However, it would be unwise for courts to loosely accept this defence in cases of HIV or AIDS as it would adversely affect public health.[89]

5. Deceit and Fraudulent Misrepresentation

Deceit is a recognized cause of action in Anglo-American jurisprudence. It consists of damage suffered by the plaintiff, based on action pursuant to the defendant making a wilfully false statement, with the intent that the plaintiff would act in reliance of it.

A person who markets any product falsely, claiming that it is a cure for AIDS, would be liable under this tort. In countries with a system for the approval of drugs, liability may stem from statutes that prohibit the sale of medications without a licence. For example, in the US, the Food and Drugs Administration should approve pharmaceutical and medical devices as safe and effective for the purposes for which they are advertised. Charges have been made against the advertising and sale of AIDS-related pharmaceuticals and medical devices.[90]

A defendant who knowingly lies or keeps silent about his or her HIV status, expecting the plainti'ff to rely on the lie or silence and causes damages to the defendant, would be liable for fraudulent misrepresentation, provided that the plaintiff justifiably did rely on the misrepresentation. The plaintiff needs to prove that the defendant knew of his or her HIV-positive status and withheld that information for the purpose of having sex with the plaintiff, for instance.[91]

REFERENCES

1. "A tort is a civil wrong for which the remedy is a common law action for unliquidated damages, and which is not exclusively a breach of contract or the breach of a trust or other merely equitable obligation", *Anglo-Saxon Petroleum co. Ltd.* v. *Damant* (1947) K.B. 794, 796; and *Philip Morris Ltd. v. Airley* (1975) V.R. 345, 347.
2. "An interest may be defined as a claim or demand put forward by a person in a civilized society", Heuston RFV, Buckley RA, *Salmond and Heuston on The Law of Tort,* 19th ed, London: Sweet & Maxwell Ltd., 1987.
3. *Ashby* v. *White* (1702) 2 Ld. Raym. 938; 14 St. Tr. 695.
4. *Chapman* v. *Pickersgill* (1762) 2 Wils: 145, 146.
5. But it may raise a presumption against the validity of such a case.
6. Schwartz, R & Grubb A. Why Britain can't afford informed consent. *Hasting's Center Report,* August, 1985.
7. *Eisener* v. *Maxwell* (1951) 1 D.L.R. 816.
8. *Kathleen K* v. *Robert B.*, 150 Cal. App. 3d 992, 198 Cal. Rptr. 273 (Cal. App. 2 Dist. 1984).

9. 29 Del. 594, 102 A. 63 (Del. Gen. Sess. 1917), 226.
10. *Baugh* v. *Delta Waters Ltd.* (1971) 1 W.L.R. 1295, 1298.
11. *Bennan* v. *Parsonnet* (1912) 83 A. 948 as reported in Mant, A. Keith *Taylor's Principles and Practice of Medical Jurisprudence*. 13th ed. Churchill Livingston, (1984).
12. *Schoendorff* v. *Society of New York Hospitals*, 211 N.Y. 125.
13. Jayawardena Hemamal, *Forensic Medicine and Medical Law*. Gampaha: Siddartha Press, 1995.
14. British Medical Association. *Hand Book of Medical Ethics*. London, 1981.
15. *Canterbury* v. *Spence*, 464 F 2d. 772.
16. *Sideway* v. *Governors of Bethlehem Royal Hospital and Maudsley Hospital Health Authority* (1985) A.C. 871.
17. Please see section on HIV infected blood and blood products under Negligence (2.2.2).
18. *Quarantine and Prevent on of Disease Ordiance* No. 3 of 1897 (Sri Lanka) is one such current example.
19. For example, sec. 330 (Wrongful restraint), sec. 331 (wrongful confinement) of the Penal Code (Sri Lanka).
20. *Blundell* v. *Att. Gen.* (1967) N.Z.L.R, 492.
21. *Glover* v. *Eastern Nebraska Community Office of Retardation*, 867 F. 2d 461 (8th cir.)
22. See supra 18.
23. Jayasuriya DC. *AIDS: Health Policy and Legal Aspects.* Commonwealth Secretariat, London, 1993.
24. *Glick* v. *Henderson*, 855 F. 2d 536 (8th Cir. 1988)
25. For example, China; Regulation of 26th December 1987, *International Digest of Health Legislation*, 1988; 39; 623.
26. *Lochgelly Iron and Coal Co.* v. *Mc Mullan* (1934), A.C. 1, at 25.
27. *Donoghue* v. *Stevenson* (1932) A.C. 562.
28. Supra note 2.
29. 543 So. 2d. 686; See also *Crowell* v. *Crowell*, 181 N.C. 66, 106 S.E. 149 (N.C. 1921).
30. A relationship which was previously formed does not cover a new ailment of the same patient that has no connection with the previous illness whatsoever.
31. A doctor is as free to select his patients as much as the patient is free to select his or her doctor and would generally not be liable under tort law (although there may be remedies under other legal theories) for refusing to treat. However, by virtue of their service contracts government doctors in some countries may be bound to treat any patient at the hospital.
32. *Maltempo* v. *Cuthbert*, 504 F. 2d 325 (5th cir 1974); *Norton* v. *Hamilton*, 92 Ga. App. 727, 89 S.E. 2d 809 (1955).
33. *Renslow* v. *Mennonite Hospital*, 67 Ill. 2d 348, 367 N.E. 2d 1250 (Ill. 1977).
34. *Blyth* v. *Birminghom Waterworks Co* (1856), 156 All E.R. 1047.
35. Scott Burris., Harlon L. Balton. *AIDS Law Today: A New Guide for the Public.* New Haven: Yale University, 1993.
36. Hall, MA, Ellman, IM. *Health Care Law and Ethics in a Nutshell*, Minnesota: West Publishing Company, 1990.
37. Metastasisof cancer and dealth as a result of the physician's failure to order relevant investigations, *Chester* v. *United States*, 403 F. Supp. 458 (W.D. Pa. 1975).
38. A two year delay in treatment-for cancer as a result of negligent diagnosis, *Trapp* v. *Metz.*, 271 N.E. 2d. 697 (N.Y. 1971).

39. Jarvis, Robert M., Closen, Michael. L, *et al.*, *AIDS Law in a Nutshell*, Minnesota: West Publishing, 1991.
40. *Morbidity and Mortality Weekly Report* 1982; 31:365-367;652-654.
41. Examples such as that the hospital was negligent in failing to offer the option of directed donation-*Kozup* v. *Georgetown Univerity*, 663 F. Supp. 1048 (D.D.C. 1987), 851 F. 2d 437 (1988).
42. Testing for some other associated infection such as Hepatitis B virus or Cytomegalo virus (CMV) as a means of excluding HIV infected blood.
43. *McKee* v. *Miles Laboratories, Inc*, 675 F. Supp. 1060 (E.D. Ky. 1987), 866 F. 2d 219 (6th Cir. 1989).
44. Collecting blood from an individual and storing it for his or her own future use.
45. An identified person known to the patient donates blood for use by a particular patient.
46. *Perlmutter* v. *Beth David Hospital*, 308 N.Y. 100, 123 N.E. 2d 792 (N.Y. 1954), 220.
47. Gostin L.O., *et al.*, "The AIDS Project: A National Review of Court and Human Rights Commission Decisions, Part 1: The Social Impact of AIDS", *IAMA*, 1990; 263 (14): pp. 1961-1970.
48. For hospitals, transfusing blood is one out of its many services whereas for blood banks, it is the main service provided.
49. *Community Blood Bank, Inc. v. Russell*, 196 So. 2d 115.
50. "Doctor was found guilty on an account of unsatisfactory professional conduct by a New South Wales Medical Tribunal after four women were infected with HIV at his surgery." *HIV/ AIDS Legal Link Newsletter*, 1994; 5, (4), Australian Federation of AIDS Organisations.
51. CDC Update: Transmission of HIV infection during invasive dental procedures—Florida. *Morbidity and Mortality Weekly Report (MMWR)* 1991; 40:377-381.
52. *Estate of Behringer* v. *Medical Center* (N.J. Super Ct.) as reported in *JAMA*, August 28, 1991, vol 266, no. 8, 1134.
53. *Rossi v. Estate of Almaraz*, No. 90344028, 1991 WL 166924 (1991).
54. 176 A. 2d 546 (N.J. Surer Court 1961).
55. *James* v. *United States*, 483 F. Supp. 581 (1980); *Mcllwain v. Willium Hosp.*, 774 F. Supp. 968 (1991).
56. *Skillings* v. *Allen*, 173 N.W. 663 (Minn. 1919); *Davis* v. *Rodman*, 227 S.W. 612 (Ark. 1921).
57. 17 Cal. 3d. 425.
58. American Medical Association Board of Trustees: Prevention and control of acquired immune deficiency syndrome: an interim report. *JAMA* 1987; 258:2097-2103.
59. AIDS policy: confidentiality and exposure. *Psychiatric News*, Jan. 15, 1988; at 27.
60. Supra 39.
61. *Holden* v. *Chief Constable of Lancashire* (1986) 3 W.L.R. 1107.
62. *The Albazero* (1977) A.C. 774.
63. Supra note 2.
64. Martha A Field. Testing for AIDS: uses and abuses, 16 *American Tournal of Law and Medicine* Vol. 33, 1990, 37-43.
65. 568 P. 2d 90 (Colo. App. 1977).
66. *Burk* v. *Sage Prods.*, 747 F. Supp. 285 (E. D. Pa. 1990); *Ordway v. Suffolk County*, 583 N.Y.s. 2d 1014, (Sup, Ct. 1992).
67. *Christian* v. *Sheft*. No. C574153, AIDS Litig. Rep. (Andrews) 2281.

68. Supra note 39.
69. *Chapman* v. *Ellesmere* (1932) 2 K.B. 431, 463.
70. 'Johnson, a New Threat to Pregnant Women's Autonomy, *Hasting's Center Report*. August 1987, 33.
71. Supra note 39.
72. Supra note 8.
73. Younger Committee (U.K), Cmd. 5012 (1972), paras. 44 and 92.
74. *Griswold* v. *Connecticut* 381 US 479 (1965).
75. For example, according to Sec. 9 of the Prescription Ordinance (Sri Lanka), no action shall be maintainable for any loss, injury or damage unless the same shall be commenced within two years from the time when the cause of action shall have arisen.
76. *Duke* v. *Housen*, 589 P. 2d 334 (Wyo. 1979).
77. 235 Neb. 457 N.W. 2d 803 (Neb. 1990).
78. Supra note 2.
79. Because of the associated stigma and discrimination of HIV persons and their families, most of them would naturally prefer that their HIV status be kept secret. A dead person may never be able to disprove a rumour that he was HIV positive. Unless the state provides this security and guarantee while they are alive (as well as after death), persons will tend to keep their known HIV status secret. Keeping an HIV-positive status secret from sexual partners and hospitals unnecessarily puts others at risk of infection.
80. Jayawardena, Hemamal. AIDS and professional secrecy. Paper presented at the *Annual Scientific Session of the College of Medical Administrators*. Sri Lanka, 1993.
81. "...whenever in connection with my professional practice, or not in connection with it, I see or hear in the life of men, which ought not to be spoken of abroad, I will not divulge, recognizing that all such should be kept secret..". Hippocratic Oath, ..supra note 14 at page 64.
82. 450 So. 2d. 858.
83. *Simonesen* v. *Swenson*, 177 N.W. 831 (Neb. 1920); *Hammonds* v. *Aetna Casualty* and *Sur. Co.*, 243 F. Supp. 793 (N.D. Ohio 1965); *Humphers* v. *First Interstate Bank*, 696 P. 2d 527 (or. 1985).
84. In *Urbaniak* v. *Newton*, 277 Cal. Rptr. 354 it was held that a physician could be liable for breach of confidentiality under the privacy clause of the California constitution..
85. *Semore* v. *Poole*, 217 Cal. App. 3d at 1103-05, 266 Cal. Rptr. at 290-92.
86. Breach of Confidence, An emerging Tort, 82 *Colum. L. Rev 1426* (1982).
87. *Chalk* v. *United States District Court*, 840 F. 2d 701 (9th Cir. 1988); *Doe* v. *Centinela Hospital*, 57 U.S.L.W. 2034 (D.C. Cal. 1988).
88. *Doe*. v. *Borough of Barrington*, 729 F. Supp. 376, 390 (D.N.J. 1990). See also *Woods* v. *White* 689 F. supp. 874, 876 (W.D. Wis. 1988).
89. As newspaper sensationalism would add to the stigmatization of the disease.
90. Supra note 47.
91. Supra, note 67.

6

HIV/AIDS Discrimination and Privacy-The Need for Legislative Protection

Helen Watchirs
Principal Counsel, HIV/AIDS Law & IHL Section
Attorney General's Department Canberra

INTRODUCTION

This chapter will focus on harnessing the power of the law in a positive and empowering way to fight the HIV/AIDS pandemic—firstly by describing the need, ways and means of enacting anti-discrimination laws, and secondly, the similar need for privacy protection. It will attempt to focus on the Asia Pacific region; most references will be to Australian national law, as this is the country with the most developed law reform programme. Anti-discrimination laws enable individuals to assert their fundamental human rights in a practical, informal, accessible way, enforceable through agencies, such as equal opportunity or privacy commissioners.

Law can have a role in complementing and assisting education and other public health measures.[1] The aim of any law reform, but especially protection against discrimination and breaches of privacy, is to facilitate full community participation and integration of people living with HIV by securing their co-operation and trust, rather than compounding stigmatization and alienation of groups who have already been rejected by society and treated in a negative, punitive way by the legal system. Minority groups adversely affected by the pandemic in the public mind[2] are homosexual men, sex workers and injecting drug users—it is just that their perceived risk behaviour (no account is usually taken of the use of safer sex and clean using) scapegoats them for the rest of the community, who want to isolate themselves through fear.[3]

With adequate education of the general population about modes of transmission, there is no excuse for ignorance breeding prejudicial attitudes, and irrational fears of infection. The creation of stereotypes comfort the majority and make them feel that HIV-infection is not a realistic possibility for them personally, and politically, and that it is not "our problem". Lobbying for law reform to provide protection for the vulnerable is important not only in terms of concrete results, but also symbolically in the binding of multi-sectoral groups, and development of group consciousness and self-esteem from achievement through adversity.[4]

NATURE OF PROTECTIVE LAWS

Anti-discrimination and privacy laws both exist in countries such as the United States, Canada, Australia and New Zealand, as well as in Europe, and can be used as models for the region with appropriate modifications to local traditions, culture, social mores, religion and legal/political systems. The benefit in having overseas models is that we can each learn from the experiences of others, as the general principles in this area of law are universal. There has been some international interest in protection of human rights in the HIV/AIDS context as demonstrated by:

- the World Health Assembly Resolution WHA41.24 of 13 May 1988, "Avoidance of Discrimination in Relation to HIV-Infected People and People with AIDS";
- the Special Rapporteur's Preliminary, Progress and Final reports to the Sub-Commission on Prevention of Discrimination and Protection of Minorities on Discrimination against HIV-Infected People and People Living with AIDS[5]
- the Paris Declaration of 1 December 1994;
- the 51st session of the Commission on Human Rights ("CHR") Resolution on the Protection of Human Rights in the Context of HIV/AIDS, adopted without a vote on 28 February 1995; and,
- the Secretary-General's report to the 51st CHR[6] in 1994—

> following a survey of individual government practice, of which only 19 responded. Although some countries had positive measures protecting human rights and preventing discrimination, there was a large gap between professed policy and actual implementation. National committees sometimes safeguarded these rights, but often their resources were inadequate to enable them to operate.

The international standing of countries may be adversely affected by ignoring the problem of HIV/AIDS discrimination. In a recent case in Australia, the Refugee Review Tribunal granted a person refugee status on the basis of his well-founder fear of persecution on the basis of being HIV-positive and belonging to a "particular social group" which his home government was unwilling or unable to protect. The discrimination was held to be so severe in this developing country in question as to amount persecution in two ways. Firstly, the lack of provision and access to medical treatment, except for identifiable HIV/AIDS healthcare facilities which would expose him to the second form of discrimination-family and community ostracism.[7] Protective laws operate by educative, rather than punitive, means with investigation, followed by conciliation. Civil remedies, however, are available to be formally determined after referral by boards or tribunals, such as interim orders to preserve the *status quo*, and damages to compensate for unjustifiable infringements.[8] These laws, often for constitutional reasons, only apply to public acts by individuals, or any acts by public authorities. This does not detract, however, from their value in sensitizing the general population to their importance by setting examples to change behaviour, and hopefully attitudes.

Although it is easy to say that discrimination and breaches of privacy should be protected against, the drafting of such legislation is usually complex in the definitions of each, and the large numbers of exception to them. The justification for these exceptions, which attempt to balance interactive rights and responsibilities will be considered in detail later in this chapter. The focus should not be lost that public health benefits in providing legislative protection against discrimination and breaches of privacy, by encouraging those at risk of infection to present early for counselling, testing, support and treatment, rather than driving people underground.

There is a close relationship between discrimination and privacy, as the ground for discrimination is often knowledge of the HIV-status of other individuals, and the reason people want their HIV-status to remain confidential is fear of discrimination. A concrete example of the inter-relationship is the prohibition in some anti-discrimination legislation on asking discriminatory questions in the first place. The question which is often asked is, why is HIV different? The approach taken in this chapter is that special HIV laws require particular justification. Sometimes general laws are sufficient, but often HIV provides the impetus to review the adequacy of protection of medical records. The need to combat the extraordinary stigma associated with HIV can sustain the momentum to achieve law reform in areas which have been languishing, not because of lack of merit in substance, but for want of political will. However, one must bear in mind that legislators are not keen to be seen having the HIV tail wagging the human rights dog.[9]

ANTI-DISCRIMINATION LEGISLATION

Anti-discrimination legislation prohibits unfair and irrelevant distinctions being made on specified grounds such as race, sex, religion and disability. The wide range of examples of HIV-related discrimination,[10] shows how important it is not to overlook any areas when drafting legislation to prohibit discrimination:

- Employment;
- Education and training;
- Accommodation;
- Superannuation and insurance;
- Provision of goods and services (e.g., medical or prison facilities[11]);
- Qualifying bodies; and professional, trade, employer or other organizations;
- Access to places and vehicles;
- Sport;
- Trade unions; and,
- Clubs or associations.

The type of treatment[12] ranges from avoidance, humiliation, harassment, rejection, denial of services, vilification to even violence. With time, there has been a second wave of HIV-related discrimination which is much more sophisticated and pre-emptive,[13] and, therefore, difficult to address because it appears to be based on scientific, actuarial[14] or other objective data, particularly in the crucial areas of employment, insurance and health care. This makes it all the more necessary to carefully draft anti-discrimination legislation that cannot be avoided by subterfuge, especially given longer productive life expectancies of HIV-infected people with growing advances in treatment.

Essential Features of Anti-Discrimination Legislation

Australia's *Disability Discrimination Act 1992, is* modelled on the *Americans with Disabilities Act 1990* (New Zealand has a similar scheme under the *Human Rights Act 1993)* and Hong Kong's Disability Discrimination Ordinance, 1995 is based on the Australian legislation. Several countries have constitutional guarantees of human rights, such as the Canadian Charter of Rights, with practical enforcement mechanisms. These legislative schemes[15] have several common features which are essential to anticipate most forms of HIV-related discrimination:

- The definition of the protected attribute of disability or impairment must be broad enough to cover asymptomatic HIV infection, and not merely AIDS, to be effective.[16] Without careful drafting, HIV-infection demonstrated by the presence of antibodies may not be covered by the legislation, as the presence of antibodies is a health response to viral infection. One successful example is "presence in the body of organisms capable of causing disease or illness" which has been used in Australia and New Zealand .[17]
- It is not only people living with HIV/AIDS who should be covered. Carers, associates,[18] and family are also discriminated against, as well as persons perceived to be infected because of their membership of stigmatized groups[19] presumed to be infected—the technical descriptions are "imputed, past and expected future" disabilities, including medical records which may be used as "markers" for HIV-infection, eg. hepatitis B, or specific STDs, such as anal gonorrhoea.
- Both direct and indirect discrimination need to be covered.[20] Direct discrimination occurs where a person treats another person less favourably than a third person would be treated in comparable circumstances, or attributes characteristics which are thought to relate generally or be generally imputed to people of a particular status, i.e. stereotypes. Indirect discrimination occurs where unreasonable conditions or requirements (e.g., mandatory HIV-testing) are applied which a substantially higher proportion of persons of a different status must be able to comply with than persons of the same status as the person complaining of discrimination. Vicarious liability should be covered to catch

employers, principals and partners. A loophole which also must be closed is the "comparability problem" whereby discriminators can argue that the disability created a difference in the way a person performed a task.[21] To prevent this, legislation must provide that circumstances will not be regarded as being materially different because the discriminator has to provide different services to the HIV-infected person.

- The problem of proving discrimination must be addressed One way is to make the fact that only one of several reasons for doing an act is discriminatory be enough to establish discrimination. A causal connection[22] rather than proof of intent[23] between the discriminatory conduct and HIV-infection should be sufficient. Persons counselling or procuring others to discriminate should be covered. Some jurisdictions have gone even further by prohibiting HIV/ AIDS vilification,[24] i.e. inciting hatred, serious contempt or severe ridicule.
- Allowance must also be made for positive discrimination, called "affirmative action" where HIV-infected people are given preference, e.g., a Californian modelling agency called "Proof Positive"[25] that employs HIV seropositive persons.
- The administrative procedure whereby complaints are lodged with an independent agency should be effective.[26] It is very important that a fast-tracking mechanism exists for cases where the complainant is terminally ill as otherwise respondents can conveniently slow down proceedings until the other party dies, thereby defeating the purpose of the complaint, and deterring others from such a pointless exercise. It is also crucial that representative complaints be able to be lodged by groups such as NGOs or trade unions on behalf of their constituents, because of the energy and time spent on cases, and also because of the possible publicity and victimization which may follow. Often remedies are only available for specific and individual instances of, rather than systemic, discrimination. It is preferable that the legislation empower agencies to investigate policies[27] and procedures which impact on large numbers of people, and order that particular practices cease in order to prevent future contraventions. In all these areas, AIDS community groups are wellplaced-to represent the interests of their

members and should be funded by governments to perform advocacy services.

Exceptions

All anti-discrimination legislation contains exceptions. Whilst disabilities are often irrelevant to most areas of public activities, in some cases they are a fair basis for exclusion, such as a person with AIDS dementia could not be expected to perform certain functions, e.g. pilot.[28] In referring to the inherent requirements[29] of a job to be performed, this test needs to be narrowed down to essential elements. A balance must be reached between the rights of the HIV-infected person with reasonable obligations being placed on employers to "accommodate", but not to the extent that unjustifiable hlardship is caused. Examples include an employer allowing an HIV-infected employee to work flexible hours in order to attend medical appointments. A more controversial example in the health care area is universal infection control (e.g., use of disposable gloves, syringes and needles, and instruments) which should make the HIV-status of care providers and clients irrelevant.[30] Using the term "reasonable"[31] in these tests means that objective and not subjective criteria must be applied, otherwise discrimination would be permissible based on coworker's, customer's or parents hysterical and irrational fears in the office, shop and school environments. There is a danger in having an exception for other legislation, as it can be even more discriminatory than administrative practice, e.g., banning HIV-infected people from marrying.

Case Studies

There has been a large amount of academic research on antidiscrimination case law, principally in the USA. This chapter will concentrate on Australian examples, but with occasional references to other countries. Australian anti-discrimination legislation was enacted gradually at the Federal level with racial discrimination in 1975, sex in 1984 and disability in 1992, and also at the provincial level.[32] A useful lesson for other jurisdictions contemplating the enactment of legislation to combat HIV/AIDS discrimination is the success in the USA, Australia and New Zealand in enacting general rather than specific grounds (such as disability), subject to exceptions. In the following cases, some have been determined by a provincial or Federal complaints body, others enforced in the courts,[33] or even settled beforehand. They represent only a small proportion of complaints actually made, and a tiny proportion of real discrimination in the community. Under the *Australian Disability Discrimination Act* 1992 (DDA), 302 complaints were received in 1993/94, nine of which related to HIV/AIDS.[34] The largest areas of complaint is employment, including superannuation and insurance, then the provision of goods, services and facilities. On average, it takes approximately 12 months before a case is even assigned for investigation.

The only HIV-related case formally determined by the Human Rights and Equal Opportunity Commission (HREOC). is X v *Department of Defence.*[35] In that case X was dismissed by the Australian Defence Force as a new recruit pursuant to a post-entry medical check where he was found to be HIV-positive. The Inquiry Commissioner found that operational deployment (which might require urgent blood donations, or blood spills from wounds during combat) was not an "inherent requirement" of employment, but merely an "incident". These alleged constraints on deployment arose from an external requirement by the employer designed to reduce HIV-transmission, and not from the physical consequences of X's disability. The decision has been appealed to the Federal Court, and no change to the ADF's HIV-policy has been announced by the Government. There is a statutory power, however, to declare "combat" and "combat-related" duties which are exempt from the Act. This decision is consistent with a decision by the Federal Court of Canada in *Attorney-General of Canada* v. Thwaites.[36]

In another case, a conciliated agreement was reached with a pathology company which refused to perform a spirometry test on a man who was HIV-positive. The settlement reached was for the company to conduct an HIV/AIDS training programme for staff, and payment of $8,000 for reimbursement of expenses and damages for injuries to feelings and humiliation of the complainant. A conciliation was also reached in a case involving a landlord's refusal to finalize a lease of premises for an HIV-positive support group. An interim determination prevented the person from taking possession of the premises occupied by the PLWA group, and eventually a lease was entered into.[37]

In Australia there are several HIV-related cases pending at present. Hearings have commenced against Swann Insurance, one of Australia's largest providers of sickness, accident and unemployment insurance. A representative complaint was made by a man who left work due to HIV illness, and the HIV/AIDS Legal Centre based in Sydney acts for six members of the class who had loan insurance and whose claims were refused.[38] A complaint has also been made against the Commonwealth Employment Service (CES) for requiring a man to disclose his HIV-status to prospective employers under its Guidelines on Jobseekers and Communicable Diseases, including HIV/AIDS. An interim determination was refused by the Human Rights and Equal Opportunity Commission (HREOC) as it was unable to prevent a practice continuing, as opposed to maintaining the *status quo* by preventing a practice being implemented.[39] In a case publicized by the media, a mother of a son who had died of AIDS complained about funeral workers refusing to carry the coffin to be opened for viewing before cremation. The funeral industry guidelines are inconsistent with health regulations which state that bodies infected with HIV should be available for viewing and transport.[40] The West Australian Government was granted a 3 month exemption by the Human Rights and Equal Opportunity Commission under the Act to develop a non-discriminatory HIV/AIDS prison policy. An HIV-positive prisoner had complained about the segregation of HIV-positive prisoners in one maximum security prison. Under the new policy HIV-positive prisoners are to be integrated into "corridor prisons", but not all these prisons have full access to all prison programmes. An interim determination was refused by HREOC in this case.

Provincial complaint bodies in Australia have also determined cases. In *Hoddy v Executive Director,* Department of Corrective Services a determination was made by the Western Australian Equal Opportunity Tribunal that HIV status was an impairment under the relevant legislation. Another complaint involving prisons has been lodged by an agent (to protect against victimization) with the Queensland Anti-Discrimination Commission. It refers to segregation, restrained movement within the prison system, lesser access to privileges, sport and employment for HIV-positive prisoners. It is hoped that the case will be resolved by conciliation.[41] Several cases have arisen involving refusal to perform medical services on gay men without prior HIV-testing. The latest case before the New South Wales Equal Opportunity Tribunal was settled by a doctor paying $22,500 in compensation and legal costs, as well as acknowledging the unlawfulness of refusing to provide services and the preferability of complying with universal infection control precautions.[42] An earlier case, *Ferguson v. Central Sydney Area Health Service* had reached the opposite conclusion, but it is explainable on the basis of the lesser state of medical knowledge at the time (1989) the incident in question had occurred.[43]

In *City of Perth and Ors v. DL Acting as Representative of All Members of People Living with AIDS (WA) Inc.* a decision of the Western Australia Equal Opportunity Tribunal[44] was upheld by the Supreme Court. It had found that the City of Perth had unlawfully discriminated against the complainant when it refused a planning application to re-zone a shop as a drop in centre for PLWA, and ordered $8,000 compensation to be paid. Five out of thirteen councillors who had voted against the application did so on the basis of the HIV status of PLWAs members, and one non-voting councillor had by his adverse public comments encouraged other councillors to refuse the application[44]. In G. v. *Lincraft*[45] an employer was found not to have discriminated on the basis of the employee's HIV-status when he was demoted from being an area manager (he stayed in this job for 18 months after notifying his employer of his diagnosis) to a lower paid position as a sales man to enable him to receive treatment. In *Jobbling* v. *Director-General, Department of Education of SA and ANOR*[46] the Equal Opportunity Commission found that a HIV-positive man had been discriminated against on the basis of his homosexuality, and his impairment was not a reason for his contract as an artist in school being cancelled. A New South Wales case was settled concerning Continental Airlines' withdrawal of an offer of employment as a reservations clerk to a man when he tested positive to HIV during a medical examination. The reason given by the employer was that it could not offer the life insurance component of its superannuation plan to HIV-positive employees. A Victorian case was also settled against the Alfred Hospital for refusing to perform laser surgery (as opposed to radiotherapy) for oesophageal Kaposi's Sarcoma because of the fear of HIV-transmission by the gastroenterology unit staff.[47]

Reports of discrimination by the government and private sector in the region are numerous. In Indonesia the Ministry of Health is investigating the dismissal of 10 HIV-positive people, and how their employers discovered their HIV-status, given the strict confidence surrounding test results at the hospital.[48] In Western Samoa a HIV-positive tourist was deported after surveillance concerning alleged drug use.[49] In the UK an airline company, Dan Air, was found to have unlawfully discriminated on the basis of sex by employing only female cabin staff, as it alleged that male flight attendants were mostly homosexual and at risk of contracting HIV. Unfortunately in anti-discrimination the UK legislation only prohibits discrimination on the basis of sex and race, and not disability.[50]

PRIVACY LEGISLATION

If the number of HIV-related discrimination complaints investigated by equal opportunity agencies represents only the "tip of the iceberg", then breaches of privacy are even more so because by their very nature. The individual concerned is often unaware of unauthorized disclosures. Information privacy protection originated in Europe through bodies such as the Council of Europe and the OECD.[51] The USA operates more through constitutional guarantees of privacy (such as the Republic of Korea and Papua New Guinea), but also with specific HIV-related data or medical records protection in local state legislation. Some countries have specific legislation dealing with health records, such as the UK *Access to Health Records Act 1990* and the New Zealand Health Information Privacy Code 1994. Privacy Commissioners have been appointed in Canada (1982) Australia (1988) and New Zealand (1991), and have been proposed for Hong Kong.[52] Both the Canadian and Australian Privacy Commissioners have issued reports and guidelines on the need for protection of HIV-related information.[53] All these schemes, however, are operative only in relation to records, and not where information is known through other means, such as oral communication, or by observation (e.g., where a person with AIDS has the easily recognizable Kaposi's Sarcoma, or hospitals use well-known coloured stickers on patient beds or wrist bands,[54] or signs such as "caution: biohazardous waste". Professional bodies have also developed ethical guidelines such as the American Bar Association's "AIDS/HIV and confidentiality ltodel Policy and Procedures".[55]

Confidentiality can be seen as a western individualized concept, not easily adaptable to some very close-knit communities where information-sharing is a basic group value. An example is the Australian surveillance scheme for recording epidemiological data on HIV/AIDS (only coded information is used), where it was proposed that in addition to basic information such as testing history, sex, age, and risk factors, information be collected on whether the person was of aboriginal descent. Some leaders of the indigenous population wanted the information to track whether the epidemic had entered its community, but public concern was raised about the increased risk of discrimination. In Fiji this has not been seen as a problem as data is broken up into two groups: Fijian and Indian populations. The danger exists, however, of discriminatory comparisons being made of the incidence of HIV-infection between ethnic groups, with blame being placed on the population with a higher prevalence.

Essential Features of Privacy Legislation

Legislative protection of privacy in the schemes mentioned above usually operates in a similar way to anti-discrimination legislation. Independent agencies, typically Privacy Commissioners, receive complaints from members of the public about breaches of legislative privacy principles by government agencies (private sector is not often regulated except in special cases such as credit records, and possibly medical records). Where cases cannot be conciliated, Commissioners can award compensation for interferences with privacy.[56]

These legislative principles cover issues such as the following:

- As to when personal information should be collected — where it is necessary to exercise a lawful function. This is the most critical point of regulation as this stops agencies from having it unnecessarily in the first place. If it should be sought indirectly from third parties (such as doctors), and what an individual should be told before being asked for it such as explaining the specific reason for its collection, the use to which it will be put, possible adverse consequences and expected disclosures to other agencies.
- The type of security measures—particularly in the case of computerized data—that should be taken to protect this information. Even simple measures for hard copy data should be taken, such as having identification codes on file covers rather than names, separating medical from administrative files, enforcing a "clean desk" policy, and locking filing cabinets with only authorized personnel having keys. Hospital practice is problematic with bedside notes being available to passers-by, rather than only clinicians with a need to know. It has been estimated that up to 75 persons have access to medical information in each case where hospitalization occurs, for the purposes of treatment, investigation, control and clerical payment procedures.[57]
- When individuals should be entitled to see his or her own records, and insist that amendments be made to them in order to make the data or information accurate, relevant (i..e., not subjective value judgments about lifestyle), complete and up to date (e.g., an initial screening HIV-antibody test may have a false-positive result, and there is

a need to show that a subsequent Western Blot test did not confirm this result. It would be better if unconfirmed test results were not collected at all, except for doctors performing the actual tests).

- The purposes for which this information can be used or disclosed, apart from the original particular purpose for which it was obtained. The various exceptions in the HIV/AIDS area will be discussed later; and
- What happens to information used for medical or social research (e.g., risk behaviour of injecting drug users etc.).

Agencies may complain that these guidelines are too onerous to administer, but, in fact, they promote efficiency, because increased client co-operation and trust should facilitate information gathering.[58] Like anti-discrimination legislation, drafting a wide definition of HIV-related information is important. In addition to whether a person is or thought to be HIV-infected, other sensitive information could be counselling in regard to risk behaviour, or a negative test result (sometimes insurance companies discriminate on this basis alone—this practice has recently ceased in the UK because of the threat of legislation).[59] The ways in which government agencies may collect HIV-related information are boundless:

- Government hospital, nursing home and medical , records;
- Personnel files, e.g., Defence, Foreign Affairs (overseas postings);
- Applications for social security, housing assistance, pharmaceutical benefits, family services etc;
- Immigration applications;
- Prisoner records;
- Court records, e.g., adoption, divorce/custody disputes;
- Counselling services for people with drug/alcohol problems or residents with intellectual disabilities;
- Compensation or superannuation claims; and
- Police records.

Exceptions

This chapter will not debate the issues of physical privacy and informed consent to testing of immigrants, prisoners and defence personnel,[60] but proceed on the basis that the information already exists. In what exceptional circumstances should it be used or disclosed for other purposes?

Informed consent is obtained from the individual—if a valid reason is given to an individual, there is often no problem with self-disclosure.

- Criminal proceedings relating to HIV transmission, such as rape or needle-bandit attacks (but not general offences relating to prostitution, drug or homosexuality) and also the other area of needle stick injuries. However, the benefits should outweigh the harm of disclosure, which in all these cases would be difficult to establish as the exposure has already occurred and the only help (limited because of the unreliability of the test result history) would be in making a decision on whether to take AZT as a prophylactic measure, given the controversy over its effectiveness and its adverse side effects (and expense, especially in developing countries).
- Special legal requirement or court order, e.g., where blood supply is found to be infected and a donor has falsely claimed to be HIV-negative. Care needs to be taken of vague legal obligations being used to justify disclosure, such as duty to warn or duty of care,[61] as only rarely is this actually the case.
- Partner notification—there should have been a serious and imminent exposure to the risk of HIV-infection, and disclosure is the only reasonable way likely to eliminate or substantially reduce that risk; the person has refused the opportunity to disclose voluntarily; and disclosure is made by a person with appropriate training and/or experience in such sensitive matters, e.g., counsellor or therapist. Any person so notified should, if it is impossible to conceal the identity of the index case, be obliged by legislation to keep this information confidential (under common law there would be no confidential relationship between the third party notified and the index case, as the information was given to a government agency).[62]

It should be noted that in having a discretion to notify partners there is no notion of "duty to warn" which could expose people in confidential therapeutic relationships to negligence actions by partners who were not notified of the risk of HIV-transmission.[63] It is unlikely that the US concept would apply in other countries such as the UK.[64] But the situation in Australia is unclear which has led to calls for a legislative protection to be given to professional care givers against actions both for breach of confidence and failure to notify partners, subject to compliance with a partner notification protocol as described above.[65]

Case Studies

This section will describe a number of HIV-related confidentiality or privacy cases which have been considered by the courts, principally in Australia, but occasionally in other countries. The most notorious Australian cases of breaches of privacy which had sustained media interest were never litigated. They concerned the HIV-status of a famous ballet dancer in Melbourne and a orchestra conductor in Sydney, who both subsequently died of AIDS. An Adelaide dentist's HIV status was leaked in January 1992 through a letter from his doctor to the Health Commission. A Sydney HIV-positive obstetrician became the focus of public attention in 1994, when a "look back" programme was conducted of 145 of his patients, none of whom were infected.[66] The cause of the death of a New South Wales Member of Parliament also became the subject of media attention in 1995.[67]

The first court cases began in 1989, such as *X v. Sattler and WA Broadcasting Services Pty.Ltd.*[68] when the WA Supreme Court granted an injunction in a defamation action to prevent a radio announcer disclosing X's identity, and his alleged transmission of HIV to a socialite. In 1990 the Royal Adelaide Hospital settled a case out of court where a patient's HIV-status was disclosed to his wife by a doctor.[69]

An investigation by the New South Wales Ombudsman found that a prison had acted illegally by posting a notice of a prisoner's HIV-status in the wing office, during the investigation of a needle stick injury to an officer which occurred in the prisoner's cell during a search. It criticized the notice as discriminatory, misleading and offensive, and implied that HIV status meant that a prisoner was inherently dangerous. The notice contravened prison regulations which only permitted limited disclosure on a need to know basis.[70]

The reference above in the discrimination case studies to the CES Guidelines on Jobseekers and Communicable Diseases is also relevant to privacy concerns. A man is contemplating a breach of confidentiality action against CES for disclosing his HIV-status to a restaurant which had offered him employment and then withdrew the offer after CES had made the disclosure.[71]

There has been a general trend in HIV-related litigation to protect the identity of the parties, but not automatically. In *DM* v. *TD* an 85 year old female patient's identity was protected by the court in an action against her surgeon for negligent transmission by cross-infection (it has been alleged it was one of four such cases on the same day of surgery). The grounds for her application were the media harassment surrounding the unique nature of the case and the deterrent effect on future litigation might amount to a denial of access to jusffce. The judge rejected these grounds but relied on precedent in cases involving blood shield legislation and medically acquired HIV, and protecting the identity of blood donors.[72] The case was subsequently settled and the doctor concerned was investigated by the NSW Medical Tribunal and found guilty of unsatisfactory professional misconduct.[73] In *Royal Melbourne New Hospital v. Matthews and Ors*,[74] a search warrant issued to police to take hospital files relating to an HIV-positive man who had been charged with conduct likely to endanger life was held by the court to be a valid exception, under the general secrecy provisions of the *Health Services Act 1988,* Victoria. Opposite conclusions have been reached in Canada and Scotland. In *Sharpe Estate v. Northwestern General Hospital*[75] a blood donor's identity was disclosed because the Red Cross owed no duty of confidentiality to its donors. However, in *AB* v. *Scottish National Blood Transfusion Service*[76] the donor's identity was protected so as not to discourage others from donating blood.

Contrary decisions have been made in other cases. However, in the *Herald and Weekly Times Ltd* v. *Barry Brown M. Jelena Popovic M. and SS* the Victorian Supreme Court overturned a suppression order preventing publication of an HIV-positive sex worker and the newspaper subsequently published her name and photograph in relation to charges of loitering with the intent to engage in prostitution. The Court held that an error had been made by the magistrate granting a suppression order under the *Health Act 1958* which empowers such orders to be made where evidence relates to HIV, and "it is necessary to do so because of many social or economic consequences" to a person if the information is disclosed. The Court held that the suppression order would infringe on the "well-being of others" as the woman had been classed a "public health risk" and relied on an interpretation provision which sets out principles to be followed in enforcing the legislation.[77]

In J *and R* v. *L and A Services Pty Ltd.,* a married couple alleged that they had acquired HIV through their employment as pathology scientists. Their application to suppress their identities was rejected by the Queensland Court of Appeal, but this decision has been appealed to the High Court.[78] In *A* v *R*, however, the NSW Compensation Court granted a suppression order to a man who alleged that he acquired HIV whilst serving as a first aid officer with a stevedoring firm because of his habit of biting his nails (surprisingly his claim was successful).[79]

In India the Bombay High Court granted an interim suppression order to prevent publication of a HIV-positive applicant's name, who is challenging a public sector corporation's decision to dismiss him on the basis of his HIV status, using the non-discrimination clauses in the Constitution of India.[80] In China the Intermediate People's Court overturned a District Court's ruling that a doctor and hospital should pay compensation to a patient for psychological pain caused by releasing details of an unconfirmed HIV test result to the patient's family, employer and the Health Department.[81]

In *Jansen Van Vuuren* v. *Kruger*[82] the South African Supreme Court upheld an appeal by an HIV-positive gay man for breach of medical confidence by his doctor. The plaintiff had obtained an express promise of confidentiality by the doctor, when he obtained an HIV-positive test result unexpectedly, while applying for life insurance. The following day the doctor had breached this confidential agreement by telling two colleagues during a game of golf, news of which then spread throughout the community. The Appeal Court rejected the trial judge's acceptance of the doctor concerns that he wished to warn his colleague against any possible "retrospective exposure" to the virus by his patient. The Appeal Court referred to the obligation of medical confidentiality and cited the UK case *X* v. *Y*.[83] In that case it was held that the public interest in preserving the confidentiality of hospital records overweighed the media's freedom to publish the identity of two HIV-positive doctors.

AUSTRALIAN EXAMPLE OF LAW REFORM PROCESSES

Deficiencies in the legal system which adversely impacted on the HIV/AIDS epidemic were fortunately recognized early in Australia. A key to successful law reform has been the relatively non-partisan approach taken by politicians, a situation facilitated by the formation of the Parliamentary Liaison Committee in 1985, consisting of Federal politicians from all major political parties.[84] A role for HIV/AIDS law reform was suggested by the Working Panel on Discrimination and Other Legal Issues—HIV/AIDS which held public hearings after being established by the Federal Government in 1989, as part of the consultative process resulting from the "Green Paper", *A Time to Care, A Time to Act: Towards a Strategy for Australia* The national HIV/AIDS Strategy, (the "White Paper") was tabled in Federal Parliament in August 1989 and recommended that a Legal Working Party ('LWP') be established as a sub-committee of the Intergovernmental Committee on AIDS (a financial and policy co-ordinating body established in 1987 in order to review legislation and propose law reform impacting on HIV/AIDS. A Privacy and HIV/AIDS Working Party was also established as a body to review the adequacy of protection given to HIV-related information by the *Privacy Act 1988* (Commonwealth).

The LWP consisted of representatives from State, Territory and Federal Attorneys-General and Departments of Health, as well as the Australian National Council on AIDS ('ANCA'). A remarkable process took place over two years, whereby an innovative, comprehensive and multi-sectoral approach was taken to ensure that protective laws responded in a rational and humane way to the challenge of the epidemic. Nine Discussion Papers, one of them on anti-discrimination legislation,[85] were produced which contained Preferred Options for law reform,in order to stimulate and focus informed discussion and public submissions. Over 300 submissions from 111 organizations and individuals were analyzed and formed the basis of the Final Report, launched by the Federal Minister of Health, Housing and Community Services in November 1992. The final report contained approximately ninety recommendations for federal and provincial law reform.

A much simpler approach was taken by the Privacy and HIV/AIDS Working Party which was established in May 1990. It reported in September 1992 and recommended voluntary Guidelines to be followed by Federal and ACT Government agencies. It consisted of representatives from the community (Australian Federation of AIDS Organisations—'AFAO'), ANCA and relevant Federal and ACT Government Departments, i.e., Health, Attorney-General's, Industrial Relations and the Public Service Commission. The existing Privacy Act which contains binding Information Privacy Principles (IPP) was reviewed in two ways. Firstly, by researching complaints received by community groups and other grievance bodies. Secondly, by administering a questionnaire to relevant agencies which handled HIV-related information, and the Privacy Commissioner's Office conducting a random audit of two respondents, by physically inspecting their work areas to assess compliance with the IPPs. The Working Party concluded that the existing IPPs were not strict enough to protect the especially sensitive HIV-related information, and drafted specific Guidelines, to be reviewed in practical operation before being recommended to be given legislative force.

In September 1993 the Federal Ministers for Justice and Health established the HIV/AIDS Implementation Working Group to monitor and facilitate implementation of the LWP Report, and later to review the privacy Guidelines. The IWG is chaired by a senior member of the Office of the Federal Minister for Justice and contains members from the Offices of the Attorney-General and the Federal Minister for Human Services and Health, the Department of Human Services and Health, the Department of the Attorney-General, AFAO, ANCA and the IGCA. The IWG is in the process of producing a Status report on the exact extent of implementation of the LWP's recommendations—about half are fully or partially implemented.

The LWP's Final Report has been viewed as a policy blueprint for uniform national law reform. The IGCA and the Australian Health Ministers Advisory Council unanimously endorsed the report's recommendations, but acknowledged that the 'in principle' adoption of the recommendations by a particular jurisdiction did not commit the government of that jurisdiction to immediate implementation of the recommendations. The priorities and needs of the various provinces differ and there are also differences in the respective legislative environments. The LWP attempted to provide the ideas, arguments and evidence to show what it believed should be done to help manage the HIV/AIDS epidemic. Responsibility for implementation of the majority of the LWP's recommendations rests with each provincial Attorney-General who has to act in consultation with relevant agencies and functionaries.

For this reason, HIV law reform has been a regular item of the agenda of the Standing Committee of Attorneys-General. Two States, New South Wales and South Australia have established their own provincial IWGs to look at the status of implementation of the LWP's recommendations.[86] The recent Evaluation of the national HIV/AIDS Strategy 1993-94 to 1995-96 recommended that all jurisdictions that have not already done so should establish their own IWG, and commented on the current status of the extent and appropriateness of implementation of the LWP Report. It found that the most active period of law reform was actually during the operation of the LWP review from 1990 to 1992, when all governments that had not already done so (except Tasmania) enacted anti-discrimination legislation. However, there was an anomaly in Tasmania enacting the *HIV/AIDS Preventive Measures Act 1993* which gave (a slightly amended version of) the Privacy Guidelines binding status, the only jurisdiction to have done so. The IWG and Privacy Commissioner's Office are currently consulting as part of a review of the Privacy Guidelines, and a similar process is taking place in Tasmania. The consultation process has revealed that the major problems are lack of awareness of and compliance with the guidelines. An example of the best practice may be found in the Department of Social Security, which has provided extensive staff training. When the review is completed in late 1995 the IWG will consider whether to recommend to the Government that the guidelines be amended before being given a legislative basis.

The evaluation also looked at discrimination and reported on four quantitative tracking surveys conducted in 1992-94 to monitor changes in knowledge and attitudes related to HIV/ AIDS and discrimination in the general community. These surveys found a gradual decrease in discriminatory attitudes towards HIV/AIDS, people living with HIV/AIDS and priority groups, with the exception of injecting drug users. In particular, discriminatory attitudes towards homosexuals have decreased dramatically. Surveys of university students in Sydney, Brisbane and Melbourne between 1987 and 1994 show a considerable decrease in the extent to which students say they would avoid social contact with gay men, bisexual men and sex workers. The evaluation also noted problems with anti-discrimination agencies dealing with formal complaints in terms of their capacity to deal with the number and range of problems, and recommended that these bodies review mechanisms for fast-tracking cases where life-threatening illnesses are involved, and provide for entertaining class actions. Consultations and submissions also suggested that the extent of discrimination against people living with HIV/AIDS has diminished since the early days of the epidemic, although areas having a low prevalence of HIV/AIDS are often identified as those in which discrimination and breaches of confidentiality, particularly by health care workers and the general community, continue in the most obvious forms. The evaluation noted that discrimination against injecting drug users and Aboriginal and Torres Strait Islander people has continued.

Accompanying practical internal reforms are also important in dealing with discrimination. A pilot project in New South Wales in two city and two rural hospitals has targeted health care workers in systematically reviewing institutional and professional matters that may have a bearing on discrimination (e.g., universal infection control, informed consent and confidentiality). It de-emphasized anti-discrimination, but in fact linked such activities to wider goals of improving service delivery and thereby made them easily integrated into routine institutional activities, and, therefore, sustainable. The interest and commitment of professionals was engaged by involving them in the review and by asking them to identify problems and solutions at a more comprehensive level than that achievable by an outsider.[87]

Whether legislation can overcome private attitudes rather than public acts is debatable. What is needed is accompanying public education not just based on scientific facts about HIV/AIDS, but challenging the structures, social institutions and groups, which can be homophobic.[88] The Australian Government has had several media campaigns,[89] one called "HIV doesn't discriminate.... People do" and a more general one on the legislation itself called "Don't judge what I can do by what you think I can't". The former reinforces the safety of everyday social contact, and uses real people giving testimonials instead of actors in order to normalize people living with HIV, showing them as friends, relations, sons, uncles, workmates, sisters, neighbours and partners. The use of real people, with informed consent of course, was controversial because of the possible discriminatory treatment which might follow. The people concerned felt that it was worth sacrificing their privacy for altruistic reasons, by making the public see "us" instead of "them". Some of these people have died since the production of these advertisements which could be a problem for some cultures including parts of Australia's own indigenous population, with taboos associated with the "spirit world" This underlines the need to be sensitive in adapting successful models from other cultures.

A process similar to the Australian law reform programme has commenced in Canada. In early 1995, Phase I of a project by the Canddian HIV/AIDS Legal Network and the Canadian AIDS Society researched and documented a set of resource documents on HIV/AIDS legal and ethical issues, and, following consultations, prioritized eight areas—one of them being discrlmination. Phase II of the project is developing a series of discussion papers and workshops on these areas.[90] Important support for this initiative comes from a network which keeps practitioners and community groups up to date on HIV/AIDS legal issues. In Australia, Legal Link has been produced since 1990 by the Legal Project of the Australian Federation of AIDS Organisations. The *Canadian*.HIV/AIDS Policy and Law Newsletter was launched by the Canadian HIV/AIDS Legal Network in October 1994.

CONCLUSION

This chapter has sought to emphasize the benefits of giving

protection against discrimination and breaches of privacy by granting people living with HIV/AIDS the respect they deserve, in terms of dignity and autonomy. The only way to support voluntary behaviour change to fight this virus is through partnership with the affected community. Whether social engineering through legislation can immediately change attitudes of the general public is not clear.[91] However, we do know that such protection backed up by education gives confidence to people living with HIV/AIDS, and can only help to create a general climate of tolerance and understanding, rather than distress and disruption.[92] There needs to be groundswell support for such law reform, as without it resentment can be felt against paternalistic "do-gooders" wanting to impose their values from above.

REFERENCES

1. See Commonwealth of Australia, *National HIV/AIDS Strategy*, August 1989, AGPS, Canberra, Guiding Principle 4, p. 24.
2. NSW Anti-Discrimination Board *Discrimination—the Other Epidemic: Report of the Inquiry into HIV and AIDS Related Discrimination,* April 1992, Sydney.
3. Kippax S., Tillet G. Crawford J. and Cregan J. *Discrimination in the context of AIDS: Disease and Deviance,* A Conceptual mapping of HIV/AIDS Related Discrimination, written for the Australian Department of Community Services and Health, Macquire University AIDS Research Unit (national Centre for HIV Social Research), July 1991.
4. Yuen N.G. "Alienation or Employment: Law and Strategies for Social Change" (1989), *Law and Social Inquiry* 551 at 552.
5. 2 August 1990, 24 July 1991 and 9 August 1993.
6. See also *Report of the Secretary-General on International and Domestic Measurers taken to Protect Human Rights and Prevent* Discrimination *in the Context of HIV/AIDS*, CHR 51, 22 December, 1994.
7. Reported by Peter Blair in 5(4), *Legal Link,* December 1994, pp 3-4.
8. Tillen G. "The Resolution of AIDS Disputes" *Australian Dispute Resolution Journal,* (1990) 12 and Thornton M. "Equivocations of Conciliation: the Resolution of Discrimination Complaints in Australia 52 (6) (1989), *Modern Law Review,* 733.
9. Watchirs H. "HIV/AIDS & the Law: The Need for Reform in Australia: (1993) I *Journal of Law* and *Medicine* 9 at p. 27.
10. See Swiss Institute of Comparative Law *Comparative Study on Discrimination Against Persons with HIV or AIDS*, Council of Europe Strasbourg 1993 and Schulman D. "AIDS Discrimination: Its Nature, Meaning and Function" 12 *Nova Law Review,* (1988) 1113.
11. *A Complainant* and *Another v. The State of Western Australia,* (1994) EOC 92-610.
12. See Quiros L. V., Discrimination against HIV-infected People or People with AIDS, *Preliminary Report* (2 August 1990) and *Progress Report* (24 July 1991), CHR, Sub-commission on Prevention of Discrimination and the protection of Minorities. E/CN4/Sub.2/199019 And E/CN, 4/Sub 2/1991/10.
13. American Civil Liberties Union *Epidemic of Fear: A Survey of AIDS*

Discrimination in the 1980 and Policy Recommendations for the 1990's, New York p. 46.

14. Trowbridge Consulting *HIV/AIDS, Superannuation and Insurance,* prepared for the Department of Community Services and Health, October 1993, Sydney.
15. Waters P. "The Coverage of AIDS-related Discrimination under handicap discrimination laws: the US and Australia compared" (1990) 12 *Sydney Law Review* 377-419. See also Tucker B.P. "The Disability Discrimination Act: ensuing rights of Australians with disabilities" 21(1) *Monash Uni Law Review* (1995) 15-52.
16. *Hoddy v. Department of Corrective Services,* (1992) EOC 92-397.
17. See also s. 3(2) *Americans with Disabilities Act 1990* and New York Human Rights Law, Executive Law, Section 292.217.
18. See *Brunner v. A.L. Attar* Dist. Ct. Harris City, Texas 295th Jud. Dis. No. 86-42628.
19. See *Proff. v. Caro* (1987) New Jersey 549 AZD 900.
20. Hunter R. *Indirect Discrimination in the Workplace* Federation press, iSydney, 1992 and CCH Australia Ltd. *Australian S New Zealand Equal Opportunity Law S Practice,* Sydney 1991 (Looseleaf service) 4-200.
21. Hunt J. in *Jamal v. The Secretary, Department of Health and Anor* (1988) EOC 92-234 and see Asto H. "Anti-Discrimination Legislation and Physical Disability: The Lesons of experience" (1990) 64 *ALJ* 113 at 119.
22. J.c.- Ferguson v. *West and Central Sydney Area Health Service and Anor* (1990) EOC 92-272 *DL (Representing the members of People Living with AIDS (WA)* Inc. & *Ors. v. City of Perth and Ors* (1993) EOC 92-510 and X v. *McHugh, Auditor General for the State of Tasmania* (1994) EOC 92-623.
23. *DL (Representing the Members of People Living with AIDS (WA) Inc.* & *Ors. v. City of Perth* and *Ors.* (1993) EOC 92-510.
24. NSW Anti-Discrimination (Amendment) Act 1994.
25. Hay D. "The Power of Positive Living" *Good Weekend* (Morning Herald) 20 May 1995, p. 32-4.
26. See recommendation 4.6 *Final Report* Legal Working Party Intergovernmental Committee on AIDS, November 1992, Department of Health, Housing and Community Services.
27. G. v. *Lincraft* (1994) EOC 92-572.
28. Testing for spatial functioning, rather than HIV, would reveal such cases.
29. X. v. *Department of Defence,* unpublished decision of Carter W.J. QC, the Human Rights & Equal Opportunity Commission, Brisbane, 29 June 1995.
30. Feldblum C.R. "Disability Antidiscrimination Laws and HIV Testing of Health Care providers: *Courts, Health Science and the Law.* Georgetown University Medical and Law Centre, (1991) Vol. 1, 2 No. 1 pp. 136-142.
31. *Woods v. Wollongong City Council* and *Ors.* (1993) EOC 92-486 and *Cocks v. State of Queensland* (1994) EOC 92-612.
32. NSW in 1977, Victoria and SA in 1984, WA in 1988, ACT and Queensland in 1992, NT in 1992. The Sex Discrimination Act of 1994 is expected to come into effect in Tasmania in the near future.
33. *Brandy v. Human Rights and Equal Opportunity Commission* (1995), 69 ALJR 191.
34. Human Rights & Equal Opportunity Commission *Annual Report* 1993-94 AGPS, Canberra.
35. (1995) EOC 92-715, Carter Hon. W.J., Brisbane.
36. T16299-3, 28 March 1994.
37. 5(3) *Legal Link* September 1994, 5.

38. *Legal Link* March 1995, 21.
39. *Id.* 14.
40. Sydney Morning Herald 10 August 1994.
41. *Legal Link* June 1995 12.
42. *G.* v. *L* (1995) EOC 92-712.
43. (1990) EOC 92-272.
44. (1993) EOC 92-510.
45. (1994) EOC 92-572.
46. (1993) EOC 92-554.
47. 4(1) *Legal Link* March 1993 2-4.
48. *Iakarta Post* 31 March 1994.
49. *Sydney Morning Herald,* 10 May 1995.
50. Harris D. & Haigh R. *AIDS: A Guide to the Law,* Routledge, London, 1990.
51. Michael J. Privacy and Human Rights: *An International and* Comparative Study, with Special References to Developments in *Information Technology,* UNESCO and Dartmouth Publishing, Paris, 1994.
52. Hong Kong Law Reform Commission *Report on the Law Relating to the Protection of Personal Data (Topic 27)* August 1994. See Madsen W. "Protecting Privacy in a Digital World: Developments in the Asia-Pacific Region *"Media Information Australia (1993)* No. 67, p. 40. Countries with data protection laws are: Japan, Sweden, Denmark, Norway, Finland, the Netherlands, France, Germany, Luxembourg, UK, Ireland, Austria, Iceland, Israel, Portugal and the USA.
53. Privacy Commission of Canada AIDS and the Privacy Act Minister of Supply and Services 1989 and *Report of the Privacy and the HIV/AIDS Working Party* Commonwealth of Australia, September 1992. See also Office of the Information and privacy Commission Ontario. *HIV/AIDS: The Need for Privacy* October 1990 Canada.
54. "Tagging condemned" 6(2), *Legal Link,* June 1995, p.4.
55. Renner S., Commission on the Mentally Disabled and Center on Children and the Law, ABA, Washington DC., 1991.
56. See Privacy Commissioner, *Federal Privacy Handbook: A Guide to Federal Privacy Law and Practice.* Redfern Legal Centre Publishing, Sydney, 1992 (looseleaf service).
57. A Llamo 'The Management of Confidentiality with AIDS Patients" in Fuenzalida-Puelma *et al.,*.(eds) *Ethics* and *law in the Study of AIDS* Pan American Health Organization Washington, D.C., 1992, p 138 at pp. 139-141. See also C. Obade" Whisper Down the Lane: AIDS, Privacy & the Hospital 'Grape Vine' 2(2) (1991) *Journal of Clinical Ethics* 133.
58. See Gostin LO *et. al.* "Privacy and Security Information in a ' New Health Care System" *Journal of the American Medical Association Vol.* 270 No. 20 (24 November 1993) 2487 and Magnusson RS "Privacy, Confidentiality and HIV/AIDS Health Care" 18(1) (1994) *Australian Journal of Public Health* 51 at 57.
59. *The Times,* 27 July 1994, p. 23.
60. See Dennis DI "HIV Screening & Discrimination: The Federal Example" in Fuenzalida-Puelma *op. cit.,* 187 & Gunderson M. *et. al., AIDS Testing* and *Privacy* University of Utah Press, Salt Lake City 1989.
61. A privilege to disclose is preferable—see Bayer R "Confidentiality & its Limits" in Fuenzalida-Puelma *op.cit.,* 145 at 146.
62. Watchirs, *loc. cit., p.* 13.
63. *Tarasoff v. Regents of the University of California* (1976) 551 P 2d 334.
64. Legal Working Party *Final Report p.* 12.

65. Legal Working Party *Final Report p.* 12.
66. 5(4) *Legal Link* December 1994, 22.
67. 6(2) *Legal Link* June 1995, 5.
68. Kenndy J. May 1989, 31.
69. *Adelaide Advertiser* March 1990, 22.
70. 5(3) *Legal Link* September 1994, 14-15.
71. 5(3) *Legal Link* September 1994, 18.
72. *H. v. Royal Alexandra Hospital for Children's CSL; Australian Red Cross* (1990) Australian Tort Reports. 80-100: E v. *Australian Red Cross Society* (1991) 27 FCR 310; *TC and Ors v. Australian Red Cross Society* (1989) WAC 335; *BC v. Australian Red Cross* Unreported. Vic SC, Cummins J. 25 February 1991. See also *PD v. Australian Red Cross Society* (NSW Div) (1993) 30 NSWLR; *PQ v. Australian Red Cross Society* (1992) Div R 191, 376 6CA.
73. *Legal Link* 5(1) April 1994, 19 and 5(4) December 1994.
74. [1993] 1VR, 665.
75. [1991] 2 OR (3d) 40.
76. (1990) SCLR 263.
77. 5(1) *Legal Link* April 1994, 21.
78. 4(4) *Legal Link* December 1993, 13; 4(2) June 1993, 7.
79. McGrath C.J., May 1992, 15.
80. 6(3) *Legal Link* September 1995, 26.
81. *Id.* 27.
82. (1993) 4 SA 842.
83. [1988] 2 All ER 648.
84. Altman DA "The Most Political of Diseases in Timewell", E. *Minichiello v. Plumber* (eds.) *AIDS in Australia.* Prentice Hall, Sydney 1992, p. 58.
85. February 1991, Department of Community Services and Health, Canberra.
86. Puplick C, *The Courage of their Convictions, HIV/AIDS: The National Strategy and the Laws of New South Wales,* Sydney, November 1993 and Sarre R *HIV/AIDS Advisory Committee Interim South* Australian Report on the Implementation of the Intergovernment *Committee on AIDS, Legal Working Party Report,* Adelaide, December 1994.
87. School of Medical Education, University of NSW, Sydney *HIV/ AIDS related Discrimination Health Care Worker Project* prepared for the National AIDS Campaign Department of Human Services and Health, August 1994, AGPS Canberra.
88. Noble J, Kippax & Crwaford J "some demographic co-relates of HIV/AIDS Discrimination 30/3" *Australian Journal of Social Issues,* August 1995, 310 at 32.
89. Lenehan Lynton Bloom Blaxland *Research into HIV/AIDS Related Discrimination v. Qualitative Research Report,* prepared for the Australian Department of Human Services and Health, October 1994, AGPS, Canberra.
90. Jurgens R "Ethics and Law in Canada" 6(3) *HIV/AIDS Legal Link* September 1995, 24.
91. See Roden R "Educating Through the Law: The Los Angeles AIDS Discrimination Ordinance" 33 UCLA (1986) 40 and Cranston IR "Reform through legislation: the dimension of legislative technique" (1979) 73 *Northwestern University Law Reveiw* 873 at 875-6.
92. Australian Federation of AIDS Organisations *HIV/AIDS Related Discrimination: PLWHA Project Report* prepared for the National AIDS Campaign, Department of Human Services and Health, December 1994.

7

Criminal Law and HIV

David Buchanan
Barristor
Sydney, Australia

There are three basic lessons about HIV/AIDS and the criminal law. The first is that there is almost no necessity for laws creating new offences. The second is that there is a need for laws inflicting penalties upon those who behave inappropriately towards people with HIV. Third, three is need systematically to examine criminal laws with a view to adjustments needed in order more effectively to deal with the epidemic and create a legal environment in which behaviour change is encouraged and respect and care for those infected and at risk is facilitated.

No New Offenses

Almost no new offences need to be created to deal with the HIV epidemic. Armed robbers who use a blood-filled syringe, whether HIV infected or not, are just as guilty of armed robbery or using an offensive weapon as those who use a stick, knife or gun. The mythical, deliberate infector is surely guilty of attempted murder, or manslaughter, or reckless act endangering life, or assault occasioning grievous bodily harm.

The usual problem is with politicians, ignorant of basic public health principles, who want to be seen to be 'doing something,' often in response to a sensationalised story in the media. They then enact quite inappropriate laws, such as one in the Australian state of New South Wales, which criminalises sexual intercourse, including oral sex, by a person with HIV unless the other party gives informed consent. The law says nothing about protected or unprotected sex. It is unenforceable, has never been prosecuted and is broken daily by the hundreds if not thousands of people with HIV who are having safe sex, particularly outside relationships. And of course the law not only fails to reinforce but, because it can operate only on those who know they have HIV, actually contradicts official government policy that people at risk for HIV have only safe sex.

An Australian territory, on the other hand (the Australian Capital Territory), has passed a law criminalising unsafe sex with a sex worker, and indeed criminalising conduct of a brothel proprietor which discourages safe sex. This is more the sort of law which is appropriate to the epidemic.

Another offence appropriate to HIV/AIDS and other blood-borne pathogens is one which imposes a penalty for knowingly making false declarations about risk behaviour history for those donating blood to the national blood pool. Such laws are not a substitute for, but work in conjunction with, systems for screening donations.

Laws Regulating those Who Deal with People with HIV

There is a need for laws to create a powerful disincentive to misconduct towards or in respect of people with HIV or at risk of infection. Such laws will be likely to include a penalty for infraction and thus constitute criminal laws.

Examples include laws requiring the confidentiality of people whose serostatus is known by reason of testing to be respected, laws making it illegal to discriminate against people with infection and their carers and associates, laws making it illegal to vilify people on the ground of their HIV, presumed HIV or status placing them at risk of HIV (e.g., homosexuality). Other instances indude strictly regulating the use and distribution of HIV test kits, respecting the wishes of people with HIV in respect of medical treatment and distribution of property both before and after death. There are numerous other examples, not all of which require penal sanction for enforcement.

Modifications to Laws Required by HIV/AIDS

There are many changes of a different kind needed to the laws of most countries in order for there to be an appropriate response to the epidemic. For example, laws which directly or indirectly penalise risk behaviours will contradict public health policy by alienating people at risk of infection from the health authorities and disempower or deter people from appropriate behaviour change and organising to look after themselves and their friends.

Laws which criminalise possession and supply of drug injection equipment should be repealed, preferable as a precursor to repeal or decriminalisation of laws regulating consumption of illicit drugs. In Australia, every state and territory has now legislated for suppliers of needles and syringes to be licensed by the local health authorities. The laws are supported by the politicians because they can see that, by contrast with developed countries without authorised needle and syringe exchange programmes, Australia has been able to keep the rates of HIV infection in the injecting drug population to remarkably low levels.

The sex industry should be decriminalised. There is a vigorous debate as to the extent to which the industry should be legally regulated after decriminalisation. Over-regulation runs the risk of playing into the hands of bureaucrats and local politicians who dislike the industry. As indicated earlier, laws which might usefully be considered are ones which empower sex workers to insist on condoms and water-based lubricant whenever they deal with their bosses or clients.

Homosexual acts should be decriminalised. Unequal or unrealistic ages of consent for homosexual sex should be lowered. (This is a different issue from the need for strict enforcement of laws against underage sex which puts girls and young women at increased risk of contracting HIV.)

Police powers to test for HIV should be strictly confined to those medical tests required for the bona fide investigation of allegations of crime. In particular, such powers should not be used for covert occupational testing of sex workers and people suspected of exposing others to HIV. Such powers should be conditioned upon the order of a judicial officer such as a magistrate after the person affected has had the opportunity to be heard on the question. Evidence laws need to be examined. An example is to prohibit the possession of a syringe as evidence in a drug case, and of condoms in a sex case.

Procedural laws may also be relevant. Consideration might be given to protecting the identity in court of people with HIV. Sentencing law must take HIV/AIDS into account where a sentence of imprisonment upon a person with HIV will involve greater hardship than if imposed upon a person without infection. Laws requiring mandatory imprisonment for offences which are not very serious of people at risk of infection plainly unduly increases the risk that more people will contract HIV by reason of being imprisoned.

CONCLUSION

All countries sooner or later must systematically examine their laws to evaluate them for their appropriateness in the light of the epidemic. A major consideration must not only be their consonance with public health policy in respect of HIV/AIDS, but also whether they will work in reality or will instead have unintended consequences of making public health programmes more difficult to implement, increasing the burden of looking after people with HIV/AIDS and contributing to the spread of the virus. Consultation with affected communities in this process is vital if the goals of such a systematic analysis are to be achieved.

8

People Living with HIV: The Law, Ethics and Discrimination

Ms. Julie Hamblin
Partner
Esworth & Elsworth Sydney,
Australia

A TRUE STORY

Let me start with a true story. This story began at 8 am on the morning of 14 February 1989, when a young man living in a coastal province of India received a visit from the police. He was asked to report to the local police station later that day. No reason was given for the request, but the man assumed that one of his friends was in trouble and had asked for his help. Upon arriving at the police station, he was taken immediately to the local hospital by two policemen and told that he must undergo a physical examination. By this time, he was quite scared as he did not know why he was being detained. His fear did not abate when he saw that six policemen were standing at the door of the casualty ward, two of them armed with rifles and the others with bamboo sticks.

The examining doctor entered the man's name in a register book. The man was able to see that on the cover of the book was written the word "AIDS". This was how he first came to know that he was infected with the human immuno-deficiency virus (HIV)—no explanation, no counselling, not even any words of sympathy or support that might suggest that this was not the end of the road.

But there was worse to come. From the hospital, the man was taken by police escort to a former TB sanatorium where he was to be detained against his will for ffie next 64 days. He was placed in a small dirty room, completely alone, not knowing why he was there or what would happen to him. He was not permitted to contact his family or friends to let them know where he was. In his own account of those first 24 hours, he said that he survived only because he had no knife or gun with which to take his own life.

Over the next few days, the reason for the man's detention gradually became clear. He had donated blood several months previously. The local hospital had tested his blood for HIV without his knowledge or consent, and had found that he was HIV positive. But instead of contacting him, the hospital informed the local police. The police had then acted in reliance on the Public Health Act in force in that province which provided for the mandatory detention of all HIV positive people. Under the Act, detention was indefinite, regardless of whether there was any actual risk of HIV transmission to other members of the public.

A month went by, and the man remained in detention. By this stage, his family and friends had been able to make representations on his behalf to the government pointing out the injustice, not to mention pointlessness, of his detention. He received extraordinary support from the people living in his home village who wrote demanding his release. Eventually, he mounted a courtchallenge to the legislation authorising his detention and, after 64 days of detention, was granted interim leave to return home ... not, however, because of any illegality in the detention provisions as such, but only because the court considered that the HIV testing procedure that had been followed was not sufficiently reliable to justify detention.

Shortly afterwards, the Act was amended, abolishing the mandatory requirement of detention of all HIV po ve people but permitting detention at the discretion of the health authorities. A court challenge mounted against the amended legislation failed.

Many of you may already have recognised that the man in this story was Dominic d' Souza. The law in question was the Goan Public Health Act which remains in force today. Dominic went on to become one of the leading advocates in India of the rights of people with HIV. He died from AIDS (acquired immuno-deficiency syndrome) in May of 1992, but his presence has been felt in many ways at this conference. Before his death he wrote:

"No matter how much I try to calm myself, I cannot help feeling desperately alone and afraid when I think that tomorrow I may meet with an accident and may require immediate medical attention. What happens then? Will anyone be willing to even take my X-ray? ... Why then do we still hear of medics refusing to even set eyes on HIVpositive persons, let alone touch or treat them ?"

"I live to take each day as it comes. I know that with God, nothing shall be impossible. I have the love of my family, neighbours and friends who will always be there to help me. I should like to put two questions to you: If you found someone you knew had AIDS, would you avoid them ? What if your brother or sister had it? "

And of course, in a very profound way, Dominic was the brother of all of us here today.

No one hearing this story can doubt that the law has a role to play in the response to the HIV epidemic. Legal issues arose at every point in Dominic's story: his blood was tested for HIV without his consent, the hospital did not disclose his HIV status to him, confidentiality was breached by reason of the disclosure to the police, and he was then detained under the Public Health Legislation. And for Dominic, the story did not end there. When he attempted to return to work, he found that his job had already been given to someone else, and his employer asked him to resign because of concern that other employees would not want to work with a person with HIV.

We have heard over and over again this week about discrimination' against people with HIV. We know that it is a deep and pervasive problem. What happened to Dominic is the reality for many people with HIV, whether they live in the United States, Australia, Asia or Africa. Ignorance about the way HIV is transmitted, unjustified fear of infection and prejudice against groups of people perceived (often wrongly) to be at risk have transcended national boundaries and differences of race and culture. No policy to address the effects of the epidemic can afford to ignore the fact that HIV threatens human rights as profoundly as it threatens public health.

HUMAN RIGHTS AND HIV

When discussing human rights in the context of the HIV epidemic, two important points need to be made. The first is one of the most important reasons why respect for human rights is so critical in the response to the epidemic. The second is a myth that needs to be dispelled.

The first point — the reason why human rights are so important in the context of HIV—arises from the fact that many of the people who have been and will be most affected by the epidemic are people who are already in a socially disadvantaged position. We have already heard this week about how the global burden of HIV infection in the years to come will be borne overwhelmingly by people in developing countries. Increasingly, inequalities of gender, race and wealth are emerging in the demography of HIV infection, with infection rates increasing disproportionately among women and even more so among poor women. The main global risk factors for HIV infection in the 1990s will not be sexual activity or drug use as such but rather social and economic dependency.

These underlying socio-economic causes of vulnerability to HIV operate in many ways. Because HIV infection is preventable, people who have access to information and appropriate preventative measures and have the means to implement these measures will in the future be able to protect themselves against infection. The people who remain vulnerable are those who are denied the means of protecting themselves against HIV because of economic need, for example, or powerlessness to control the basis upon which their sexual relationships take place. Many factors come into play here, including poverty, geographical isolation, inadequate health care and health education, and cultural values that compel certain practices that expose some members of the community to the risk of HIV transmission.

> The fact that those now most at risk of HIV infection are those who are already socially and economically vulnerable means that the need to incorporate human rights concerns into HIV policy has a particular resonance.

For women, the social and economic obstacles to avoiding the risk of HIV infection are particularly great. Their position within families and societies means they are often not free to make their own decisions about their sexual relationships or to insist upon measures, such as the use of condoms or fidelity on the part of their partner, that would reduce the risk of exposure to HIV. Cultural expectations in relation to marriage and childbirth and the absence of means of economic support outside the family unit compound the difficulties for women to avoid exposure to the virus.

The fact that those now most at risk of HIV infection are those who are already socially and economically vulnerable means that the need to incorporate human rights concerns into HIV policy has a particular resonance. Similar issues arise in relation to drug users, gay men and sex workers, for whom discrimination and social stigmatisation were already pervasive problems before the HIV epidemic arrived on the scene. What this means is that these people, more than any, need protection against the abuse of their rights threatened by the HIV epidemic. As Justice Michael Kirby has said, human rights matter most when they are most under threat.

So there is a special need, a special responsibility, to honour the rights and needs of these people. Moreover, the fact that these human rights are so much under threat presents unique challenges to effective policies for preventing the further spread of HIV.

This leads to my second point: the myth that needs to be dispelled.

Too often, the HIV policy debate is characterised as an inevitable conflict between public health and individual rights. Policies that infringe individual rights, such as forcible HIV testing or detention are defended on the basis of an overriding need to protect public health. But an effective response to the epidemic demands a more complex understanding. This is not to say that there will never be conflicting values or interests because of many of the necessary measures may represent profound challenges to prevailing cultural beliefs and practices. However, an effective response to the HIV epidemic requires, above all, a recognition by all individuals, the infected and the uninfected, and by communities and governments that they have a common interest in working together to do whatever is necessary to contain the spread of HIV in order to ensure the survival of their families and societies. The emphasis in our response to the epidemic must be on this community of interest rather than on the potential conflicts.

We now have a decade of experience with the HIV epidemic and with a range of different policies that have attempted to reduce the spread of HIV. We know what works and what does not. We know that alienating people with HIV from society, making them feel they have nothing to gain by protecting themselves or others, breeds helplessness, indifference and lack of respect for other people. These are perfect conditions for the spread of the virus and will undermine any efforts to encourage the voluntary behaviour changes that are necessary to prevent the spread of infection. In contrast, policies and laws that reduce the stigma attaching to HIV infection and build the self esteem of people with HIV or at risk of infection can create the environment of mutual trust, support and colaboration that is critical to bringing about and sustaining behaviour change.

The coalition of interest that is required must include people living with HIV. Their collaboration is fundamental to effective HIV policy interventions - not only because of the immediate need to prevent further transmission of the virus but also because people who are already living with HIV can be powerful agents for behaviour change. No one who heard Bill O'Loughlin speak yesterday can doubt that.

Respect for the rights of people with HIV must exist if this necessary collaboration is to be achieved. There must be a sense within each community that all its members, both those directly affected and those not yet affected, are equally valued and supported. Only within a supportive environment that respects individual worth will people have the courage to acknowledge publicly that they may be infected or at risk of infection and thereby to take the first step towards changing the behaviours that place them and others at risk.

So let us dispel the myth that there must be an inevitable conflict between individual rights and public health. And let us also dispel the myth that respect for human rights can be a gloss to be added to other aspects of HIV policy. It must pervade our whole thinking and experience of this epidemic if we are to be able to respond effectively. How do we convince our policy makers of this? Of course we can argue that respect for human rights has an inherent value of its own, and we would hope that this argument—would be compelling. But if we cannot persuade our HIV policy makers on this ground alone, we have to convince them that, as an HIV prevention measure, respect for human rights works.

THE LAW AND HIV

So what does this mean for legal policy on HIV?

Clearly, the law has an important impact on how the HIV epidemic is experienced in any country. This became evident very early on in the epidemic because many of the people affected, such as sex workers, gay men and drug users, were already the target of punitive legal provisions. Moreover, the fear generated by the epidemic has meant that responses relying upon punitive, restrictive models of law have been common. Dominic's case is just one example of many.

In this way, the law has been an important part of the backdrop against which the experiences of people with HIV have been lived and intervention strategies have been implemented. Of course it is only one element of many that go to make up this backdrop, but it has been a critical element–in both a practical and symbolic sense.

So we know that the law matters in the context of this epidemic. The more important and the more difficult issue is to identify the way forward if we are to use (or, on occasions, not use) the law constructively and appropriately in our response to HIV.

In many ways, the principles that should guide legal policy on HIV are very simple. There are four points that I would like to leave you with today.

A Protective and Supportive Legal Framework

The first point, I hope, is obvious. The law can and must be used to establish a protective and supportive framework for people affected by the epidemic and not a punitive one. This is a critical element of the environment I described earlier, the environment of collaboration and mutual support that emphasizes the community of interest between the infected and the uninfected and between governments and individuals. Only in such an environment can we be confident that our efforts to reduce the transmission of HIV and care for those affected will have optimum effect.

> The laws that we do not need are the laws which discriminate against peopk with HIV, which distance them from their communities and which nske it less likely that these people with share in the common.interest to reduce the effects of the epidemic.

Creating a supportive legal environment can involve both negative and positive legal interventions. The negative interventions arise from the need for absence of law in some contexts. The laws that we do not need are the laws which discriminate against people with HIV, which distance them from their communities and which make it less likely that these people will share in the common interest to reduce the effects of the epidemic. Examples of such laws are:

— Laws that make homosexuality a criminal offense.
— Offenses relating to drug use and prostitution that have the effect of making it harder to reach drug users and sex workers with HIV care and prevention measures.
— Laws restricting the availability of condoms and needles and syringes.
— Censorship and broadcasting laws that restrict the dissemination of safe sex information.

— Laws that permit HIV testing without consent or the detention of people with HIV.
— Immigration and travel laws that restrict the movement of people with HIV between countries.

These laws have no place in a sensitive and sensible response to the epidemic and need to be repealed.

Then there are the positive legal interventions–the ones that can actively promote the supportive environment I have described. These legal interventions include:

— Human rights laws that give legal effect to rights such as the right to privacy, the right to protection against unlawful search and seizure and rights to protection against unlawful detention.
— Anti-discrimination laws that will provide redress in the event of discrimination in employment, housing, access to health care etc., against people with HIV or their family or friends.
— Legal provisions that protect the confidentiality of a person's HIV status.
— Laws compelling a person' s consent to be given before HIV testing is undertaken.
— Laws that encourage appropriate workplace practices, e.g. infection control procedures and HIV education for employees.

These are just a few examples of many. The thrust of this approach to legal policy on HIV must be to use the law not as a weapon but as a protective instrument that respects the worth of all individuals and reinforces co-operative efforts to deal with the effects of the epidemic.

Ethics and Law

It has become common in the context of HIV policy to talk about ethics and law in the same breath. This is done for obvious reasons because the ethical dilemmas that arise are invariably played out in legal terms. Nonetheless, the blurring of the distinction between law and ethics can sometimes obscure the fact that tensions may exist between ethical imperatives and legal obligations. It is therefore worth considering the interaction between law, ethics and HIV.

We like to think that ethics and law do go hand in hand. As a lawyer, I know that this is not true, and I imagine that most of you do not need a lawyer to tell you that. With some of the very complex dilemmas that arise with HIV—such as whether to tell the wife of a man with HIV that she is at risk—the existing law is not a sufficiently subtle mechanism to deal with the problem. Existing legal principles may be inadequate to mediate all the different interests involved and may lead to inappropriate and anomalous results.

The potential inadequacy of existing law does, however, provide us with an opportunity. Because so many of the legal issues thrown up by the HIV epidemic are new, the development of new legal principles and solutions will be required. There is therefore an opportunity to direct the law in the way we want it to go, that is, to have ethics drive law reform and not the other way around. If one takes the case of whether to disclose a man's HIV status to his spouse, for example, the legal principles governing this decision may well be uncertain and any judge called upon to decide the case will almost certainly be less well equipped to arrive at an informed view than those of us in this room today. There is therefore a real possibility that careful and informed ethical debate can guide the direction of the evolution of law in this area. Appropriate ethical guidelines may even mean that the law will not need to become directly involved. At the very least, such guidelines will assist in shaping the law in the best way possible.

The Law as an Instrument of Behaviour Change

My third point is one that I propose tentatively because it is a complex and controversial issue and, in many ways, a dangerous issue. It is, however, an issue that needs to be explored if we are to use the law to its full potential in the response to the HIV epidemic. The point to which I am referring is the notion that the law can be used actively as an instrument to bring about changes in personal behaviour.

In order to understand this point, it is necessary to appreciate the complex interdependence between the law and the society within which it operates. While, on the one level, the law is a product of prevailing social and cultural values within any community, it can also be instrumental in defining, reinforcing and, in some cases, actively promoting certain values and practices. By either condoning or outlawing certain forms of behaviour or expressions of cultural values, the law can be a powerful instrument for shaping or reinforcing these behaviours or values.

I do not want to overstate the extent to which the law can be used to bring about behaviour changes. Certainly, legal coercion has rarely been effective in the past in changing personal behaviour, and there is no reason to think that the HIV epidemic will be any different. It is possible, however, that used in combination with other measures, some forms of legal intervention can be used actively to bring about change.

One example of this is the experience with laws requiring brothel owners to insist upon condom use by their clients. On a practical level, such a law is difficult if not impossible to enforce, and its immediate direct impact is therefore questionable. However, there is some evidence that such a law can assist in encouraging condom use, if only because it makes it easier for prostitutes to insist upon condom use by their clients. The legislation can be an instrument for bringing about behaviour change in this way.

Looking beyond the immediate reach of HIV policy, it is possible also to envisage other ways in which the law could be used, albeit indirectly, to reduce vulnerability to HIV exposure. Where poverty and economic dependency lead to vulnerability to HIV, such as where the sale of sex is a person's only source of income or where women are denied economic rights independently of the family unit, laws that address these issues–for example, through changes to land ownership or credit regulation–may assist other efforts to change the behaviours that spread HIV. Where women are unable to protect themselves against the virus because of their unequal position within relationships, or in communities, laws such as those dealing with rape within marriage and the age of marriage or sexual consent, which uphold the independent rights of women, may increase the options for women in the context of the epidemic.

It is important to explore these creative ways in which the law may be able to be used actively in the response to the HIV epidemic.

> While, on the one level, the law is a product of prevailing social and cultural values within a community, it can also be instrumental in defining, reinforcing and, in some cases, actively promoting certain values and practices.

Mobilize the Lawyers

The last point I want to leave you with is a critical one. You have to find ways of mobilizing the lawyers in your countries to take up these issues. It is not that there are not lawyers willing to take up social issues such as this. It is just that most lawyers think HIV does not have much to do with them. Or, if they do, they can' t see that the law has much to do with HIV. You would be surprised how often I am asked what I, as a lawyer, are doing working in the field of HIV. I know from my own work in this region that if you go and talk to lawyers about HIV, it is very easy to generate interest and enthusiasm. We all need to find ways to tap this resource of lawyers within our own countries. We need to have lawyers who are prepared to argue for appropriate law reform on HIV, to give legal advice to people affected by the epidemic and to take test cases to court where necessary. Only by having an informed group of lawyers can we ensure that the legal issues associated with the epidemic will be tackled properly.

We have had a wonderful response this week to the UNDP proposal to establish an HIV legal network in this region. We need to find ways of carrying on this momentum. We know that the law can be used constructively and positively in the response to the HIV epidemic. What is important at this stage is that we do not waste this opportunity.

9

Law, Ethics and HIV: Strategies for Ethical and Effective Policy

Ms. Julie Hamblin
Partner
Elsworth and Elsworth Solicitors Sydney,
Australia

INTRODUCTION

A decade into the HIV epidemic, there is now a need, more than ever, to ensure that effective and appropriate strategies are put in place to reduce the spread of the virus and to address the consequences of the epidemic. This need is nowhere stronger than in the Asian and Pacific region. In these countries, the epidemic was not immediately apparent in the early 1980s when the world first became aware of AIDS. In the intervening years, however, HIV has spread rapidly in the region, and no country remains untouched. We now know that the effects of the HIV epidemic in this part of the world will be as devastating as those already visible in parts of Africa unless effective measures are implemented without delay.

The fact that the HIV epidemic has emerged in Asia and the Pacific later than some other parts of the world presents some opportunities for HIV policy in the region. Countries in Asia and the Pacific can draw upon the understanding and experience that has grown out of the first decade of the epidemic. They can know from the outset that the effects of the sector, and that any effective policy on HIV must encompass many dimensions both in its understanding of the epidemic and in the scope of its operation.

Among the many dimensions that must be integrated into the response to the HIV epidemic, the legal, ethical and human rights aspects are of central importance. This is particularly so because of the complex dynamics within any society or culture which give rise to difficult questions about rights, responsibilities reducing the impact of the epidemic.

HIV, Culture and the Socio-economic Patterns of the Epidemic

Unlike many epidemic diseases in the past, HIV is not spread by mere casual contact between individuals. As is now well known, the virus is transmitted only through direct exposure to the bodily fluids of an infected person, as can occur during sexual intercourse, from sharing needles and syringes or during pregnancy from an infected woman to her child.

An understanding of the scientific basis of transmission, however, provides little insight into the social, economic and cultural factors within any society that determine the patterns of vulnerability to HIV infection. Increasingly, the global patterns of vulnerability to HIV indicate that the people most likely to become infected are those who, by reason of their social or economic position, are unable to protect themselves against infection.

These underlying socio-economic causes of vulnerability to HIV operate in many ways. In the first place, basic information about HIV and how to prevent transmission may be denied to people, particularly in developing countries, through poverty, geographic isolation and poor amenities. Even where knowledge about the epidemic is available, the ability of individuals to act on this information in order to protect themselves against infection may be seriously limited. The pattern of sexual relationships is frequently prescribed by culture, social roles and expectations and economic need. Changing these patterns in order to prevent transmission of HIV will involve addressing deeply-rooted social and cultural practices, as well as the economic factors which may underpin and reinforce them.

For them, the obstacles to avoiding the risk of HIV infection are particularly great. Their position within families and societies means they are often not free to make their own decisions about their sexual relationships or to insist upon measures, such as the use of condoms or fidelity on the part of their partner, that would reduce their risk of exposure to HIV. Cultural expectations in relation to marriage and childbirth and the absence of means of economic support outside the family unit compound the difficulties for women to avoid exposure to the virus. For these women, as for many poor or disadvantaged people of any gender or race, the main risk factors for HIV are inequality and powerlessness within their relationships and societies.

The implications of this for strategies to respond to the HIV epidemic, and particularly for legal policy, are critical. The changes that are required to prevent the spread of HIV demand changes to fundamental patterns of social and economic interaction at both the individual and the communal level. They clearly transcend what can be achieved by coercive interventions by governments. Rather, a social contract is required that can acknowledge the existence of different values and interests within any one society, but at the same time allow those differences to be bridged to the extent necessary to respond effectively to the HIV epidemic. This depends upon there being a recognition by all individuals, the infected and the uninfected, and by communities and governments that they have a common interest in working together to do whatever is necessary to contain the spread of HIV in order to ensure the survival of their families and societies.

As a consequence, strategies to bring about the necessary behaviour changes are most likely to be effective if they occur in an environment that emphasizes this common interest, demonstrated by support for infected people rather than alienation and by a respect for the interests and needs of each person affected by the epidemic.

Whether such an environment exists will depend upon many factors, including culture, tradition and religion, each of which may in any society militate either in favour of or against a supportive environment for HIV strategies. One of the most important of these determining factors, however and one of the factors most amenable to change, is the existing legal framework of rights and responsibilities.

The HIV Epidemic and the Law

Too often, analyses of the interaction between the HIV epidemic and the law focus only on legislation that is directly applicable to health policy, such as public health legislation. In fact, the impact of the law on the pattern and consequences of the epidemic is much more complex than these analyses suggest, and will touch upon HIV policy in a multitude of ways.

In the first place, there are the legal rights and duties that impact directly upon individuals affected by the HIV epidemic and determine what these individuals, infected or uninfected, can legally do or have done to them. Many examples can be found of these direct legal provisions. They include:

— whether and, if so, in what circumstances, individuals can be compelled to undergo testing for HIV;
— how the test is to be carried out, such as whether the individual must be informed that the test is to be undertaken, whether he or she may refuse the test, and whether counselling is permitted or required;
— what steps can be taken by government authorities in the event that a person is found to have HIV—whether restrictions or sanctions, such as quarantine, can be imposed on that person;
— what notification requirements exist in relation to AIDS and HIV infection, and what consequences will these have for infected people;
— whether there are legally-recognised rights of privacy or obligations of confidentiality to guard against unauthorised disclosure of a person's HIV status;
— whether a person with HIV will be permitted to continue working and will be protected against discrimination in the workplace;
— what access to education, training and health care will be available for infected people and will this be legally sanctioned or required;
— are criminal or civil sanctions available for use against people who transmit the virus to others.

In these ways, the law has an immediate and self-evident impact on the HIV epidemic. It determines rights and duties as between infected individuals and other members of the community and as between individuals and the state.

In more subtle ways, though, the law can have an equally pervasive yet indirect impact on HIV/AIDS policy by influencing the background or context within which the policy response to the epidemic takes place. It can be instrumental in shaping the environment for all aspects of HIV policy and, by promoting an environment of support, co-operation and collaboration—an "enabling environment"—can be used actively to give maximum effect to other HIV strategies aimed at encouraging the behaviour change necessary to prevent the spread of the virus.

Experience teaches us that reducing the stigma attaching to

HIV infection, and building the self-esteem of people with or at risk of infection, create the conditions necessary for mutual trust, support and collaboration in effecting and sustaining the behaviour changes needed to stem the epidemic. Conversely, alienating people from society, making them feel they have nothing to gain by protecting themselves or others, breeds helplessness, indifference and contempt for self and others: perfect conditions for the spread of HIV.

The law can contribute to the desired "enabling environment" on both a practical and symbolic level. At the practical level, the law will determine whether people with HIV or those at risk of infection are subject to punitive measures such as compulsory testing and detention or whether they have strong, legally enforceable protection against discrimination or breach of confidentiality. In this way, it will be the test of whether HIV policies can truly be said to be based on principles of collaboration and trust. At the symbolic level, these legal measures set the tone for society's response to HIV. They make a statement about whether our response to infected people should be based on understanding and support or on rejection, and by either condoning or condemning certain forms of response, they can actively promote the attitudes that will enable policies on HIV to have the best effect.

The laws that go to make up this legal environment are many and varied. Some may relate specifically to HIV, while others will be more general in their focus. Some have consequences both in the direct ways already discussed and also as part of the general environment within which HIV policy is implemented. Among the types of laws that are relevant, whether because they encourage or discourage the desired responses, are:

— laws that prohibit discrimination against people infected with HIV in employment, housing, access to medical treatment, association with others and the provision of services;
— human rights instruments that recognise the rights of infected people, such as equality rights, rights of privacy and rights of access to health care, and provide legal mechanisms for upholding these rights;
— laws that impose criminal sanctions on activities that involve a risk of HIV infection, such as homosexuality, prostitution and drug use, and are therefore likely to alienate the people concerned;
— laws that protect the confidentiality of a person's HIV status;
— laws that were not intended to deal with HIV but which can

be used indirectly to implement HIV policy without explicit acknowledgement of this intention, e.g., internal security laws;

— laws that restrict access to measures to prevent HIV transmission, for example, laws that regulate the availability of condoms and needles and syringes, or laws that restrict the advertisement of condoms or the publication of safe sex messages;

— laws that require the free and uncoerced consent of individuals to HIV testing, thereby recognising the right of all people to decide for themselves whether to be tested;

— laws that encourage the provision of information about HIV and its modes of transmission, for example, by requiring employers to implement appropriate workplace policies on HIV.

Looking beyond the immediate reach of HIV policy, it is possible also to envisage other ways in which the law could be used, albeit indirectly to reduce vulnerability to HIV exposure. Where poverty and economic dependency lead to vulnerability to HIV, such as where the sale of sex is a person's only source of income or where women are denied economic rights independently of the family unit, laws that address these issues—for example, through changes to land ownership or credit regulation—may assist other efforts to change the behaviours that spread HIV. Where women are unable to protect themselves against the virus because of the unequal position within relationships and communities, laws such as those dealing with rape within marriage and the age of marriage or sexual consent, which uphold the independent rights of women, may increase the options for women in the context of the epidemic.

While one could debate the extent to which changes of this kind can be effected through legal measures, it is nonetheless important to keep these broader considerations in mind when formulating strategies on HIV and the potential role of the law. They demonstrate that there is scope for creative approaches to HIV legal policy that go beyond the traditional ambit of infectious disease control.

Questions for Legal Policy on HIV/AIDS

Because effective legal policy on HIV requires an appreciation of the socio-economic and cultural contexts of the epidemic and the many different levels at which the law can operate, it follows that there are certain questions that should underpin any formulation of legal policy in the context:

— What will be the impact of the policy, both on infected people and others? Have the interests of all people affected by the policy been appropriately weighed and reconciled to the greatest extent possible?
— Does the policy accord with the requirements of appropriate ethical principles, international law and the Global Strategy on AIDS?
— Has consideration been given to both the direct and the indirect consequences of the proposed legal measure? Is there a risk that the indirect consequences will be counter-productive or obstruct other HIV/ AIDS policy objectives?
— Can the policy objective best be achieved by legal or non-legal means (e.g., by non-binding policy or by encouraging voluntary cooperation)?
— What is the main thrust of the proposed intervention? Does it aim, for example, to punish or proscribe certain forms of behaviour or to protect individuals against abuses of their rights?
— Does the proposed intervention take account of the context within which HIV is spread and the social, economic, cultural and religious factors which may lead individuals to be exposed to the virus? Does it cut across prevailing culture and values? If so, will this impede or enhance its effectiveness?

To ensure an appropriate legal response to the HIV epidemic in the context of existing law, attitudes and culture and potentially divergent views about what measures are required, there needs to be input from a range of different perspectives. These perspectives include those of policy-makers, people infected with HIV and their advocates, lawyers in private practice, community-based organisations, the business sector and academic lawyers

10

HIV/AIDS-Related Ethical Principles

Ms. Susan Timbarlake
World Health Organisation, Geneva

Ethical Principles that should Guide the International, National, Community and Individual Response to HIV/AIDS

Compassion

Compassion requires that people respond to the suffering of others, including those with HIV/AIDS, with sympathy, mercy and a willingness to help.

Solidarity

Solidarity requires that people come together to respond to the suffering, as well as the injustice, caused by HIV/AIDS.

Responsibility

Responsibility means that every individual, community, institution and nation must act responsibly towards HIV/AIDS to prevent its spread and to care for those infected and otherwise affected.

Tolerance

Tolerance requires respect for the equal worth, dignity and

autonomy of people affected by HIV/AIDS, including those with different beliefs, opinions, and life styles.

Information

All individuals and communities should have available to them the information necessary to make good and necessary decisions about health, including how to avoid infection with HIV/AIDS and how to cope with its consequences.

Empowerment

All people should have the ability to protect themselves from infection by being able to refuse unsafe sex and to cope with HIV/AIDS if they or someone in their family is infected.

Ethical Principles that should Guide Policy Formulation and Implementation in HIV/AIDS Health Pollcy

Well-being/Benef icence

HIV/AIDS policies should be designed for the general good, and the benefits of the proposed policy should be weighted against the harms. There should be no infliction of harm on people, including those living with HIV/AIDS or suspected of it.

Equity/Distributive Justice

The burdens and benefits of HIV/ATDS policy should be distributed equitably among the population. No groups or individuals should be discriminated against in the context of HIV/AIDS. All people and groups should be treated fairly and equally and have equal access to available information, prevention methods and treatment.

Respect for Persons

Individuals have the capacity and the right to make choices and decisions about their bodies, personal integrity, and actions as long as they do not diminish rights of others, and should be free from unjustified interference by others, including in the context of HIV/ AIDS. People of diminished autonomy who are dependent or vulnerable should be protected against discrimination.

Confidentiality

People have a right to keep confidential any information which is highly personal and the divulgence of which could be detrimental for them, including information about their HIV/AIDS status. Professional ethics requires that professionals (lawyers, health care workers, insurance, social workers) maintain strict confidentiality concerning all personal information obtained from clients in the context of their professional work.

Obligation to Treat

Medical ethics requires that health professionals must treat, to the best of their ability, all persons seeking their medical attention without discrimination and without prejudice based on the origin or nature of the patient's illness, including HIV/AIDS.

Informed Consent

Respect for the integrity and autonomy of the individual means that informed consent should be obtained before the administration of medical tests, drugs, treatment or participation in research, including those that are related to HIV/AIDS.

Elements of Informed Consent

The individual must be a competent individual who has the capacity to make decisions. S/he must have received all necessary information, and arrived at a decision without coercion, inducement or intimidation. If s/he does not have capacity to give free consent, s/he should be protected by supplementary measures or authorized representatives.

Information Essential to Informed Consent

Information concerning HIV/AIDS testing, treatment and research should be explained in a language the individual will understand. All benefits/risks/problems/alternatives should be fully explained. No information should be withheld that would cause a reasonable person to refuse. The person should understand that they are free to refuse and/or withdraw at any time without penalty. The degree to which confidentiality can be maintained should also be explained to the person.

General Sources and Further Reading: "Declaration at Dakar", UNDP, 1994; *International Ethical Guidelines for Biomedical Research Involving Human Subjects*, CIOMS, 1993; "The Rights and Humanity Declaration and Charter on HIV/AIDS". Rights and Humanity, 1992.

11

AIDS and Ethics

Prof. Ronald Bayer,
School of Public Health Columbia University, New York, U.S.A.
Prof. Lawrence O.Gostin
Department of Law Georgetown University, U.S.A.

AIDS, the first serious epidemic disease to strike advanced industrial nations in more than a generation, has posed an extraordinary array of ethical challenges. Most of these challenges also confront the less developed nations. Among the issues that have drawn attention are: the duty of the state to prevent the spread of the disease; the obligation of physicians to care for those who are in need; the limits and significance of medical confidentiality; the obligation to seek informed consent before testing and commencing treatment; the functions of counselling infected individuals about their duties to partners and of assisting women who are infected as they are compelled to make reproductive decisions; the clash between the cannons bf research and the cannons of care; the limits of acceptable underwriting by insurance companies; the rights of individuals with costly medical conditions to emigrate; and, finally, the obligations of the advanced industrial nations to less developed nations.

Despite the extraordinary context of the epidemic during the past decade, what is striking about the issues that have been pressed to the fore is that they are not all new. What is new is the intensity of the discussions, the broad participatory nature of the debate, the political forces called into play, the demands they have made, the solutions they have sought to fashion, and the extent to which efforts have been made to shape an international consensus on the ethics of prevention and care. More strikingly, AIDS has provided the occasion for a rethinking of the traditions of public health in the light of human rights concerns.

As a lethal illness spread in the context of the most intimate relationships and as a public health threat, AIDS has forced us to confront questions regarding the appropriate role of the state in limiting morbidity and mortality. In so doing it has required a reconsideration of the ethical limits on state power in the face of a grave social threat. As a disease of the socially vulnerable, HIV infection and AIDS have compelled us to face issues involving the role of the state in protecting the weak in moments of social stress. As a disease that has affected large numbers of poor individuals without adequate health insurance or who live in nations with limited health care systems, AIDS has required us once again to consider what justice demands, in terms of the protection of individuals against the costs associated with illness. Thus the roles of government in advancing the public health, defending the weak, and assuring access to health care have all been called upon by the AIDS epidemic.

In this chapter, three broad topics will be considered: the ethics of prevention and protection; the ethics of research; and the ethics of care. The special issues raised by the ethics of screening are treated in a separate chapter in this publication. The discussion is based upon the experience of the United States and other advanced industrial democracies, but the broad issues have relevance for all nations confronting the AIDS epidemic.

The Ethics of Prevention and Protection

AIDS is a blood-borne, sexually transmitted disease. As such it is transmitted by infected persons to those who are infected during sexual intercourse, homosexual or heterosexual, through needle sharing by drug users and by pregnant women to their foetuses. Early on in the epidemic, infection was also transmitted through blood transfusions and to those dependant on clotting factor for haemophilia. That is no longer a problem in advanced industrial nations, although it lingers on as a challenge in less developed nations. Nevertheless, AIDS is pre-eminently a behaviourally transmitted disease. In the absence of a vaccine, transmission of HIV infection can only be interrupted through modifications in behaviour. Those who are infected must wear condoms during sexual intercourse. Those who are uninfected must do so to protect themselves against the risk of infection. Intravenous drug users must not share needles. The risk of paediatric AIDS can be eliminated completely only if infected women do not bear children (although the risk can be radically reduced through the use of AZT during pregnancy and delivery).

It is these biological facts that provide the foundations for public health strategies designed to prevent AIDS. It is these facts that raise profound questions about the moral responsibilities of those with HIV infection to behave in ways that limit the prospect of spreading a lethal disease; and of the state to shape policies that will facilitate the radical modification of sexual and drug using behaviour.

Before turning to these issues it is necessary to note a matter of overarching importance in a discussion of the ethical issues posed by a pandemic like AIDS: the extent to which the ethical norms that should inform AIDS policies can be considered transnational; the extent to which such norms are so culture-specific that they can only be used to judge policies and practices within given societies. While we cannot engage with the broader theoretical issues implicated in this matter (universalism versus relativism) in the context of this chapter, it is important to recognize some of the most fundamental questions posed by AIDS prevention efforts: should cultural views that subjugate women and restrain their freedoms to protect themselves in sexual relationships be tolerated in the name of cultural differences? Should cultural conservatism about homosexuality, drug use, commercial sex work, or sex education affect AIDS prevention programmes such as needle exchahge, explicit sex education, or condom availability? Should Western liberal views about the pre-eminence of individual liberty and autonomy govern public health policies on testing and confidentiality?

These questions take on special significance in light of the fact that a central tenet of efforts to encourage the adoption of behaviours that will limit the spread of HIV infection is that they be culturally sensitive.[1] Two arguments are typically made on behalf of the centrality of cultural sensitivity. The first is pragmatic and instrumental; the second is ethical. The pragmatic-instrumental claim asserts that AIDS prevention efforts that are not culturally sensitive will be ineffective. They will fail because they will not reach their intended audience, will not be understood by those who are reached, and will not be accepted by those who understand. They may, indeed, provoke outright opposition.

A second claim on behalf of cultural sensitivity, less often made explicitly but nevertheless of central importance, is ethical. The basic principle of ethics that individuals should be treated with respect and that their dignity should not be violated is by extension applied to cultures. Cultural sensitivity is thus required of us by the ethics of pluralism. A failure to respect the cultural integrity of others is almost characterized as an imposition of the values of the dominant and powerful on the subordinate and marginal. The insistence on cultural sensitivity is premised on an egalitarian ethos, on the ethos that should inspire public policy in a multicultural democratic society. Both arguments have great merit. Yet the claims on behalf of cultural sensitivity may, in fact, be overstated. The demands of AIDS prevention may necessitate a confrontation with cultural norms that sustain patterns of behaviour which foster the spread of HIV.

Among the bitterly fought issues raised in the context of AIDS prevention has been the question of whether education should stress the moral responsibilities of those who are infected or the importance of self-protection for the uninfected. Of greater moment in the developed nations has been the political controversy provoked by the centrality of educating gay men and drug users about how they should modify their behaviours to protect themselves and others. Social conservatives opposed to homosexuality and all extramarital sex have objected to the "legitimization" of what they take to be immoral behaviour in the name of public health. Indeed, efforts have been made to impose restrictions on the language and content of messages designed to inform and shape AIDSrelated behaviours. Similarly, those who view drug use as morally reprehensible have opposed educational efforts designed to instruct intravenous drug users about how they might continue to use drugs without placing themselves at risk of a lethal infection. They have opposed the distribution of sterile injection equipment through needle exchange programmes and the lifting of restrictions on the sale of injection equipment to drug users.

Such opposition, in the name of morality, has paradoxically imposed limits on the state's first ethical responsibility in the context of the AIDS epidemic: to protect the vulnerable. It is no accident that those who bore the burden of that failure were already socially vulnerable.

In developing nations the epidemiological pattern of HIV is very different from that which prevails in western Europe and North America. Heterosexual behaviour is the dominant mode of HIV transmission. The central ethical challenges posed by this fact are the importance of broad condom education for men and women and the provision of condoms at prices that are affordable. Candour in sexual education has often met with conservative resistance, paralleling in a way the experience in economically advanced nations. As important, the pattern of HIV transmission compels a confrontation with the subordinate status of women which denies them the capacity to control their own sexual lives. Here we have underscored the most troubling dimensions: as long as women are subordinate, they will not be able to protect themselves against HIV; but to end that subordination will require far-reaching social changes. Whether such changes can occur at a pace that is compatible with the threat by HIV remains an open question.

Historically, as nations confronted the challenge of the epidemic disease, they tended to rely on policies that were marked by an authoritarian perspective. Indeed, traditional public health practice in Europe and North America centred on mandatory case finding, reporting the cases to public health registries, contact tracing, compulsory treatment, and at times quarantine and isolation. Both the nature of the infections threats with which public health officials had to deal and prevailing conceptions of the appropriate relationship between the individual and the state dictated the shape of public health practice. AIDS has provided the occasion for a challenge to the traditional approach to public health practice.

In the United States as well as in the other nations bound by the liberal tradition, ethical considerations, pragmatic concerns, and extraordinary efforts on the part of AIDS service organizations have contributed to the adoption of public health strategies to control the spread of HIV infection that may be broadly defined as voluntaristic—stressing mass education, counselling, and respect for privacy.[2] Indeed, both in the United States and elsewhere what might be termed "HIV exceptionalism" has dominated public health policy.[3] A focus on voluntarism has also informed the policies put forth by the Global Programme on AIDS of the World Health Organization. That in turn has helped to shape policies in nations around the world. This general consensus has affected policies on discrimination, the protection of confidentiality, and the use of the coercive powers of the state to restrict those whose behaviours are thought to pose a risk of HIV transmission.

Discrimination and Public Health

Because AIDS represented the first major infectious threat with which advanced industrial societies had to contend in almost a generation, and because the causative agent was not identified until three years after the first case report, it is not surprising that it provoked considerable social anxiety. How was it spread? Who posed a risk? Who was endangered? That AIDS was a disease of socially marginal, and not infrequently despised, individuals only intensified the urge toward discrimination. Employers, landlords, school personnel, and even the staff of some health-care institutions evidenced a willingness to exclude those with the new disease. With the discovery of HIV, and the development of a test that could detect antibodies to the virus, the potential scope for discriminatory activity increased, despite the epidemiological evidence about how infection was spread.

In the United States, the Centers for Disease Control moved swiftly to contain the irrational impulse toward exclusion. (Those efforts were mirrored by the Global Programme on AIDS). At the end of 1985, guidelines to prevent the spread of HIV infection in schools[4] and the workplace[5] were issued. Early in 1986, detailed guidelines for health care workers on preventing the spread of infection while engaged in invasive procedures were published.[6] In each instance, the goal was to convey the information, to provide protection, and to prevent panic. The message was clear: HIV could not be casually transmitted, and so there were no public health grounds for exclusion of infected individuals who otherwise were capable of performing their expected functions. There were thus no grounds for mandatory testing for HIV. In the context of the health-care setting, universal blood and body fluid precautions would protect workers not only from HIV, but also from the far more infectious hepatitis B. In the absence of any significant risk, there was no possible ethical foundation for discrimination against persons with HIV. Indeed, the absence of demonstrable risk and the irrational nature of discriminatory practices imposed on the government a positive ethical duty founded on the principle of justice to protect those at risk from discriminatory actions.

The situation in health care has not been so clear-cut. The 'unresolved question of the appropriate response to HIV-infected clinicians has continued to fester, even in actions that have by and large sought to protect the rights of people with HIV. Debate on this matter has been driven by the single, still unexplained case of a Florida dentist to whom the only cases of HIV infection in patients linked to a clinician have been traced.

Some have argued that although professionals have a moral duty to assume some risks - especially those that are quite small—

in caring for their patients, patients do not have an equivalent duty to expose themselves to even small risks when being cared for.[7,8,9] Dismissing as irrational those who would deny all infected health-care workers, whatever their functions, the right to engage in clinical work, many have asserted that physicians whose invasive work can place their patients at some risk ought not to engage in those procedures. But the logic of this perspective leads to troubling conclusions. If those who know themselves to be infected with HIV have professional duties not to place their patients at (remote) risk, are there correlative institutional obligations to identify the infected, to exclude them from certain functions? Are they obligated to screen health-care workers, and if so, at what frequency? Might concern about protecting patients provide the basis for mandatory screening and surveillance after so much effort to forestall such programmes? And if screening were to be adopted, what would be the impact on an anxious social climate?

In thinking about these issues it would be useful to underscore the apparent tension between the ethics of informed consent and the ethics of protecting the vulnerable from discrimination. The ethics of informed consent has increasingly been shaped by a commitment to the view that patients should be able to determine, for themselves, the level of risk that is acceptable in the context of medical practice. Such a view rejects the "objective" standard of the reasonable person or the physician in determining which risks should be revealed to a patient for his or her consideration. The ethics of anti-discrimination practice and policy is profoundly different. It rejects subjectivity; views it as the fount of irrationality. From that perspective, personal views about risk cannot override the rights of those with particular disabilities to work. A refusal, for example, to hire a person with limited hearing loss because of a belief that such an individual would represent some remote theoretical risk would never be countenanced under prevailing conceptions of the rights of those with disabilities. Thus the understanding of the problem posed by the HIV-infected surgeon or dentist will very much depend on whether it is defined essentially as one that implicates the ethics of informed consent of the ethics of disability rights.

Confidentiality and its Limits

There is perhaps no ethical issue involving AIDS that has received more attention than that of confidentiality. That gay men and those who have spoken on their behalf have placed such great stress on confidentiality should come as no surprise. A history of oppression and the existence of anti-sodomy laws have made the protection of privacy a critical feature of the struggle for social survival. But the call for the protection of confidentiality has come as well from those vested with the responsibility for public health, including the World Health Organization,[10] the Council of Europe,[11] and the US Centers for Disease Control and Prevention.[12] For them the protection of confidentiality was critical to the strategy to encourage mass behavioural change and to the goal of encouraging people to come for testing and counselling.

The legal safeguards that nations have adopted, reflecting a variety of ethical considerations, however, are highly variable. An international survey of AIDS legislation undertaken for the World Health Organization in 1991 found that 33 countries had specific confidentiality provisions relating to HIV/ AIDS. Indeed, countries may have quite different cultural conceptions of privacy.[13] In the North and West, privacy is defined as the right of an *individual* to limit access by others to some aspect of the person. Accordingly, the contemporary cultural expectation, reflecting important changes over the past several decades, is that medical information about the person is kept confidential and cannot be disclosed even to family members without the person's permission. In parts of Africa and the Far East, however, privacy is not understood in the same way. In many societies, matters of disease and death are seldom individual concerns but affairs of the family or even the entire community. In many traditional societies, too, issues of health and medicine—even death itself—become public. Thus, confidentiality—as a one-to-one exchange between clinician and patient—rarely exists. Here, in a stark way, the tension between cultural particularism and the claims of ethical universalism are made clear.

But even in the developed nations of the northern and western hemispheres, the principle of confidentiality has required modification in light of pressing public health necessities. The principle of confidentiality is never absolute and has always been subject to limits.[13] In many nations, a central responsibility of public health officials has been to record the names in special registries of those with certain diseases. In part, such reporting has been deemed necessary for purposes of epidemiological surveillance. On other occasions, reporting has been thought of as crucial to adequate follow-up to ensure that individuals with communicable conditions are appropriately treated. Finally, such reporting has been central to contract tracing.

Each of these public health functions has been used as a justification for requiring the reporting of the names of individuals with AIDS and HIV infection. Given the threat posed by the epidemic such nominal reporting of AIDS cases has, in general, not been subject to ethical challenge. In some nations, however, efforts have been made to achieve goals of reporting without the use of names, thus revealing the extraordinary sensitivity of confidentiality in the AIDS epidemic. More common has been the controversy over the reporting of people with HIV, without the manifestations of AIDS. In some nations, only the latter is reportable.

Where reporting by name does occur, the ethics of confidentiality dictate that the identity of those with AIDS be shielded from unwarranted disclosure. The reporting of names is justified on public grounds alone, and thus no disclosure to those who may have other reasons to want to know the identity of individuals with AIDS or HIV is ethically justifiable. Those who are responsible for public health registries have a special obligation to protect the integrity of the lists created by reporting requirements.

But what of the role of confidentiality in the clinical setting? What are the moral responsibilities of a physician when an HIV-infected patient refuses to inform identifiable, unsuspecting past or current partners about the dangers of infection. In the United States a central legal doctrine emerged out of the widely discussed *Tarasoff*[15] case, which held that under certain circumstances a clinician has an affirmative duty to warn or protect unsuspecting targets of his patient's violent intentions. That case need not detain us here. What is crucial is the underlying ethical principle that confidentiality, while critical, is not the only ethical value. Indeed when vulnerable unsuspecting persons are placed at risk it may be imperative to breach confidentiality.

In the context of HIV, concern has centered on two very different situations: the possibility that an individual unknowingly infected by a past partner might act as unwitting agent of transmission to yet others or might lose the opportunity to commence early therapeutic intervention; in the case of an individual who has not disclosed his or her infected status to a current partner, the focus has been on the possibility of preventing the transmission of HIV. As these issues were considered, it became clear that the process of warning past sexual partners did not require the identification of the source of potential infection. No public health goal would be served by breaching the cloak of anonymity of the index case. Where an infected individual refused to warn a current partner, the situation posed graver difficulties. It was not possible to provide any effective protective warning without identifying the source of risk.

Informing the dispute about how it might be best to proceed has been a deep concern about the consequences that couid well follow were it to be widely believed that physicians would routinely breach confidentiality when presented with a patient who refused to warn past or current partners about the risk of HIV infection. Would the consequence be a reduction in clinical candour? Would patients be discouraged from seeking to know their HIV status? Would they be less accessible to the efforts of clinicians to convince them of the importance of warning those who might be at risk? In sum, would breaching confidentiality to warn unsuspecting individuals result in a net loss from the perspective of public health?

Beginning in the latter part of 1987, a number of efforts were made in the United States to resolve the issues associated with the warning of unsuspecting third parties. At the end of 1987, the American Medical Association issued a broad set of statements on the ethical issues posed by the AIDS epidemic.[16] In that document the AMA addressed the issue of warning in a forthright manner. Physicians were to try to convince patients of their obligation to warn the unsuspecting. If they failed in that task, they were to seek the intervention of public health officials. Only if public health officials refused or were unwilling to take on the responsibility of warning was it the obligation of the physician to act directly.

When the Presidential Commission on the HIV Epidemic addressed this issue in mid-1988, it too endorsed the notion that physicians should have the right to breach confidentiality in order to warn the unsuspecting, despite the centrality of confidentiality to its overall strategy.[17] Reflecting, however, a commitment to professional autonomy, the Commission held that the decision about whether to breach confidentiality was to remain with the physician and was not to be imposed as a matter of law. That too was the stance of a wide spectrum of public health officials, including the Association of State and Territorial Health Officials,[18] who chose to speak of a "privilege to disclose" rather than a duty to warn. The lingering ethical question is whether such a strategy meets the moral challenge clinicians face when confronted with patients who may threaten the lives of their partners. This issue has been the source of enduring controversy in nations such as Denmark,[19] Sweden[20] and The Netherlands.[21]

Coercive Controls

The question of how to respond to individuals whose behaviour represents a threat to unknowing partners has inevitably provoked discussion of the public health tradition of imposing restrictions on liberty in the name of communal welfare. The spectre of mass quarantine has haunted all such discussion. Only Cuba has sought to quarantine all individuals with HIV-infection.[22] In other nations the focus has been on the more limited case of individuals whose behaviours have placed others at risk of HIV. Even such limited efforts have provoked concern because of fears that they would lead to egregious intrusions upon privacy and insidiously impose deprivations of freedom.

In the United States, fierce opposition has surfaced to all efforts to bring AIDS within the scope of state quarantine statutes. Nevertheless, more than a dozen states had done so between 1987 and 1990, typically using the occasion to modernize their disease control laws to reflect contemporary constitutional standards which detail procedural guarantees, and to require that restrictions on freedom represent the "least restrictive alternative" available to achieve a "compelling state interest."

Despite the intensity of the debate that has surrounded this issue, the only empirical study of the use of power of isolation in the United States has found that state health departments have almost never exercised the authority granted by statute.[23] During 1981-90 only 10 cases were documented, and in virtually every case the duration of confinement has been very brief. Far more common has been the use of public health authority to warn individuals that their behaviour posed a risk. Such warnings have often been accompanied by "cease and desist orders." Public health efforts to isolate the small numbers of individuals deemed to pose a behavioural threat to "an unsuspecting partner" have occurred in other countries, typically focusing on prostitutes. Sweden provides a number of such cases.

The enactment of statutes criminalizing behaviours linked to the spread of AIDS or the application of general criminal law to such cases has paralleled the political receptivity to laws extending the authority of public health officials to control individuals whose behaviour posed a risk of HIV transmission.[24]

What are the ethical foundations of such statutes? Criminal law serves to express a society's profound abhorrence of certain behaviours. In so doing, the law threatens to punish individuals who violate certain social norms. It may also serve as a deterrent. Some acts are universally the subject of criminal law. Murder, for example. Other acts are crimes only in certain societies. The enactment of criminal statutes that prohibit the wilful and knowing infection with HIV of an unsuspecting sexual partner would clearly fall within the morally acceptable use of criminal law. But the enactment of such statutes has often served ends that raise profound ethical questions. To seek to punish acts that cannot possibly result in the spread of AIDS—spitting, for example—serves only to underscore the penchant for repressive measures in the face of complex social problems.[25]

Whatever the allure of such measures and of the rediscovery of traditional public health approaches in the effort to combat the spread of HIV infection, it remains clear that the future course of the AIDS epidemic will be determined by the creation of a social and institutional milieu within which radical voluntary changes in behaviour can occur and be sustained. Educational campaigns and counselling programmes most effectively undertaken by groups linked to the populations at risk, not repressive measures, remain the centre-piece of that preventive effort.

The Ethics of Research

The HIV epidemic has provided the circumstances for the emergence of a broad and potent political movement that has sought to reshape radically the conditions under which research is undertaken in the United States. The implications for research in other nations with important pharmaceutical efforts are clear. The role of the randomized clinical trial, the importance of placebo controls, the centrality of academic research institutions, the dominance of scientists over subjects, the sharp distinction between research and therapy, and the protectionist ethos that has informed research ethics since the end of the World War II have all been brought into question.

Although scholars concerned with the methodological demands of sound research and ethicists committed to the protection of research subjects have played a crucial role in the ensuing discussions, both as defenders of received wisdom and as critics, the debate has been driven by the articulate demands of those most threatened by AIDS. Most prominent have been groups such as the People With AIDS Coalition and ACT-UP, organizations made up primarily of white, gay men. But advocates of women's, children's and prisoners' rights have also made their voices heard. What has been so stunning and disconcerting to some, and exciting to others, has been the rhythm of challenge and response. Rather than the careful exchange of academic arguments, we have been witness to the mobilization of disruptive and effective political protest.

The threat of death has hovered over the process. "The shortage of proven therapeutic alternatives for AIDS and the belief that trials are, in and themselves, beneficial have led to the claim that people have a right to be research subjects. This is the exact opposite of the tradition starting with Nuremberg-that people have the right *not* to be research subjects.[26] It is this striking reversal that has resulted in a rejection of the model of research conducted at remote academic centres, with restrictive (protective) standards of access, and strict adherence to the "gold standard" of the randomized clinical trial. Blurring the distinction between research and treatment—"A Drug Trial is Health Care Too"—those insistent upon radical reform have sought to open wide the points of entry to new "therapeutic" agents both within and outside of clinical trials; have demanded that the paternalistic ethical warrant for the protection of the vulnerable from research be replaced by an ethical regime informed by respect for the autonomous choice of potential subjects who could weigh, for themselves, the potential risks and benefits of new experimental treatments for HIV infection. Thus demands have been made that women be enrolled in trials in greater numbers; that prisoners and drug users be granted access; that children be included in trials at a much earlier point than had been considered acceptable. Moreover, the revisionists have demanded a basic reconceptualization of the relationship between researchers and subjects. In place of protocols imposed from above, they have proposed a more egalitarian and democratic model in which negotiation would replace scientific authority.[27]

The reformulation of the ethics of research that has begun under the impact of AIDS has implications that go far beyond the epidemic of HIV disease since the emerging new conceptions and standards could govern the conduct of the entire research enterprise. Protagonists, who have been locked in often acrimonious debate, foretell very different consequences of the changing social standards of research. Proponents of the new ethos hold out the prospect of a revised regime that is both respectful of individual rights and the requirements of good science. Critics, on the other hand, have warned that the blurring of the distinction between research and treatment can only harm the desperate. "It is not compassionate to hold out false hope to terminally ill patients so that they spend their last dollars on unproven 'remedies' that they might live longer."[28]

A different set of issues is raised by the question of research in less developed countries, particularly international collaborative research initiated by investigators in the advanced industrial nations. A body of scholarship has evolved in relation to the ethics of international collaborative research. The Council of International Organizations of Medical Sciences has issued ethical guidelines for both biomedical and epidemiological research that are highly influential. These guidelines require ethical review of research proposals both in the country of origin and in the host country. They require consent of the research subject, a favourable benefit-to-burden ratio, confidentiality, and compensation for subjects who are harmed within the research.

Perhaps the most important and controversial issue in international collaborative research is the need to build infrastructure in the host country and to make the fruits of the research available to people in that community or similarly situated populations. The central ethical question is: to what extent does the principle of distributive justice require that therapeutic interventions developed in the course of such research be made available to subjects in their communities?

The issue is especially relevant to the conduct of vaccine trials. For epidemiological reasons, it has been argued that countries in Asia and Africa represent ideal settings for investigation into possible preventive vaccines. Large numbers of infected persons, and the tragically high incidence of infection, make nations in Asia and Africa ideal for the determination of vaccine efficacy. But no vaccine trial would be ethical—assuming that issues of consent could be resolved—if there was no assurance that a successful vaccine would be provided by international agreement, despite the potential cost. Such agreements must precede the conduct of vaccine trials.

The Ethics of Care

For almost four decades, health care workers in America, as well as in other advanced industrial societies, were largely shielded from what had been the routine experience of those who had in prior eras worked with the sick—the acquisition of their patients' infections and sometimes lethal diseases. Though never as total as many had come to believe, this invincibility was psychologically ruptured by the intrusion of AIDS, beginning in 1981. AIDS forced physicians and health care workers to consider the possibility that theirs was indeed a "dangerous trade."[29]

Early in the history of this epidemic, anecdotal reports began to surface about hospital aides leaving food trays at the doors of those who were sick, and of nurses, physicians, and dentists refusing to treat patients with the new disease. As noted earlier in this chapter, the Centers for Disease Control confronted such behaviour by publishing in late 1985 and 1986 a series of reports in *Morbidity and Mortality Weekly Report* that sought to provide guidance for sound infection control practice and rational social policy.

Confronted with the challenge represented by the threat of patient abandonment, those committed to stanching the emerging trend turned to history[30] in the hope that an unambiguous lesson on responsibility of physicians would emerge. Physicians had, after all, been called to respond when epidemics were more common, when morbidity was awesome. For those who had hoped to discover a univocal message from the chronicles of the past, the turn of history proved a disappointment. Although some physicians had stayed behind to care for their patients, many had fled. At times they did so in order that they might attend to their fleeing patrons, sometimes simply to protect themselves. Perhaps most significant as a reflection of the extent to which many physicians refused to remain with those afflicted in earlier plagues was the need to make arrangements for the care of the sick through the special institution of the "plague doctor". Employed by local merchants and the political elites, these physicians took up where others had failed.[31]

If history provided no clear guidance, what of the codes of ethics that have expressed the aspirations of the guilds and associations of medical practitioners? Remarkably, such codes had been silent on the duty of physicians to treat in the time of epidemics. In the United States, the AMA code of 1847 was unique in its forthright assertion of such a responsibility. "And when pestilence prevails, it is their duty to face the danger and to continue their labours for the alleviation of suffering, even at the jeopardy of their own lives." This provision remained in the code until 1957, when a revised and shortened statement eliminated the stipulation that must certainly have seemed an anachronism. After all, the era of epidemics had come to an end in the advanced industrial world.

But remaining in the code was a provision—first incorporated into the AMA's statement of professional responsibility of 1912—which in the absence of a strong assertion of a duty to care was to be a source of great confusion when AIDS confronted American medicine. "A physician shall, in the provision of appropriate patient care, except in emergencies, be free to choose whom to serve."

Amending the blunt articulation of an unencumbered professional freedom, the AMA's Judicial Council has ruled that refusals to treat on the basis of race, religion, or creed were unethical. In November 1987, in the seventh year of the AIDS epidemic, the Council ruled that "A physician may not ethically refuse to treat a patient whose condition is within the physician's current realm of competence solely because the patient is seropositive." In so doing, the AMA joined the American Nurses Association, which had a year earlier denounced discrimination against patients with AIDS.

Some philosophers attempting to struggle with this issue, stressed the importance of a *social* responsibility to guarantee each HIV-infected individual access to health care; the responsibility of the health care *professions* as collective entities to provide appropriate care to those in need, rather than the responsibility of each individual health care worker to treat. In short, some argued, if somewhat reluctantly, that as along as the needs of the HIV infected were met, there might be no sound ethical grounds for insisting that each health care worker share in the responsibility.

Others have argued for a more universal obligation. Thus did physician-philosopher Edmund Pellegrino state, "to refuse to care for AIDS patients, even if the danger were greater than it is, is to abnegate what is essential to being a physician."[32]

For many who have stressed a universal obligation to treat, it is clear that the relatively low risk of infection has been central. Were the risks of HIV transmission very much greater, it would have required an ethics of heroism to insist that each health care worker bear the responsibility of assuring adequate and appropriate health care to the infected. Given the level of risk entailed in the face of HIV infection, even among surgeons and obstetricians, those who stress the obligation to treat argue that it was not heroism but more straightforward duty that is involved.

The issue-of access to care is not, however, primarily raised by the spectre of physician abandonment. Rather, it centres on the problem of access to care on the part of the poor.

In the United States, which unlike other economically advanced nations does not guarantee access to care on the part of its citizens, the striking contrast between important clinical advances in the care of those with HIV infection and the social organization of American medicine led the National Commission on Acquired Immune Deficiency Syndrome to warn, in a December 1989 report to the President,[33] that medical breakthroughs would "mean little unless the health care system can incorporate them and make them accessible to people in need." The existence of a medically disenfranchised class meant that for many, access to care was almost solely through the "emergency room door of one of the few hospitals in the country that treats people with HIV infection and AIDS."

The issue of how to assure access to care and, more importantly, the question of what level of care to provide in nations that are poor and that can provide only rudimentary health care services poses very difficult ethical questions. No simple answers are possible in situations where so many pressing health care needs go unmet. A basic ethical principle would require that those with HIV disease not be discriminated against because of that fact; that they receive no less than other gravely ill persons. Ultimately, the choices made within conditions of severe constraints make clear how the resolution of pressing human needs in the less developed nations will require support and assistance from economically advanced nations.

AIDS and the World

AIDS links, in a grim way, the most advanced technological societies, like the United States, with the poorest nations of Africa, Asia and Latin America. The vast proportion of HIV infection in the world exists outside North America and western Europe. In the next decade the already stark contrast will become even sharper. In the face of the social catastrophe now making itself felt, it will be critical to confront the question of what the rich nations of the world owe the poor as the latter confront the issues of prevention and treatment. The social, economic and political realities of general assistance to the Third World cannot be ignored as we confront the AIDS pandemic. The basic fact is that advanced industrial world does very little to meet the needs of the Third World, in terms of food, health care or other basic goods.

It is all too easy to imagine development of expensive therapeutic agents that will be reserved for those who fall ill as a result of HIV infection in the advanced industrial societies but which will not be available to those similarly placed in Third World nations. The use of AZT during pregnancy poses a paradigm challenge.[34] Here is a therapy that could radically reduce HIV transmission. It is in the less developed world that paediatric AIDS poses so significant a problem, yet the cost of AZT places it out of reach to those in need. As noted above, if and when a vaccine were to be developed, will it be made available to those most in need? And who would pay the cost of production and distribution for those nations too poor to bear the cost?

AIDS, because of its dramatic features, underscores the limitations of our capacity to conceive of and act upon notions of shared responsibility across national boundaries. At stake, of course, is the question of justice and the global distribution of resources.

CONCLUSIONS

To recognize the extent to which efforts to control AIDS will call forth sharp ethical and social controversies is not, however, the end of the analysis. It is, in fact, just the beginning. Which values—with what impact on the lives of men, women and children, with what implications for democratic social life, with what likely consequences for the further spread of HIV infection—should guide us? This is the critical ethical question raised by the epidemic.

NOTE

[Ed.: The text of a 'Statement on HIV Infection and AIDS—The Ethical Considerations' issued by the General Medical Council of the United Kingdom in May 1993 is reproduced as Annexure E.]

REFERENCES

1. Bayer R. AIDS prevention and cultural sensitivity: are they compatible? *American Journal of Public Health* 1994; 84:6.
2. Bayer R. *Private Acts, Social Consequences: AIDS and the Politics of Public Health.* 2nd ed. New Brunswick, NJ: Rutgers University Press, 1991.
3. Bayer R. Public health policy and the AIDS epidemic: an end to HIV exceptionalism. *New England Journal of Medicine* 1991; 324: 1500-4.
4. Centers for Disease Control. Education and foster care for children infected with human T-lymphotropic virus type III/lymphadenopathy-associated virus. *Morbidity and Mortality Weekly Report* 1985; 34:517-21.
5. Centers for Disease Control. Recommendation for preventing transmission of infection with human T-lymphotropic virus type III/lymphadenopathy-associated *virus* in the workplace *Morbidity and Mortality Weekly Report* 1985; 34:681-6, 691-5.
6. Centers for Disease Control. Recommendation for preventing transmission of infection with human T-lymphotropic *virus* type III/lymphadenopathy-associated virus during invasive procedures. *Morbidity and Mortality Weekly Report* 1986; 35:221 -3.
7. Gostin L. HIV-infected physicians and the practice of seriously invasive procedures. *Hastings Center Report* 1989;19:32-39
8. Daniels N. HIV-infected health care professionals: public threat or public sacrifice? *Milbank Quarterly* 1992;3:42.
9. Glantz *et al.* Risky Business: setting public health policy for HIV infected health care professionals. *Milbank Quarterly* 1992;43:80.

10. World Health Organization. International Consultation on AIDS and Human Rights (Geneva, 26-28 July, 1989, UN Doc. HR/ AIDS/1989/3.
11. Council of Europe. Committee of Ministers Recommendation No.R(89) 14. On Ethical Issues of HIV Infection in Health Care and Social Settings (Adopted by the Committee of Ministers on 24 October 1989).
12. Centers for Disease Control. Recommended Additional Guidelines for HIV Antibody Counseling and Testing in the Prevention of HIV Infection and AIDS (30 April 1989). Mimeo.
13. Gostin, LO. Informed consent, cultural sensitivity, and respect for persons. *Journal of the American Medical Association* 1995;274:844-5.
14. Dickens BM. Legal limits of AIDS confidentiality. *Journal of the American Medical Association* 1988;259:3449-3451.
15. *Tarasoff V Regents of the State of California.* 17 Cal. 3d 425, 551p. 2d 334, 131 *Cal.Rptr.* 14 (Cal) 1976.
16. American Medical Association. Prevention and control of acquired immunodeficiency syndrome. *Journal of the American Medical Association* 1987;258:2097-103.
17. Report of the Presidential Commission on the Human Immunodeficiency Virus Epidemic 1988. Washington, DC.
18. Association of the State and the Territorial Health Officials. *Guide to Public Health Practice: HIV Partner Notification Strategies.* Washington DC: Public Health Foundation 1988.
19. Albaek E. Denmark: AIDS and the political 'pink triangle'. In: Kirp D and Bayer R, ed. *AIDS in the Industrialized Democracies: Passions, Politics and Policies.* New Brunswick, NJ:Rutgers University Press, 1992:381.
20. Henrikkson B and Ytterberg H. Sweden: the power of the moral(istic) left. In: Kirp and Bayer, eds. *AIDS in the Industrialized Democracies: Passions, Politics and Policies.* New Brunswick NJ:Rutgers University Press, 1992:317-38.
21. Van Wijngaarden J. The Netherlands: AIDS in consensual society. In: Kirp and Bayer R, eds. *AIDS in the Industrialized Democracies: Passions, Politics and Policies.* New Brunswick, NJ:Rutgers University Press, 1992:252-80.
22. Bayer R and Healton C. Controlling AIDS in Cuba. *New England Journal of Medicine* 1989;320:1022-24.
23. Bayer R and Fairchild—Carrino A. AIDS and the limits of control: public health orders, quarantine, and recalcitrant behaviour. *American Journal of Public Health* 1993;83:1471 6.
24. Gostin LO. The AIDS litigation project: a national review of court and Human Rights Commission decisions, part I: the social impact of AIDS. *Journal of the Americal Medical Association* 1990;263:1963.
25. Field MA and Sullivan, KM. AIDS and the criminal law. *Law Medicine and Health Care* 1987;15:(1-2):46-60.
26. Levine C. Has AIDS changed the ethics of human subjects research? *Law, medicine and Health Care* 1988;16:167-73.
27. Dubler N, Levine C and Levine R. Building a new consensus: ethical prineiples and policies for clinical research on HIC/AIDS. *IRB* 1991:13:1-17.
28. Annas G. Faith (healing), hope and charity at the FDA: the politics of AIDS drug trials. *Vdlanova Lauo Review* 1989;34:77197.
29. Arras J. The fragile web of professional responsibility: AIDS and the duty to treat. *Hastings Center Report* 1988. Special Supplement, April-May.
30. Zuger A and Miles SH. Physicians, AIDS and occupational risk: historic traditions and ethical obligations. *Journal of the American Medical Association* 1987;258;1924-8.

31. Fox D. The politics of physicians' responsibility in epidemics: a note on history, *Hastings Center Report* 1988. Special Supplement, April-May.
32. Pellegrino E. Altruism, self-interest and medical ethics. *Journal of the American Medical Association* 1987;258;1939-40.
33. National Commission on AIDS. Report. 1 November 1989.
34. Bayer R. Ethical challenges posed by Zidovudine treatment to reduce vertical transmission of HIV (editorial. *New England Journal of Medicine* 1994; 331:1223-5.

12

HIV Screening: The Ethical Issues

Prof. Ronald Bayer
School of Public Health
Colombia University New York, U.S.A.
Prof. Larry O.Gostin
Department of Public Health
The John Hopkins University U.S.A.

INTRODUCTION

From the outset the test developed to detect antibody to the AIDS virus—and first used on a broad scale in blood banking—was mired in controversy.[1] Uncertainty about the significance of the test's findings and about its quality and accuracy provided the technical substrate of disputes that inevitably took on a political and ethical character, since issues of privacy, communal health, social and economic discrimination, coercion and liberty were always involved. How would the test be used outside the context of blood banking? Would groups at increased risk for AIDS be encouraged to take the test? How forceful would such encouragement be? How would those who agreed to be tested be counselled about the test's significance for themselves and others? Would and could the results be kept confidential? Would voluntary testing be a prelude to compulsory screening? What would be the consequence of testing for the right to work? To go to school? To obtain insurance? To bear children? To remain free? Each of these questions would force a confrontation over the fundamental matter of the relationship between the defence of privacy and the protection of the public health; over the roles of voluntarism and coercion in the social response to the threat of AIDS.

Out of the controversies that whirled about the antibody test there emerged a broad voluntarist consensus. Except for clearly circumscribed circumstances, testing was to be done under conditions of voluntary, informed consent, and the results were to be protected by stringent confidentialiy safeguards. In the United States, to underscore the importance of protecting the privacy of tested individuals the option of anonymity was made broadly available. This consensus was supported by gay leaders,[2] civil libertarians,[3] bioethicists,[4] public health officials[5] and by professional organizations representing clinicians.[6] But as broad as the consensus was, it was also fragile, based as it was on differing interests and commitments.

In this chapter five broad issues will be addressed: screening and behavioural change, screening for clinical purposes, screening for safety, screening in blinded seroprevalence studies, and changing technologies in screening.

Screening and Behavioural Change

Even before the screening of the blood supply had commenced in mid-1985 it was clear that the new antibody test would be enlisted in the effort to achieve the overriding public health goal of mass behavioural change. What was the matter of deep dispute and what has remained a matter of controversy was how much of a role. For public health officials who faced the daunting challenge of affecting the most intimate behaviours and for whom the legacy of other health promotion campaigns gave little reason for optimism, the test seemed a technology that could motivate the desired changes. Those who tested positive could be counselled about the urgency of behavioural changes to the prevention of the spread of HIV. Those who tested negative could be counselled on the importance of self-protection. Opponents of too great a reliance on testing—often representatives of the gay community and of civil liberties groups—were fearful of the social consequences of being identified as infected with HIV. It was mass education and individual counselling they argued, that were crucial. From this perspective testing with all of its technical uncertainties was too costly and too dangerous.

Over the past several years the bitter edge has all but vanished from the dispute. Public health officials have recognized that an extraordinary change has taken place in the behaviour of gay men, for example, a change that could in no way be directly linked to the availability of testing. Representatives of those most at risk have come to recognize that for some mass campaigns of education have been insufficient to motivate behavioural change, that the more direct and targeted efforts associated with test-linked counselling are necessary. What remains a matter of controversy is how aggressively to press for testing among those groups where the degree of behavioural change thus far attained gives cause for concern, even alarm—intravenous drug users and their sexual partners, for example.[7] In many developing countries, where patterns of transmission powerfully affect the heterosexual population, testing of women, particularly sex workers, has resulted in sharp controversy.

Contributing to the always fragile consensus on testing for behavioural change has been a recognition on the part of public health officials of the need to win the confidence of those most at risk for HIV infection. To the fears that the confidentiality of test results would be breached, thus exposing the infected to stigma and discrimination, public health officials have often responded by embracing the cause of confidentiality and legislation to protect the social and economic rights of individuals with HIV infection. What ethics required because of the duty to respect the dignity of each individual, the public health demanded as well. Absent careful assurances of confidentiality and protections against irrational discrimination, it would be impossible to encourage those at risk to come forward for testing.[8,9,10,11]

Screening for Clinical Purposes

Early in the history of the epidemic, when medicine was all but impotent before the opportunistic diseases that afflicted those with HIV infection, the question with which some patients and many of their advocates confronted those who proposed antibody testing was, "Of what benefit will a positive finding be for me?" Furthermore, this was not a test like any other typically employed by clinicians and typically covered by the broad general consent implied in an agreement to be treated.

Rather, it was argued, the antibody test was for social and psychological reasons more like those invasive procedures for which special consent was required. Faced with such challenges, and the undeniable reality of social stigma associated with HIV infection, physicians, their professional associations and public health officials agreed that an exact standard of consent for HIV testing was appropriate: specific informed consent was to be sought from patients or their surrogates. To many clinicians, however, such requirements represented an unacceptable intrusion into the therapeutic relationship, a hurdle designed to impede sound diagnostic work.

The early history of HIV testing in developed countries may still apply in the developing world, where effective treatment is still beyond the reach of much of the population. What purpose, critics may ask, is served by requiring impoverished people to be tested when there is little personal benefit that may accrue?

Now that there have been some remarkable advances in the capacity of medicine to control the life-threatening illnesses faced by HIV-infected individuals in the North and West, given the hopes of physicians and researchers for the prophylactic use of therapeutic agents like Zidovudine may slow the progression of HIV disease, that other medications may prevent pneumocystis pneumonia, and given the range of clinical trials for which the infected may be eligible, the picture for patients is very different from that which had prevailed just a short time ago. Under such circumstances it is possible to answer the question, "Of what benefit will a positive finding be for me?" quite differently than in 1985. It is possible to respond, "Though we are nowhere close to a cure for HIV infection, there are many interventions that may extend your life if we move aggressively." Under such circumstances pressure has begun to mount on the part of clinicians to loosen the requirements for specific informed consent before testing occurs. In short, clinicians have begun to assert that the time has come to return AIDS to the "medical mainstream".

Although it is possible to appreciate the impatience expressed in this perspective, it is important at this juncture to resist the pressure for routine unconsented testing.[12] In the first place, as much as the clinical picture has begun to change, there is no definitive therapeutic course for HIV-infected but otherwise asymptomatic individuals. At the same time the possibility of stigma and of discrimination remains an ever present threat to the social wellbeing of the infected. Given these conditions the arguments for specific informed consent remain as pertinent as they ever were. But even were the clinical picture to improve dramatically the moral grounds for insisting on informed consent before HIV testing would not change. It is an established principle of medical ethics that competent adults have the right to determine whether or not to undergo treatment, whether or not to terminate treatment already begun. Certainly, the principle that limits the paternalistic authority of the physician to order therapies in the interest of the patient extends to the authority to order those tests that would serve as the basis for commencing treatment.

But if respect for the autonomy of the patient requires that physicians exercise restraint, the physician's ethical responsibility to provide appropriate care and the principle of beneficence, now require that physicians routinely offer HIV antibody testing in those circumstances *where therapies are available and accessible to* patients at risk, either geographically or socially. Only by routinely offering such tests can patients be given the opportunity to learn whether or not they are infected. Only then can they exercise their right to choose whether or not to begin therapy or enter available clinical trials. In urging patients to undergo testing physicians must clearly define the risks associated with being identified as infected and the benefits that may be associated with treatment. An attempt to persuade a patient by exaggerating current therapeutic possibilities or the advantages that might follow from participating in clinical trials entails a deception that deprives the individual of the right to make a fully informed decision in the face of a very difficult situation.

More complex still is the question of whether the current situation justifies the routine or mandatory screening of infants born to mothers at increased risk for HIV infection.[13] In more developed countries pediatricians have for some time now asserted that the early identification of infected newborns provides an opportunity to initiate aggressive intervention, including the prophylactic administration of drugs to prevent pneumocystis pneumonia. Others have been more sceptical of what can be done. They have argued that the long-term benefit to infected children of early clinical intervention is by no means clear. What the test does is to identify the existence of an infected mother. Certainly, before such identification is permitted to occur without consent it should be necessary to demonstrate more than a theoretical benefit to the infant.

This debate takes place against a background of widely accepted mandatory or routine testing of newborns to permit the identification of those in need of special treatment. Screening in these instances is held to represent a legitimate exercise of the states power to protect the vulnerable. Screening for PKU is paradigmatic. Early identification is critical so that a special dietary regime can be initiated. The failure to undertake such a therapeutic intervention can be catastrophic for the child. A definitive diagnostic test, a definitive therapeutic intervention, an imperative to act quickly—these are the conditions that provide the empirical and moral grounds for the routine screening of newborns without first seeking parental consent.

None of these conditions prevail in the case of HIV. There is, therefore, no basis for mandatory newborn screening. That the current test is, in fact, a test of the mother makes the argument against unconsented testing all the more compelling. Were a therapy for such infants available the clinical foundation would exist for making a claim on behalf of the vulnerable child. Such a claim might well be sufficient to establish the grounds for testing without prior parental consent.

Despite the enormous attention devoted to the question of newborn testing in the late 1980's and early 1990's, that issue will, in all likelihood, be superseded by pressure to identify HIV-infected pregnant women.[14] That pressure will stem from a remarkable research finding in early 1994 that showed a radical reduction in HIV transmission from infected pregnant women to their foetuses when AZT was administered during pregnancy and delivery and to the newborn for six weeks after birth. In the wake of this finding, obstetricians and pediatricians began to assert that the regime surrounding testing should be liberalized so that all infected women could be identified and offered treatment. Some have called for mandatory testing during pregnancy, using as a model testing for syphilis and hepatitis B.[15] While rejecting mandatory treatment as ethically unacceptable and practically impossible, advocates of mandatory screening have asserted that women who learn of their HIV infection will be more likely to accept voluntary treatment. More common, many physicians have asserted that the stringent requirements of informed consent with pretest counselling should be replaced with a strong recommendation to undergo testing with an informed right of refusal. Such proposals explicitly seek to shift the burden of decision—making to those women who would reject HIV testing.[16] The foundation for such a shift, it is argued, is the benefit for the foetus which might have been infected had its mother not been identified and offered AZT treatment. Here, as in the case of mandatory screening, there is an assumption that while women might be reluctant to undergo testing, they will, once they know they are infected, undertake therapies designed to protect the children they will bear.

Despite such proposals, the posture of the United States Public

Health Service has been steadfastly voluntarist.[17] The result of ongoing consultations among broad constituencies, this rejection of mandatory testing or near-mandatory testing has been premised on the assumption that when fully informed of the benefits of AZT treatment during pregnancy, the vast majority of women at risk will accept voluntary HIV testing. Non-coercive testing would, it is asserted, provide the context of a therapeutic alliance conducive to the commencement of treatment with AZT during pregnancy.

Much will depend on whether the assumptions of the Public Health Service prove correct. If most infected women are identified, and if the rate of vertical HIV transmission declines dramatically, it is less likely that mandatory measures will be adopted. If, however, that does not turn out to be the case, the voluntarist approach will be difficult to sustain.

Screening for Safety

Because AIDS represented the first major infectious disease with which advanced industrial societies had to contend in almost a generation, and because the causative agent was not identified until three years after the first case reports, it is not surprising that it provoked considerable social anxiety. How was it spread? Who posed the risk? Who was endangered? That it was socially marginal and not infrequently despised individuals who appeared to be epidemiologically at increased risk only intensified the urge towards discrimination. Employers, landlords, schools and even some health care institutions evidenced a willingness to exclude those with the new disease. With the discovery of HIV, and the development of a test that could detect antibody to the virus, the potential scope for discriminatory activity increased, despite the epidemiological evidence about how infection was spread.

The World Health Organization,[18] Council of Europe, and international AIDS organizations[19] have long opposed exclusion of persons with HIV infection in the workplace, schools, and other public places. Anti-discrimination provisions have been among the earliest and the most consistent pronouncements of the Global Programme on AIDS.

In the United States, the Centers for Disease Control moved swiftly to contain the irrational impulse towards exclusion. At the end of 1985 guidelines to prevent the spread of HIV infection in schools and the workplace were issued.[20] Early in 1986 detailed guidelines on preventing the spread of infection when health care workers were engaged in invasive procedures were published.[21] In each instance the goal was to convey information, to provide protection, to prevent panic. The message was clear HIV could not be casually transmitted and so there were no grounds for exclusion from school and workplace of infected individuals who were otherwise capable of performing their expected functions. In the context of the health care setting, universal blood and body fluid precautions would protect workers not only from HIV but from the far more infectious hepatitis B. Screening would only provide illusory protections.

Although there are still shameful occurrences of efforts to exclude or isolate school children with AIDS or HIV infection, and although cases of discrimination by employers continue to occur, they are almost universally deplored as irrational, unscientific and ethically retrograde.

The situation in health care has not been so clear cut. The relatively few cases of transmission that have occurred as a result of needle sticks, and the even smaller number of transmissions linked to blood splashes, have provoked distress among health care workers, especially among surgeons, obstetricians, nurses and emergency room personnel.[22] Persons whose work regularly brings them into contact with their patients' blood have felt vulnerable. On rare occasions they have asserted the right to refuse to care for the infected.[23] Far more frequently, such clinicians have publicly challenged the adequacy of the recommendations for universal blood and body fluid precautions. Instead, they have demanded the right to know whether or not their patients are infected, and the right to screen on a routine or mandatory basis for HIV infection. The level of vigilance demanded by the threat of a lethal infection could not, they have argued, be maintained at all times. The conflict between public health officials who have declared that universal precautions are sufficient, and clinicians who have asserted that they are not, has not abated; indeed, it has intensified. A deep fissure has thus emerged, rupturing the broad alliance which had existed within the medical profession.

In many less developed countries, there is inadequate sterilization of instruments and lack of gloves and equipment necessary for effective infection control. Health care workers claim the right to protect themselves and their patients, urging that infection control equipment must be a priority.

Paralleling this debate has been the unresolved question of the appropriate measures to protect patients from HIV-infected clinicians. Debate on this matter has been driven by the single, still unexplained case of a Florida dentist to whom the only cases of HIV infection in patients linked to a clinician have been traced. Some have argued that although professionals have a moral duty to assume some risks—especially those that are quite small—in caring for their patients, patients do not have an equivalent duty to expose themselves to even small risks when being cared for. Dismissing as irrational those who would deny all infected health care workers, whatever their functions, the right to engage in clinical work, many have asserted that physicians whose invasive work can place their patients at some risk ought not to engage in those procedures. But if those who know themselves to be infected with HIV have such professional duties, are there correlative institutional obligations to identify the infected, to exclude them from certain functions?[24] Are they obligated to screen health care workers and, if so, at what frequency? Might concern about protecting patients provide the basis for mandatory screening and surveillance after so much effort to forestall such programmes? And if screening and surveillance were to be adopted, what would be the impact on an anxious social climate?

Seroprevalence Studies

When the Centers for Disease Control announced that it would begin to undertake blinded seroprevalence studies in order to track the course of HIV infection in the United States, the media assumed that the stage had been set for a bitter confrontation between public health officials and the proponents of civil liberties, gay rights, and medical ethics. In fact, no such conflict occurred.

Those who had proposed the studies made the following arguments: Samples drawn from gay men at testing sites, from blood donors, and recruits to the armed forces did not provide an adequate base for determining the prevalence of infection in the general population. Nor did such samples provide a very good base for determining the level of infection among those most at risk. Selection bias was inevitable. Only with blood drawn for other purposes in hospitals and clinics would it be possible to develop accurate epidemiological data—data critical to an understanding of the course of HIV infection, to the evaluation of preventive interventions, to the planning for needed health care and social services. But would such efforts represent a violation of the moral norm of voluntariness, and would they represent an unacceptable intrusion upon privacy?

From the perspective of those concerned about the protection of individual rights and for whom the threats of stigmatization and discrimination in the face of the AIDS epidemic were of deep concern, these were critical questions. Neither voluntariness nor privacy seemed threatened by the proposed seroprevalence studies. The blood being subject to analysis had been drawn for other purposes presumably with consent. Because the samples were to be stripped of identifiers, because the findings produced could not be linked to particular persons, and because the data produced could not only be statistical, no threats to privacy were posed.[25]

Ironically, what *few* objections were made to blinded seroprevalence studies came not from those concerned about individual rights but from some public health officials and clinicians. It was precisely the features of blinded seroprevalence studies that recommended them to those concerned about privacy that such opponents found most disturbing. Stripping samples of identifiers made it impossible to link results and persons, made it impossible to inform the infected about their own serological status, about the hazard they might inadvertently pose for others. These objectives were not significant. Yet to public health officials and those who studied the ethical issues posed by the AIDS epidemic the overall benefits of blinded seroprevalence studies seemed, on balance, to provide a warrant for them.

Remarkably, the rather unimpeded conduct of such studies in the United States was not repeated in Europe. In Great Britain a forceful assault on the ethics of such surveillance by those who saw such studies as entailing an unacceptable invasion of privacy was joined by public health concerns about the conduct of investigators that would not permit investigators to inform the infected. Finally, some in the Ministry of Health argued that the quality of the data produced by studies would in fact be poor. It was only at the end of 1988 after a protracted debate that a decision at the highest levels permitted Great Britain to pursue a research course first undertaken by the United States and strongly supported by the WHO Global Programme on AIDS.[26]

Strikingly, as the epidemiological benefits of blinded seroprevalence studies have become ever clearer, controversy has surfaced in the nation where the broad scale application of the approach faced virtually no opposition. In 1995 in the United States, a broadly based political challenge to blinded seroprevalence studies involving newborns was launched. How, it was argued, could one justify the failure to inform a mother that her child was potentially infected with HIV? Did not the prospect of early therapeutic intervention render such efforts ethically unacceptable? Was this not but a latter-day version of the infamous Tuskegee syphilis experiment in which poor African-American men were denied the knowledge that they had syphilis because of the desire to trace the natural history of the disease? (Begun at a time when there was little that could be done for individuals with syphilis, the experiment continued through the 1960's, two decades after discovering that penicillin could cure syphilis). Could the justification of blinded seroprevalence at a time of therapeutic impotence be carried over to a period marked by a commitment to early intervention?

So forceful was this challenge that the CDC was compelled to suspend its funding for such efforts. At a deeper level the challenge does raise an important ethical question about the point at which the ethical justification for blinded seroprevalence may need to be resisted as the therapeutic picture changes.

Changing Testing Technologies

A striking departure from the conventional approach to HIV testing has been proposed in some developed countries, one that would permit individuals to obtain a blood sample in the privacy of their homes, send it to a laboratory where it would be analyzed, and then obtain the results by telephone after entering a unique code number. Those who were negative would receive this information by a recorded statement that would include information about the importance of safer sex. Those who tested positive would receive the results from a telephone counsellor. The proposed sale of over-the-counter HIV test kits would radically change the role of health professionals at critical junctures in the testing process.

The proposed test kits, which have been under review by the Food and Drug Administration, raise a number of questions: Would they be used by people at risk for HIV infection who thus far have not been tested? Would those tested suffer because they would not receive face-to-face counselling? How would such testing affect public health practices?[27]

When first proposed in 1987 home-access HIV testing met with virtually unanimous opposition. The American Medicine Association, the Centers for Disease Control and Prevention (CDC), and the gay community all denounced the idea as threatening the foundations *of* America's formal HIV-testing policy, predicated on the importance of pre- and post-test counselling. With so forceful a public reaction, it is not surprising that in 1989 the Food and Drug Administration prevented marketing of the test, expressing scepticism about "whether a lay person can reliably and safely perform the test and interpret the results without benefit of medical advice and professional counselling.[28]

The reconsideration of home testing has been made possible by a profound shift in the political climate and by refinements in the ability to offer counselling by telephone. No longer is there a solid wall of opposition from the people engaged in public health, medicine, research, gay activism, and service to patients with AIDS. Support—some cautions, some enthusiastic—has come from those who in the past viewed home-access testing as anathema.

The conflict over the home-access HIV test raises some public policy issues unique to AIDS and other issues that touch on matters with even broader implications—the role home diagnostic techniques should have in the evolving practice of medicine and the extent to which federal regulatory bodies should protect people from technically accurate devices that may produce psychologically burdensome results.

The challenges posed by such home access testing are limited in terms of the worldwide HIV epidemic, because of the quite obvious extent to which home telephones are a rarity in parts of Africa and Asia where the epidemic is raging. But the challenge does open up a profound question about the extent to which individuals should be permitted to discover their HIV status without the guidance of medical professionals at every important juncture of the process.

The home access test challenges the traditional model in a limited way. But future technologies may permit for home testing in a way that poses a much more fundamental challenge. The future holds out the possibility of a true home test—like the pregnancy test—that would permit an individual to discover in the privacy of his or her home, without a laboratory, without a telephone counsellor, his or her HIV status. Such tests would, in principle, be more widely accessible. Such home HIV tests will pose profound ethical and policy questions that have yet to be addressed—issues of the extent to which individuals should have the right to undertake such self-diagnosis, the extent to which the harm that might befall such individuals as a result of such self-diagnosis provides the warrant for limiting access to such tests for both reasons of paternalism and the common good

CONCLUSIONS

The HIV test, a simple technological device, has been the subject of ongoing controversy because what it reveals has such profound significance for both individuals and the communities within which they live. The issues posed by the HIV test may change as the therapeutic context changes, and as the technologies of testing themselves undergo transformation. But what cannot change is the enduring necessity of careful analysis of the ethical and social implications of policies designed to guide the use of the test. By their very nature, such policies compel us to consider matters of privacy, dignity and social welfare. As such they compel us to confront the most important questions of ethics and human rights posed by the AIDS pandemic.

REFERENCES

1. Bayer, R. *Private Acts, Social Consequences: AIDS and the Politics of Public Health.* New York: The Free Press, 1989.
2. American Association of Physicians for Human Rights (November 12, 1985). Mimeo.
3. Northern California Branch, American Civil Liberties Union: AIDS and Civil Liberties. San Francisco. Northern California Branch, ACLU, March 1986.
4. Bayer R. Levine C., Wolf S.M.: HIV antibody screening: an ethical framework for evaluating proposed programs. *Journal of American Medical Association* 1986, 256:1768-74.
5. Association of State Territorial Health Officials: ASTHO Guide to Public Health Practice: HTLV III Antibody Testing and Community Approaches. Washington DC: Public Health Foundation, 1985.
6. American Medical Association: *Report of the Council on Ethical* and Judicial *Affairs: Ethical Issues Involved in the Growing AIDS Crisis,* Chicago, 1987.
7. Coates, T.J., et al. AIDS Antibody Testing: Will It Stop the AIDS Epidemic? Will It Help People Infected With HIV? *American Psychologist,* 1988, 43:859-64.
8. Centers for Disease Control: *Recommended Additional Guidelines* for HIV *Antibody Counseling and Testing in the Prevention of HIV Infection and AIDS* (April 30, 1987). Mimeo.
9. Surgeon General's *Report on Acquired Immune Deficiency Syndrome,* Washington, D.C. 1986.
10. Institute of Medicine and the National Academy of Sciences: *Confronting AIDS.* Washington, D.C: National Academy Press, 1986.
11. *Report of the Presidential Commission on the Human Immunodeficiency Virus Epidemic.* Washington, D.C: 1988.
12. Levine C. and Bayer R. "The Ethics of Screening for Early Invention in HIV Disease," *American Journal of Public Health* (December 1989), Vol. 79, No. 12, pp. 1661-67.
13. Bayer R., "Womens Rights, Babies' Interests: Ethics, Politics, and Science in the Debate of Newborn HIV Screening," in *HIV Infection in Women,* H. Minkoff, J. DeHovitz, and A. Duerr, eds., (New York: Raven Press, 1995), pp. 293-307.

14. Bayer R., "Ethical Challenges Posed by Zidovudine Treatment to Reduce Vertical Transmission of HIV" (Editorial), *The New England Journal of Medicine* (1994) Vol. 331, No. 18: 1223-25.
15. Hoffman C. and Munson R., "Ethical Issues in the Use of Zidovudine to Reduce Vertical Transmission of HIV", (letter to the Editor), *The New England Journal of Medicine* (1995), Vol. 332, No. 13:891.
16. Minkoff H. and Willoughby A., "Pediatric HIV Disease, Zidovudine in Pregnancy, and Unblinding Heelstick Surveys: Reframing the Debate on Prenatal HIV Testing, *Journal* of *the American Medical Association,* October 11, 1995, Vol. 274, No.14:1165-68.
17. Recommendations of the US Public Health Service Task Force on the use of Zidovudine to reduce perinatal transmission of human immunodeficiency virus. *MMWR* 1994:43 (RR-11):1-20.
18. World Health Organization, Consensus Statement from the Consultation of AIDS in the Workplace, Geneva, 27-29 June, 1988, WHO/GPA/INF/88.7.
19. World Health Assembly, (40th), Global Strategy for the Prevention and Control of AIDS. 15 May 1987. WHA, 40/26. World Health Assembly, (41st), Avoidance of Discrimination of Relation to HIV-Infected People. WHA, 41.24, May 13, 1988.
20. Centers for Disease Control: Recommendations for preventing transmission of infection with human T-lymphotropic virus type III/lymphadenopathy-associated virus in the workplace. *MMWR* 1984, 34:681-86, 691-95.
21. Centers for Disease Control; Recommendations for preventing transmission of infection with human T-lymphotropic virus type III/lymphadenopathy-associated virus during invasive procedures. *MMWR* 1986, 35:221-23.
22. Centers for Disease Control: Update: Acquired immunodeficiency syndrome and human immunodeficiency virus infection among health care workers. *MMWR* 1988, 37:229-39.
23. *New York Times,* November 9, 1987.
24. Gostin L., "HIV-infection physicians and the practice of seriously invasive procedures", *The Hastings Center Report* 19:1:32-39 (1989)
25. Bayer R., "The ethics of blinded seroprevalence testing," *Amercian Journal of Public Health* (1993), Vol. 83, No. 4.
26. Bayer R., Lumey L.H. and Wan L., "The American, British and Dutch responses to unlinked anonymous HIV seroprevalence studies: an international comparison," *AIDS (UK)* (April 1990). Reprinted in *Law, Medicine* and *Health Care,* (Fall-Winter, 1991) Vol. 19, No. 3-4.
27. Bayer R., Stryker J. and Smith M., "Testing for HIV Infection at Home," (Sounding Board). *The New England Journal of Medicine* (1995) 332:1296-99.
28. Banned at home: Food & Drug Administration ruling on AIDS test. *Time.* April 18, 1989-26.

13

Drug and Vaccine Trials: Scientific, Ethical and Legal Considerations

John Dunne
Former Director
Division of Drug Management and Policies
World Health Organisation Geneva, Switzerland

The generalized application of experimental scientific medicine to biomedical research is a product of the present century. Many fundamental discoveries were made before this time, but the sustained progress subsequently achieved in patient care and preventive medicine owes much to the application of scientific principles to the clinical assessment of drugs and vaccines. The following analyses of these principles draw from and update previous reviews undertaken by the author.[1, 2]

The Philosophy and Design of the Clinical Trial

New forms of treatment rarely lead to dramatic, self-evident advances in medicine. They may also be dangerous even if beneficial. Before they can be used with confidence, their value must be adequately established by clinical trial. Fifty years ago judgments were almost always based on uncontrolled clinical impression alone, but now the controlled trial enables evaluations to be made more efficiently and more accurately. Two principles underlie its success: reduction of bias, and controlled comparison of clinical measurement.

Accommodating Variation and Reducing Bias

Many factors apart from treatment influence the response of a patient to disease. Age, genetic factors, and general physical and psychological health are obvious factors that influence the prognosis. The effect of treatment cannot, therefore, be determined with certainty in one or several individuals, but the response of groups of patients treated in different ways can be meaningfully compared. Provided these groups are not inherently different, overall differences in their responses can be ascribed to the effect of treatment.

Biased as well as random errors of measurement can occur during the course of a trial. Indeed, bias is frequently induced by the trial situation. The clinician may develop prejudice for or against a treatment. This can, perhaps unconsciously, affect his assessment of the progress of those receiving it. Should those patients detect in him an increasing or waning enthusiasm for the treatment, their response can be modified. Double-blind techniques are designed to avoid these difficulties. However, schemes which require both the doctor and the patient to be ignorant of the identity of the prescribed treatment have obvious dangers if adequate safeguards are not used:

— the clinician should know the identity of all the competing treatments and the dosage schedules used in the trial;

— he should be aware of, and seek in each patient, the known toxic effects of each of the competing treatments;

— if he is at any time concerned at a patient's progress and is reluctant to continue treatment with an unidentified preparation, he should be free to withdraw the patient from the study. If he does so, he should be able to discover immediately which treatment that patient (and that patient alone) was receiving.

Ethical precepts demand that the best available treatment is used as the standard for comparison. Only when no established competitive treatment exists can a placebo be used. The ideal placebo preparation, which must be pharmacologically inert and have no known non-psychological therapeutic value, should match the active treatment in form, size, colour, texture and taste. A good match is particularly important when it is planned to give each patient consecutive courses of each treatment.

These preparations serve two purposes. Not only are double-blind evaluations of new treatments often made possible when no standard therapy exists, but both the treated group and the control group can be managed in an identical manner and be seen at the same intervals. In this way the true effect of a treatment can be distinguished from a factor associated with it in the trial. A fair trial is much more difficult to devise when standard placebo techniques cannot be used.

Patients are admitted to a controlled trial only if they conform to relevant pre-arranged criteria. In this way variation among patients which might obscure the effect of treatment can be reduced. However, as the criteria for admission become more restrictive, the application of the results becomes more limited, and the problem of obtaining enough suitable patients for the trial becomes greater.

Systematic bias in the composition of the different groups is avoided if each patient has an equal chance of entering any treatment group on admission to the trial. This is the basis of random allocation of treatment which cannot be done haphazardly but only in accordance with a previously prepared plan. Whatever the technique used, it is essential that the clinician cannot be influenced in his decision to admit a patient by knowledge of the treatment he or she will receive.

Selecting an Efficient Design

When there is concern that variation between the available patients might obscure the effects of treatment, the danger may be controlled by gathering similar patients into subgroups or strata. The number of patients allotted to each treatment in each of these strata may be equalized at frequent intervals by keeping separate randomization lists. When the results are analyzed, systematic differences in the responses of the subgroups are sought. If such differences cannot be demonstrated, or are small compared with those between the treatment groups, the sub-groups can be ignored in the ultimate analysis. Stratification of patients can be based on age, sex, prognosis, previous treatment or any other factors that might influence the response to treatment. A refinement of this procedure is to match pairs of patients on similar criteria. One member of each pair is allocated to each treatment group.

In most trials the response of each patient to treatment is evaluated by comparing data obtained before and after the treatment was started. When the disease process is chronic and no permanent cure is available it may be possible to evaluate and compare each patient's response to a series of different treatments. Such "within-patient" comparisons reduce extraneous variation, but there are difficulties and drawbacks to using a patient as his own control. It is difficult and sometimes unethical to withdraw a treatment to which a patient is responding well.

The interpretation of "within-patient" responses can be complex: spontaneous fluctuations may occur in the severity of the disease; the first treatment may have changed the course of the illness; its effects may have extended into the subsequent period of treatment; it may gain apparent advantage because the response of the patient was most obvious during the transition from "no treatment" to "treatment". The analysis may be more reliable if a rest period can be interposed between each period of treatment, or if the sequence of treatments is arranged in a block design so that each treatment is preceded equally often by every other treatment.

A further difficulty arises when the patients are asked which treatment they prefer. Different oral preparations should be easily distinguishable, but identifying qualities such as colour or taste may themselves be of therapeutic importance. If all oral preparations are prepared in the same form and in each of two contrasting colours, colour becomes a variable which can be allocated independently of treatment. Its own contribution to the response of the patient can be determined separately. In this way different treatment periods can be distinguished and the double-blind design will not be impaired; indeed, it may even be enhanced.

Occasionally it is necessary to obtain information about several variables, each of which can be altered independently. For example, the effects of two drugs, each administered by two alternative routes, may be compared using each at two dose levels. The aim of factorial design is to allocate the competing treatments among the patients using the possible combinations of the three variables (drug, dose and route of administration) in such a way that as much information as possible is obtained from the sample about the effect of each of the variables, and their various combinations, upon the response of the patients.

This type of design can also be used for comparisons of three or more treatments which might have additive effects when used in pairs. Some patients are treated with a single drug and others with pairs. If the design is efficient, the combinations and sequences of treatments used give more information about interactions than could be obtained from a larger sample of patients receiving only pairs of treatments.

Designs in which two or more drugs are compared at several dose levels involve complex sub-grouping of patients. The analyses are complicated and missing data present difficult statistical problems. Treatment schedules in which each patient's dose may be adjusted throughout the trial have advantages. The clinician has greater freedom of action, and the trial conditions approach those of routine practice. Single dose schedules are fallible because the dose decided upon may be too low to give optimum responses. Should this happen, (and it is questionable whether one arbitrary dose can ever be optimal for every patient in a trial), information is confined to the relative potency of the treatments at the doses used rather than their potential efficacy.

Posing the Right Questions

Precautions need to be taken to ensure that the services of patients and staff involved in a trial are not wasted. The clinical issue must be clearly defined at the outset. One or two fundamental questions should be posed and the trial planned to provide decisive answers to them. Attempts to pose too many questions can complicate and possibly compromise the design so that no reliable results are obtained.

In general, the problem is to establish the relative worth of two or more competing treatments. Some factors which normally influence choice of treatment are not easily measured in a trial. One drug may occasionally be associated with a serious adverse effect. Another may have been shown in animal studies to have a teratogenic potential. If so, the criteria by which success is measured in the trial, no matter how well they are chosen, are not the only appropriate considerations.

The criteria by which the progress of patients will be judged may be difficult to select. They should at once be subject to objective measurement and, at the same time, of relevance to the patient. So-called "surrogate" variables are frequently measured in default of a variable directly demonstrative of clinical benefit: changes, for instance in blood pressure in hypertension, renal function in diabetes, radiographs in rheumatoid arthritis, or CD4 counts in HIV infection. It is mandatory in these situations, however, to review the strength of the evidence supporting the use of the proposed surrogate as an indicator of clinical responsiveness. The association should never simply be presumed as self-evident.

Determining the Size of the Trial

Before the trial starts it is essential to define, however arbitrarily, the margin of superiority demanded of a treatment before it is to be preferred to its competitors or to a placebo preparation. This definition has two uses: it ensures that conclusions derived from the study are directly relevant to clinical practice, and it allows an estimate to be made of the minimum number of patients required to compare the treatments. If too few patients were admitted the results might be inconclusive and the work wasted. If too many were admitted an unnecessarily large number might receive an inferior treatment.

Since, in the majority of trials, the sample size is fixed at the outset and no data are analyzed until the experiment is complete, it is essential to estimate the "optimum" sample size beforehand. In every case this estimate will be dependent upon: the least difference between the effects of the treatments which would be regarded as clinically useful; the stability of the criteria used for assessing the response to treatment; the level of statistical significance at which the null hypothesis will be rejected; and the power of the experiment (or the probability of detecting the smallest difference regarded as important between the two treatments, if it exists).

An important disadvantage of the fixed sample size trial is that the results cannot be continuously examined. Although it might seem expedient and ethically correct to monitor results throughout the trial the practice has serious drawbacks. It greatly increases the risk that a difference between the effects of two treatments will be accepted as important when it really is not, and this creates the danger that the trial will be closed prematurely on unreliable findings. In an attempt to resolve this problem, modified statistical methods have been designed that permit continuous monitoring.[3] Such sequential trials are concluded either as soon as one treatment shows a significant superiority or when it is evident that neither treatment has an important advantage.

The sample size required for a sequential trial is usually smaller than that needed for a fixed sample size trial of equal power. However, quantitative differences between responses cannot be measured by the sequential approach which offers little advantage unless the response time of each patient is short compared with the rate of admission of new patients to the trial. When the responses are measured over months or years the fixed sample methods are usually preferred.

Deciding whom Should be Admitted

The greater the variation between patients in a trial, the greater is the danger that the effects of treatment will be obscured. However, a usefully representative and large enough sample of patients can only be obtained by permitting some variation. This must be controlled, and the rules or criteria by which patients are selected will depend on:

- — the population of patients towards which the research is directed;
- — the need to exclude particular groups of patients; and,
- — the number of patients available for study.

The first consideration defines the target population. Is it appropriate to confine the trial to patients of one sex, one age group or one race? Should the state of the disease be defined by its aetiology, by its morbid anatomy or its chemical pathology; by the signs or symptoms to which it gives rise; or by a combination of some or all of these criteria? If a prophylactic measure is to be tested how is the population at risk to be defined?

The second consideration narrows the field further. It excludes two groups of patients who would otherwise be eligible for the trial. First, there are those who are likely to respond typically to the treatment. These are patients who are known to be resistant to available alternative treatments, and those whose previous behaviour marks them as uncooperative. Secondly, there are patients who would be exposed to additional hazards in a trial. Patients with incidental disease, particularly of the liver or kidneys, may not be able to metabolize or excrete drugs efficiently and dangerous interactions might occur between the trial drugs and those they are already receiving. The possibility of inducing teratogenic effects during a pregnancy should always be considered.

The third consideration is of great practical importance. An adequate number of patients must be admitted to a trial for it to succeed. Abandonment of a trial is most commonly caused by a lack of suitable patients. Even careful predictions made on the basis of records of a particular hospital service or clinic for the preceding year or so, are apt to prove over-optimistic when the trial is started. The criteria for admitting patients, therefore, should not be unnecessarily restrictive. Good trial design will accept extraneous variation and minimize its effects.

Some Pitfalls and Fallacies

It is neither sufficient to assume that patients take their drugs as prescribed, nor that those who are uncooperative are randomly distributed among the different treatment groups. A drug which is unpleasant to take or which causes frequent toxic effects will never be a popular remedy. Whenever possible, checks should be made on drug consumption, either through "pill checks" or detection of markers in the urine.

Almost inevitably some patients will default from the trial. It cannot be assumed either that these patients defaulted through an unconnected circumstance or that they represent a random selection of the patients admitted. They may be cured; they may be dead or they may prefer to remain untreated. In any case, the conclusions drawn from the trial could be modified or even inverted by knowledge of the missing patients' fate. Attempts must be made to discover the reason for their withdrawal.

At the end of a trial it may be apparent that a greater proportion of patients responded well to one treatment than to another. It is not logical to conclude that the "better" treatment has an all round superiority, and that this is the treatment of choice for all patients. Indeed, if "within-patient" comparisons were made it is likely that a few responded better to the "inferior" treatment. With regard to the minority group a feature of their disease or some other factor may have modified their response. When variables other than treatment are likely to influence the response, it may be possible to measure their influence by a form of multifarious analysis. A successful trial allows treatments to be placed in order of preference: it does not necessarily indicate that the less generally effective treatments should be discarded.

Ethical and Legal Considerations in Therapeutic Trials

Consideration is required in both developed and developing countries as to whether prevailing legal provisions and administrative arrangements ensure that the human rights and welfare of subjects involved in medical research are adequately considered and protected through the operation of the ethical principles set out by the World Medical Association in the Declaration of Helsinki.[4] In the final resort, however, the ethical conduct of this research is the responsibility of the investigator.

The following principles reflect those established in the Declaration of Helsinki. They draw extensively upon proposed international guidelines that were drafted by the author and subsequently published in 1982 after wide international consultation under the aegis of the Council for International Organizations of Medical Sciences.[5] Since that time these guidelines, which were updated in 1993,[6] have been used to guide the work of WHO's Secretariat Committee on Research Involving Human Subjects in reviewing research protocols under consideration within the organization for financial support or other forms of sponsorship.

The Assessment of Benefits and Risks

Few developing countries command the resources or expertise in toxicology, pharmacology and clinical assessment to support the complex regulatory apparatus now considered mandatory for new drug development in industrialized countries. However, it is essential that drugs of potential value against diseases endemic in these countries be tested within the populations at risk. Community interests must always be accommodated in planning such investigations, but developing countries faced with such responsibilities should have recourse to international advisory bodies for technical support and assistance. Decisions concerning the investigation and subsequent use of specific drugs need to be based on local judgment and experience, and directed to practicable options rather than unattainable ideals. An axiom of undertaking research on new drugs in developing countries is that, whenever feasible, a new treatment shown to be of value to the community should remain available to it after it has been tested.

In many instances, particularly in countries where new approaches are still urgently needed to alleviate an inadmissible burden of microbial and parasitic infection, both the disease under investigation and the treatment of the candidate may carry material risk. Without a full assessment of these risks no investigation involving human subjects is warranted. Proposed interventions must be justifiable in terms of the declared objectives. The experimental design must offer every practicable safeguard to the subjects and ensure that a statistically valid result will be obtained efficiently from the smallest possible number of subjects.

Subjects who are otherwise beyond the reach of organized medical care should benefit from the treatment of incidental illness. Monitoring the possible occurrence of unanticipated adverse effects associated with treatment also assumes high priority. When trials are prolonged and conducted under double blind conditions, patients interests are served by defining in advance circumstances that would justify termination of the trial or a break in the coding, and by arranging for a biostatistician to oversee trends and to alert the investigator on any reason to conclude the trial prematurely.

The Principle of Informed Consent

The essence of the Helsinki Declaration is that biochemical research can be legitimately undertaken only if any inherent risks to the subject are consonant with the importance of the objective. At all times concern for the interests of the subject must prevail over the interests of science and society. Studies may be conducted only by scientifically qualified persons and under the supervision of a clinically competent medical person. Risks and benefits must always be carefully assessed beforehand and be based both on adequate laboratory and animal experiments and a thorough knowledge of the scientific literature. Moreover, if the hazards are found to outweigh the potential benefits of the research, the study should be stopped immediately.

The Declaration distinguishes between non-therapeutic research conducted on healthy volunteers and clinical research conducted on patients. Clinical research—a term which embraces therapeutic trials—is sanctioned "only to the extent that it is justified by its potential diagnostic or therapeutic value to the patient". Every patient, it is emphasized, should be assured of the best proven diagnostic and therapeutic management, and the refusal of a patient to participate in a study must never interfere with the doctor-patient relationship.

To protect the rights and welfare of all subjects two fundamental requirements are imposed: firstly, an obligation to present the research protocol to an independent peer review body, or ethics review committee, for clearance; and, secondly, a need to obtain freely-given informed consent from each person approached to participate in a study, once it has been cleared. It is instructive to discuss the principles of informed consent first, since the need for peer review results from the limitations and flaws inherent in the concept of consent.

Informed consent implies a willingness on the part of a prospective subject to take part in a trial after receiving a full description of all proposed interventions, together with an explanation of the objectives, the possible benefits and risks, and assurance of the right to abstain or withdraw from participation at any time without fear of prejudice. No alternative basis exists for protecting the freedom of choice of the individual and ensuring that clinical research finds acceptance with the public at large.

The Limitations of Informed Consent

Notwithstanding its importance, individual informed consent is always vulnerable to abuse; in some circumstances it is flawed and occasionally, in community studies, it may be impractical. Whenever it is given it is axiomatic that it should protect the interests of the subject, and not reduce the legal liability of the investigator. Relevant information should be presented objectively, in a form that is understandable to the patients, and without omission or under-emphasis of dissuasive facts. No inducement that exceeds reasonable compensation for services rendered should be offered to elicit collaboration.

Ideally, each potential research subject should possess the intellectual capacity and insight to provide valid informed consent. In reality, however, few potential subjects are able fully to comprehend the implications of involvement. In some communities the very concept of experimental evaluation of therapy is alien and inconsistent with cultural precepts. In these circumstances participation in research is passive and uncomprehending. Consent can then signify no more than innate confidence in the judgment of the investigator. The intermediary of a trusted community leader can be valuable in these circumstances, at least to make it clear that participation is entirely voluntary and that subjects are free to abstain or withdraw at any time from the experiment.

Other important groups of patients—notably young children, and mentally handicapped persons—do not have the mental capacity to comprehend even these essentials. In legal terms, they are regarded as incompetent to provide valid consent. Yet, to totally debar their involvement in medical research would impede these groups from benefitting in full from the achievements of modern medicine. Not only is informed consent of a parent or other legal guardian a mandatory requirement for the involvement of such individuals in medical research: the willing co-operation of the subject should also be sought whenever this is feasible. Older children, in particular, should be regarded as capable of offering meaningful collaboration, although this must be backed by formal consent provided by the parent or other legal guardian.

It is evident that children should never be the subjects of research that might equally be well carried out on adults,[7] nor should they be involved in research holding no potential benefit for them, unless with the objective of understanding physiological or pathological conditions peculiar to infancy and childhood. On the other hand, their participation is indispensable for research on diseases of childhood and other conditions, including malnutrition, diarrhoea and malaria, to which children are particularly susceptible.

Ultimately, drugs or vaccines intended for children need to be tested on children. There is no merit in unduly delaying such tests when these are appropriate: marketed drugs may otherwise be used in children without the benefit of knowledge obtained from appropriately designed clinical studies. Under no circumstances, however, should tests in younger subjects be contemplated until all reasonable steps have been taken to establish the safety and efficacy of the intervention in adults.

Special consideration should always be given to the way that consent is obtained from members of the armed forces, subordinate members of hospital or laboratory staff, or other junior members of a hierarchically-structured group. Every precaution should be taken to ensure that willingness to volunteer is not influenced by expectation, justifiable or not, of adventitious benefit.

Where research is undertaken on a community basis—as, for example, when supplements are added to staple foods on a pilot basis—individual consent on a person-to-person basis may not be feasible. Similarly, in large scale trials designed to study the efficacy of new prophylactic agents, individual consent may not be practicable. In such cases, particular care is required to ensure that all other measures embodied in the Helsinki Declaration are implemented to protect the interests of everyone involved. Whatever the circumstances, the ethical considerations and safeguards applied to research on individuals must be translated, in every possible respect, into the community context: The ultimate decision to undertake such research will rest with the responsible public health authority. Inherent in this responsibility is a duty to inform the community concerned, using all appropriate means, of the aims of the research, the advantages expected from it, any possible hazards or inconveniences, and the right of dissenting individuals to withhold participation.

Informed consent offers an imperative but imperfect safeguard to protect subjects from undue risk. Its limited application and its vulnerability render it inadequate as an exclusive means of protecting the human rights and welfare of research subjects, and it fails most decisively when the population from which the subjects are drawn is most vulnerable.

The Need for Expert Evaluation of Safety

Patients may be exposed, even in the best of circumstances, to risks that could not reasonably have been foreseen. Unanticipated adverse events may become apparent during the course of a study; others may only become evident much later. Such risks can and should be minimized by ensuring that any new drug or vaccine released for clinical trial has undergone extensive preclinical assessment and preliminary testing on volunteers. But since risk can never be completely excluded, provision for compensation should be available in the rare event of personal injury. Even when each of these safeguards is in place, and when the intention is to proceed strictly on the basis of valid informed consent, both the subjects and the investigator should have assurance that the research protocol has been reviewed and sanctioned by representative and, when appropriate, lay opinion.

The development of new drugs and vaccines is the function of the research-based pharmaceutical industry. The granting of marketing licences for these products on the basis of documentation provided by the manufacturer is a responsibility of government. Most national drug regulatory authorities rely for these assessments on multi-disciplinary advisory committees that include leading clinicians, clinical pharmacologists, pharmacologists, toxicologists, pathologists, pharmacists and statisticians. Other countries at present lack resources to formulate independent assessments of technical data according to the procedures and standards now considered mandatory in the most highly developed countries. In the short term, these countries must remain dependent on free and efficient exchange of relevant information internationally and on advice from technically competent international agencies.

There is marked variation in the extent to which governments of industrialized countries control pre-marketing clinical trials. In the relatively infrequent event that early trials need to be undertaken in a developing country, assurance should be available that the use and safety of the product in this context has been considered and cleared either by the regulatory authority in the country of manufacture or by an internationally competent group convened under the aegis of an international health agency. In every case, the government of the country in which the trials are proposed should be given prior notice of the plans in good time by the main sponsor.

Reports of serious and even fatal injury to subjects volunteering to participate in therapeutic research are on record, but they are rare. In fact, subjects enrolled in clinical trials are in a favoured situation in that they are likely to be under close observation by experienced investigators who are alert to detect early signs of untoward reactions. Such oversight can rarely be provided in routine medical practice.

There should be understanding, none the less, that any serious adverse event that occurs within the context of a clinical trial will be reported promptly to the competent national drug regulatory authority. In the wake of a recent and unprecedented clinical study in which five drug-related deaths occurred, the US Food and Drug Administration now requires that:

- before a clinical trial may be started, the sponsor must provide a written description of the specific measures that will be taken to monitor the safety of the product in question;
- specific adverse effects that need to be reported immediately to the sponsors by the investigators must be discussed and listed in the trial protocol, and the nature and length of subsequent medical follow-up of subjects who participated in the trial must be described;
- each suspected adverse effect must be immediately evaluated by the investigators and sponsors to establish as precisely as possible whether it was causally related to the administration of the product; and
- at the request of the FDA, and in addition to statutory reporting obligations, sponsors may be required to prepare a comprehensive report on information generated in any specific study that bears upon any aspect of the safety of the drug under investigation.

The Right to Compensation for Injury

Any subject involved in medical research who may suffer injury as a result of their participation should have entitlement to financial or other assistance sufficient to compensate them fully for any temporary or permanent disability. In the case of death, the dependents should be eligible for appropriate material compensation. Experimental subjects should never, in giving their consent to participation, be required to waive their rights to compensation in the case of injury; nor should they be required to show negligence or lack of a reasonable degree of skill on the part of the investigator.

Provision for providing such compensation should be settled before the study is undertaken. The responsible company is generally required to accept liability fc· any defect in the quality of a product that is attributable to a fault in manufacture. However, the manufacturer may contest any responsibility for an adverse effect that results from using the product in any way that does not conform with the purposes for which it is intended. In these circumstances, appropriate insurance may need to be arranged, as a condition of clearance during peer review, by the principle investigator, the institution to which that person is attached, or by one or more sponsors of the study.

In some countries a system of insurance against risks, financed either by public or private funds or both, has been created to cover this contingency. The injured party is not required to show fault in respect of the investigator or the sponsor of the trial. The only requirement that is applied is provision of circumstantial evidence of a casual relationship between the investigation and the injury. When studies are sponsored by pharmaceutical manufacturers, the manufacturers themselves are still expected to assume full responsibility for any injury consequent upon the subject's involvement in the trial. Such precautions are particularly necessary in the case of externally sponsored research involving subjects who are not protected by any system of social security.

The Principle of Peer Review

Provision for peer review of protocols for clinical trials is influenced by political institutions, national organization of medical practice and research, and the degree of autonomy accorded to medical investigators. Whatever the circumstances, there is broad acceptance that responsibility exists within society to ensure:

— all drugs and devices under investigation in a clinical trial meet adequate standards of safety;

— compensation will be provided in the rare event of causally related injury; and,

— the provisions of the prevailing version of the Helsinki Declaration are applied.

Ethics review committees have now been widely established. However, their size, composition and terms of reference vary within broad limits. Two principles generally determine representation:

— committees must command the technical competence and judgment to reconcile the physical and psychological consequences of participation with both the welfare of the subjects and the objectives of the investigation; and,

— they should accommodate respected lay opinion in a manner that provides effective representation of community as well as medical interests.

It is not possible to draw a clear dividing line between scientific review and ethical review: an experiment on human subjects that is scientifically unsound is *ipso facto* unethical in that it may expose subjects to risk or inconvenience to no purpose. Normally, therefore, ethics review committees consider both scientific and ethical aspects of a proposal. If a review committee, having considered the protocol and any relevant decisions taken by national drug regulatory authorities or other authoritative bodies, finds the proposal scientifically sound, it will then consider whether any known or possible risk to the subject is justified by the expected benefit and, if so, whether the proposed procedure for eliciting informed consent is satisfactory.

These assessments are most effectively and conveniently conducted by ethics review committees operating at local or regional level. Peripheral committees, operating on an institutional or regional basis, are inherently better placed through awareness and understanding of local factors, not only to assess the ethical aspects of individual studies but also to retain oversight of their implementation, whether by monitoring specific aspects, receiving progress reports or requiring further periodical review.

Although organization of ethical review committees has been determined in many countries by official policy, professional organizations have a responsibility to recommend appropriate standards of operation and to assume a harmonizing role. In particular, representative bodies of pediatricians, psychiatrists and other clinical specialties are uniquely qualified to address some of the problems inherent in informed consent.

Not least, sponsoring agencies and the governing bodies of institutions in which clinical research is undertaken have a strong vested interest in developing and maintaining acceptable ethical standards. The success and rigour of the review process is dependent upon their commitment to it. They share responsibility for requiring evidence of independent committee review as a mandatory precondition for providing the funding and facilities required to undertake the research.

Terms of Reference of Review Committees

The general responsibilities of locally-constituted committees to the review process are three-fold:

— to verify that all proposed interventions and, particularly, the administration of drugs under development, have been assessed by a competent expert body as acceptably safe to be undertaken in human subjects for the purposes in question;

— to ensure that all other ethical considerations arising from the protocol are satisfactorily resolved both in principle and in practice; and,

— to exclude any real or perceived conflict of interest in exercising these judgments.

The last of these requirements demands that any members of the committee who could benefit professionally or personally from implementation of the study should declare their interest and withdraw from all discussion or assessment of the project.

Collectively, the committee needs to possess the experience and the competence to discern whether the protocol provides the following assurances:

— the objectives of the research are directed to a justifiable advancement in biomedical knowledge that is consonant with prevailing community needs;

— the interventions are justifiable in terms of these objectives; the required information cannot be obtained from animal models; and the study has been designed with a view to obtaining this information from as few subjects as possible who will be exposed to a minimum of risk and inconvenience;

— the responsible investigator is appropriately qualified and experienced, and commands facilities to ensure that all aspects of the work will be undertaken with due discretion and precaution to protect the safety of the subjects;

— adequate preliminary literature research and experimental studies have been undertaken to define, as far as practicable, the risks inherent in participation;

— every effort will be made to inform prospective subjects of the objectives and consequences of their involvement, and particularly of identifiable risks and inconvenience;

— any arrangement to delegate consent has adequate justification, and appropriate safeguards will be instituted to ensure that the rights of subjects will be in no way abused, and that provision has been made to compensate subjects in the event that injury is incurred; and

— appropriate measures will be adopted to ensure the confidentiality of data generated in the course of the research.

Ethics and External Sponsorship

Research activities in developing countries are frequently sponsored—and sometimes administered and conducted—by external agencies including international organizations or funding agencies, foundations, research councils, universities and research-based pharmaceutical companies.

Support from these sources is essential if required research is to be fostered on an adequate scale in the developing world but external sponsorship carries certain implications that require careful preliminary assessment:

- — the investigation may be oriented more to external interests rather than local needs;
- — foreign investigators and sponsors may not possess adequate insight into local mores, beliefs, customs and legal systems;
- — the absence of any long-term commitment to subjects involved in the research, and withdrawal of outposted personnel on completion of their task, may result in local disillusionment; and
- — lack of accountability may deprive subjects of any form of compensation for incidental injury.

To overcome or alleviate these difficulties, externally sponsored research should be undertaken with the active collaboration—or through the agency—of an established local institution. At the same time tangible commitment can be offered to the host country by using the opportunity to introduce improvement in related services and to train locally recruited medical scientists.

Medical manpower is a scarce and extremely valuable resource in developing countries. The diversion of highly-trained doctors into research is justifiable only when the objectives are clearly attuned to important matters of immediate local relevance.

Ethics and HIV Trials: A Learning Curve

The advent of HIV infection and its subsequent dramatic incursion into the sexually active population of countries in both the developed and developing world has provoked many questions that have forced a re-examination of the basic principles and ethical implications of clinical drug assessment.

Anxiety to ensure that promising new anti retroviral drugs became accessible to everyone in need of them at the earliest possible opportunity has given rise to pressure for "accelerated approval" by drug regulatory authorities. Enrollment into HIV drug or vaccine trials can stigmatize volunteers in a social environment where submission to HIV diagnostic tests is sufficient cause to raise a health insurance premium. Questions of conscience and confidentiality arise over the handling of HIV serological results. Does the physician hold a responsibility or not to inform the patient when the test is positive? In either case, what are the implications for the patient, the family and other sexual contacts? What social disadvantage accrues to a volunteer who becomes HIV positive not as a result of infection, but as a consequence of administration of a test vaccine? What are the broader criteria that need to be considered in determining the design and location of a large scale vaccine trial?

These questions defy authoritative answers, but they typify the emotional overlay that tends to intrude when new approaches to treating and protecting individuals vulnerable to HIV infection are under assessment. They also impose pressures on the research community to produce tangible results. Increasingly, however, it seems that the established framework of scientific and ethical precepts provides the most efficient and secure mechanism for developing the drugs and vaccines that are so desperately needed to control this disease. The short history of AIDS research is punctuated with examples of optimism generated by inconclusive evidence followed by redressment of early expectations. Anxiety to deliver promising therapies without delay to a population of patients desperate for reassurance has on several occasions led to miscalculation and disillusionment which, if continued,—will erode confidence in medical science.

Assessment of Antiviral Substances

Initial enthusiasm for the antiviral drug, zidovudine, arose from the results of a single, prematurely-terminated trial which indicated that it protected patients from opportunistic infections and death over a period of some 20 weeks.[9] Zidovudine had already been shown markedly to inhibit the replication of human immunodeficiency virus *in vitro.*[10] These findings were heralded as a major landmark in suppressing the disease. Continuation of placebo treatment was regarded as unethical, and a resounding success was claimed for the concept of the accelerated clinical trial.

Few at the time challenged the inference that short-term suppression of the virus would presage suppression in the longer term. Thus, antiviral therapy first with zidovudine, and latterly with other nucleoside analogues, became the cornerstone of management of symptomatic HIV infection—notwithstanding early concerns about potential toxicity and development of resistance.[11]

Eight years later it has become evident that, at best, treatment with zidovudine achieves no more than some two years extension of survival time when treatment is started after the diagnosis of AIDS.[12] There remains the possibility that starting treatment in the asymptomatic phase of HIV infection might have greater effect, but most trials have indicated that—even though decline in CD4 cells may be slowed—this has little, if any, influence on overall survival time.[13,14,15] Indeed, some commentators have concluded that prophylaxis and treatment of *Pneumocystis carinii* pneumonia are more important in extending life than antiretroviral therapy.[16]

However, it would be premature to formulate a definitive judgment on the value of zidovudine, or antiviral therapy in general, on the basis of this evidence. Within the past year, two important findings have been reported that provide hope for more effective management of HIV infection.

Firstly, a randomized, placebo-controlled study has indicated that zidovudine therapy administered during the primary phase of infection (confirmed by a febrile illness, history of possible exposure, presence of antigenemia and lack of HIV antibodies) substantially increases the CD4 count and is likely to ameliorate the clinical course of the disease.[17] Among 77 patients who started treatment during or very shortly after the initial febrile illness, 8 patients within the placebo group, but only one of the treated patients, developed minor opportunistic infections (oral candidosis, herpes zoster, and oral hairy leukoplakia) over the next 15 months.

It has been pointed out[18] that a rationale for early antiretroviral intervention is evident: newly infected persons generally harbour a relatively homogeneous population of HIV-1.[19] During the subsequent explosive phase of viral replication[20,21,22] many variants are generated by mutation[23] any one of which, through substitution of a single base, may result in resistance to antiviral agents.[18] The finding that zidovudine administered alone exerts a clinically detectable effect at this stage of the disease is seen as particularly encouraging since— like the other available nucleoside inhibitors of reverse transcriptase, didanosine, zalcitabine, and stavudine—it is a relatively weak antiretroviral agent.[24]

Other inhibitors of HIV-1 protease still under development[25,26] are claimed to have a potency to lower plasma viraemia that is more than 10-fold greater.[21,22] Meanwhile, preliminary clinical data recently generated in three separate studies on the response to treatment with zidovudine in combination with one[27, 28] or two other protease inhibitors[29] indicate that these regimens offer the possibility of increased survival to previously untreated patients, even when they have relatively advanced symptomatic disease. The largest of these trials—an European/Australian multicentre study involving over 3000 patients— was stopped prematurely when it was shown that death rates were approximately one third lower among patients receiving two antivirals (zidovudine with either didanosine or zalcitabine) compared with those receiving zidovudine alone.

Secondly, persuasive evidence has been reported from two trials within the past year to show that zidovudine is of value in reducing the risk of vertical transmission of HIV-1 infection from mother to child.[30, 31] It is estimated that 15 per cent to 30 per cent of children born to HIV-infected women in the United States are infected before or during delivery.[32] Zidovudine therapy throughout the last trimester of pregnancy coupled with intravenous infusion of zidovudine during labour and postpartum treatment of the infants has been shown to prevent some two-thirds of the expected infections. As yet, the relative importance of each of these phases of treatment remains uncertain. It may well prove far easier to resolve the residual questions generated by this remarkable technical advance than to devise national policies that provide adequate assurance of confidentiality to the mothers and, at the same time, assure the possibility of protecting their endangered children.[33, 34]

Assessment of Vaccines

A similar interplay between considerations of science, ethics and pragmatism, determines the clinical development of vaccines.

Early in the course of HIV infection both cell-mediated immune responses and production of neutralizing antibodies are well preserved. Immunogenic epitopes in the outer envelope of the virus have been shown in animals to stimulate antigen-specific clones of cytotoxic T lymphocytes which, by a lytic action, provide a measure of immunity.[35] It is possible that, in some cases, human infection is aborted at this stage.[36,37,38]

Classical approaches to the development of vaccines, including the use of killed viruses, have been essentially abandoned to avoid any possibility of infection of the recipient by viable genetic material. However, hopes of developing a protective vaccine were raised when neutralizing antibodies to specific glycoproteins in the envelope of the virus were shown to protect primates from infection with homologous virus-infected cells.[39–42] Unfortunately, plans to develop a live vaccinia virus genetically engineered to express an HIV virus envelope glycoprotein were shelved following highly promising initial studies in human volunteers, presumably because of concerns regarding liability for any presumptive consequential injury[43].

Although these glycoproteins vary markedly in different strains of HIV[44–46]—at least eight distinct HIV-1 subtypes have been identified[47]—they have remained the primary focus for vaccine development.[48–51] Preliminary studies in seronegative volunteers have shown that subunit preparations containing epitopes from strains dominant in the United States and Europe can produce neutralizing antibodies, not only to these strains, but to other widely prevalent strains.[5l, 52]

Since 1988, some 1,400 HIV-negative volunteers have participated in trials involving 12 subunit vaccines.[53,54] These studies were designed to assess immunogenicity and safety rather than efficacy. However, a major setback occurred when it was reported that, of 10 subjects who acquired HIV infection subsequent to their enrollment in the trials, 8 had received an active vaccine.[55,56]

These infections cannot be directly attributed to the vaccines, none of which contained viable virus material. However, commentators were quick to speculate that immune changes induced by the vaccine might have rendered recipients more vulnerable to HIV infection. The evidence on which these doubts are based is both speculative and tenuous. Formal statistical tests are of little help: no more than three individuals who received any one vaccine subsequently became infected. In each case high-risk sexual behaviour was reported, and preliminary evidence indicates that at least some of these subjects may not have received the full recommended immunizing dose.[56]

It has been suggested that a candidate vaccine might prevent AIDS without preventing infection, in which case infection may be a misleading surrogate for activity[57]. Such a mode of action is plausible, given that some HIV-patients have remained asymptomatic for many years after initial infection[36–38]. The possibility also exists that false security among vaccines may lure them into high risk behaviour. Whereas it is a truism that direct, indirect, behavioural, and biological effects all determine vaccine efficacy,[57] what is desperately needed is a vaccine that offers secure and reliable primary protection against HIV infection. Anything less will divert massive sums of money from competing projects over periods of many years during which time the prospect of total failure remains open.

This much is evident from the fact that these few cases have been sufficient to tip the scales of judgment against conducting large-scale trials of the existing vaccines in the United States.[58] An ethical dilemma has arisen from a crisis of confidence.[59] There is concern that public opinion would be unimpressed by a vaccine shown to protect only 30 per cent to 50 per cent of persons who are immunized; there is doubt whether the 4500 volunteers required to show whether the vaccines are effective at this level could be recruited; and, given this situation, there is reluctance to invest US$ 20 million annually for a minimum of 4 years in order to demonstrate such a modest effect.

In those countries suffering the greatest burden of HIV infection and where the prevalence of the disease continues to rise most steeply, the prospect of a delay of several years in full-scale preventive vaccine trials is viewed with dismay. Contingency plans have consequently been put in hand by the Global Programme on AIDS to undertake such trials where they are most needed, provided appropriate conditions are met. The Global Programme, it is emphasized, should take the initiative to promote the development of appropriate and affordable vaccines world wide, and should explore every mechanism to make future vaccines accessible to everyone in need of protection.[60]

Note:

[Ed.: The text of the 'International Ethical Guidelines for Biomedical Research Involving Human Subjects (prepared by the Council for International Organizations of Medical Sciences (CIOMS) in Collaboration with the World Health Organization (WHO) in 1993' is reproduced in Annex G, and the 'World Medical Association Declaration of Helsinki on Recommendations Guiding Physicians in Biomedical Research Involving Human Subjects' is reproduced in Annex H].

REFERENCES

1. Dunne, J. Designing a clinical trial. *Hospital Medicine,* London, January 1967.
2. Dunne, J. Drug safety control: pre-clinical requirements for clinical studies in the United Kingdom. *Gazzetta Sanitara,* 1972, 21: 154-157.
3. Armitage, P. *Sequential Medical Trials.* Blackwell, Oxford, 1960.
4. World Medical Association Declaration of Helsinki Recommendations guiding physicians in biomedical research involving human subjects. Adopted by the 18th World Medical Assembly, Helsinki, Finland, 1964 and amended by the 29th Assembly, Tokyo, Japan, 1975, the 35th Assembly, Venice, Italy, 1983 and the 41st Assembly, Hong Kong, 1989.

5. Council for International Organizations of Medical Sciences Proposed International Guidelines for Biomedical Research Involving Human Subjects. CIOMS, Geneva, 1982.
6. Council for International Organizations of Medical Sciences International Ethical Guidelines for Biomedical Research Involving Human Subjects. CIOMS, Geneva, 1993.
7. New requirements for pediatric labelling. *WHO Drug Information,* 1995, 9: 32.
8. Reporting adverse effects: new FDA rules. *WHO Drug Information,* 1994, 8: 212.
9. Fischl, M., Richmann, D., Grieco, M. *et al.* The efficacy of azidothymidine (AZT) in the treatment of patients with AIDS and AIDS related complex: a double-blind, placebo-controlled trial. *New England journal of Medicine,* 1987, 317: 185-191.
10. Mitsuya, H., Weinhold, K., Furman, P *et al.* 3'-azido-3'deoxythimidine (BW A509U): an antiviral agent that inhibits the infectivity and cytopathic effect of human T-lymphotropic virus type III/lymphadenopathy-associated virus in vitro. *Proceedings of the International Academy of Sciences, USA,* 1985, 82: 7096-7100.
11. Erice, A., Balfour, H. Resistance of human immunodeficiency virus type 1 to antiretroviral agents: a review. *Clinically Infectious Diseases,* 1994, 18: 149-156.
12. Lundgren, J., Phillips, A., Pedersen, C. *et al.* Comparison of long-term prognosis of patients with AIDS treated and not treated with zidovudine. *Journal of the American Medical Association,* 1994, 271: 1088-1092.
13. Hamilton, J., Hartigan, P., Simberkoff, M. *et al.* A controlled trial of early versus late treatment with zidovudine in symptomatic human immunodeficiency virus infection: results of the Veterans Affairs Co-operative Study. *New England Journal of Medicine,* 1992, 326: 437-443.
14. Concorde Coordinating Committee. Concorde: MRC/ANRS randomised double-blind controlled trial of immediate and deferred zidovudine in symptom-free HIV infection. *Lancet,* 1994, 343: 871-881.
15. Volberding, P., Lagakos, S., Grimes. J. et al. A comparison of immediate with deferred zidovudine therapy for asymptomatiz HIV-infected adults with CD4 cell counts of 500 or more pecubic millimeter. *New England Journal of Medicine,* 1995, 333: 401-407.
16. Osmond, D., Charlbois, E., Lang, W. et al. Changes in AIDS survival time in two San Francisco cohorts of homosexual men, 1983 to 1993, *Journal of the American Medical Association,* 1994, 271: 1083-1087.
17. Kinloch de-Loes, S., Hirshel, B., Hoen, B. *et al.* A controlled trial of zidovudine in primary human immunodeficiency virus infection. *New England Journal of Medicine,* 1995, 333: 408-413.
18. Ho. D. Time to hit HIV, early and hard. *New England Journal of Medicine,* 1995, 333: 450-451.
19. Zhu, T., Mo, H., Wang, N. *et al.* Genotypic and phenotypic characterization of HIV-1 in patients with primary infection. *Science,* 1993, 261: 1179-1181.
20. Coffin, J. HIV populations dynamics in vivo: implications for genetic variation, pathogenesis and therapy. *Science,* 1995, 267: 483-489.
21. Ho, D., Neumann, A., Perelson, A. *et al.* Rapid turnover of plasma virions and CD4 lymphocytes in HIV-1 infection. *Nature,* 1995, 373: 123-126.
22. Wei, X., Ghosh, S., Taylor, M. *et al.* Viral dynamics in human immunodeficiency virus type 1 infection. *Nature,* 1995, 373: 117 122.
23. Preston, B., Poiesz, B., Loeb, A. Fidelity of HIV-1 reverse transcriptase.

Science, 1988, 242: 1168-1171.

24 Cao, Y., Ho, D., Todd, J. *et al.* Clinical evaluation of branched DNA signal amplification for quantifying HIV type 1 in human plasma. *AIDS Research and Human Retroviruses,* 1995, 11: 353 361.

25. Vacca, J., Dorsey, B., Schleif, W. *et al.* L-735, 524: an orally bioavailable human immunodeficiency virus type 1 protease inhibitor. *Proceedings of the National Academy of Sciences, USA,* 1994, 91: 4096-4100.

26. Kempf, D., Marsh, K., Denissen, J. et al. ABT-538 is a potent inhibitor of human immunodeficiency virus protease and has a high oral bioavailability in humans. *Proceedings of the National Academy of Sciences, USA,* 1995, 92: 2484-2488.

27. Combination superior to zidovudine in Delta trial. *Lancet,* 1995, 346: 895.

28. Study shows two drugs are best for HIV infection. *British Medical Journal,* 1995, 311: 827.

29. Triple therapy effective in HIV. *Pharmaceutical Journal,* 1995, 255: 175.

30. Boyer, P., Dillon, M., Navaie, M. *et al.* Factors predictive of maternal-fetal transmission of HIV-1: preliminary analysis of zidovudine given during pregnancy and/or delivery. *Journal of the American Medical Association,* 1994, 271: 1925-1930.

31. Connor, E., Sperling, R., Glber, R. *et al.* Reduction of maternal infant transmission of human immunodeficiency virus with zidovudine treatment. *Nezo England Journal of Medicine,* 1994, 331: 1173-1180.

32. Davis, S., Byers, R., Lindegrin, M. Prevalence and incidence of vertically acquired HIV infection in the United States. *Journal of the American Medical Association,* 1995, 274: 952-955.

33. Minkoff, H., Willoughby, A. Pediatric HIV disease, zidovudine in pregnancy, and unblinding heelstick surveys: reframing the debate on prenatal HIV testing. *Journal of the American Medical Association,* 1995, 274:1165-1168.

34. Chrystie, R., Wolfe, C., Kennedy, J. *et al.* Voluntary, named testing for HIV in a community based antenatal clinic: a pilot study. *British Medical Journal,* 1995, 311: 928-931.

35. Koup, R., Ho, D. Shutting down HIV. *Nature,* 1994, 370: 416.

36. Clerici, M., Giorgi, J., Chou, C. *et al.* Cell-mediated immune response to human immunodeficiency virus (HIV) type 1 in seronegative homosexual men with recent sexual exposure to HIV-1. *Journal of Infectious Diseases,* 1992, 165: 1012-1019.

37. Rowland-Jones, S., Nixon, D., Aldous, M. *et al.* HIV-specific cytotoxic T-cell activity in an HIV-exposed but uninfected infant *Lancet,* 1993, 341: 860-861.

38 Langlade-Demoyen, P., Ngo-Giang-Huong, F., Oksenhendler, E. Human immunodeficiency virus (HIV) nef-specific cytotoxic T lymphocytes in noninfected heterosexual contact of HIV-infected patients. *Journal* of *Clinical Investigation,* 1994, 93: 1293-1297.

39. Berman, P., Gregory, T., Riddle, L. *et al.* Protection of chimpanzees from infection by HIV-1 after vaccination with recombinant glycoprotein gp120 but not gp 160. Nature, 1990, 345: 622-625.

40. Girard, M., Kieny, M., Pinter, A. *et al.* Immunization of chimpanzees confers protection against challenge with human immunodeficiency virus. *Proceedings of the National Academy of Sciences, USA,* 1991, 88: 542-546.

41. Fultz, P., Nara, P., Barre-Sinoussi, F. *et al.* Vaccine protection of chimpanzees against challenge with HIV-1 infected peripheral blood mononuclear cells. *Science,* 1992, 256: 1687-1690.

42. Mannhalter, J., Pum, M., Wolf, H. *et al.* Immunization of chimpanzees with the HIV glycoprotein gp 160 induces long-lasting T-cell memory. *AIDS Research and Human Retroviruses, 1991,* 7: 485-493.
43. Cohen, J. Is liability slowing AIDS vaccines? *Science,* 1992, 256:168-170.
44. Leigh Brown A. Sequence variability in human immunodeficiency viruses pattern and process in viral evolution. AIDS, 1991, S (suppl. 12): 35-42.
45. Kusumi, K., Conway, B., Cunningham, S. *et al.* Human immunodeficiency virus type I envelope gene structure and diversity in vivo after co-cultivation *in vitro. Journal of Virology,* 1992, 66: 875-885.
46. Mascola, J., Louwagie, J., McCutchan, F. *et al.* Two antigenically dinct subtypes of human immunodeficiency virus type I: viral genotype pretLicts neutralization serotype. *Journal of Infectious Disezses*, 1994, 169: 48-54.
47. Myers, G., Korber, B., Wain-Hobson, S *et al.* A compilation and analysis of nucleic acid and amino acid sequences. Human retroviruses and AIDS, 1994. Los Alamos National Laboratory, Los Alamos, New Mexico, USA.
48. Dolin, R., Graham, B., Greenberg, S. *et al.* The safety and irnmunogenicity of a human immunodeficiency virus type 1 (HIV-1) recombinant gp160 candidate vaccine in humans. *Annals of Internal Medicine,* 1991, 114: 119-127.
49. Fast, P., Walker, M. Human trials of experimental AIDS vaccines. *AIDS,* 1993, 7(suppl 1): 147-159.
50. Belshe, R., Clements, M., Dolin, R. et al. Safety and immunogenicity of a fully glycosylated recombinant gp160 HIV 1 vaccine in low risk volunteers. *Journal of Infectious Diseases,* 1993, 168: 1387-1395.
51. Schwartz, D., Gorse, G., Clements, M. *et al.* Induction of HIV 1 neutralising and syncytium-inhibiting antibodies in seronegative recipients of HIV-1MN rgpl20 subunit vaccine. *Lancet,* 1993, 342: 69-73.
52. Belshe, R., Graham, B., Keefer, M. et al. Neutralizing antibodies to HIV-1 in seronegative volunteers immunized with recombinant gp120 from the MN strain of HIV-1. *Journal of the American Medical Association,* 1994, 272: 475-480.
53. Cohen, J. The HIV vaccine paradox. *Science,* 1994, 264: 1072-1074.
54. National Institute of Allergy and Infectious Diseases. Scientific review supports expanded clinical studies of two candidate HIV vaccines. National Institutes of Health, Bethesda, MD. 29 April 1994.
55. National Institute of Allergy and Infectious Diseases. HIV infection in vaccine trial volunteers. National Institutes of Health, Bethesda, MD. June 1994.
56. Belshe, R., Bolognesi, D., Clements, M. *et al.* HIV infection in vaccinated volunteers. *Journal of the American Medical Association,* 1994, 272: 431.
57. Scaper, C., Fleming, T., Self, S., Rida, W. Statistical issues in the design of HIV vaccine trials. *Annual Reviews of Public Health,* 1995, 16: 1-22.
58. National Institute of Allergy and Infectious Diseases. NIAID advisors recommend continuing but not expanding at this time ongoing trials of two candidate HIV vaccines. National Institutes of Health, Bethesda, MD. June 1994.
59. Macilwain, US puts large-scale AIDS vaccine trials on ice as 'premature'. *Nature,* 1994, 369: 593.
60. Meeting report: Scientific and public health rationale for HIV vaccine efficacy trials. Vaccine Development Unit, Global Programme on AIDS, World Health Organization, Geneva, 13–14 October 1994.

14

HIV/AIDS-Related Human Rights

Ms. Susan Timberlaka
WHO Geneva, Switzerland

In the context of HIV/AIDS, protecting human rights both safeguards human dignity and promotes public health because it helps to:

* get the message on how to avoid infection to most people
* work with people to encourage them to avoid risky behaviour
* provide people a supportive environment and health care that will help avoid infection, or cope, if infected.

Human Rights relevant to HIV / AIDS are:

* Non-discrimination and equality before the law
* Right to life
* Right to health
* Right to liberty and security of persons
* Freedom of Expression
* Freedom from inhuman or degrading treatment or punishment
* Freedom of movement
* Right to privacy
* Right to marry and found a family
* Right to education
* Right to work
* Right to an adequate standard of living
* Right to social security, assistance and welfare
* Right to seek and enjoy asylum

* Right to share in scientific advancement and its benefits
* Right to participate in public and cultural life

How do some of the relevant rights apply?

For prevention of the spread of infection among the general population, the following rights should be protected so that people will come forward for HIV/AIDS information, education and means of protection and will avoid risky behaviour:

Non-discrimination

* Protected against discrimination if seek help or are HIV+

Right to privacy

* Protected against mandatory testing
* HIV status kept confidential

Right to liberty and freedom of movement

* protected against imprisonment, segregation or isolation in a special hospitalward

Right to education/information

* access to HIV/AIDS prevention education and information

Right to health

* access to health care prevention services, including STD services and condoms.

For prevention of spread to vulnerable groups (women, children, minorities, indigenous people, poor people, migrant-workers, refugees, sex workers, drug-users, men having sex with men), these groups should have equal access to available HIV/AIDS preventiont information, education, health care and condoms, should not be subject to isolation where applicable; and should participate in the formulation and implementation of HIV/AIDS policy that affects them.

Non-discrimination/equality before law

* same access as others to available services

Rights to education and health

* same access to available HIV/AIDS prevention education and information, and health care services, including STD services and condoms

Freedom from cruel, inhuman and degrading treatment

* right to be free from coerced unsafe sex

Right to participate in public life

* participate in the formulation and implementation of HIV/AIDS policy

For those living with HIV/AIDS or otherwise affected by it, the following rights should be protected:

Non-discrimination and equality before law

* right not to be mistreated on the basis of health status, i.e., HIV +

Right to health

* right not to be denied health care/treatment because HIV + status

Right to liberty and security of person

* right not to be arrested and imprisoned because HIV + status

Right to marry and found a family even if HIV +

Right to education

* right not be thrown out of school if HIV +

Right to work

* right not to be fired if HIV +

Right to social security, assistance and welfare

* right not to be denied these benefits if HIV +

Right to freedom of movement if HIV +

Right to seek and enjoy asylum if HIV +

Human Rights can be Restricted for the Public Health or to Protect the Rights of Others, but the following criteria must be satisfied:

Rights can be restricted only if restriction is

* prescribed by law (not arbitrary)
* necessary (pressing social need)
* in a democratic society (product of consensus)
* for a legitimate aim (public health or rights and freedoms of others)

Restriction must:

* be proportional to achieving the aim
* be the least restrictive means available
* actually achieve aim

Restrictions of Human Rights in the context of HIV/AIDS do not achieve the aim of Public Health and often are neither proportional nor the least restrictive means available.

15

Human Rights and HIV/AIDS

HUMAN RIGHT	APPLICATION TO HIV/AIDS	PUBLIC HEALTH RATIONALE
NON-DISCRIMINATION EQUALITY BEFORE THE LAW	(1) promote access of disadvantaged groups to HIV prevention and caw programmes	(1) prevention/care efforts should reach all, including those difficult to reach
	(2) prevent discrimination against HIV + or those suspected in employment, travel, health care, education, social assistance	(2) almost no threat of transmission in these settings
PRIVACY	(1) prevent mandatory testing	mandatory teseng:
	(2) prevent routine or hidden tests	(1) can never reveal identity of all HIV +
	(3) ensure confidentiality	(2) may involve false test results
	(4) ensure informed consent before tests, treatment or research	(3) drives people away from prevention/health care efforts
		(4) results in psyche trauma if no counselling
		(5) involves diversion of resources better spent on education/health care

LIBERTY	(I) prevent arrest/detention on account of HIV status alone	detention/isolation
	(2) prevent isolation or segregation in administrative setting on account of HIV status alone	(1) no public health rationale; does not prevent spread (2) is costly and impracticable since life
FREEDOM FROM INHUMAN/DEGRADING TREATMENT	(I) promote measures to protect against sexual violence/sexual coercion	(1) any coerced sex increases risk of transmission
	(2) prevent compulsory isolation or segregation of prisoners HIV +	(2) no public health rationale for isolating presoners; more useful to make available information, dean needles, bleach and condoms
	(3) prevent forced abortion/sterilization of HIV + women	(3) only I out of 3 babies born to HIV + other infected; must less if AZT used
FREEDOM OF MOVEMENT	(1) prohibit testing of returning nationals	(1) excluding does not prevent spread as HIV b already present
	(2) prohibit testing of entering foreigners	(2) exclusion gives false sense of security
	(3) regarding cost of care, HIV/AIDS be treated the same as comparable disease	(3) better to use resources on education/security
FREEDOM FROM FORCED SERVITUDE	(I) prevent trafficking in women, men or children	(1) any coerced sex increases risk of transmission
	(2) prevent forced prostitution or involuntary servitude for sexual purposes	(2) difficulty of access for prevention and care
	(3) prevent harmful traditional practices, e g, manage of minors, wife inheritance, female genital mutilation	(3) harmful traditional practices can increase social and/or biological vulnerability

{Cont.} HEALTH	(I) promotional access for disadvantaged, vulnerable groups to HIV health prevention and care programmes	(1) prevention/care should reach all people, including those difficult to reach
	(2) prevent discrimination against HIV + persons in health care	(2) if use universal precautions, little risk of transmission
	(3) promote confidentiality in health care setting	(3) should maintain confidence in health care
	(4) promote blood safety through screening of all blood, body parts and fluids	
EDUCATION/ INFORMATION	(1) prevent equal access for disadvantaged, vulnerable groups to HIV prevention education/information	(1) prevention/care should reach all people, including those difficult to reach
	(2) prevent discrimination against HIV + people in access to education facilities	(2) virtually no risk of transmission in educational setting with basic precautions
WORK	(1) prevent pre-employment or during employment mandatory testing	(1) almost no risk of transmission in work place with basic precautions
	(2) prevent Isolation or termination due to HIV status	(2) HIV + person can and should be productive for long time according to health needs
	(3) ensure reassignment/accommodation	
	(4) ensure same employment policies for HIV / AIDS as for any comparable disease	
	(5) ensure confidentiality in work place	
SOCIAL SECURITY	(1) promote equal access of women to social security and other available benefit in case of termination of marriage/employment	(1) women should have alternative to relationships that threaten them with infection; and to support, if husband dies

	(2)	prevent discrimination for HIV + people In access to social security	(2)	HIV + people need means of support
SEEK AND ENJOY ASYLUM	(1)	prohibit revealment on basis of HIV status	(1)	no public health rationale to deny asylum
	(2)	promote humane/generous grant of asylum for HIV + persecution	(2)	refugee cannot return home to
FAMILY	(1)	prevent pre-marital mandatory HIV	(1)	HIV + married people can practice
	(2)	prevent prenatal mandatory HIV testing	(2)	only I in 3 babies born infected if mother infected, much less if AZT used
	(3)	provide information/counselling regarding risks/prevention		

16

AIDS and Human Rights

(Report of an International Consultation on AIDS and Human Rights, Geneva, 26-28 July 1989)

A. THE PUBLIC HEALTH RATIONALE FOR PREVENTING AIDS RELATED DISCRIMINATION

At the end of the 1980s–the first decade to know of AIDS-the world faces three interconnected epidemics the epidemics of human immunodeficiency virus (HIV) infection, of HIV-linked disease, acquired immunodeficiency syndrome (AIDS), and of social, cultural and political reaction to HIV and AIDS. This third epidemic threatens increasingly to overshadow and overwhelm the epidemic of HIV and AIDS. Myths about HIV and AIDS persist, generally involving fears about casual contact. According to surveys throughout the world from 10 per cent to 30 per cent of people still believe that HIV can spread through a handshake and that it is not safe to ride a bus or share a workplace with an infected person. Also, sadly, the twisted bring forth their twisted ideas, spreading their talk of "secret germ warfare", massive ever ups" and "AIDS conspiracies". This is harmful, for an African Minister of Health recently reported that such myths have reduced condom use because of the rumour that condoms have been contaminated with HIV. Finally, assaults on the rights and dignity of HIV-infected people continue to increase involving work, education, housing and travel, even in countries which have thus far steadfastly resisted such discrimination.

Over two years ago, the foundation was laid for an international programme of concerted action and common purpose-the programme Global AIDS Strategy. The Global AIDS Strategy provides a practical framework for national efforts, literally around the world, and for international programme. World Health Organization Global Programme on AIDS is active in over 150 countries, providing financial and technical support for planning, training and implementing in the field. National AIDS programmes have been developed rapidly, with great energy and local creativity; such programmes now exist in most countries and should be established in all of the world's 187 countries and areas by the end of 1989 or early 1990.

As of 1 November 1990, 298,914 cases of AIDS have been reported to the WHO. However, because of extensive under -recognition,, under-reporting and delays in reporting, WHO has estimated that by the and of 1990, over 800,000 AIDS cases in adults, and over 400,000 cases in infants and children will have occurred globally since the start of the pandemic, for a combined global total of over 1,200,000 cases. Furthermore, as of late l990, about 8 million to 10 million people are estimated to be infected worldwide with HIV of whom, 3 million are women in the reproductive age group The incidence of heterosexually transmitted HIV infection appears to be increasing rapidly, particularly in developing countries.

WHO has projected that by the year 2000, a cumulative total of 5 million to 6 million AIDS cases in adults may have occurred, and 15 million to 20 million adults cumulatively HIV-infected. Consequently, the number of infants born HIV-infected since the start of the pandemic may reach 10 million by the end of this century. The majority of these infants and children will either have progressed to and died of AIDS, or have died of another disease whose severity may have been accentuated because their immune systems were crippled by HIV infection. Thus, by the year 2000, AIDS and HIV infection in infants and children may lead to child mortality rates increasing as much as 50 per cent over the present levels in regions where heterosexual transmission of HIV predominates. Moreover, by the year 2000, more than 10 million infected young children are likely to be threatened with orphanhood, as a result of the death of their mothers or both parents due to AIDS. This escalating burden of adults, infants, and children with AIDS and other HIV-related ill health will require continued and increasing solidarity from the entire international community.

Therefore, whether considering the cumulative number of AIDS cases worldwide, or the numbers of HIV-infected people, it is anticipated that the decade of the 1990s will be more serious, and perhaps much more serious than that we have experienced during the 1980s.

To convert the initial effort of the 1980s into strong and resourceful programmes to deal with HIV infection and AIDS during the 1990s will therefore, require sustained energy and commitment. Yet the epidemics of HIV and AIDS are but two of the three we will continue to face. The third epidemic of social, cultural and political reaction and response may be as important to our future as the virus itself.

In many countries, there is evidence that behavioural changes have occurred or are occurring which will help prevent HIV infection. After several years of experience in many countries, it is clear that, regardless of the cultural and social context, three elements have been present wherever positive behavioural changes have occurred First, locally relevant and targeted information and education has been provided by credible sources. Secondly, the information and education has been linked with those health and social services needed in order to support and strengthen behaviour change. Finally, the entire programme has been imbued with the them of support. A supportive social environment is a necessity, not a luxury. These are the principles which emerge from experience and they can bo adapled to any setting or culture. Unfortunately, wherever information remains inadequate, inaccurate or frankly misleading, where needed health and social services do not yet exist, or where the entire effort is undermined by a discriminatory and punitive social environment in these places, prevention has not yet been given a chance.

The World Health Organization has taken a series of strong and proactive stands to help protect the right of, and prevent the rights of, and prevent discrimination against, persons infected with human immunodeficiency virus (HIV). This position was reinforced by the 41st World Health Assembly, which adopted a resolution on 13 May 1988 entitled "AIDS: Avoidance of Discrimination in Relation to HIV-infected People and People with AIDS".

This resolution starts by urging WHO member states to "foster a spirit of understanding and compassion for HIV-infected people and people with AIDS through information, education and social support programmes[11]. Experience With national AIDS programmes has suggested that as public information and education increases in quantity and quality, irrational fears about HIV and its transmission tend to diminish. Nevertheless, while people may understand that HIV cannot be spread through casual contact, the specific and individual instance of an HIV-infected child in a school or an

HIV-infected adult in the workplace can still provoke unwarranted but substantial anxiety and can unveil deep-seated prejudices. Consequently, the World Health. Assembly resolution urges WHO's 167 Nation Member States "to protect the human rights and dignity of HIV-infected people and people with AIDS and of members of population groups, and to avoid discriminatory action against and stigmatization of them in the provision of services, employment and travel". In addition, Member States are urged "to ensure the confidentially of HIV testing and to promote the availability of confidential counselling and other support services to HIV-infected people and people with AIDS".

There is a strong and clear public health rationale for this emphasis on protecting the human rights and dignity of HIV-infected persons, including people with AIDS. HIV spreads almost entirely through identifiable behaviour and specific actions (sexual intercourse and intravenous drug use) which are generally—though not always—subject to individual control. In most instances, HIV transmission involves the behaviour of two persons; a change in behaviour of either the HIV-infected or the uninfected person will be sufficient to prevent HIV transmission. However, it must be remembered that HIV is transmitted mainly through behaviour which is private secret, often hidden and, in some societies, illegal.

Therefore, if HIV infection, or suspicion of HIV infection, leads to stigmatization and discrimination (e.g. loss of education or employments, persons already HIV infected, and those who are concerned they may be infected, will actively avoid detection and contact with health and social services will be lost. Those needing information, education, counselling or other support services would be "driven underground". The person who fears be or she may be infected would be reluctant to seek assistance but of fear of being reported—with severe personal consequences. The net result would be to jeopardize seriously educational outreach and thereby exacerbate the difficulty of preventing HIV infection.

For these reasons, discrimination may endanger public health; stigmatization may itself represent a threat to public health. The World Health Assembly resolution, therefore, directs WHO "to stress to Member States, and to all other concerned, the dangers to the health of everyone of discriminatory action against and stigmatization of HIV-infected people and people with AIDS and members of population groups". Protecting the human rights and dignity of HIV-infected people, including people with AIDS, and members of population groups, is a necessity for effective public health programmes to prevent and control HIV/AIDS. It is not a question of the "rights of the many" or the "rights of the few"; the protection of the uninfected majority depends upon and is inextricably bound with the protection of the rights and dignity of the infected person. Therefore, as the World Health Assembly has identified this issue as critical to the success of national and international AIDS prevention programmes, the protection of the rights and dignity of HIV-infected persons has become an integral part of the Global AIDS Strategy.

Around the world, these is evidence of growing complacency, among some peoples and governments and growing fatalism among others. Complacency invites marginalization—of groups or nations—and could tragically reduce the commitment of human and financial resources at this critical moment in national AIDS programme development. Fatalism can lead either to passive hopelessness or to proposals for simplistic and extreme solutions.

For this reason, solidarity is a transcendent and dominant need in the 1980s, we have learned and we have taught that discrimination and stigmatization of HIV-infected people must be prevented—for the sake of all. More recently, we have discovered that beyond the limited concept of anti-discrimination there is a more positive and active quality—a respect for human rights and dignity—a spirit of active tolerance. Yet even beyond anti-discrimination and tolerance, there is a higher call—to solidarity.

Solidarity is at once a personal and a universal manner, for it raises the fundamental question of "what is the self"' and what is the "other" One of the glories of our era is that we have witnessed the birth of global solidarity—imperfect, struggling yet nevertheless real—in the creation of the United Nations, in the concern about nuclear war, in the growing worldwide resolve to protect the environment, and in AIDS.

We must practise the wisdom that refuses to separate the condition of the few from the fate of the many. We must prevent emotional negligence and indifference to the fate of peoples and nations. We shall continue to face painful and intractable aspects of life and society: complacency, ignorant, fear, discriminant, prejudice and hate; abandoned children;. prostitution of boys and girls, men and women; drug injection; the suffering of those who ; are infected and ill and those who live with them and death itself. Concerned with AIDS, we are drawn to solidarity. This solidarity gives us confidence to continue to look into the face of AIDS—and known that we will not turn away.

As we mature as individuals, our innate feeling of personal immortality evolves into an awareness of our mortality, and this helps us in our search for understanding. And at some time we accept our common humanity, and this knowledge also helps us better to understand. Are we—is this world— now mature enough, now wise enough—to accept that the deepest meaning of solidarity requires that we consider ourselves as if we too were infected with HIV—that we are all—on a human level—seropositive?

WHO believes it will be essential for non governmental and governmental human rights organizations to play an active and proactive role. Such organizations particularly at the locally and national levels, must help prevent discrimination against HIV-infected persons, persons with AIDS, or high risk population groups. An informed and alerted human rights network; can help protect public health and promote the human rights and dignity of all persons, including those with HIV/AIDS.

The human rights network will continue to require clear, accurate and up-to-date information on HIV infection and AIDS. The World Health Organization, which has been given the mandate to direct and co-ordinate the global fight against AIDS, stands ready to continue providing the human rights network with useful and reliable information upon which all effective public health and human rights action related to AIDS must depend. At the national level, organizations concerned with human rights must:

— link with AIDS-related organizations, NGO and governmental organizations: and
— work with national AIDS Committees to help broaden understanding and seek effective alliances against AIDS-related discrimination.

The Global Programme on AIDS is committed to this task. We must break new ground and work together—to fight against AIDS—to protect human rights and dignity.

While many tragedies and struggles leave no visible trace once they are past we know that AIDS is the 1980s has altered us—in our world, in our countries, in our countries—and in our hearts. From our experience in the decade now passing, we know that we, and those who think and work and believe as we do, will not simply survive—we will prevail. For finally, it is the commitment and strength of individuals hundreds and thousands of individuals—whose humanity and whose acts of solidarity illuminate the world—and our future.

B. THE HUMAN RIGHTS RATIONALE FOR PREVENTING

AIDS-related Discrimination

AIDS is a global problem hence it demands a global response. This response has been provided by the global strategy for prevention and control of AIDS, adopted by the World Health Assembly and endorsed by the limited Nations General Assembly. The Global AIDS Strategy has been universally accepted as the policy-framework for, the worldwide effort to combat AIDS. This strategy includes promotion and protection of human rights, thus for the first time in history a strategy against a disease includes promotion and protection of human rights. Protection of human rights, especially protection against discrimination has been stressed first by the World Health Assembly and then by the Commission on Human Rights and other global, regional and national human rights bodies as the core principle in the application of human rights to HIV/AIDS and all the other health issues.

AIDS is also a global challenge of unprecedented scope. In the field of human rights, it has threatened to undermine universal respect of human rights. Therefore, the Secretary-General of the United Nations, in his speech at the General Assembly on 20 October 1987, said that our fight against AIDS "is also a fight against fear, against prejudice and against irrational action born of ignorance. For these are the causes of some of the most critical violations of human rights".

The need for a co-ordinated response and concerted action by all parts of the United Nations has been postulated by the General Assembly in all its resolutions concerning AIDS. This Consultation has been a result of the co-operation of the Centre for Human Rights and the WHO Global Programme on AIDS. In 1988 the Centre started carrying out its co-ordinating role in addressing human rights aspects of HIV/AIDS. The Secretary General requested the Centre to start collecting information on legislation and practices of countries, particularly on discrimination and the danger it entails. The Centre's role of acting as the secretariat to the human rights treaty bodies has included an increased attention to HIV/AIDS. A briefing on HIV/AIDS was held at the meeting of all the chairpersons of the human rights treaty bodies in October 1988. States' reports on the right to health, submitted under the International Covenant on Economic, Social and Cultural Rights, increasingly include descriptions of national AIDS policies, laws and practices. The

Human Rights Committee has also included AIDS-related issues in the consideration of States' reports under the International Covenant on Civil and Political Rights.

The United Nations human rights bodies have introduced HIV/AIDS related human rights on their agenda. In August 1988, the Under-Secretary General for Human Rights. Mr. Jan Martenson, suggested to the members of the Sub-Commission on the Prevention of Discrimination and Protection of Minorities that they should address human rights problems raised by HIV/AIDS. The Sub-Commission considered AIDS and human rights in 1988, and asked Mr. Luis Varela Quiros, one of its members, to prepare a concise note on the methods whereby the Sub-Commission could study AIDS and human rights. In 1989, Mr. Varela Quiros was appointed the Special Rapporteur on this subject. In the same year, the Commission on Human Rights adopted resolution 1989/11 on non-discrimination in the field of health. This resolution reaffirms that non-discrimination should apply throughout the field of health to all people in all circumstances.

The importance of human rights stems from the fundamental principle that society in all its activities must respect the basic dignity of the human person. Moreover, stigmatization of and discrimination against people who are HIV positive and those with AIDS form an obstacle we have to combat first to be able to combat the disease itself. The Secretaries-General of the United Nations emphasized in his speech on World AIDS Day, 1 December 1988, "our determination [is] that the world should make war *against AIDS* and *not* against *people* with AIDS".

One might say that we have learned from past experience how not to react to disease but not how to act. Typical reactions were often fear and rejection rather than measures needed to contain and control diseases, not to mention the respect of human rights of those affected by the disease. It is sufficient to remind ourselves that not long ago the death penalty was applied against persons whose only "crime" was a fatal or contagious disease. Punishment was used as if disease were a crime. Segregation, expulsion or detention of the sick was also frequent. The institution of quarantine has survived for centuries, and is sometimes proposed without a public health justification, as now in the case of AIDS. Plague barriers were used between countries in the 18th century, preventing passage for all except those with a certificate of good health. Similar certificates have been introduced today in the case of AIDS. There have been proposals to use old leper colonies for the interment of HIV-infected persons and people with AIDS. Such reactions testify to the fact that some of the fear and rejection that we know from history has survived. Conventional views die hard, and it is still sometimes heard that AIDS is a self-inflicted disease hence those affected should be punished and isolated rather than helped and supported.

Responses to AIDS have shown us that racism and racial discrimination are still unfortunately a long way from being eradicated. Racist interpretations of the origins and transmission of AIDS, and discriminatory practices applied with the pretext of combating AIDS, have to be combated.

AIDS-related discrimination has not been confirmed to the grounds, of race and provenance. Open discrimination against HIV-infected persons has been reported often. Discriminatory practices also target persons suspected of possible infection with HIV, and a wide circle of those subsumed under the notion of "high-risk groups". Rather than by their own behaviour, people have thereby been categorised according to the presumed risk that their belonging to, or identification with, a group entails. "High-risk groups" have been defined on the grounds of sexual preference, lifestyle, or racial or national origin. Such categorizations entail the narrowing of the range of rights the person belonging to them can exercise. Prostitutes or drug addicts, regularly exposed to rejection and stigmatizations, are often being victimized by repression and exclusion under the pretext of combating AIDS. This is not only an attack on basic human dignity but also it undermines efforts to reach these people and solicit their co-operation in combating AIDS which is Indispensable in the strategy to prevent and control AIDS.

Such limitations of human rights have sometimes been justified by the false dilemma between the "rights of the few" and the "rights of the many". It has long been recognizeed in human rights that trade-offs undermine their very basis. In fact, international human rights law sets very strict conditions for restrictions in the enjoyment of human rights. Thus one cannot respect some rights at the expense of others, nor can one respect the rights of some while denying that others have equal rights. To justify AIDS-related discrimination a conflict was claimed to exist between the rights of the "uninfected majority" and the rights of those infected with HIV or ill with AIDS. Consequently, the rights of persons infected with HIV and AIDS patients were restricted or denied altogether. This dees not represent a conceptual conflict between rights of some and rights of others, but between the recognition of human rights of all human beings and their denial.

Virtually all human rights are touched upon in the responses to AIDS and this raises complex problems. The scope of human rights which seems to have been jeopardized by various responses to AIDS is large indeed.

Most importantly, AIDS threatens human life. The right to life is the fundamental right and the obligation to protect it reaches far beyond prohibititions of international or arbitrary killings. The right to life entails the obligation of governments and of the international community to undertake al' the appropriate measures, to the utmost of their resources, to protect human lives. Difficult choices have been imposed on policy-makers by the transmission of the HIV infection through activities which are illegal in many countries, such as intravenous drug use. The spread of infection through the sharing of needles by intravenous drug users prompted some governments to supply safe injecting equipment to protect lives which would have otherwise been jeopardized. Though the free supply of sterile needles has not made the abuse of drugs, or access to them, easier, such actions have been criticized because of their negative effects on the programmes to curb drug abuse.

The right to life and the principle of non-discrimination are cornet-stones of international human rights law. Numerous restrictions on human rights and fundamental freedom have already been enacted in a number of countries on the grounds of the protection of public health. The protection of public health is recognized to be among the legitimate grounds for the restriction of human rights. Limitations placed upon privacy, freedom of movement or individual liberty are sometimes dictated by the need to protect public health. The requirements which such restrictions have to satisfy are determined in international human rights law. WHO has declared on many occasions that such restrictions are not necessary in the case of HIV/AIDS, that there is no public health rationale for the imposition of quarantine, isolation or compulsory screening or testing. The human rights bodies are now faced with the task of examining the legitimacy of these restrictions and their compatibility with existing human rights standards.

The protection of privacy has been jeopardized by the introduction of compulsory screening and testing, and by the establishment of registers of HIV-infected persons. This has often led to restrictions of the right to work, to freedom of movement and residence, even to access to health care for HIV-infected people.

Moreover, HIV-infected persons have sometimes been

deprived of their liberty. This may develop into indefinite detention, and even deprivation of their liberty for the rest of their lives. The United Nations human rights bodies have been dealing with legal safeguards against arbitrary and unlawful detention and these now need to be examined in the context of HIV/AIDS. If HIV-infected persons are placed in detention this may constitute administrative detention without charge or trial in violation of the existing human rights norms.

International migration and travel have been severely affected by responses to HIV/AIDS. These include restrictions on the freedom of movement, exclusion of HIV-infected persons from certain countries, or the use of compulsory tests to deport, exclude or detain HIV-positive persons, usually but not exclusively non-citizens. These measures raise a range of human rights issues, and necessitate tackling the complex area of the rights of aliens. Though these restrictions have often been invoked on public health grounds, WHO is consistently repeating that there is no public health rationale for them. No screening of international travellers can prevent the introduction or spread of HIV infection. Moreover, these measures may breach the nondiscrimination principle and violate the rights of those targeted by them.

Children who got the infection from their mothers, most often before they were born, represent a challenge to our ability to respond to their needs while recognizing their rights. The number of children born infected with HIV is expected to increase to 10 million by the year 2000, but our response has not yet matched the challenge this perinatal transmission of HIV poses. Transmission of HIV from infected mothers to their children brought up dilemmas in a wide area of our work, from family planning to maternal and child health care and to the recently adopted Convention on the Rights of the Child.

Combating AIDS is not confined to the circle of medical experts, scientists, government officials and health personnel. Everybody needs to be involved in the programme to prevent and control AIDS. The Global AIDS Strategy is based on the prevention of the further spared of HIV infection, using information and education as the main instruments to achieve changed and responsible behaviour. The challenge of AIDS has revealed the necessity of strengthening primary health care, and of setting up the basic infrastructure where it does not exist. An unprecedented international mobilization and co-operation in the past couple of years has demonstrated the ability of the international community to act. This assistance for the prevention and control of AIDS has reached an unprecedented level and is still increasing. It is carried out through technical assistance to all the developing countries which need and request it. As human rights have been included as a complement and reinforcement of public health principles, assistance provided within the Global AIDS Strategy has included promotion of human rights. Our Programme of Advisory Services and Technical Assistance in Human Rights has recently been further expanded to include the subject-matter of HIV/AIDS and human rights.

The importance of promoting human rights in the area of health cannot be over-emphasized. AIDS presents a challenge because responses to it have affected all human rights and fundamental freedoms; thereby it also represents an opportunity to reaffirm and reinforce human rights standards as they relate to HIV/AIDS and to the entire field of health.

C. HIV/AIDS AND HUMAN RIGHTS: POINTS FOR CONSIDERATION

The participants considered the breadth of the ethical and human rights issues raised by HIV/AIDS, and of the international human rights instruments and standard relevant to this subject. They considered for example the relevance of the International Covenant on Economic Social and Cultural Rights as well as the International Convent on Civil and Political Rights, the International Convention on the Elimination of All Forms of Racial Discrimination and the Convention on the Elimination of All Forms of Discrimination against Women, and other relevant instruments, including the numerous conventions and recommendations adopted under the auspices of the International Labour Organisation.

The participants were assised by a background paper which outlined some, but by no means all, of the human rights issues raised by HIV/AIDS.

I

1. AIDS represents an urgent worldwide problem with broad social, cultural, economic, political, ethical and legal dimensions.
2. The Global AIDS Strategy developed by WHO and endorsed by United Nations General Assembly has three objectives:
   (a) to prevent HIV infection;

(b) to reduce the personal and social impact of HIV infection;

(c) to unify national and international efforts against AIDS.

3. In the realization of these three objectives, human rights must be respected and discrimination must be prevented.
4. International human rights instruments, including regional arrangements and treaties, and the decisions of courts and bodies established thereunder, provide a framework within which measures to limit the spread of HIV should formulated.

II

The following measures are among those which appear consistent with international human rights standards:

A. With respect to the right to marry and to found a family, the provision of pre and post-marriage information on HIV/AIDS and counselling of a non-directive, non-coercive nature, and the other or voluntary HIV tests to marriage candidates, soon to comply with international human rights standards.

B. Measures based on the explicit, free and informed consent of the persons concerned seem to comply with international human rights standards; for example;

(a) the voluntary testing of individuals for HIV infection, anonymously or otherwise, with stringent safeguards for confidentiality.

(b) the counselling of individuals, both before and after they are tested;

(c) voluntary treatment to mitigate the effects of HIV infection;

(d) voluntary modifications of the behaviour of HIV-infected individual, designed to prevent the transmission of the virus.

III

The following measures should be reviewed in the light of relevant international human rights standards;

(a) the mandatory testing of any individuals (other than voluntary donors of blood, semen, or other issues or organs) for HIV infection, however selected;

(b) the compulsory registration of HIV-infected persons;

(c) the mandatory collection, strong and processing by a public authority of identifiable personal information about HIV-infected persons or those with AIDS without protecting the information concerned by the strictest rules of medical confidentially or by anonymity;

(d) the disclosure of the results of HIV tests to third persons (including health professionals without the patient's consent) or permitting the improper discovery of such results by third persons (see below; point K);

(e) enforced admission to a hospital or hospice of such persons (see below, point J);

(f) compulsory isolation, quarantine or internment in a colony of such persons removed from the rest of society (see below; point J).

IV

A. Discrimination on the grands of HIV/AIDS in areas such as access to education, employment, housing, has to be examined from the viewpoint of applicable international human rights standards.

B. The right to marry and found a family may be affected by:
   (a) compulsory HIV tests for persons who wish to marry;
   (h) mandattory abortion for or sterilizations of HIV-infected women;

C. HIV/AIDS also affects the rights of children. Particular issues which need to be examined include, inter alia;
   (a) the rights of children to information and education to enable them to protect themselves and others against HIV infection;
   (b) the difficulties of providing care and support for HIV-infected children or children from HIV-infected families, especially those who lose one or both parents.

D. HIV/AIDS also raises special concerns about human right; of women. These include, inter *alia*
   (a) vulerability of women to HIV infection because of this disadvantaged position in the family and society;
   (b) issues related to pregnancy in the context of HIV/AIDS;
   (c) feminization of poverty and its relationship to prostitution

E. The right of HIV-infected people and those with AIDS to public social.security, social and medical assistance, or social welfare services needs to be analysed from the viewpoint of applicable international human rights standards.

F. The right to freedom of movement has been affected:
  (a) when the entry into a country of its own nationals is conditional ran their taking an HIV test, or obtaining negative result;
  (b) when the entry of aliens who would be otherwise admissible has been restricted on the grounds of HIV/AIDS status.
  (c) when the entry of aliens has been restricted on HIV/AIDS grounds, this interferes with their enjoyment of other rights guaranteed to them by the applicable international human rights standards.
  (d) by cases of expulsion on the grounds of HIV/AIDS status only;
  (e) by cases of restrictions of liberty of movement within the territory of a State or the freedom to choose a residence for nationals or for aliens lawfully within that territory.

G. The denial of admission attendance or exclusion from school of sorneone solely on the ground that he or she is HIV infected needs to be examined from the viewpoint of international human rights standards relating to education.

H. The denial of work, or refusal of employment or dismissal of an employee solely on the ground that he or she is-or is suspected of being—HIV infected needs to be examined from the viewpoint of international human rights standards relating to work and of the public health rationale for any restrictions considered. Compulsory or routine pre-employment or post-employment HIV testing need particular attention.

I. The right to privacy of the individuals needs to e examined in the following circumstances:
  (a) when the prevalence of HIV in the existing population is estimated by unlinked asonymous keeping. This is an epidemiological technique whereby samples of blood specimen that have been take from individual for other legitimate purposes is made completely anonymous ("unlinked") so as to make it impossible to relate the sample back to the individual from whom it was taken;
  (b) when AIDS or HIV infection is made a notifiable disease by law, provided that the information reported is either wholly anonymous in the first place, or is protected by

the strictest compliance with rules of medical confidentiality—that is, that it would only be released either anonymously, or with the express and informed consent of the person to whom it relates.

K. The following measures which sometimes appear necessary to protect the rights of others may be considered provided that the person concerned is counselled, refuses to co-operate, and all persuasion failing, that the least restrictive measure is applied and, where relevant, a procedure for its revocation established. These measures included, for example:

(a) in the case of a high degree of risk of the transmission of HIV, informing the person at risk of the patient's known HIV status, provided that the circumstances in which this is allowed are either clearly defined by law or can be legally justified;

(b) the application of restrictive measures against an HIV-infected person who refuses to take preventive measures so as not spread the infection.

D. INTERNATIONAL CONSULTATION ON AIDS AND HUMAN RIGHTS (Geneva, 26-28 July 1989)

Background Document

1. Introduction

1.1. The World Health Organization, which has as its primary function under Article 2 (e) of its Constitution to act as the directing and co-ordinating authority on international health world, has a particular concern in the interests of public health, that AIDS and HIV infection should be approached from a social as well as a medical point of view. The protection of the rights and dignity of HIV-infected persons and persons with AIDS is an integral part of the WHO Global AIDS Strategy.

1.2. WHO is therefore seeking a consensus to affrin at this protection is offered by the existing international human rights instruments, which should consequently govern the public health policies and practices with government; might wish to adopt in order lo limit the spread of HIV infection and AIDS within their populations.

1.3. AIDS is essentially a matter falling within the specialized expertise of medical science and public health and therefore within the direct remit of WHO. The protection of human rights is one of the main purposes of the United Nations under its Charter and hence directly concerns WHO as a specialized agency (Articles 56 and 5). The human rights provisions of the Charter of the United Nations are elaborated in the International Bill of Human Rights as well as in over first other instruments. These are interpreted and supervised by the United Nations as well as other responsible bodies. It is the purpose of this document to outline and propose a resolution to some of the important human rights questions.

2. Definitions

2.1. The term human immunodeficiency virus (HIV) is used for the virus that causes AIDS (acquired immunodeficiency syndrome). HIV has replaced earlier names for the virus (HTLV-III, LAV) and in this document includes all related viruses (HIV-I and HIV-II). The term aids refers either to the specific clinical entity, the acquired immunodeficiency syndrome, or to the entire spectrum of pathological manifestations associated with HIV infection, and is so used in this document.

2.2. HIV-infected persons include al individuals, regardless of their clinical status, who are infected with HIV, as shown by confirmed positive serological tests.

3. HIV/AIDS

3.1 The epidemic of AIDS is a global health problem of extraordinary scale and extreme urgency. It represents an unprecedented challenge to the public health services of virtually every country in the world.

3.2. AIDS is caused by a newly recognized retrovirus called human immunodeficiency virus (HIV). One of the primary targets of HIV are T4 helper cells, a subpopulation of lymphocytes that are essential to the body's defence against disease. HIV infects and kills T4 helper cells, thus disrupting communication within the cellular and humoral immune system and progressively disabling the body's defence against disease.

3.3. At the present stage of the HIV pandemic, asymptomatic infection with HIV is far more common than AIDS. But HIV infection can progress and result in a wide range of adverse clinical manifestations. Clinical classification of disease associated with HIV infection includes AIDS-related complex (ARC), full-blown AIDS, including, HIV-neurological disease.

3.4. HIV has been isolated from blood, semen, vaginal secretions, saliva, tears, breast milk, and urine and is likely to be present in other body fluids, secretions, and excretions. However, despite this wide distribution, extensive laboratory and epidemiological studies indicate that only blood, semen, and vaginal/ cervical secretions are important in the transmission of HIV. These studies have repeatedly documented only three routes of HIV transmission: sexual, by heterosexual or homosexual intercourse; parenteral, by blood products including transfusion of unscreened blood and the use of inadequately sterilized syringes and needles; and parenteral, from an infected mother to her foetus or infant. There is no evidence to suggest that HIV can be transmitted by other routes, such as respiratory or enteric routes, or by casual person-to-person contact in any setting, including household, social, work, school or prison environments. There is very small risk of transmission possible through participation in sports, especially combative sports with direct body contact and other sports where bleeding may be expected to occur. There is no evidence that HIV transmission involves insects, food, water, toilets, swimming pools, sweat, tears, shared eating and drinking utensils or other items such as secondhand clothing or telephones. After infection, most persons develop detectable antibodies against HIV within the first three months.

3.5. The incubation period between infection and the development of AIDS is long (an average of 8 years). Because HIV infection is presumably lifelong, the risk of illness may continue throughout the infected person's life. While infected persons may be a sympromatic for long periods, they are nevertheless capable of transmitting HIV. Infected persons are likely to be highly infectious to others at the earliest moments of infection, before the immune system has been fully activated and particularly before antibodies are detected, as well as during the symptomatic period. Owing to the long incubation period, the number of reported AIDS cases provides at best an inaccurate and at worst a misleadingly optimistic view of the real extent and intensity of HIV infection. Therefore, even if transmission were to cease immediately, clinical cases of AIDS would constitute a major and increasing public health problem for years to come.

3.6. WHO estimates that between 5 million to 10 million persons are currently infected with HIV. The cumulative number of AIDS cases globally may exceed one million by 1991. At present these cases cannot be prevented from occurring because most will occur among persons already infected with HIV. In addition, reticence in reporting cases from some areas as well as under-recognition and under-reporting to national authorities have meant that the number of reported AIDS cases represents only a fraction of the total number of cases. Who considers the number of countries officially reporting cases (151 as of August 1989) to be more indicative of the geographical extent of the HIV pandemic than the number of reported cases, and more relevant to an assessment of its scope.

3.7. Although the modes of HIV transmission are constant, four broad yet distinct global epidemiologic patterns of HIV infection can be recognized.

3.8. In the first pattern (I). Most cases occur among homosexual or bisexual males and urban intravenous drug users. Heterosexual transmission is responsible for only a small percentage of cases, but it is increasing. Transmission due to blood and blood products occurred between the late 1970s and early 1980s, but has now been largely controlled, at least in developed countries, through the self-referral of persons with known risk factors or behaviour and by routine blood screening for HIV antibodies; inadequately sterilized injection equipment, other than that used by intravenous drug users, is not a significant factor in HIV transmission. The male/female sex ratio ranges from 10:1 to 15:1. Mother-to-infant transmission does occur but the number of HIV-infected infants is low owing to the relatively low number of women currently infected. The overall prevalence of HIV infection in the general population is estimated to be less than 1% but it has been reported to exceed 50% among persons who practise high-risk behaviour, such as men with multiple male sex partners and intravenous drug users. This first pattern is typical for industrialized countries with a large number of reported AIDS cases, including North America, most western European countries, Australia and New Zealand.

3.9. In the second pattern (II), most cases occur among heterosexuals. The male female ratio is approximately 1:1, and as a result mother-to-infant transmission is common. Intravenous drug use and homosexual transmission are either nonexistent or occur at a very low level. Because of the high number of HIV-infected women, perinatal transmission is common. In a number of countries it is estimated that the prevalence of HIV infection in the overall population is more than 1%, and that in some urban areas up to 25% of certain segments of the young and middle-aged adult population (15-49 years of age) are infected. Transmission through contaminated blood remains a significant problem in countries that have not yet implemented nationwide blood donor screening. In addition, the use of inadequately sterilized needles and syringes, or any other skin-piercing instruments, is considered an important public health problem. This second pattern is currently observed in sub-Saharan Africa and parts of the Caribbean.

3.10. In the third pattern (II), extensive spread of HIV commenced around the late 1970s or early 1980s. Initially, the Burden of HIV infection was more or less confined to homosexual men with multiple sexual partners, self-injecting drug users sharing injection equipment, as well as recipients of HIV-contaminated blood or blood products. In the middle to late 1990s, increasing transmission among heterosexuals with multiple sex partners has been noted to the extent that the latter mode of HIV transmission. As a result, the male/female ratio of recent HIV infection has been found in some pattern I/II areas, the predominant mode of HIV transmission. As a result, the male/female ratio of recent HIV infection has been found in some patter I/II areas to be close to equal. As more heterosexual transmission occurs, an increasing number of paediatric AIDS cases resulting from transmission from an infected mother to her foetus or infant can be expected in these areas.

3.11. those areas where HIV has only been introduced in the early to mid-1980s or early 1980s. Initially, the burden of HIV infection was more or less confined to homosexual men with multiple sexual partners, self-injecting drug users sharing injection equipment, as well as recipients of HIV-contaminated blood or blood products. In the middle to late 1980s, increasing transmission among heterosexuals with multiple sex partners has been noted to the extent that the latter mode of HIV transmission has increasingly become, in pattern I/II areas, the predominant mode of HIV transmission. As a result, the male/ female ratio of recent HIV infection has been found in some pattern I/II areas to be close to equal. As more heterosexual transmission occurs, an increasing number of paediatric AIDS cases resulting from transmission from an infected mother to her foetus or infant can be expected in these areas.

3.11. Those areas where HIV has only been introduced in the early to mid-1980s form the fourth pattern (III). Only a small number of AIDS cases have so far been reported from these areas (Eastern Europe, the Far East, the Near and Middle East, North Africa. Southeast Asia. and most of the Pacific). Cases have been recorded among homosexuals/bisexuals and self injecting drug users; heterosexual transmission and transmission through blood transfusion or blood products have also occurred. Cases have mostly occurred in persons who have travelled to higher prevalence areas or those who could have acquired the infection from such persons.

3.12. Testing for HIV infection is carried out through HIV antibody assays. The techniques used, when performed by experienced technicians, are very accurate in detecting antibodies either to the whole virus or to its subcomponents. However, the ideal of 100% sensitivity (all true positives correctly identified) and 100% specificity (all true negatives correctly identified) will not be achieved in practice.

3.13. Depending on the sensitivity and specificity of the particular test used. HIV tests may thus sometimes produce a "false positive" result-that its, appear to show that a patient is HIV positive when he or she has not in fact been infected by the virus; or they may produce a "false negative" result- that is, appear to show that a patient is HIV negative when he or she has in fact been infected by the virus and has already started to develop antibodies. The earliest tests produced a high proportion of false positives and also some false negatives, because they could not detect the early production of antibodies. The best tests currently in use give accurate results in over 99% of cases if performed by experienced technicians.

3.14. In developed countries the cost of HIV tests is significant but not prohibitive. But in a country lacking resources, it may be so high that testing many people could absorb a substantial part of the resources available for health services, and in extreme cases distort the health budget, which may result in an increase in the number of premature deaths from other causes. However, the cost of tests has decreased substantially during the past years and may become even lower.

4. WHO-The Global AIDS Strategy

4.1. In late 1985, as the global scope and impact of HIV infection and AIDS was just being discovered, WHO initiated the development of the global strategy for the prevention and control of AIDS. This strategy was reviewed, revised and discussed widely in 1986 and served as the basis for initial WHO action against AIDS. The Global AIDS Strategy was then unanimously approved and adopted as the foundation for global action by the World Health Assembly (Geneva, May 1987), the Venice Summit of the Heads of State or Government (Venice, June 1987), the Economic and Social Council of the United Nations (Geneva, June/July 1987), the United Nations General Assembly (New York, October 1987) and the World Summit of Ministers of Health on Programmes for AIDS Prevention (London, January 1988). Thus the Global AIDS Strategy has been supported by every nation, the human and financial resources required to begin implementing this strategy have been mobilized, and the result has replaced the chaotic anxiety of the early 1980s with the structured, purposeful and increasingly powerful work of national and international AIDS prevention and control.

4.2 The Global Strategy establishes basic principles for national and international AIDS prevention and control, based firmly upon knowledge of HIV virology and epidemiology and is derived from broad and practical experience with programmes to control infectious diseases. Therefore the Global AIDS Strategy provides the necessary framework, within which each country can develop its own detailed programme.

4.3 The Global AIDS Strategy has three objectives:

(a) To prevent HIV infection;
(b) To reduce the personal and social impact of HIV infection;
(c) To unify national and international efforts against AIDS.

4.4. The first objective is straightforward and clear: as drugs to cure HIV infection are not available, as infection with HIV is likely to be lifelong, and given its extremely serious personal and social consequences, it is essential to prevent new HIV infections. The second objective involves support and care for those who are already HIV-infected, regardless of whether they are presently healthy or have developed illnesses associated with HIV infection, including AIDS. The support and care of HIV-infected persons is not only humane, it is vital for the success of prevention and control programmes. The third objective arises directly from the special and global nature of this problem and reflects the realities of the modern world, in which AIDS cannot be controlled in any country unless it is controlled in every country.

4.5. In the realization of each of these objectives, human rights must be respected and discrimination must be prevented. There is no public health rationale to justify isolation, quarantine or other discriminatory measures based solely on a person's infection status. Therefore discrimination against HIV-infected persons threatens not only human rights, but effective prevention of the spread of HIV. We have seen all over the world that as people are informed about AIDS, panic and groundless fears recede. As leaders speak knowledgeably and clearly about AIDS, public confidence and commitment increase and illusory and simplistic solutions to the problems of AIDS are rejected.

5. The Public Health Rationale

5.1. In resolution WHA 41.24, adopted on 13 May 1988, the Forty-first World Health Assembly requested the Director-General to take all measures necessary to advocate the need to protect the human rights and dignity of HIV-infected people with AIDS, and of members of population groups. The resolution stressed to the Member States and all others concerned the danger to the health of all of discriminatory action against and stigmatization of HIV-infected people and people with AIDS as well as members of population groups. A similar statement is included in the London Declaration on AIDS prevention.

5.2. There is a strong and clear public health rationale for this emphasis on the protection of the human rights and dignity of HIV-infected persons, including people with AIDS. In fact the World Health Assembly has stated that this policy is critical to the success of national and international AIDS prevention programmes. Therefore the protection of the rights and dignity of HIV-infected persons is an integral part of the Global AIDS Strategy.

5.3. The first objective of the Global AIDS Strategy is to prevent HIV transmission. HIV spreads almost entirely through identifiable behaviour and specific actions (sexual intercourse, self-injecting drug use) which are generally - though not always-subject to individual control. In most instances, HIV transmission involves the behaviour of two persons; a change in behaviour of either the HIV-infected or the uninfected person will be sufficient to prevent HIV transmission. However, it must be remembered that HIV is transmitted mainly through behaviour which is private, secret, hidden from society and illegal in some societies.

5.4. For these reasons, the following are critical elements in the design of programmes to prevent HIV infection:

(a) The keystone of HIV prevention is information and education, as HIV transmission can be prevented through informed and responsible behaviour;

(b) Each person, HIV infected or uninfected, must bear in mind his responsibility not to put himself or other persons at risk of infection with HIV;

(c) In addition to information and education, specific health and social services will be required to support risk-reducing behaviour changes.

5.5. If HIV infection or suspicion of HIV infection leads to stigmatization and discrimination (e.g. loss of employment or housing forced separation from family), persons already infected and those who an afraid that they may be infected will avoid contact with health and social services.

5.6. This contact is difficult even without discrimination, because the activities that create the highest risk for HIV transmission are intensely personal, private, and therefore usually hidden. Some of this behaviour is also disapproved of, or even illegal in some countries, which increases the likelihood of its being hidden, so the person concerned may already be experienced in avoiding detection. Fear of being reported or previous experience with breaches of confidentiality may well lead those most in need of information, education, and social services to distance themselves from the support that is available and to be less trusting of those who offer support. In this manner, educational outreach is weakened and the difficult task of preventing HIV infection is further complicated. In addition, as persons belonging to groups in which high risk activities are concentrated are often important participants in promoting behaviour change among their peers, to sever contact with them is to lose vital for the prevention and control of HIV infection and AIDS.

5.7. The same concept applies to the provision of care to those who are infected or ill with HIV. If persons who are infected or ill do not seek the best available information or health or social support, then both the individual and society suffer, because of the resulting inability of the public health services to provide the necessary assistance.

5.8. To present HIV infection effectively, persons whose behaviour increases their risk of exposure to HIV must be informed, educated and provided with health and social support. Persons suspected or known to be HIV-infected should remain integrated in society to the maximum possible extent and be helped to assume responsibility for preventing HIV transmission to others. Exclusion of these persons would be unjustified in public health terms and would undermine the public health programme to prevent HIV infection.

5.9. For those reasons, discrimination endangers public health, stigmatization itself represents a threat to public health. In summary, protecting the human rights and dignity of HIV- infected people, including people with AIDS, and members of population groups, is not a luxury- it is a necessity. It is not a question of the "rights of the many" against the "right of the few"; the protection of the uninfected majority depends upon and is inextricably bound with the protection of the rights and dignity of the infected persons.

5.10. The solution is to inform and educate not only the individuals with high-risk behaviour about prevention of HIV infection, but also the general public, health workers, people in the workplace and others in a position to create discrimination.

5.11. WHO believes that it will be essential for governmental and non-governmental organizations working in the human rights field to play an active and proactive role in this area. Such organizations, particularly at the national and local levels, must help prevent discrimination against HIV-infected persons, persons with AIDS or stigmatized population groups. An informed and alert human rights network can help through information and education about HIV and AIDS and through promotion of the human rights and dignity of all persons.

5.12. The policy of avoiding and overcoming AIDS-related discrimination also has a firm base in international human rights law and encompasses all human rights and fundamental freedoms and restrictions or limitations thereto. The Universal Declaration of Human Rights defines rights that are now being threatened by discriminatory reactions to AIDS, including the rights to housing, employment, education, access to medical care, and freedom of movement.

5.13. Furthermore, the Declaration states categorically that "everyone is entitled to all the rights and freedoms set forth in this Declaration, without distinction of any kind". Conventions and other human rights instruments that have been based on the Universal Declaration echo this principle of non-discrimination while giving legal substance so the specific rights that are their particular focus.

5.14. In the context of HIV/AIDS and human rights, a point needing special attention is the acceptance under international law that individual rights may be limited if to do so is genuinely in the interests of the community. General welfare, public health and rights and freedoms of others are three distinct grounds for restricting human rights, and a range of human rights and fundamental freedoms can be restricted invoking these grounds if respect for the principle of non-discrimination is maintained. In the interpretation and application of human rights law, restrictions on public health grounds are a rare exception. The vital importance of the public health rationale for avoiding AIDS-related discrimination is that it demonstrates not only that it is unnecessary to impose general limitations on human rights, but that it is likely to be counter productive to do so. It is important that "public health" not be used as a pretext to limit human rights unless based on a true public health rationale. An isolated example of individual rights being justifiably limited would be the extreme situation where one individual deliberately and purposefully set out to infect another. However, this has not been shown, anywhere, to be a sufficiently serious public health problem to warrant a general limitation on fundamental freedoms. International law and public health policy are therefore in agreement on the need for non discrimination and the protection of human rights and dignity.

6. Human Rights

6.1. The preamble to the Constitution of WHO declares that "the enjoyment of the highest attainable standard of health is one of the fundamental rights of every human being without distinction of race, religion, political belief, economic or social condition". This notion is also contained in Article 12 of the International Covenant on Economic, Social and Cultural Rights, where States parties to the Covenant recognize the right of everyone to the enjoyment of the highest attainable standard of physical and mental health and undertake steps to achieve the full realization of this right, including the prevention and control of epidemic diseases and the creation of conditions which would assure medical service and medical attention to all in the event of sickness.

6.2. Both the World Health Assembly and the International Conference on Primary Health Care held in Alma-Ata, USSR, in September 1978 have proclaimed the right to health in the context of "Health for All by the Year 2000" and WHO's principal effort towards the achievement of this right has been through its programmes. This can only be done through public health measures based on biomedical progress and an atmosphere of public comprehension. As the WHO Constitution itself declares that the right to health must be without discrimination, the member States of WHO have already accepted this principle in their mutual relationships.

76.3. Human rights in relation to health are covered by a wide spectrum of international instruments in addition to the WHO Constitution and the International Covenant on Economic, Social and Cultural Rights. In addition to the International Bill of Human

Rights, which includes the above Covenant, other instruments expressly cover the prevention of discrimination, human rights in the administration of justice, employment policy and social welfare, progress and development; all of which relate to concerns raised by HIV/AIDS. These instruments, in turn, involve other international organizations, particularly the human rights bodies of the United Nations family, as well as non-governmental organizations and other actors. WHO is seeking a broad coalition of all concerned for the purpose of bringing together the strengths of their disciplines to reaffirm the sound basis in international law for the prevention of discrimination and the protection of the rights that are threatened in the context of AIDS.

6.4. The International code of human rights law is laid down in a series of instruments, which, in addition to those already referred to, include; the United Nations Charter and other instruments adopted under the aegis of organizations of the United Nations family; regional instruments, including the American Declaration on the Rights and Duties of Man, the American Convention of Human Rights, the European Convention for the Protection of Human Rights and Social Charter as well as others covering specific rights in greater detail.

6.5. Apart from these instruments, there are other human rights of international purport, covering such matters as human experimentation and biomedical ethics. These issues will not be dealt with in this document, since they do not lend themselves to any solutions by the application of the existing norms and guidelines, and may therefore be better dealt with in other forums.

6.6. The international code of human rights law declares and protects some 40 to 50 different rights, each specifically defined, "for everyone... without distinction of any kind, such as race, colour, sex, language, religion, political or other opinion, national or social origin, property, birth or other status". Among these are:

(a) The right to life;
(b) The right to health;
(c) The right to liberty and security of person;
(d) Freedom from inhuman or degrading treatment or punishment;
(e) The right to freedom of movement;
(f) The right to privacy;
(g) The right to marry and to found a family,
(h) The right to work;
(i) The right to education;

(j) The right to social security, assistance and welfare.

6.7. The legal enforcement of this code, in the conventional sense of the term, leaves much to be desired, in the absence of a single compulsory jurisdiction with such powers. Nevertheless, methods for the monitoring and supervision of international human rights instruments are being developed by human rights bodies whose decisions are, in practice, followed by the States concerned. More than half of the world's sovereign States are bound by the two international Covenants and accept the jurisdiction of the supervisory organs which they establish. An increasing number of these States allow individual complaints to be directed to the Human Rights Committee established by the International Covenant on Civil and Political Rights.

6.9. In the code, certain rights are absolute, such as freedom from torture or inhuman or degrading treatment or punishment, and may not be derogated from under any circumstances even in time of war or of public emergency. Other rights are couched in the language of limitations and restrictions, in order to define their boundaries. In such case, the code declares a "core" right and hen proceeds to state that there shall be no interference with or restriction or limitation of this right unless provided for or prescribed by law and necessary in a democratic society for the protection of one or more of the specified public interests. Detailed conditions have been elaborated through the examination of States' reports, United Nations studies and the work of special rapporteurs.

6.10. Article 29 of the Universal Declaration of Human Rights contains the fundamental provision concerning restrictions of human rights. Individual articles of the two Covenants effectively apply and develop this general provision and indicate the fields in which exceptions may be permitted, for example, Articles 4, and 8.1 (a) of the international Covenant on Economic, Social and Cultural Rights and Articles 4,12.3, 13,18.3.21 and 22.2 of the International Covenant on Civil and Political Rights. The list of exceptions includes such items as national security, public order, safety and morals, the general welfare and the protection of the rights and freedoms of others. Most importantly, "public health" or what we may term here the "public health exception" is included as a measure restricting the exercise of a right or freedom with the intention of removing or reducing a claimed danger to public health.

6.11. Such a provision must not be understood, however, as taking away with one hand what has just been given with the other.

The existing case law has been unanimous in holding that any State wishing to justify and interference with, or limitation or restriction of, any declared "core" right has the burden of proving affirmatively that the restriction was: (a) prescribed by law, (b) necessary, (c) in a democratic society, (d) for the protection of one or other of the legitimate interests of society.

6.12. In the light of the above, we can consider the problems which the current and prospective spread of HIV/AIDS are likely to present in the context of human rights and what options may exist for their resolution. In doing so, account will need to be taken of the time span covering the post-war development of international human rights law.

6.13. At the time of the adoption of the Universal Declaration, in December 1948, shortly after the entry into force of the WHO Constitution, biomedical science was considerably less evolved than it is today. Isolation and quarantine remained a conventional technique for attempting to contain the international spread of disease, although many had already criticized such measures as largely illusory and ineffective. Indeed, had the HIV/AIDS pandemic occurred at the time, it would have been impossible with the technology of the period to identify the causative agent. Measures to prohibit discrimination against disabled persons were not introduced into the code until 1975 and there are still no express provisions covering the rights of the sick in relation to discrimination, save as regards

medical service and medical attention. With this in mind, the provisions of the code as a whole should be viewed in the light of present-day knowledge, that is to say that the public health exception should be viewed in the light of present-day knowledge, that is to say that the public health exception should be taken as applicable only in the light of actual medical justification and not merely as a means of assuaging unreasonable public fears and condemnations.

7. HIV/AIDS and Human Rights

7.1. In the Guidelines for the Development of a National AIDS prevention and Control Programme, WHO has stated the following:

Personal and public reaction to AIDS throughout the world has been of considerable depth and extent. Fear of AIDS and stigmatization of different groups (homosexual men, haemophiliacs, female prostitutes) have become common. Wherever those free from HIV feel threatened by those infected with HIV, especially where the latter are perceived to belong to a defined group such as homosexual and drug addicts, there may be calls for marking out and isolating those infected... As the toll of clinical diseases rises, there will be increasing pressure on the authorities to take further action and adopt approaches that may or may no be effective or have any rational justification.

7.2. In fact, what is critical for the control of any such infection is not whether it is endemic, epidemic, or (in the extreme case) pandemic, but how the infective vector travels from one person to another, for how long any given person is liable to remain infectous and whether at any given time there are any means either for protecting another person from the infection, or for combating the infection once he or she has acquired it.

7.3. HIV/AIDS bears little resemblance to previously known infections diseases. Unlike the vectors of other diseases, HIV is not transmitted through droplet infection, insect or other parasite infestations, polluted water or ordinary social contact. Morever, infected persons fall essentially into three groups: the sexual partners of infected individuals, those who receive contaminated injections or transfusion, and the babies of infected women. Where the incubation period - that is, the time between infection and the moment that the infected person begins to present unidentifiable symptoms - of most of the more common infectous diseases is measured in days or, at most, weeks, that for AIDS may be several years, during all of which time the carrier is potentially infectious.

7.4. The result of measures which do not reflect these considerations would be that those persons needing information, education, counselling or other support services would be driven underground". The person who fears he may be infected would be reluctant to seek assistance out of fear of being reported - with severe personal consequences. The net result would be to seriously jeopardize educational outreach and thereby exacerbate the difficulty of preventing HIV infection.

Policy options

7.5. WHO has reported that no region of the world is now free from AIDS. With no vaccine or cure yet available, all governments are therefore faced with the task of indentifying and adopting measures which offer a realistic prospect of limiting its spread within their populations. From the viewpoint of their impact on human rights, such measures may be most conveniently grouped into three categories:

(a) Measures which do not lend themselves easily to an

examination within the general human rights context, and are better dealt with individually;

(b) Measures which may have adverse effects and therefore can only be implemented with the explicit, free and informed consent of the individual concerned;

(c) Measures entailing some degree of direct or indirect compulsion.

7.6. Measures in the first category, which are not dealt with here, include the following:

(a) Research into the pathophysiology of the disease, its modes of transmission and the development of vaccine and curative drugs;

(b) Ensuring the safety of blood for transfusions, blood products for use in treatment, semen for artificial insemination, and other cells, tissues and organs for transplantation;

(c) Preventing the re-use of needles, syringes and other skin-piercing or invasive equipment without proper sterilization;

(d) Making safety devices, such as condoms, more widely available, especially to persons who practise high-risk behaviour;

(e) Facilitating access to sterile needles and syringes;

(f) Health information, education and promotion programmes, directed either at the general public or at groups particularly are risk- such as prostitutes of either sex, their clients, self injecting drug user, and homosexual and bisexual men.

7.7. Such measures raise legal and ethical issues, a number of which have been dealt with by WHO's Global Programme on AIDS in global and regional consultations and through consensus statements emerging therefrom.

7.8. Measures requiring explicit consent include:

(a) The voluntary testing of individuals for HIV infection either anonymously (that is, without being required to give a true name, or any other identifying particulars), or with stringent safeguards for confidentiality;

(b) Counselling of individuals, both before and (if the result is positive) after they are tested;

(c) Voluntary treatment to mitigate the effects of infection, or to achieve modification of their behaviour which they themselves desire; thus, for example, it should be "the responsibility of any athlete participating in a combative sport with direct body contact who has a wound or other skin lesion to report it immediately to a responsible official, and to report for medical attention, or of persons who know they are HIV-infected to seek medical counselling about further participation in sports".[1] These measure are recommended by public health experts. Provided that they are undertaken completely voluntarily- that is, after a full explanation of all the possible consequences, and with the explicit, free and informed consent of the person concerned, obtained without the application of any illicit pressures, whether in the form of promises or of threats - there can be no objection to them on human rights grounds. Therefore these need not be further considered herein.

Measures entailing compulsion

7.9. Compulsion may take many different forms. The most obvious is the use, or the threat of use, of direct force. But making an act (e.g. refusal or failure to undergo an HIV test) criminal is also a form of compulsion; as are express or implied threats of any kind- such as that the person concerned will be deprived of some benefit if he or she does not submit to the desired procedure. It is this group of measures which carries clear risks of violating human rights.

7.10. If we set aside extreme measures, such as the screening of a whole population for HIV antibodies, declared by WHO to be "unnecessary and unrealistic", we are left with a group of measures which may be feasible in practice and could therefore be realistically considered by public authorities, in order to impose some kinds of restriction on actual or potential HIV infected persons so as to minimize the likelihood of their passing their infection on to others. These restrictions, which are considered below, could be of several kinds.

7.11 Before any restriction can be imposed, one needs to identify the persons concerned. This can only be done by some kind of screening, either for one or more attributes regarded as indicators of probable infection, or by testing directly for actual infection. All the remaining measures therefore necessarily entail a direct or indirect assessment of the seropositivity of the persons concerned and the reporting of the result to someone else - as, for example by establishing registers of such persons, by making HIV infection a notifiable disease, or by compulsorily tracing and informing the sexual partners of HIV-infected persons.

7.12. Since it would never be possible in practice - let alone justifiable on either public health or human rights grounds - to carry out compulsory screening of the entire population of even a small nation, such screening has in practice concentrated on previously specified groups. For example:

(a) Persons thought to be at special risk of both acquiring the infection and passing it on to others, such as prostitutes of either sex, their clients, self-injecting drug users or homosexual or bisexual men;
(b) Persons - whether citizens or aliens - seeking entry at a frontier, port, or airport;
(c) Hospital patients;
(d) Persons wishing to marry;
(e) Prisoners;
(f) Persons engaged in various particularly sensitive occupations.

7.13. Restrictions which might be contemplated for those found to be HIV-infected include the following:

(a) Quarantine, isolation or detention;
(b) Refusal of entry into a country;
(c) Denial of marriage, employment, housing, social services, attendance at educational or other establishments, or of some other benefit.

It is necessary to distinguish here between those restrictions which constitute a denial of human rights, such as the right to marry, and those which do not constitute a denial of a human right, such as entry into a country for aliens. In the case of the former, the specific human right denied may be invoked, while with respect to the latter the best and often the only way to seek remedy is to seek the application of the principle of non-discrimination.

Testing the legitimacy of policies

7.14. The remainder of this document considers the legitimacy of the various permutations and combinations of these measures in different circumstances by reference to the international code of human rights law.

7.15. Where the code allows any restrictions of any of the human rights which in seeks to protect, such a restriction will only be considered justifiable under the following condition.

Testing the legitimacy of policies

(a) If determined by law;
(b) If necessary in a democratic society;

(c) If necessary for the protection of a "legitimate aim " which falls within one of the categories specifically listed in the relevant provisions of the applicable instrument.

7.16. The second of these requirements in turn entails that (a) there must be a "pressing social need"; and (b) the restriction must be "proportional", weighed both against its adverse effects on the persons on whom it is imposed and against the public interest in the free exercise of the right concerned.

7.17. For the first requirement- "determined by law" - the State concerned must enact, by the procedures normally required for that purpose under its constitution, legislation which satisfies the necessary criteria; the law concerned must be sufficiently accessible, clear and precise for the ordinary individual to be able to regulate his or her conduct accordingly. He or she must be able- if necessary with appropriate advice - to foresee, to a degree that is reasonable in the circumstances, the consequences which a given action might entail. It is hereafter assumed that any restrictions on human rights imposed by public authorities for the purpose of limiting the spread of HIV among their populations will satisfy this test.

7.18. The next question will be whether the restriction is designed to serve a "legitimate aim " for the protection of which restrictions on the right under consideration may be allowed in appropriate circumstances. Only two are relevant in the present context: the protection of the rights and freedoms of others and the protection of public health.

7.19. Among the rights and freedoms of others the most important one that needs to be considered here, at least so long as there is no cure for AIDS, is the right to life. Apart from the question of the sanctioning of certain forms of conduct in order to protect this right, in relation to AIDS this right can only impose on a State the obligation to take what measures it reasonably can to prolong the lives of its inhabitants where this can be done at a cost that is reasonable, both in terms of resources and restrictions on other human rights.

7.20. Since AIDS, once the full clinical syndrome has developed, is almost invariably fatal and since there is at present no known cure for it, every new HIV infection is a potential fatality and thereby threatens the right to life of the person infected. Accordingly, every measure which succeeds in reducing the spread of HIV will not only serve " the protection of public health", but will automatically serve to protect the right to life. If follows that it will be enough consider such measures under the aspect of the protection of public health and that it will be unnecessary to consider them separately from the point of view of the protection of the right to life, and so (with few exceptions) of "the protection of the rights and freedoms of others".

7.21. The final criterion for testing the legitimacy of such measures is proportionality of the balance between the benefits to be expected, their adverse consequences for the persons concerned, and the public interest in the free exercise of the right being restricted. All these need to be considered in light of the degree and the kind of a "pressing social need" presented to the Government of the State concerned.

7.22. This balance will therefore be the principal focus of any consideration of the human rights at issue. For this purpose, any views already expressed by responsible and reputable public be important, though not necessarily conclusive. These views may of course change hereafter, in light of the advancing knowledge and experience of the public health aspects of AIDS. The same human rights considerations apply to decisions of the international organs competent to interpret and apply human rights law. So far no case specifically about AIDS has been decided, and there are few in which restrictions upon human rights on public health grounds have been considered. Nevertheless, the examination of States' reports on the implementation of human rights treaties enables the human rights bodies to assess the compatibility of national laws and practices in the area of AIDS with the existing human rights standards.

8. Rights and Freedoms

8.1. The following analysis of HIV/AIDS-related measures in relation to human rights and freedoms is grouped under these main headings, which are not necessarily exclusive:

(a) The right to privacy;
(b) The right to liberty and security;
(c) The right to freedom of movement;
(d) The right to marry and to found a family;
(e) The right to work;
(f) The right to education;
(g) The right to social security, assistance and welfare;
(h) Freedom from inhuman or degrading treatment of punishment;
(i) The right to equal protection of the law;
(j) Public emergencies.

8.2. These rights and freedoms appear sometimes under virtually identical definitions and at others under different definitions in the international human rights instruments. For certain of them, such as the right to work, or the right to social security, assistance and welfare, the precise meaning of the formulation is controversial, or the circumstances under which the benefit is to be obtained not specified. Nevertheless, they are sufficiently general to serve as indicators for the consideration of measures taken on account of AIDS which might entail adverse consequences for the human rights of individuals.

A. The right to privacy

8.3. Under this heading is considered the impact of measures designed to limit the spread of HIV by screening for potential or actual HIV infection.

8.4. Several possible measures would necessarily entail interferences with the individual right to privacy, which the State concerned would need to justify under the established criteria. These measures include:

(a) Mandatory testing for HIV infection;
(b) Compulsory registration of persons considered likely to be infected with HIV, but who have not been tested;
(c) Mandatory collection, storage and processing by public authorities of personal information about those who are suspected of being infected or have been tested;
(d) Making AIDS, or HIV infection, a notifiable disease;
(e) Disclosure of test results, or of other personal information, to third parties;
(f) Criminalization of behaviour thought to be conducive to the spread of AIDS.

Routine screening

8.5. The WHO position on routine screening is the following:

Routine screening of high-risk groups (homosexuals and heterosexuals with multiple sexual contact and intravenous drug users), of other groups (military personnel, international travellers and hospital patients) and as a prerequisite for marriage is of little use in controlling or slowing down the AIDS epidemic.[2]

8.6. In any case, a negative HIV test gives no guarantee that the person tested is not a carrier of the virus: he or she might acquire the infection the following day, or night indeed have already become infected, but not yet have seroconverted.

8.7. Public health experts appear so far to have been unanimous in rejecting mandatory HIV screening as an efficacious means for reducing the spread of this infection- except in the case of voluntary donors of blood, semen, or other cells, tissues or organs. Some countries do not apply the "informed consent" requirement for blood donors, at least not in the way that "informed consent" is generally understood. In the view of the experts, efforts to compel testing would be counter-productive: knowledge that a test would be required would simply deter those who most need to be educated and counselled from seeking medical advice: HIV infection would effectively be driven underground, when the most pressing need is to bring it to the surface.

8.8. Instead, public health experts recommend a less coercive, and in their view more efficacious, alternative, namely increasing the availability of voluntary testing, together with a broadly based information and education campaign aimed at encouraging the abandonment of high-risk behaviour. The purpose is to identify infected persons- who might not otherwise change their behaviour because they do not know they present a risk- so they can be intensively counselled not to engage in behaviour that might be dangerous to others.

8.9. It is pertinent to note that the Committee of Ministers of the Council of Europe, explicitly taking into account the European Convention on Human Rights, has recommended that "there should be no compulsory screening (for HIV infection) of the general population nor of particular population groups" and that "health authorities should instead invest resources in the setting up of sites... for voluntary testing..."[3]

8.10. In the light of all these considerations it seems unlikely, in present circumstances, that any scheme for mandatory screening would satisfy the test of being "necessary in a democratic society" for the mandatory screening would satisfy the test of being "necessary in a democratic society" for the protection of public health; the interference with the right to privacy, and the severe adverse consequence which would flow it to the individuals concerned, and to society at large through he limitation placed on the right to privacy, would appear to outweigh any public health benefits which could reasonably be expected - if indeed any exist.

Compulsory registration of suspected HIV carriers

8.11. Manifestly, the entry of one's name on a register maintained by a public authority of what would effectively be regarded as a list of potential dangers to the community would be a grave violation of a person's privacy. Further, in order for such a measure to be effective, it would need to be enforced by law.

8.12. Such a measure could not pass the stringent tests implied in the phrase "necessary in a democratic society" without overwhelming evidence of its efficacy in public health terms. Coming from reputable public health experts. So fare as is known no such evidence exists. The State concerned would also need to show that no measures existed which had less dramatically adverse consequences for the persons concerned, or for society generally, or could be expected to have similarly beneficial results for public health. That burden too would be decidedly difficult to discharge.

Mandatory collection and storage of information

8.13. Scheme which include the mandatory collection, storage, and processing by a public authority of personal information about individuals suspected of or tested for HIV infection (including, for example, test results, and answers to questions about sexual activities, partners, and drug use) would involve a clear interference with the right to privacy- unless the information was protected by the strictest rules of medical confidentiality or by complete anonymity at the time of collection, so that it could never be traced back to an identifiable individual.

8.14. In order to justify such an interference, the State concerned would need once again to establish proportionality with a legitimate aim. In the case of mandatory collection and storage of information, however, it is not immediately clear what aim would be served.

8.15. If the collection is made by reference to identifiable individuals, and its purpose is to impose restrictions on some or all of them, then its establishment and maintenance would only be justified if both: (a) the obtaining of the information, by testing or by the creation of registers of potentially "dangerous" individuals, could be justified in its own right, which is unlikely to be the case; and (b) the restrictions themselves could be justified independently.

8.16. If, however, the only purpose of such information gathering would be to ascertain HIV prevalence or to study the epidemiology of HIV infection, this can be achieved far less intrusively by using only anonymous samples. Public health experts are in any case agreed that the assurance of anonymity is more conducive to securing compliance with testing schemes, and thereby make the information more reliable.

AIDS or HIV infection as a "notifiable disease"

8.17. Collecting and storing information is a consequence of making AIDS of HIV infection a "notifiable disease". There are two possible variants:

(a) To require notification to a public authority of all cases of AIDS or HIV infection as and when they become known, without any identifying particulars from which the patients could be traced, or else subject to the strictest rules of medical confidentiality; or

(b) Require medical practitioners, by law, to report to a public authority of all cases of the disease which they encounter among their patients, in what would otherwise be a breach of medical confidentiality- that is, with identifying particulars, and without adequate guarantees of confidentiality thereafter.

8.18. Here precisely the same considerations apply as in the general case considered in the previous Section. If identifying details are to be recorded, this clear interference with the right to privacy would have to be specifically justified, in the face of the accumulating evidence that it would deter some - perhaps many - possible HIV carriers from coming forward to be tested, knowing that their condition, if they were found to be HIV -infected would deter some- perhaps many-possible HIV carriers from coming forward to be tested, knowing that their condition, if they were found to be HIV-infected would be identifiably reported to a public authority.

8.19. However, if the entire scheme were subject to the strictest compliance with the general rules of medical confidentiality - or, better still, entailed only anonymous notification from the outset- there would be no obvious objections.

Disclosure of information

8.20. A policy permitting or requiring the disclosure of the results of HIV tests to third persons without consent, or which permits the improper discovery by third persons of those results, also amounts to an interference with privacy.

8.21. In order to justify such a policy, the State concerned would need to show that it was necessary for the protection of the rights of other (e.g. the patient's sexual partner(s), or his or her medical attendant, dentist, or other health workers) or, more generally, for the protection of public health. However, the available evidence suggests that such a policy is not effective. Ever since special clinics were established in many countries at the beginning of this century to deal with sexually transmitted diseases, it has been recognized that a guarantee of confidentiality is an indispensable condition for encouraging people to seek treatment, and thus reduce the spread of these diseases.

8.22. This is particularly true in the case of AIDS, where one wants to prevent infected persons from "going underground", out of the mainstream of health care and education. Current health practice is to protect the privacy of the infected individual and to maintain the strictest confidentiality concerning his or her medical records.

8.23. Breach of confidentiality might, be warranted in exceptional circumstances - where, for example despite counselling and advice, the patient continues to have unprotected sexual intercourse with his or her partner, having been warned by the doctor both of the dangers of doing so and of the doctor's intention to make the disclosure if the patient does not; of if the patient is a health worker and is consistently negligent in observing routine hygiene precautions, or fails to follow medical advice about his or her work. If doctors were allowed to breach confidentiality in such circumstances, this would of course have to be defined with sufficient precision to comply with the requirement that the interference with privacy be "in accordance with the law".

Criminalization of behaviour

8.24. In some jurisdictions, consideration has been given to the imposition of penal sanctions on persons exposing other to HIV, whether intentionally or recklessly. Such action might be taken under the general criminal law, laws relating to sexually transmitted disease, or under specially adopted legislation.

8.25. Such prosecutions would have an impact on privacy rights and their application would pose difficult problems of proof, but might be held to be justifiable on the grounds of the protection of public health, or of the rights and freedoms (and especially the right to life) of others, provided that the offence could be defined sufficiently precisely to meet the requirements of legal certainty and foreseeability. It is an elementary proposition not only of international human rights law, but of virtually all domestic legal systems, that the ingredients of any criminal offence must be sufficiently precise for any person contemplating the commission of a particular act not to be in any doubt as to whether or not that act is criminal.

8.26. Accordingly, the definition of any such offence would have to specify clearly how the accused may be held accountable. This would necessitate proving the following:

(a) The accused knew that he or she was HIV infected;
(b) The accused knew that his or her actual conduct carried a substantial risk of infecting another person;
(c) It was this conduct which in fact infected that other person;
(d) The other person did not give knowing consent to the risk of being infected.

8.27. WHO believes that such cases will be rare. Few human beings set out intentionally to kill another and it cannot be assumed that HIV-infected persons will act irresponsibly. The important point is that voluntary compliance, voluntary control, voluntary behaviour change and voluntary testing must constitute the policy to control the spread of HIV. This approach has been effective and must be continued.

B. The right to liberty and security

8.28. In order to determine whether the protection of the international human rights instruments applies to the deprivation of liberty, account must be taken of a whole range of criteria such as the type, duration, effects and manner of implementation of the measure in question.

8.29.Once there has been a lawful deprivation of liberty, mere modifications of the conditions of detention- such as isolation imposed on a prisoner as a disciplinary measure - will not be regarded as constituting independent deprivations of liberty. Such treatment may, however, raise an issue of compliance with the right not to be subjected to inhuman or degrading treatment (see below).

8.30. The following possible public health measures would appear to involve a deprivation of liberty:

(a) Compulsory quarantine, e.g. by enforced confinement or isolation in a hospital or hospice;
(b) Compulsory internment in a colony removed from the rest of society.

8.31. Such measures would then have to satisfy the test that they are not arbitrary, but are taken on a ground, and in accordance with a procedure, established (or prescribed) by law.

8.32. In order to justify the measures under consideration, the State concerned would have to establish:

(a) In the case of compulsory blood testing, that it was necessary to prevent the spread of HIV infection;
(b) In the case of detention, both that the individual concerned

has the infection and that his or her detention was necessary for the prevention of its spread.

8.33. The views of public health experts on the effectiveness of compulsory blood testing as a measure to prevent the spread of HIV infection have been set out above and do not need to be repeated here suffice it to say that they make it extremely doubtful that such a measure could be justified under international human rights law.

8.34. WHO has expressed the firm view that detention of any kind is not warranted for the prevention and control of the spread of AIDS:

There is no public health rationale to justify isolation (or) quarantine... based solely on the fact that a person is suspected or known to be HIV spreads almost entirely through identifiable behaviour and specific actions which are subject to individual control. In most instances, the active participation of two people is required for HIV transmission, such as in sexual intercourse and in sharing contaminated needles or syringes... HIV infection is not spread through casual contact, routine social contact in school, the workplace or public places, nor through water or food, eating utensils, coughing or sneezing, insects, toilets or swimming pools.[4]

8.35. Moreover, WHO has adopted, within its recommended strategy for the prevention of the spread of HIV, the following principle:

Persons suspected or known to be HIV transmission to others. Exclusion of persons suspected or known to be HIV infected would be unjustified in public health terms and would seriously jeopardize educational and other efforts to prevent the spread of HIV.[5]

8.36. There would appear to be no public health justification for a policy of compulsory segregation or isolation of prisoners who are known or suspected to be HIV infected or who have AIDS, either in a separate unit or in single cells. If such restrictions are imposed on the prisoner's already limited liberty, they are not to be considered as independent deprivations of liberty, but ought to be considered under the right to liberty Moreover, they may be open to challenge on the ground that they amount to inhuman or degrading treatment.

8.37. There may be an exception in the case of a genuine emergency- for example if someone known to be, or suspected on cogent grounds of being infected with HIV is found bleeding copiously and so presents an acute risk of infecting others, and is unable to take care of himself or herself.

8.38. Another exception might be conceivable in the case of a person so disturbed or embittered by the knowledge of HIV infection that, despite intensive counselling, he or she insists on deliberately infecting others.

8.39. In either of these cases, such a person's detention might be justified, in the one case until the immediate emergency is over, and in the other until there is no further risk of conduct likely to infect others. However, it should be noted that in the case of any detention, all the relevant international instruments require strict judicial control: the detainee must be entitled to take proceedings before a court in which the lawfulness of this detention can be decided without delay (or "speedily"), and release can be ordered if the detention is not lawful.[6]

C. The right to freedom of movement

8.40. Freedom of movement comprises an interrelated cluster of issues: Entry into a country; abode and movement within a territory; expulsion from a country and leaving a country. Each of these is regulated differently as between nationals of the State concerned and aliens (i.e. non-nationals).

8.41. The present text deals with the first three in order to assess the extent to which, if at all a State might legitimately impose controls on entry into its territory of those who are HIV infected, restrict their movement within the country, or permit or require their expulsion from it.

8.42. The right to enter a country is confined to nationals of the State concerned; nowhere in any international human rights treaty has any State accepted an express obligation to allow aliens to enter its territory.

8.43. For nationals, the right to enter is absolute and not subject to any restrictions. It could not, therefore, be legitimate for a State to make the entry into the country of its own returning nationals conditional on their taking an HIV test, let alone on obtaining a negative result.

8.44. By contrast, States enjoy a wide discretion over the entry of aliens. The choice of grounds for exclusion is largely a matter for decision by each State. This does not, however, mean that there are no restrictions on a State's ability to control entry for purposes of work, travel, or immigration. Rules of general international law have made a limited impact on this broad power, in particular by affirming the principle of non-discrimination.

8.45. For states, further restrictions are derived from specific treaty obligations, as for example in health matters under WHO

Internationa' Health Regulations or, more generally, in respect of other rights guaranteed under other aspect of other rights law, such as respect for family life.

8.46. It is not the case, therefore, that the entry of all aliens into a country could be made contingent upon production of a certificate of freedom from HIV infection, or submission to an HIV test. Such a requirement could only be imposed in such cases where the State could establish that it was necessary for the protection of public health.

8.47. WHO has stated: Since HIV infection is already present in every region and in virtually every major city in the world, even total exclusion of all travellers (foreigners and citizens travelling abroad) cannot prevent the introduction and spread of HIV.[7]

Hundreds of millions of persons cross international borders each year, by boat, air, rail, motor vehicle and foot, and any screening programme for international travellers would present immense problems.

8.48. The freedom to choose a residence within the territory of a State and to move about freely within that State is guaranteed to nationals and aliens alike, but may be restricted on the usual grounds, including public health. It complements the protection afforded by the right to liberty of the person.

8.49. Any such restriction would have to be strictly justified as being necessary in a democratic society for the protection of public health. However, public health experts have counselled against the introduction of such measures, and thereby their necessity has been called into question.

8.50. The protection against expulsion from a country afforded by international human rights law is more limited and differs in certain significant respects between the various instruments. As regards the protection afforded to aliens, most provide that an alien lawfully in the territory of a State may be expelled therefrom only in pursuance of a decision reached in accordance with the law.

8.51. Under the provisions of the Covenant on Civil and Political Rights, the alien must be given the opportunity to submit reasons against his or her expulsion and have his or her case competently reviewed, the public health exception not being a reason for the non-application of these safeguards.

D. The right to marry and to found a family

8.52. A policy of mandatory premarital HIV testing, coupled

with a denial of a marriage licence if either person prove to be positive, would be a measure interfering with the substance of the right to marry as protected by the international human rights instruments, as indeed would any prohibition of marriage for persons known to be, or suspected of being, HIV infected. The question would then arise whether such a policy could be justified as being "necessary" to reduce either the sexual or the perinatal transmission of the HIV virus. Although these might well be regarded as legitimate aims, it seems exceedingly doubtful that preventing HIV-infected persons from marrying would be an effective means for achieving them.

8.53. For many people today not being married does not bar sexual activity. Even where there are ample opportunities for marriage, a substantial proportion of sexual activity takes place outside it. With marriage barred for some, that proportion could only increase, and probably involve more sexual partners.

8.54. There is no reason to suppose that prohibiting marriage would be an effective means of preventing the transmission of the HIV virus to children. An increasing number today are born outside marriage. Indeed, measures have already had to be taken, at national and international levels, to ensure that they are not discriminated against by comparison with children born to married parents. There is evidence that the great majority of children infected with AIDS are born to unmarried parents.

8.55. WHO has stated the following: "Routine screening .. as a prerequisite for marriage is of little use in controlling or slowing down the AIDS epidemic"[8]

8.56. One of the most serious questions which arises in the context of AIDS is whether it could ever be justifiable for a government to adopt a policy which imposed restrictions on procreation for those identified as HIV-infected.

8.57. The wording of the international provision concerning the right to found a family makes it clear that it must be read subject to the same qualifications as those outlined above for the right to marry-namely that national laws may regulate the exercise of this right, but may not impair its substance. Clearly, therefore, public authorities would not be entitled to interfere with the founding of a family by, for instance, adopting a policy of ordering mandatory abortions or sterilizations - unless this was "necessary" in order to achieve a legitimate aim, and strictly proportional to it.

8.58. Such a policy would presumably have the two-fold aim of seeking to protect the health of both the mother and the unborn child. While these might be legitimate aims, it seems clear for the following reasons that such a policy would be quite unjustifiable.

8.59. As regards the health of the prospective mother, it appears to be the case that the immune system weakens during pregnancy, and physicians are therefore concerned that pregnancy may increase the risk that women who are already infected with HIV will develop full clinical AIDS. However, the need to protect the person concerned from herself could not be considered to be of sufficient weight to justify a measure of this nature, particularly in the case of an individual of full age and in possession of her mental faculties.

8.60. As for the unborn child, perinatal transmission of HIV has been found to occur during pregnancy, delivery, and perhaps also soon after birth. The extent of the risk of transmission by these means is not yet known with any certainty. However, even if it proved to be high, this could not justify such gross violations of human rights as compulsory abortions or sterilizations, contrary to the woman's express wishes, any more than one could every attempt such a justification in cases of genetically transmitted diseases.

E. The right to work

8.61. The relevant international instruments provide that everyone has the right to an opportunity to gain his of her living by work which he or she freely chooses or accepts. States have an obligation to take appropriate steps to safeguard this right and /or to protect it effectively.

8.62. The United Nations Committee on Economic, Social and Cultural Rights, interpreted the relevant provisions of the Covenant to include an effective guarantee against arbitrary dismissal as an integral element of the right to work.[9]

8.63. To the extent that some forms of discrimination in this field are permissible, the question becomes whether the ground for the discrimination is objectively relevant to the efficient and proper performance of the duties of the employment.

8.64. If follows that if an applicant for a job were refused employment or an employee were dismissed solely on the ground that he or she was - or was suspected of being -HIV infected, this would constitute an interference with his or her right to work, unless it could be established that the absence of infection was a bona fide and necessary occupational qualification or that the infection would clearly and substantially affect job performance.

8.65. For example, there might be no interference with the

right to work if someone who was HIV infected were not employed in a position requiring travel to countries which bar those who are infected. Nor might there be such an interference is persons were not employed because they were already displaying some symptoms of fully developed AIDS and their prognosis was such that they would either not be in the position long enough or would not be in sufficiently good health to be able to carry out the normal duties of the employment. However, in any case of this kind the situation would be no different if such persons were suffering from any other disease affecting their performance at work. As WHO and the International Labour Organisation (ILO) have pointed out:

Pre employment HIV/AIDS screening as part of the assessment of fitness to work is unnecessary and should not be required.. There should be no obligation of the employee to inform the employer regarding his or her HIV/AIDS status.[10]

8.66. As for overt HIV-related symptoms manifesting after someone has been employed WHO and ILO state:

If fitness to work is impaired by HIV related illness, reasonable alternative working arrangements should be made... HIV infection is not a cause for termination of employment. As with many other illnesses, persons with HIV- related illnesses should be able to work as long as medically fit for available, appropriate work.[11]

8.67. Next, the question arises whether the risk of HIV infection leading to neuropsychiatric disorders might be a sufficient reason to avoid employing infected persons in some exceptionally sensitive occupations, such as train drivers or commercial pilots, on the grounds that their faculties might become impaired and thereby put other people's lives at risk. WHO concluded the following:

....governments, employers and the public can be assured that based on the weight of available scientific evidence, otherwise healthy HIV-infected individuals are no more likely to be functionally impaired than uninfected persons. Thus, HIV screening of healthy persons would be useful infection is not spread through water or food, (or) eating utensils".[13]

8.69. The question then arises as to what extent measures may be taken which would interfere with the right to work of a person with HIV/AIDS where his or her ability to perform the work in question is not at issue. Here the analysis is a familiar one: any restriction or limitation on the right to work must be prescribed by law and be necessary in a democratic society for one of the specified purposes.

8.70. In the context of AIDS, there is - in the context of the protection of the rights and freedoms of others - a particular purpose for which restrictions might be imposed on the right to work, namely the right of all workers to safe and healthy working conditions. Could this be invoked to justify refusing to employ, or dismissing, someone who is HIV infected (or who refuses to reveal whether he or she is HIV infected) on the grounds that his or her presence constitutes a danger to fellow workers?

8.71. In the views of public health experts, such a measure would not meet the test of necessity. WHO and other public health experts have emphasized that there is no risk of infection where there is no direct contact with the blood, semen, or vaginal secretions of infected individuals. Because few jobs outside the provision of health services involve contact with these body fluids, other employees are therefore sale from infection whilst at work. WHO has stated:

HIV infection is not spread through casual contact (or) routine social contact in the workplace. [14]

In the vast majority of occupations and occupational settings, work does not involve a risk of acquiring or transmitting HIV between workers, from worker to client, or from client to worker.[15]

8.72. The risk of employees coming into contact with such infected body fluids is likely to arise only from accidents and their treatment. According again to the public health experts, in a situation requiring first aid the standard precautions taken to reduce the risk of transmitting other blood-borne infections, including hepatitis B. will be equally effective against HIV.

8.73. Finally, the question whether health workers should be treated as a special case needs to be addressed. Consideration has already been given to the special risks to which they may be exposed in acquiring HIV infection: We must now consider the risks of their transmitting it.

8.74. Clearly, those who are routinely involved in invasive procedures- for example medical and dental surgeons, nurses inserting cannulae or even just giving injections or taking blood samples- present a special risk of transmitting HIV to their patients if they themselves carry it, and if they do not observe the routine precautions designed to prevent any blood-borne infections from which they suffer from being transmitted.

8.75. However, health workers are themselves uniquely aware of this risk and how it is best avoided - e.g. by withdrawing from particular aspects of their work which embody such a risk- and are generally highly responsible people. Indeed, there is not a single reported case of health worker infecting a patient with HIV.

Accordingly, the circumstances in which it would be justified to interfere with the right to work of an HIV-infected health worker would have to be quite exceptional, e.g. if he or she were consistently negligent in observing the routine precautions or failed to follow medical advice about his or her work.

F. The right to education

8.76. Access to education, flowing from the right thereto, implies that measures governing conditions of such access be both for a legitimate purpose and proportionate to the achievement of that purpose. A health policy prohibiting children infected with HIV from attending school would clearly constitute an interference with their right to education.

8.77. The reasonableness of exclusion of children infected with HIV from school is highly questionable. Public health experts have been unanimous in stating that, based on all present evidence, there is no risk of transmitting HIV in school. WHO states: HIV infection is not spread through... routine contact in schools" (emphasis in the original).[16]

8.78. They state further that (as in the case of accidents occurring at the workplace) accidents at school- where, for example an infected child is cut, sick, or incontinent- can be dealt with safely by following standard hygienic procedures.

8.79. Accordingly, it is recommended that HIV infection should not be a factor taken into account by education authorities with respect to school admissions, transfers, attendance, or their powers of exclusion from school.

8.80. There may, conceivably, be some exceptional cases, as for example children who are so developmentally delayed or neurologically handicapped as to lack control of their body secretions. In such cases, it might be legitimate to take this fact into account, together with known information about the HIV serological status, when assessing the child's educational needs.

G. The right to social security, assistance and welfare

8.81. As regards social security, ratification of ILO Convention NO. 102 Concerning Minimum Standards of Social Security of 28 June 1952 entails, inter alia, that a State must have a system which provides benefits in respect of at least three of the following:

(a) Medical care;

(b) Sickness;

(c) Unemployment;
(d) Old age;
(e) Employment injury;
(f) Family;
(g) Maternity;
(h) Invalidity;
(i) Survivorship.

At least one of these must be unemployment, old age, employment injury, invalidity or survivorship.

8.82. It follows that a system may be a genuine system of social even if some risks (e.g. sickness and maternity benefits) are not covered.

8.83. The question then arises whether a government could legitimately stipulate that if employees were dismissed because they had AIDS or took sick leave because of sickness attributable to AIDS, they could be denied unemployed or sickness benefits to which they would otherwise be entitled. It seems clear that it could not. The guarantee applies to all workers. Accordingly, if a social security system provides for the payment of benefits in case of unemployment or sickness, it could not exclude persons with AIDS from that protection.

8.84. To so do would constitute an interference with the individual's enjoyment of this right, which would have to be justified as being necessary in a democratic society for the protection of the rights and freedoms of others or for the protection of public health. It is not evident how this exacting test could be met, as there is no apparent link between curtailing the rights of persons with AIDS to social security, enhancing the protection of the rights and freedoms of others, and protecting public health.

8.85. The second component of the right to social security is social and medical assistance. The right is accorded to all those persons- without distinction- who do not have adequate resources of their own. It would therefore not be permissible either to deny social or medical assistance to an individual who meets the relevant economic criteria for it, or to limit the amount of that assistance, solely on the ground that he or she has AIDS. Again, such measures would constitute an interference with the individual's enjoyment of this right.

8.86. The third element is social welfare services. In this connection, the question arises whether it would be permissible for social workers to withhold their services from a person with AIDS and his or her family on the ground that, in providing those services, they run the risk of becoming infected. In seeking the answer, one must bear in mind that one of the tasks of social workers in the face of the challenge posed by AIDS must be to assist those affected y the disease and their families to cope with it, to adjust to their new situation, and to make the necessary modifications to their lifestyles. Failure to provide that assistance would therefore constitute an interference with the rights of the individual and his or her family to benefit from social welfare services.

8.87. As to whether such a withholding of services could be justified on the ground of being necessary to protect the health of the social workers, this has been dealt with above in connection with the right to work. The answer is that could not; social work entails no contact with blood, semen, or vaginal secretions, and public health experts have made it clear:

In the vast majority of occupational settings, work does not involve a risk of acquiring or transmitting HIV between workers, from worker to client, or from client to worker.[17]

H. Freedom from inhuman or degrading treatment or punishment

8.88. A State's obligation here is absolute and there are no qualifying clauses of any kind. As a result, any failure by a State to comply with its obligations in respect of any one of these modes of conduct amounts to a violation of this prohibition; no question of justification can ever arise.

8.89. The question has been raised as to whether the compulsory segregation or isolation of prisoners with AIDS or HIV infection might amount to a breach of this prohibition. Clearly, such a measure would not constitute "torture" although it might amount to inhuman or degrading treatment.

8.90. While the compulsory segregation or isolation of prisoners with AIDS or HIV infection would probably not constitute "inhuman" treatment, it might well, depending on the circumstances, amount to "degrading" treatment, especially bearing in mind that public health experts have said they see no need for it. Principles of medical ethics relevant to the role of health personnel, particularly physicians, strengthen the protection of prisoners and detainees against torture and other cruel, inhuman and degrading treatment or punishment.[18]

I. The right to equal protection of the law

8.91. This right derives from the principle of equal protection of the law without discrimination and the prohibition of discrimination in law or in practice in any field regulated and protected by public authorities. It is thus concerned with the obligations imposed on States in regard to their legislation and the application thereof.

8.92. There could be circumstances in which a law which discriminated against people with AIDS or HIV, or which gave them less protection than it gives to others, could constitute a violation of this right even is no other human right of the persons concerned were being denied or abridged as a result.

8.93. The areas to which this principle could be applied will vary from one country to another and will depend on the matters which are regulated by law, such as access to public housing or the granting of licences for various activities.

8.94. It follows that an individual with AIDS or HIV may only be subjected to differential treatment in any field regulated and protected by law if it can be established that the distinction has a legitimate aim (i.e. an objective and reasonable justification) and that the means employed are proportionate to that aim.

8.95. The only imaginable legitimate aim would be the protection of public health. However, public health experts throughout the world are on record as saying that this aim is best pursued by not discriminating against those who are infected with HIV, or people with AIDS. To take just two examples:

Discrimination against, and stigmatization of, HIV-infected people and people with AIDS and population groups undermine public health and must be avoided.[19]

The avoidance of discrimination against persons known or suspected to be HIV infected is important for AIDS prevention and control: failure to prevent such discrimination may endanger public health.[20]

8.96. It is difficult to see how discrimination against persons with AIDS or HIV-infected persons in respect of any of their legal rights, or their protection by the law, in any field regulated by public authorities could be justified as a measure proportionate to the legitimate aim of seeking to limit the spread of this infection.

J. Public emergencies

8.97. A State may not simply declare a public emergency in order to seek to justify measures that would otherwise be a breach of its international obligations. Whether such an emergency exists is, ultimately, a matter for objective assessment by the international supervisory organs in the human rights field, as is the question whether the measures taken by the State did or did not exceed those "strictly required by the exigencies of the situation".

8.98. The question then arises whether the prevalence of AIDS within a country could ever be so high as to amount to 'a public emergency threatening the life of the nation" and so entitle the government of that country to introduce drastic measures to suspend the human rights of its inhabitants. It is difficult to imagine such a situation in the case of a disease which does not have the dramatic virulence of, say, a medieval outburst of bubonic plague; the effects of the disease would have to involve the entire nation and threaten the continuance of its whole organized life.

8.99. However, even if one could imagine a scenario where AIDS threatened the survival of an entire nation, one can only speculate what considerations would need to be weighted in the balance. Much would of course depend on whether, by then, any efficient vaccine or cure had been found . If it had, there would certainly be powerful arguments for administering it, if necessary by compulsion- perhaps even if this entailed some incidental risk to the health of a few.

However in the absence of a vaccine or cure, it is difficult to see how even the most drastic measures could help to prevent the further spread of a disease and thereby justify derogations on the ground of a public emergency.

9. Conclusions

9.1. The following is a summary of the conclusions that may be drawn from the preceding sections.

9.2. Those public health measures designed to counter the spread of HIV infection which do not entail adverse consequences for any individuals are unobjectionable on human rights grounds.

9.3. The following measures may have adverse consequences but would be acceptable on human rights grounds provided that they are undertaken completely voluntarily- that is, only after a full explanation of all the possible consequences, and with the explicit, free and informed consent of the persons concerned, obtained without the application of any illicit pressures, whether in the form of promises or of threats. These are:

(a) Voluntary testing of individuals for HIV infection, either on an "anonymous" basis (that is, without the requirement that the person give their true name), or with stringent safeguards to ensure confidentiality:

(b) Counselling of individuals, both before and (if the result is positive) after they are tested;

(c) Voluntary treatment to mitigate the effects of infection or to achieve modifications of behaviour.

9.4. The following measures would, in present circumstances, constitute interference with the right to privacy of the individuals concerned, and would not be justifiable under international human rights law on public health (or any other) grounds. These are:

(a) Mandatory testing of any individuals (other than voluntary donors of blood, semen, or other tissue or organs) for HIV infection, no matter how they are selected;

(b) Compulsory registration of suspected HIV carriers;

(c) Mandatory collection, storage and processing by a public authority of identifiable personal information about persons with AIDS or HIV-infected persons, by making either or both of these a "notifiable disease" by law - without protecting the information concerned by the strictest rules of medical confidentiality or, better still by anonymity;

(d) Disclosure of the results of HIV tests to third persons (including health professionals) without consent, or permitting the improper discovery of such results by third persons.

9.5. The following measures, while entailing some interference with the right to privacy, might be justified on public health grounds:

(a) In exceptional circumstances, informing someone at risk of a patient's known HIV-infected status, even in breach of medical confidence- e.g. where the patient refuses, despite counselling and advice, to take the necessary precautions to avoid passing on the infection to a known sexual partner, or if the patient is a health worker and is consistently negligent in observing routine hygienes precautions, or fails to follow medical advice about his or her work-provided the circumstances in which this was allowed are clearly defined by law;

(b) Making it a criminal offence for an HIV-infected person knowingly or recklessly to infect others. Provided that the offence could be defined sufficiently precisely to meet the requirements of legal certainty and foreseeability.

9.6. The following measures would not constitute interference with the right to privacy of the individuals concerned:

(a) Estimating the prevalence of HIV infection in existing populations by testing fractions of samples taken from individuals, with their consent, for other purposes, and which have been so completely anonymised as to make it impossible to relate them back to the individuals from whom they were taken;

(b) Making AIDS or HIV infection a "notifiable disease" by law, provided that the information reported is either wholly anonymous in the first place or is protected by the strictest compliance with the general rules of medical confidentiality - that is, that it could only released either anonymously or with the explicit and informed consent of the person to whom it relates.

9.7. The following measures would entail violations of the right to liberty and security, and could not be justified on public health (or any other) grounds:

(a) Compulsory blood tests;
(b) Compulsory isolation or quarantine, e.g. by enforced admission to a hospital or a hospice;
(c) Compulsory internment in a colony removed from the rest of society.

9.8. The following measures, measures hey entail violation of the right to liberty and security, might be justifiable on public health grounds, provided that the person detained has the right to have the lawfulness of his or her detention tested initially, and thereafter periodically, by an independent judicial tribunal:

(a) Detention in an emergency of an individual known, or suspected on cogent grounds, to be HIV infected while he or she presents an acute risk of infection to others and is unable to take case of himself or herself;
(b) Detention of an individual while he or she is deliberately trying to infect other with HIV.

9.9. As for the right to freedom of movement, it would not be legitimate for a State:

(a) To make entry into the country of its own returning nationals conditional on their taking an HIV test, let alone on their obtaining a negative result;
(b) To restrict, on AIDS/HIV grounds, the entry of aliens whom it is bound to admit by some specific treaty;
(c) To restrict, on such grounds, the entry of aliens where this would interfere with their enjoyment of other rights guaranteed to them under international human rights law, such as the right to family life;
(d) To restrict on such grounds, either for nationals or for aliens

lawfully within its territory, liberty of movement within that territory or the freedom to choose a residence.

9.10. The expulsion of an individual on the grounds of AIDS OR HIV infection would be a violation of the right to freedom of movement if done outside the provisions of the relevant international instruments. Most importantly, the principle of non-discrimination ought to be applied.

9.11. The human right to equality before the law and to the equal protection of the law would render it illegitimate to discriminate against individuals on the grounds of AIDS or HIV infection not only in respect of their specifically protected rights, but also in any other fields legally regulated by public authorities.

9.12. To justify the suspension - and not merely the various restrictions and limitations discussed in this paper - of any of the human rights and fundamental freedoms guaranteed by international law, there would have to be a "public emergency threatening the life of the nation" on such a scale as to involve the entire nation, and to threaten the continuance of its whole organized life. Even in such a situation, it is difficult to imagine what suspensions of human rights could be justified in the absence of a vaccine or cure.

9.13. Prohibition of marriage for persons known to be HIV infected would be an interference with the substance of the human right to marry, and could not be justified on any grounds.

INTERNATIONAL CONSULTATION ON AIDS AND HUMAN RIGHTS

Final Document

1. Inter-Disciplinary Meeting

The United Nations Centre for Human Rights (the Centre), with the technical and financial support of the World Health Organization Global Programe on AIDS (who/GPA), convened a Consultation of experts at the United Nations Office at Geneva from 26 to 28 July 1989. The Centre's initiative was taken in the context of the World Public Information Campaign on Human Rights launched by the General Assembly of the United Nations on 10 December 1988. The WHO support was offered in the context of the global strategy for the prevention and control of AIDS and in accordance with World Health Assembly resolution WHA 41.24 on the avoidance of discrimination in relation to HIV-infected people and people with AIDS. The purpose of the Consultation was to bring together exerts in the fields of law, religion, ethics, human rights, public policy and public health to discuss aspects of human rights, including various forms of discrimination in relation to the human immunodeficiency virus (HIV) and acquired immunodeficiency syndrome (AIDS).

The inter-disciplinary meeting represented the first such coming together of the disciplines mentioned under the aegis of the Centre and with the support of WHO/GPA. Its primary objectives were to promote a better understanding of the human rights dimension of HIV/AIDS and to explore possible guidelines which might assist compliance with international human rights standards in decisions regarding law, administrative practice and policy. The Consultation also intended to give fresh emphasis to the importance of respect for human rights in the global struggle against AIDS. The participants welcomed the initiative to hold the Consultation. Several participants noted the need to strengthen the understanding of health issues amongst human rights specialists and of human rights among public health specialists. The initiative in convening the Consultation was especially welcomed because of the particular relevance of HIV and AIDS for human rights as reviewed and discussed during the Consultation. While the present Consultation was concerned principally with those rights protected by the International Covenant on Civil and Political Rights and the International Covenant on Economic, Social and Cultural Rights, it was recognized that there were many other aspects of human rights which were important for the Global AIDS Strategy (for example, the rights protected under the International Convention on the Elimination of All Forms of Racial Discrimination, the Convention on the Elimination of All Forms of Discrimination against Women, the relevant ILO conventions, and regional conventions on human rights). Some participants expressed the hope that the relevance of these rights to the Global AIDS Strategy would be emphasized in the appropriate context.

2. The AIDS Pandemic

The Consultation received expert advice from the Director of GPA, Dr. Jonathan Mann, concerning the present known status and projected future course of the AIDS pandemic in all parts of the world. It noted that the latest WHO figures at 1 July 1989 involved approximately 168,000 cases of AIDS reported from 149 countries. It noted that WHO estimated that this represented only a proportion of actual cases of AIDS and that between five million and ten million people were probably already infected with HIV. The available statistics indicate that HIV infection continues to spread rapidly. The World Health Organization, with constitutional responsibility to direct and co-ordinate international health work, developed the Global AIDS Strategy which has been universally adopted as the guide for global AIDS prevention and control. WHO's central role in the global effort against AIDS was formally recognized by the World Health Assembly (resolutions WHA 42.33, WHA 41.24 and WHA 40.26), ECOSOC (resolutions and 1987/75) and the General Assembly (resolutions 43/15 and 42/8).

The Deputy Director of the Centre, Mr. Kwadwo F. Nyamekye, in an opening statement, drew the attention of the participants to the two basic issues considered by the Centre to be vital to this problem:

(a) The issue of discrimination and the danger of the creation of new minorities and new structures of discrimination; and

(b) The rights of everyone to equitable access to health care and facilities.

He reviewed the efforts of WHO, other components of the United Nations system and the Centre, in identifying and dealing with the human rights aspects of this issue. He pointed to the intent of the Sub-Commission on Prevention of Discrimination and Protection of Minorities in the relationship between human rights and AIDS, and the co-operation between the Centre and WHO in that regard.

A background document, AIDS and Human Rights, was placed before the Consultation. It was introduced by the Chief of the External Relations Section of the Centre, Mr. John Pace.

Closing statements were made to the Consultation by Dr. Mann and by the United Nations Under-Secretary-General for Human Rights. Mr. Jan Martenson. Mr. Martenson underlined the complex nature of the problems involved and expressed the hope that the Consultation would facilitate the task of policy-makers as well as legislators. The Centre for Human Rights, in coordination with WHO/GPA, would be prepared to extend technical assistance and advice in the field of human rights. Mr. Martenson stressed the importance of strengthening national infrastructures for the promotion and information. The world Public Information Campaign would be most useful in this regard and the proceedings of the Consultation would be published within this context.

3. HIV/AIDS and Human Rights

The participations discussed the features of the social response it HIV/AIDS which present special risks of breach of human rights, particularly discrimination. They emphasized that a thorough understanding of the facts of HIV/AIDS was essential to sound ethical analysis and good public policy. Without exhausting all of the specially relevant features of HIV/AIDS, the participants noted in particular:

(a) There is no present cure for AIDS, and available palliative treatment is expensive and not readily available in all parts of the world;

(b) There is at present no vaccine against HIV;

(c) In many less economically developed countries, systems for screening blood and blood products are still non-existent or inadequate as a result of economic constraints;

(d) The consequences of infection by the virus are life-threatening;

(e) The virus has been identified relatively recently, and has quickly spread and is still spreading in many parts of the world;

(f) There are relevant limitations in the tests developed to determine whether a person who has been exposed to HIV has, in fact, been infected. In particular, the tests produce a proportion of false negative and false positive results;

(g) Becasue most of the tests so far used detect antibodies which develop after infection with the virus, there is a "window period" between the time of infection and the time of a positive test result which makes present HIV antibody tests an incomplete assurance that a person whose test result is negative is in fact free from infection with HIV;

(h) In some parts of the world, HIV has principally affected minorities who are already the subject of discrimination, stigmatization and legal sanctions. These include, in particular, persons engaged in prostitution, homosexual activity and intravenous drug use and heterosexual men and women infected with HIV/AIDS has increased the special risks of their further marginalization and of deprivation of their basic human rights;

(i) As demonstrated by centuries of effort in all parts of the world, behaviour modification in drug-taking and sexual activity cannot be achieved solely through the use of law;

and

(j) Persons infected with HIV typically do not become sick for years and even decades after exposure, during which time they may be able to continue to lead useful and full lives but may-unknowingly in most cases- infect others.

The participants noted that the most effective means currently available to prevent the spread of HIV was to promote positive behaviour among persons infected with HIV and those at risk of exposure to infection. In some societies, the behaviour which contributes to the spread of HIV is regarded as immoral or illegal. Yet success in stemming the further spread of HIV depends upon winning the confidence and co-operation of such persons in order to be able to provide them with information, education and support to promote changes in their behaviour. However, discrimination or stigmatization may discourage them from seeking relevant services. It was for this reason, amongst others, that the World Health Assembly stressed the need to assure respect for the human rights of HIV-infected persons and those with AIDS and also those at risk, or apparent risk, of exposure to HIV. There is, thus, a clear public health rationale for protecting people from discrimination. It was also for this reason that the centre, within the context of the World Public Information Campaign for Human Rights, took the initiative of convening the Consultation.

The participants recognized the risk of the adoption of measures which are not based upon a sound understanding of the features of the virus and its modes of transmission based on both the understandable fear and concern which the epidemic causes to individuals, Governments and public health officials. Already some such measures have been adopted in several countries. In the opinion of the participants, the past history of oppressive and ineffective responses to infection and disease serves as a warning to the international community of the particular risks of discrimination and loss of human rights in the face of the HIV/AIDS pandemic.

The participants recalled the unprecedented efforts of the international community, particularly under the aegis of the United Nations, to produce a body of international human rights law expressing universal human rights standards. These standards are specifically relevant and applicable to persons with HIV/AIDS and also relate to the right of others to health, including access to information necessary in order to avoid exposure to HIV and the risk of AIDS. Provisions in binding international human rights instruments and in declarations, resolutions of the General Assembly and other sources were reviewed by the participants. In this review, the participants also had before them the background document (HR/aids/1989/1), and the study by the late Mr. Paul Sieghart "AIDS and Human Rights- A U.K. Perspective" (British Medical Association Foundation for AIDS; London, 1989).

The attention of the participants was drawn to applicable provisions of fundamental human rights. The participants recognized that the fundamental rights of one individual were sometimes affected by the assertion of the fundamental rights of another. The achievements of a proper reconciliation between their respective rights requires knowledge, judgement and a careful balancing of the applicable rights with special care to avoid the risk of discrimination or the unjustifiable loss of basic human rights by the one in the name of protecting the human rights of the other.

In the past, departures from respect of universal human rights have sometimes been justified by an appeal to he exception applicable in some cases for measures required to achieve a legitimate aim of society. In the context of HIV/AIDS, the protection of the rights and freedoms of others and the protection of public health are frequently mentioned. But the participants stressed that an exemption from observance of universal human rights could not be justified simply by claiming that a measure was required for "public health" reasons. The participants stressed that international human rights law was significantly more precise than this. It was also necessary, in each case, to establish that the exception was provided for with precision:

(a) By a specific law which is accessible and which contains foreseeable standards as opposed to administrative policy or individual discretion not based on legal rules;

(b) By such a law which in the circumstances could be shown to be strictly required to achieve a legitimate purpose of society for which a pressing social and need could clearly be shown; and

(c) In measures strictly proportional to the achievement of the pressing objective so defined and to any harm inflicted, and which are the least intrusive and restrictive measures available.

Some participants expressed the view that a reconsideration of the "public health" exception in certain human rights instruments was required by a consideration of the particular dangers to human rights demonstrated by certain measures described as being for "public health" purposes. Other participants thought it sufficient to stress the fact that universal human rights continue to apply and that the exception for "public health" is strictly limited in the ways referred to above.

4. General Observations

The participants then turned to a consideration of:

(a) The audience to which the special concerns about the respect for human rights in the context of HIV/AIDS needed to be particularly addressed;

(b) The particular concerns that should be addressed given the necessary constraints of their meeting; and

(c) The form in which future initiatives to protect human rights in the context of HIV/AIDS should be expressed.

The participants laid emphasis upon the need for education in international human rights standards at the following levels:

(a) The components of the United Nations system;

(b) Other international, regional and iter-governmental bodies;

(c) Member States to which the relevant international instruments were expressly addressed;

(d) Non-governmental organizations and community groups; and

(e) Individuals.

Although it was recognized that in many of the above there was a full appreciation of applicable human rights standards, and that important progress in this regard had been made, this has not always been the case. In the past the content of such human rights standards may either not have been known or understood by public health officials or was regarded as not applicable due to the exigencies of public health Likewise, the point was made that, in the past, legal advisers may not have always been aware of the needs of public health. The participants considered that it was important to bring home to officials in all relevant national and international agencies, concerned with developing and implementing HIV/AIDS policy, the importance and the relevance of international human rights standards to their tasks. In many cases, such standards have been specifically accepted by Member States and therefore must be complied with in the context of HIV/AIDS.

The participants also drew attention to the importance of translating human rights standards, in international instruments and elsewhere, to actual observance when they were most needed. In this context, they stressed the necessity of education in human rights, the work of non-governmental and governmental agencies, and the need to provide for the enforcement of human rights by international supervisory bodies or in independent courts or tribunals. In addition, anti-discrimination legislation could provide individual redress where this is justified and assist community education in replacing fear and ignorance with knowledge and elighement. The fulfillment of the right to health information and education about HIV/AIDS and the means of preventing the spread of HIV was emphasized as an indispensable first step in self-protection and the protection of others.

As to the general concerns of the participants, the following in particular were noted:

(a) The participants observed that the Global AIDS Strategy developed by WHO and endorsed by the General Assembly of the United Nations had accepted, from the outset, the imperative necessity, in the realization of its objectives, for the respect of the human rights of all those concerned including the prevention of discrimination against HIV-infected persons with AIDS or persons at risk, or thought to be at risk, or exposure to HIV. The participants endorsed the strategy of WHO/GPA in this regard. In their view, no other strategy would be consistent with observance of internationally accepted human rights standards. Moreover, no other strategy would, for the reasons already referred to, be likely to succeed in the prevention and control of HIV/AIDS.

(b) The participants believed that the United Nations World Campaign on Human Rights provided an important channel through which relevant information and education could be promoted. The work, which was initiated in the United Nations Sub-Commission on Prevention of Discrimination and Protection of Minorities, could provide a useful basis upon which applicable health and human rights priorities could be identified. In this regard, it was necessary that the Centre and WHO/GPA continue to work closely together;

(c) Although human rights are, by their nature, universal, the participants recognized that there was room for legitimate differences of view about the interpretation of some rights, their applicability in particular situations and the relevance to them of some cultural differences. Different views of the meaning of provisions of international standards which have not yet been interpreted by the relevant bodies are, in part, an inescapable aspect of the ambiguity of language which gives rise to opportunities for judgement and choice of meaning. Nevertheless, the global challenge of AIDS and its international character draws new attention to the universality of human rights standards and to the fact that they are inherent in people as human beings. Human rights must be respected as an attribute of the uniquely precious value of each human life and not just because they are laid down by law or because their observance promises greater success in combating AIDS;

(d) Although the human rights of all need to be observed and protected, the features of the AIDS pandemic and the urgent necessity of its containment call particular attention to the need for protection of the human rights of those especially at risk of exposure to HIV so that they will be empowered to protect themselves. By so doing, they are enabled to fulfil their responsibility to protect others. In different parts of the world this includes the special need to ensure the protection of the human rights of persons engaged in both female and male prostitution, male homosexual activity, intravenous drug use, and the protection of heterosexual men and women infected with HIV;

(e) The participants considered that; in the context of HIV/AIDS, special attention should be given to the human rights of women. There are certain factors relating to the reproductive role of women and their subordinate position in society which render women particularly vulnerable to infection. The subordination of women may vary in degree in different societies, but its nature remains the same. Women typically lack equal access to education, health, training, independent income, property and legal rights. This affects both their access to knowledge about AIDS and the measures that may be taken to prevent transmission of HIV infection, as well as their ability to protect themselves from infection.

There was considerable amongst participants about the desirability, in the current circumstances of HIV/AIDS, of the elaboration, by the Commission on Human Rights, of a relevant international instrument specifically addressed to the human rights problems raised by HIV/AIDS, including the need for measures to prevent and redress discrimination. Upon this subject, the views of the participants differed. In summary, without exhausting the opinions expressed, those who opposed such an initiative expressed the views that:

(a) It would require the devotion of much time and resources in circumstances of urgency where there were already applicable provisions;

(b) It ran the risk of isolating HIV/AIDS from its proper conceptual setting as a matter of health care and social justice or as an illness or disability and of thereby promoting the further marginalization of persons with HIV/AIDS;

(c) It ran counter to the current tendency to resist the expansion of international human rights law, in order to allow concentration upon the implementation of the law already adopted, of which there was a great deal that was clearly applicable to HIV/AIDS; and that

(d) It ran the risk, by re-opening debates on the specific topic of HIV/AIDS in present circumstances, of undermining the welcome strategy of WHO concerning human rights and HIV/AIDS and providing an outlet for ill-informed fears and prejudice.

On the other hand those who favoured such a course referred to the following considerations, amongst others:

(a) The existence of particular and specific international human rights instruments addressed to particular and specific problems of which HIV/AIDS is undoubtedly as important and challenging as many;

(b) The evidence of the benefit to the advancement of respect for human rights in the existence of human rights laws, both national and international;

(c) The stimulus given to the enactment and effective implementation of national and local or provincial laws and the adoption of policies by the achievement of international instruments dealing with particular issues of importance for human rights;

(d) The focus which such an instrument would provide to individuals and advocacy groups working towards preventing or redressing discrimination;

(e) The opportunity which such an instrument would present to strengthen the protection of the human rights of persons suffering from all forms of ill-health or disability;

(f) The assistance given to the national and local or pvoincial political process in the protection of the human rights of unpopular or stigmatized minorities by the existence of an instrument representing the consensus of the international community; and

(g) The probability that the challenges to human rights in the context of HIV/AIDS would become more pressing and serious with the global spread of the epidemic.

The participants invited international, intergovernmental and regional bodies concerned as well as national governments, in the light of these considerations, to consider whether there was need for new human rights instruments concerning HIV/AIDS at the international and national levels.

5. Specific Observations

The participants noted that the fundamental basis of human rights law and standards is the recognition of the equal worth and dignity of every man, woman and child and that this is reflected in the principle of non discrimination. As the Secretary-General of the United Nations has stressed, the common fight of humanity is against HIV/AIDS, not against those persons with HIV/AIDS.

In the context of HIV/AIDS, the participants stressed the particular importance of the obligation to respect the rights to information and education, and the fight to the highest attainable standards of physical and mental health, as well as the need to prevent discrimination at the local, national and international levels.

The rights to information and education require that every individual should have access to accurate and up-to-date information about HIV/AIDS, not against those persons with HIV/AIDS.

In the context of HIV/AIDS, the participants stressed the particular importance of the obligation to respect the rifhts to information and education, and the right to information and education, and the right tot he highest attainable standards of physical and mental health, as well as the need to prevent discrimination at the local, national and international levels.

The rights to information and education require that every individual should have access to accurate and up-to-date information about HIV/AIDS, the means by which HIV is spread and how best they might protect themselves and others from infection. The contents of such educational material and the means by which it is disseminated will necessarily vary in different cultural environments.

It was further recognized that particular attention needs to be given to ensuring that such information reaches the most disadvantaged sectors of society such as those who are illiterate.

In addition, it was noted that experience already gained in educational projects aimed at combating the spread of HIV has indicated that the most successful projects are those in which the inherent dignity of the members of the target group has been recognized. Projects were more likely to be effective where members of the population concerned were actively encouraged and empowered to design and implement their won educational projects.

The right to everyone to the enjoyment of the highest attainable standards of physical and mental health requires, amongst other things, that persons should be entitled to equal access to those health care and welfare services which are available.

Another factor to be recognized is that the right to health care including measures to prevent the spread of HIV, is restricted in some States by lack of resources on the parat of the individual, community or State. The full realization of the highest attainable state of health, as well as the limitation of the spread of HIV, requires assistance to individuals, and the support of the world community to less economically developed countries.

Whilst recognizing the efforts being made by Governments and international bodies to prevent and control the spread of HIV, the participants noted that some of the policies proposed or implemented on the grounds of protecting public health raised very serious ethical and human rights issues. The participants were not able to consider all of the relevant issues. However, they noted, for example the inequality of resources available in the fight against the spread of HIV, the need for a more equitable distribution of presently available drugs; the need for compliance with strict ethical and human rights principles with respect to vaccine and drug testing and the future need for an equitable distribution of effective drugs and vaccine which might be discovered. This Consultation specifically examined existing human rights standards relation to a number of areas of particular concern, need further detailed and wide consultation and will form the basis of ongoing work on HIV/AIDS and human rights.

6. HIV/AIDS : Harmonizing Public Health and Human Rights

The participants expressed their appreciation of he initiative of the Centre and WHO in promoting the Consultation on the interrelationship of AIDS and international human rights standards. They expressed the hope that this Consultation and its outcome would result in other such joint initiatives concerning the interaction of human rights, law, ethics, health law and policy in connection with HIV/AIDS and also with other health issues. In all areas of health the observance of human rights is essential. But in the context of HIV/AIDS, as the Consultation demonstrated, there are particularly urgent concerns. The most urgent of these is to remind those formulating relevant policies of the existence and terms of the applicable international human rights standards.

The participants strongly endorsed continued close co-operation between the Centre and WHO/GPA to harness the potential of both bodies in developing practical programmes aimed at furthering the results of this Consultation.

Observance of international human rights standards in the context of HIV/AIDS is not only legally required, but pragmatically useful to the prevention and control of AIDS and a moral imperative of humanity.

The participants emphasized that it is important to recognize expressly their consensus and not just differences in relation to issues raised by HIV/AIDS. All of humanity can unite in endeavors to combat the spread of HIV and to support persons with AIDS. All share the common objective to prevent the further transmission of HIV.

Recommendations

The participants recommended that the Centre for Human Rights and WHO/GPA transmit this statement to the following bodies with a request to place this item on their agenda and to consider what action should be taken to protect the human rights of persons at risk or affected by HIV/AIDS:

(a) Each of the four human rights treaty bodies (the Human Rights Committee, Committee on Economic, Social and Cultural Rights, Committee on the Elimination of Racial Discrimination, and Committee on the Elimination of Discrimination against Women);

(b) Each regional human rights treaty body (the European Commission on Human Rights, Inter-American Commission on Human Rights, and the African commission on Human and Peoples' Rights).

The participants recommended that Governments ensure that measures relating to HIV/IDS and concerning persons already infected conform to international human rights standards, and that they re-examine the measures already in force for the protection of human rights in the light of the particular issues raised by HIV/AIDS.

The participants recommended to WHO/GPA, in collaboration with the Centre for Human Rights, that it prepare an distribute practical information to national AIDS programmes on the international human rights instruments which are relevant to measures relating to HIV/AIDS and on the importance of the need to comply with these instruments.

The participants recommended to the Centre for Human Rights that in collaboration with WHO/GPA, it prepare and distribute relevant information to international, regional and national human rights organizations on AIDS, the Global AIDS Strategy, and on the need to ensure vigilantly that measures relating to HIV/AIDS are in conformity with human rights standards.

References

1. Consensus Statement from Consultation on AIDS and sports (WHO, Geneva, 1989).
2. AIDS Diagnosis and Control: current' situation (WHO, Geneva, 1987), p.3.
3. Guidlines for the Drawing up of a Public Health Policy to Fight AIDS, Appendix to Recommendation No. R (87) 25 concerning a Common European Public Health Policy to Fight the Acquired Immunodeficiency Syndrome.
4. Social aspects of AIDS Prevention and Control Programmes (WHO, Geneva, 1987).
5. Ibid.
6. International Covenant on Civil and Political Rights, Art. 9 (4); European Convention on Human Rights, Art. 5 (4): American Convention on Human Rights. . 7 (6).
7. Statement on screening of international travellers for infection with HIV (WHO, Geneva, 1987).
8. AIDS diagnosis and control; current situation (WHO, Geneva, 1987). p. 3.
9. See, for example the Committee's consideration of the Report submitted by the Netherlands: "Without a fundamental guarantee against arbitrary dismissal the right to work would be meaningless" (Summary records of the Committee on Economic, Social and Cultural Rights, E/C.12/1987/SR.5.p.3).
10. Statement from the Consultation on AIDS and the Workplace (WHO, in association with ILO, Geneva, 1988).
11. Ibid.
12. Statement on Neuropsychological Aspects of HIV infection (WHO, Geneva, 1988).
13. Social Aspects of AIDS Prevention and Control Programmes (WHO, Geneva, 1987)
14. Social Aspects of AIDS Prevention and Control Programmes (WHO, Geneva, 1987).
15. Statement from the Consultation on AIDS and the Workplace (WHO, in association with ILO, Geneva, 1988).
16. Social Aspects of AIDS Prevention and Control Programme (WHO, Geneva, 1987).

17. Statement from the Consultation on AIDS and the Workable (WHO, Geneva, 1988).
18. Statement from the Consultation on Prevention and Control of AIDS in Prisons (WHO, Geneva, 1987). para. C.A, and General Assembly resolution 37/194.
19. World Summit of Ministers of Health. London Declaration on AIDS Prevention. 28 January 1988. 20 Social aspects of AIDS Prevention and Control Programmes (WHO, Geneva, 1987).

17

Public Health Versus Individual Rights

David Buchanan
Barrister, Sydney, Australia

The traditional response to any public health threat is based upon the ethic that the rights of the infected or at-risk individual must be sacrificed to the rights of the wider community. In the context of HIV/AIDS, this has sometimes been expressed in the aphorism that "a virus has no rights."

It should come as no surprise that this is the usual response to the HIV/AIDS epidemic. First, medical practitioners see themselves as the logical source of authority in controlling the response to HIV/AIDS, and most were trained in medical schools before the advent of the notions of preventive and community medicine. Second, the fact that HIV/AIDS, like other major public health problems, tends to be a condition of the oppressed, stigmatised and marginalised in our communities, is taken as 'authority' for the proponents of fundamentalist religions to dictate the terms of the community response.

The premise upon which the classic conundrum of community versus individual rights is based is, of course, that the two sets of entitlements are opposed to each other. The lesson of HIV/AIDS is that the interests of the wider community depend upon respect for the rights of the affected individual.

In many countries, the notion the civil liberties or human rights should be respected for no better reason than that they are an important human value often fails to appeal. Politicians and those who put them in power are more interested in what will work and what will save money. Facts that impress political decision-makers much more than human rights for their own sake: the HIV/AIDS epidemic threatens the economies of regions and countries; that caring for those ill with AIDS costs infinitely more than preventive measures in the first place; that coping with generations of survivors of the epidemic causes massive social dislocation.

In other words, for every suggestion of the need to advance a particular human rights value in relation to HIV/AIDS, it is necessary at the same time to demonstrate how doing so willreduce the spread of HIV and/or will save money in the short to long term.

There is no society in which sex workers, injecting drug users, male homosexuals and women are not marginalised, stigmatised and generally disempowered. The experience of a number of countries in responding to HIV/AIDS is that removal of legal and social disabilities, if not the empowerment of these groups, is critical to a country's ability to deal with HIV/AIDS.

Empowerment can mean different things in respect of different groups, in different regions, but in every case it means respecting individuals for the person they are, and giving them the same ability to control life and social, cultural and economic condition as is possessed by the dominant groups in society.

In Australia, the government has supported the organisation by sex workers of professional or trade union groups. This has given sex workers the power to deal with their bosses and clients so as to enforce the safe sex ethic. Given the choice, sex workers will always prefer to enforce safe sex because it protects not only them but their industry and reputation. The consequence in Australia is that in a country in the region with the longest history of HIV/AIDS, there has yet to be reported a case of infection contracted from an Australian sex worker.

The stereotypical view of injecting drug users is that their only motivation is the source of their next fix. In practice, resourcing needle users and ex-users to organise outreach programmes has demonstrated that drug users are just as capable as others of taking control of their life and caring for their peers as other groups.

In developed countries, the experience has been that where gay men see themselves at risk from HIV, they organise groups to promote safe sex activities and to care for members of their communities who get sick from AIDS. Government resourcing of such groups in Australia has been cited as a significant factor in the massive decline in infection spread which has occurred amongst gay men since the early days of the epidemic.

In the case of all three sections of society, sex workers, injecting drug users and men who have sex with men, it is the decriminalisation of their behaviour, rather than criminalisation, which has contributed to an environment in which they both are able and want to protect themselves, their peers and those in the rest of society with whom they deal. It has been a recognition that the best way to changing risky behaviour and caring for the infected is to give the necessary resources to the affected groups for them to design and implement their education and care programmes.

To accord respect to infected and at-risk individuals and communities is to engender self-esteem and empower people to deal with the problem in ways best suited to their own situations. Economic rights such as the right to work are as important to avoiding needless loss of productivity through discrimination against the infected as they are to people such as women at risk of infection through lack of economic power to control their own life. Information rights are important to the spread of understandable knowledge about how to avoid infection. Rights to self-expression and to organisation are important not just for preventive education but also for giving those affected a feeling of power over their life. Guarantees of confidentiality encourage people at risk to talk with health care workers and others about risks of and dealing with infection. Protection from discrimination generally and according full social and civil rights operate to combat social, cultural and religious stigma. This in turn prevents the spread of infection and encourages a caring ethic by reducing alienation and fear amongst at-risk and infected groups.

Migration questions tend to figure prominently in considerations of 'balancing' the rights of the individual and those of the community. But in truth, mobility rights are just as significant a contributor to a cost efficient response to HIV/AIDS as other human rights. First, preventing migration or entry of people with HIV never succeeds in preventing the introduction of the virus to a country. Even quarantine by an authoritarian regime has been seen to fail to prevent the epidemic. Second, it is costly. When resources are taken away from peer education programmes for affected groups and diverted to testing, there will always be a net increase in spread of infection.

Respect for Individual Rights is Tritical to Combuting HIV/AIDS

It is the Australian experience that when governments and the medical profession deal with affected groups as equals, when there is a partnership between government, the health care industry and affected communities, then those most at risk of spreading or countracting the virus and those with the greatest need for health and treatment care are put in the position of being able to do so themselves. Contrast with countries with comparable cultures and levels of development teaches us that where affected groups are marginalised, they go further underground, there is massive denial on all sides, and in the space of only a few years the virus silently explodes into a far less controllable social, economic and public health calamity.

18

Public Health Versus Individual Rights: The Case of Singapore

Wilfred Ong
Counsel
Singapore Corporation
Singapore

INTRODUCTION

There are few laws, policies and regulations which have been enacted specifically to deal with AIDS in Singapore although some pre-existing laws, policies and regulations are equally applicable to AIDS and related matters. Invariably, these instruments have been defended as being necessary in the interest of "public health."

The only example of a law enacted specifically to deal with AIDS is the recent amendment to the Infectious Diseases Act (Cap 137 1985 Ed) (hereinafter referred to as the IDA).

Infectious Diseases Act

S20A of the IDA empowers the Director of Medical Services to order any infected person to undergo counselling and "to comply with such precautions and safety measures as may be specified by the Director." S20A (2) spells out a maximum fine of $10,000 and/or a jail term of up to two years for failure to comply.

S20B had been lifted out from some Australian statutes (which have been abandoned in some Australian states), and requires an infected person to reveal his serostatus to his sexual partner and to obtain his consent. Any person who contravenes this provision is liable to a maximum fine of $10,000 and/or a jail term of up to two years.

S20C criminalises the donation of blood by a person who knows he is infected and (as a catch-all provision perhaps) does "any act which is likely to transmit or spread AIDS to another person or cause another person to be infected." The punishment is similar to the ones enumerated above.

AIDS has also been gazetted in Schedule 1 of the IDA, which lists the infectious diseases which are covered by the Act. Therefore, other provisions available in the IDA for dealing with infectious diseases are also equally applicable to infected persons. These include S6 and S14 of the IDA. S6(3) reads, "any person who is aware or who suspects that any other person is suffering . . . or is a carrier of an infectious disease shall forthwith give notice in the prescribed form to the Director." Characteristically, S6(6) shifts the onus of proving that a person being charged under this provision did not know of the existence of the disease, to himself, since he is automatically presumed to have known. "Any person" means exactly what it says— including family members, spouses, children, colleagues, etc. S14 empowers the Director to "order the removal of any person who is a case or carrier or contact, or is suspected to be a case or carrier or contact of an infectious disease, for detention and isolation in a hospital or in any other suitable place for such period as the Director considers necessary." The Director is also given powers of arrest under S16 for any breach of isolation orders issued under S14. Although we have inherited these laws on quarantine from the British, it is in theory anyway, equally applicable to PLWHAs.

Blood Transfusion

Every blood donor is required to complete a statutory declaration before he donates blood in Singapore. He must affirm, *inter alia,* that he has not had "unprotected sex (i.e., sex without using a condom)" with a prostitute in the last six months from the date of donation OR have "if male, engaged in any sexual activity with another male since 1978." Two persons so far have been prosecuted for allegedly having made a false declaration.

Immigration Laws

Every work permit holder in Singapore is now required to

undergo HIV tests u'nder newly promulgated regulations or if he wishes to renew his work permit.

Guidelines Issued by the Singapore National Employers' Federation

The basic prermises upon which the SNEF guidelines are formulated include, *inter alia*, the premise that HIV infection is generally contracted outside the workplace, and is therefore the responsibility of the infected employee. Apart from occupational health hazards like asbestosis, silicosis, mosothelioma and noise-induced-deafness, many other illnesses which are normally covered under company health-plan policies are not necessarily proved to be work-related either, e.g., cancer, heart and liver ailments, etc.

This is the first comprehensive statement issued by the SNEF in response to AIDS in the workplace. Although generally enlightened, some guidelines leave much to be desired:

(a). e.g., termination of an infected employee is permissible if "a number of employees are still unwilling to work with the HIV-infected employee despite efforts made to assure them that HIV infection cannot be spread through casual work contact . . . " Surely the individual and his dependants' right to livelihood is more important than collective ignorance.

(b). e.g., in the event of a transfer to lighter work, it is advised that companies who have a policy of maintaining similar terms of employment for such employees may do so for HIV-infected employees, taking into account factors like "whether the infection was contracted inadvertently . . .", etc.

(c). e.g., if employers exclude medical expenses arising from self-inflicted injuries or disease caused by "misconduct," they need not bear the expenses for the treatment of AIDS. Even on a sympathetic case-by-case basis, employers may want to pay for their infected employees, taking into account for "whether the infection was contracted inadvertently ...", etc.

Actual Effects of Laws Enacted in the Name of Public Health

Under the IDA, S20A' s penal sanction may not achieve its noble aims of ensuring compliance with the directives of the Director since it may deter infected persons from coming forward to be identified and to have his lifestyle legislatively regulated. S20B has a whole host of problems:

a. e.g., satisfying strict evidentiary burdens (and thereby affecting enforcement as well;
b. discouraging those most at risk from testing and thus acquiring knowledge of their serostatus (since it pays to be ignorant of one's serostatus under this provision); and
c. embeds a false sense of security on the uninfected that legislative action has been taken to "protect" them, thus conferring some form of psychological immunity on them. This deluded sense of immunity would only detract from the central theme of any effective AIDS educational strategy of ensuring that EVERYBODY takes precautions and to treat all unfamiliar sex partners as being potentially infectious.

S6 of the IDA infuses fear of family betrayal and discourages an infected person from seeking much needed emotional support from his family and loved ones. It goes without saying, the powers of isolation and detention under Ss14 and 16 are also a strong deterrent to infected persons coming forward to be identified and treated.

The existing Blood Transfusion Questionnaire, drafted to screen our blood supplies, is particularly misleading. It seems to imply that homosexual sex between men, no matter whether protected or not, penetrative or non-penetrative, since 1978 is intrinsically unsafe whereas heterosexuals who had unprotected sex with prostitutes more than six months ago are considered "safe" and may donate blood. This irresponsibe misinformation cannot be justified by any medical evidence today and merely forments prejudice against homosexuals by perpetuating the myth that homosexuals are intrinsically more predisposed to AIDS. Not only does this attitude alienate homosexual individuals further beyond the reach of epidemiologists, but it also fosters a sense of denial and complacency among heterosexuals who are made to feel they are less at risk.

The impact of the new regulations under the Immigration Act requiring all work permit holders in Singapore to be tested periodically is not only an expensive exercise, but again singles out a particular group of people and subjects them to discrimination. This has the same adverse effect when any individual group is singled out for a particular treatment.

The guideline by SNEFwas clearly designed to shift the burden of health care cost away from the employers, at the expense of the individual HIV-infected employee. Without any strong guarantees of protection from being dismissed solely on the grounds of being infected, these otherwise healthy individuals live in fear of revealing their medical condition to anyone. Some experience such a state of denial that they only present themselves for treatment when it becomes too late and when AIDS sets in. By adopting a "fault" approach in assessing whether an employee deserves optional health care benefits, it raises ethical questions on which employers should choose between to dispense their health-care largesse. If for AIDS, then why not for other ailments? Then again, many other illnesses, to some extent or another are "self inflicted", e.g., smoking, over-eating, lack of exercise, stress-related illnesses due to one's quick temperedness, etc. Where do you draw the line? Does this sanctimonious approach serve a long-term interest in the control of the spread of the disease? How far can you go to encourage people to confront this disease when it is very much weighted against the employees to find out their serostatus or to come forward for treatment and counselling?

It is obvious, therefore, that the rneasures above which have been enacted to "protect public health" in one way or another do not protect public health in the long run. HIV is mainly transmitted by unsafe sexual practices in Singapore. Personal behaviour has not always been a model subject for legislative control. Sexual behaviour is the most difficult of personal behaviour to control. It is a complex web entangled with emotion, taboos, religion, morals, and social-cultural norms. Some of the basic aims of epidemiological control are:

(a). Reaching out to and gaining the trust of target groups in order to contain the spread of the disease through encouraging those at risk to come forsvard for counselling, testing and treatment, and to organise grassroots peer education groups;

(b). To educate the uninfected—to break down their sense of denial, to get them to take precautions, and to help themselves by helping the infected to feel integrated and not isolated.

Those laws cited above are antithetical to these objectives. It must be understood that the protection of individual interests is synonymous with protecting public health, in the long run. It is said that the most effective laws to change personal behaviour are, ironically, those laws that help and not penalise the target group.

Why is Public Health Protection Being Pitted Against Indvidual Rights?

The first and foremost reason is probably official ignorance. Those in positions of authority and influence are not infalliable and sometimes fail to keep abreast with current AIDS epidemiology. Since officials are only human and AIDS involves human sexual behaviour, personal beliefs and values are sometimes infused into their professional responsibilities and judgment.

Short-sighted and ambitious politicians have been known to sacrifice long-term gains for short-term gratification in order to appease their constituents. Playing to the tune of popular ignorance and misconceptions can sometimes win votes.

It is also far more expedient and less complicated to install "instant protection" for the public by curbing the rights of the infectious and dangerous HIV/AIDS bogeyman. This is infinitely easier than establishing a comprehensive education effort and social overhaul that has all the ingredients politicians fear most—cost, controversy and only long-term gains.

Singapore's political culture; with its implicit acknowledgement of Confucian ethics, places what it perceives to be the community interest above all else. If you make exceptions to extend the individual rights of those infected, there is the fear of the floodgates opening in the other areas as well.

How Do We Oversome this Problem?

Those concerned with the disease should try to convince politicians that AIDS would affect issues which politicians prioritise. In other words, speak their language. Understand what are issues which would strike a chord with politicians and couch your advocacy in those terms. If politicians are concerned with dollars and cents, couch your advocacy in terms of the economic losses that AIDS would bring about in the future and support this stand by detailed studies.

Special efforts should also be made to constantly educate and update officials and politicians on AIDS epidemiology. There should be a greater and more enthusiastic participation by those in positions of authority in regional and international dialogues and conferences so that a more macro perspective of the AIDS pandemic would be appreciated.

It would be futile to merely ease restrictions on the rights of infected individuals without simultaneously educating the public.

Constant reinforcement of public opinion would gradually win the support of the public for such measures, while simultaneously eroding the myths surrounding PLWHA by integrating the infected with the uninfected.

Lastly, greater participation by PLWHAs would put a face to the epidemic which many yet view with an air of abstract nonchalance. Society's sense of individual vulnerability would be greatly enhanced if PLWHAs were more visible since the public would then realise it could happen to any of them. Once there is public support to deal with the infected humanely, changes will follow.

19

Public Health, HIV and the Law: Why Individual Rights Matter?

Ms. Julie Hamblin
Partner
Ebsworth & Elsworth
Sydney, Australia

INTRODUCTION

Consider the following examples:

- A policy is introduced requiring all migrant workers returning home to be tested for HIV. The government keeps a register of the names of those who test positive, which is available to potential employers of the workers.
- The director of a prison decides to test all prisoners for HIV. Those who test positive are to be housed separately from the other prisoners and denied access to the prison's recreation yard.
- In an attempt to prevent the spread of HIV, a law is passed making prostitution a criminal offence. Any sex worker convicted will receive a prison term of several years.

One would like to think that these are not common examples in reality, but unfortunately the opposite is the case. Frequently, punitive measures such as these are seen as necessary to deal with the risk of HIV infection.

If one questions the wisdom of these measure by pointing to

the need to demonstrate care and compassion for people with HIV, and their families and carers, the response all too often is: But what about the rights of the rest of the community? Does not the need to protect public health come before the rights of infected individuals?

These peoole would seek to sugest that we have two competing interests - the interests of people with HIV and the interests of everyone else. Because it is believed that the interests conflict, it is suggested that one most choose between them, and the more compelling interest is often said to be this notion of 'public health'. It is used to justify all sorts of harsh, punitive measures that are abusive of the individuals who are affected by the epidemic.

This notion of a conflict between public health and individual rights is one of the great myths of the HIV epidemic. Those people who see decisions about policies on HIV as being decisions between the rights of the individual on the one hand and public health on the other are making a grave mistake.

We need to understand why this approach is so misconceived and to move beyond this one dimensional approach to HIV policy if we are to respond effectively to the epidemic.

At the outset, it must be made clear that in rejecting the myth of the conflict between public health and individual rights, it is not suggested that there are no conflicts or tensions in the way we respond to the HIV epidemic. The epidemic has thrown up enormously difficult ethical problems which defy any simple 'right' solution. It is exactly this complexity which makes any simple notion of 'public health' an inadequate principle for guiding HIV policy.

In explaining why it is a myth to say there is an inevitable conflict between the rights of the individual and the rights of the community in the context of the HIV epidemicj four points must be made.

1. The False Distinction Between 'Us' and 'Them'

Any argument that there is a conflict between 'public health' and the rights of the individual must rest upon the assumption that, in the HIV epidemic, there are two distinct group—'us' and 'them'.

In other words, there is a group of people infected with HIV ('them') and then there is the rest of the community whose own personal behaviour does not place them at risk, who would therefore normally be untouched by the epidemic, and who have a 'right' to be protected from the actions of others.

We know this is not true. It is not true anywhere in the world, but particularly not in many parts of Asia where HIV infection is spreading faster than anywhere else in the world.

Everyone will be affected by the HIV epidemic. There is no 'them'. It is only 'us'. Everyone in the world will be affected in one way or another by the epidemic.

The word 'affected' has been chosen very carefully. Not everyone will be infected, but we all will be affected. We will see someone we love die, we will have to care for a person with AIDS, we will see children left without parents ....

So the notion of a group of infected individuals separate from and in conflict with 'the community' or 'the public' is fundamentally flawed.

2. The Elements Necessary to Prevent the Spread of HIV

The spread of HIV is preventable and we know how. There are two basic prerequisites:

— Each individual must take responsibility for protecting himself or herself and others from infection.

— Each community must take responsibility for empowering its members to take steps to prevent HIV from spreading.

The way HIV is spread—primarily through sexual contact—means that individual behaviour is the key: how people interact with each other and whether their sexual lives risk spreading HIV. So decisions made by individuals about their own lives will determine whether the spread of HIV can be contained.

But individuals don't live in a vacuum. They live within a community, and their choices about their own individual lives (and, therefore, their risk of exposure to HIV) are very often limited or determined by the community within which they live. For example:

- The position of women means they often cannot make their own decisions about their sexual lives; they cannot, for example, compel their husbands to remain faithful to them or to use a condom.
- There are cultural traditions which are very difficult to resist, such as wife inheritance or other patterns of sexual interaction.
- Economic circumstances may limit choices, such that a woman has no source of economic support outside her family other than sex work.

So individuals cannot by themselves bring about the changes that are necessary to respond to the HIV epidemic. They must take responsibility, but they must also have the support of their communities, collectively, to enable them to exercise this responsibility.

3. Partnership and Shared Responsibilty

It follows from this that there must be a sense of partnership and shared purpose between individuals and between each individual and his or her community if that community is to be able to deal with the epidemic.

This partnership must transcend any simple division between the infected and the uninfected. We are all affected and we must all support each individual in our community in measures to deal with HIV, just as they must support us in our own personal measures to protect ourselves and others.

What does this mean for the notion that there is a conflict between the rights of infected individuals and public health? It means that it is simply wrong.

And if this misconception leads to measures such as compulsory HIV testing, breach of privacy and discrimination, it is dangerously wrong. Because what hope will there then be that the people who suffer as a result of such measures will have a shared sense of the need to protect themselves and others and will be empowered to do so?

On the contrary, they will be disempowered, alienated from their communities, and left without the emotional resources and support which might enable them to join in and take responsibility for their community's response to the epidemic.

4. The Role of Criminal Law

Where a person knows he or she is infected with HIV and continues, despite the best available counselling and support, to behave in a way that place others at risk, there is always going to be an argument that this form of behaviour is criminal and should be punished.

In the vast majority of countries, existing criminal law on murder, manslaughter, assault or causing harm to others covers this situation very adequately—no new legislation is necessary to deal with such cases.

But the possible application of criminal law in this way is a side issue in the context of the HIV epidemic. To focus on criminal law as the main legal mechanism for dealing with HIV involves the fundamentally wrong assumption that the deliberate, malicious spreading of HIV is the main problem.

Obviously, the opposite is the case—the overwhelming majority of people who transmit HIV to others do not even know they are infected. And even where people suspect they might be carrying the infection, all kinds of other social forces come into play. There have been cases, for example, of women who believe they may have HIV but are nonetheless not able to resist pressures from their families to remarry, even though this may risk spreading the infection to the new husband.

These values and practices are not going to be changed simply passing a law making them a criminal offence. As stated already punitive laws are not only useless; they are actively harmful.

So while there may be a tiny number of exceptional cases where the transmission of HIV may constitute a criminal offence, we must not allow this to sidetrack the debate. Existing criminal law is perfectly adequate for these cases; in fact, HIV raises no new legal issues in this area. But criminal law has little relevance for the real challenges involved in dealing with the HIV epidemic.

Does this mean that law, and legislation generally, has no relevance for the response to the HIV epidemic at all?

This is not so, because the law can play roles other than a punitive one. In particular, there is a great need in the face of the HIV epidemic for protective laws which respect the rights and needs of people affected by the epidemic, and which reinforce efforts to build the necessary partnerships.

These are much more fruitful avenues to pursue when considering the law and HIV than to look to punitive measures found in criminal law.

CONCLUSION

To return to the question posed at the beginning: How should the issue of individual rights be addressed in the face of the HIV epidemic?

It is entirely possible (for many countries have done this already) that as a result of policies on HIV, we will live in a society where compulsory HIV testing is the norm, where no one is informed of their HIV status, where people with HIV are rejected and discriminated against, where they lose their jobs, and where they are denied any respect or privacy.

But let us consider two questions: First, even where the justification for these measures is said to be a need to protect public health, we all need to ask whether we would want to live in such a society. And second, could we really say that such a society is healthy?

20

Health Law Versus Individual Rights in Developing Countries

Akshoy Rekhi
Attorney, New Delhi
India

The spread of HIV in the last decade has changed many of the features of the existing health care system, particulary in respect to its finances. Health care, to begin with, has always been expensive. The United States of America, for example, with its vast military presence all over the world spends much more on health care for its citizens than what it does on maintenance of its defence forces, due mainly to governmental support on research and development. In developing countries the scenario is similar, though the nature of burden is different. The burden put on the state exchequer is mainly due to two different set of reasons. The first set is comprised of actual expenses incurred in providing health care, which is enormous due to factors such as large population, unhygenic living conditions, poverty resulting in malnutrition and ill health, illiteracy, etc. The second set of expenses includes training of health care professionals, providing expensive health facilities at almost no cost to the individual and providing drugs at subsidised rates.

The HIV epidemic is proving to be a great financial burden on the state, as people with HIV require more medical facilities and for a longer duration of time. Under such circumstances a strategy has to be worked out that assures, at the least, that the *status quo* as per the present provision of health care is maintained. This is easier said than done, as developing countries with their high inflation rates and an ever increasing population leave no room for any extra financial burden on the state of the kind that the spread of HIV is posing.

The first response to the HIV epidemic by most of the developing countries was to wash their hands of the problem. This was done by simply holding the individual with HIV responsible for his own condition, on the pretext that "life style" contributes to HIV infection, and hence the responsibility is that of the individual and not the state. Therefore, any extra burden executed by the spread of HIV is entirely to be borne by the individual. The only step taken by the state was to create barriers in the further spread of HIV by using traditional methods like quarantine and social ostarisation. This response was the natural outcome of the characteristrs on which the health care system has evolved in the developing countries. These characterstics are:

(a). The public health care system is elitist in nature;

(b). The system caters primarily to the needs of the dominant group;

(c). The health needs of the masses are considered the product of ignorance and traditionalism of such masses and therefore fall within the class of self-inflicted losses, with which the state may sympathise but would do little to ameliorate;

(d). Extensive use of criminal law is made to avoid the spread of infections and contagious diseases as well as to maintain adequate standards of delivery;

(e). The modern western-oriented system of medicine is considered the preferred system but the indeginous systems are also allowed to survive, though they are never integrated in the main flow. This results in streams of different medical systems that flow together but whose waters never mix;

(f). The public health system is conceived in a top-down mold. The state is considered the dispenser of health but the recipient is not recognised to have a right to good health, and therefore, economic considerations are always paraded first as excuses for the negligence of the state;

(g). The maintenance of the public health system is considered a social good to which individual rights must give way and no effort is made to make the system responsive to claims of individual liberty.

These traditional public health characteristics have now come in direct conflict with recent constitutional developments in India where the notion of liberty, equality and freedom of speech has been interpreted in a much broader sense by the courts in the last two decades. Issues like professional misconduct are likely to be taken much more seriously and their scope will be widened to include breach of confidentiality and discrimination since these are all signs of the growing emphasis on individual rights. The HIV epidemic has put forth the neccessity to review the whole health care system and to develop a different format than the way it had progressed earlier. In India there is a need to integrate the recent constitutional developments on individual rights to the field of health care in order to continue the fight against HIV and also to save the public health care system from crumbling under its own weight.

21

Human Rights, HIV Infection and Women

Prof. Rebecca J. Cook
Faculty of Medicine and Centre for Bioethics
University of Toronto, Canada

I. INTRODUCTION: HISTORY OF HUMAN RIGHTS LAW

Some authorities claim that human rights lie at the very origins of international law.[1] The earliest records of legal dealings among peoples, traceable to relations among the city states of classical Greece, emphasized the need to respect the rights that individuals enjoyed under Natural Law by virtue of their human status. The respect paid to the protection of diplomatic representatives of other city states upon the outbreak of war reflected their entitlement to human rights. Anthropologists tracing the evolution of law, and its contribution to order, have interpreted law, including the laws of warfare, as a means of limiting violence and savagery and of preserving the respect that individuals owe to each other through the common bond of their human status.

The historic rules of humanitarian intervention provided exceptions to the otherwise absolute claims of national sovereignty. The concept of sovereignty among nations governed the international legal order defined by Natural Law principles and endorsed by European religious authorities during the formative phase of modern international law. The sovereign equality of members of the community of nations precluded one nation from intervening in the domestic affairs of other nations. If'a state dealt inhumanely in its territory with the nationals of another state, however, the national state had legal rights of humanitarian intervention. The historic laws of war among states, more ancient than the laws of peace, required confinement of hostilities to combatant forces of hostile nations, and provided immunity from attack for their civilian populations on grounds of humanity.

The limitation of humanitarianism under the legal doctrine of sovereignty was that international law provided no supervision of a state's treatment of its own nationals. International law regulated the rights by which a state could claim that individuals and populations were its nationals, for instance on territorial acquisition and transfer between states, but when an individual's nationality was not legally contested, that individual's subjection to the sovereign power of his or her nation state within its territory was complete. Nations whose treatment of individuals fell short of the perceived standard of civilization maintained by the historic European nation states might be considered not to be members of the community of nations whose practices furnished the content of international customary law, but recognized members were free from the scrutiny of others concerning treatment within their territory of their own nationals.

Women's special needs of international protection were recognized at the beginning of the present century through a series of international agreements. Their aim was not to liberate women within their homes, but rather to protect them in industry outside the home, and to protect them from sexual and other personal vulnerability that might diminish the integrity of family units. The International Convention Respecting prohibition of Night Work for Women in Industrial Employment, of 1906, was the first of a series of international conventions, supported by the International Labour Office, protecting women in the workforce, which was reinforced by other conventions reflecting humane protection of women such as the Convention concerning the Employment of Women Before and After Childbirth, of 1919. Similarly, the International Convention for the Suppression of Traffic in Women and Children, of 1921, was the first of a series of international conventions reflecting humane and moral concerns for protection of women and families. These treaties were open to adoption by states as an act of sovereign authority but were not binding, as is international customary law, on states that did not adopt them (see V, below).

The conclusion of World War II marked a turning point in international tolerance of states' absolute sovereign authority over their own nationals, and over individuals who had become stateless by declarations of governments of territories from which they had fled and who were therefore not amenable to protection under the laws of humanitarian intervention. The conduct of Germany and of administrations in other countries collaborating in the German war effort regarding their Jewish and other nationals, gypsies and homosexuals, culminating in policies for their extermination, was considered a violation of any powers that could legitimately be claimed by even sovereign authorities. Such conduct constituted punishable crimes against humanity committed by governmental and military leaders and those exercising powers derived from sovereignty.

To recognize the violation of humane and civilized conduct that had recently been evidenced, the United Nations, created in 1945, drafted the Universal Declaration of Human Rights in 1948. The document was entitled a "Declaration" to confirm that it was not attempting to create new law, but simply to declare the international law on human rights that existed before, and that had been violated in events preceding the Declaration and inspiring its expression in concrete language in 1948. Being a declaration, the 1948 text was not itself legally binding. However, to give direct legal force and definition to the spirit of the Declaration, a series of international conventions was implemented that has formed the modern international basis of human rights law. These legal instruments have provided a set of human rights principles now so widely accepted as to be understood in many regards to have become international customary law, which is legally binding on states without their express acceptance or ratification.[2] The modern international legal order requires governments to respect international customary law in their international and domestic affairs as a condition of their legitimacy as governments capable to be recognized as such.

II. INTERNATIONAL FOUNDATIONS OF HUMAN RIGHTS LAW

Modern international human rights law is founded on international, regional and subject-specific conventions inspired by the Universal Declaration of Human Rights. The general conventions are the International Covenant on Civil and Political Rights (the Political Covenant) and the International Covenant on Economic,

Social and Cultural Rights (the Economic Covenant). The regional conventions are the European Convention on Human Rights, the American Convention on Human Rights and the African Charter on Human and Peoples' Rights. The leading specialized conventions are the International Convention on the Elimination of All Forms of Racial Discrimination (the Race Convention), the Convention on the Elimination of All Forms of Discrimination against Women (the Women's Convention) and the Convention on the Rights of the Child (the Children's Convention).

These conventions have all established committees to monitor state compliance with their provisions through mandatory, periodic state reports, and some committees receive complaints of violations that individuals make against states. The treaty committees may conduct investigations and deliver opinions on complaints of state violations. The committees can also offer guidance to states on the scope and content of obligations arising under the terms of each of the articles of the conventions.

Leading provisions of the various conventions relevant to HIV infection and the maintenance of health can be identified by reference to named rights under their particular articles (see IV below). It is important to observe the functional interdependence of individual rights in view of the socio-economic and cultural dimensions of women's health status.[3] The importance of applying all human rights to improve women's status within societies and thus their negotiating power within sexual relationships was underscored by the Platform for Action adopted by the Fourth World Conference on Women in Beijing in 1995 (the Beijing Platform for Action). It explained that:

> "[t]he human rights of women include their right to have control over and decide freely and responsibly on matters related to their sexuality, including sexual and reproductive health, free of coercion, discrimination and violence. Equal relationships between women and men in matters of sexual relations and reproduction, including full respect for the integrity of the person, require mutual respect, consent and shared responsibility for sexual behaviour and its consequences."[4]

Some rights may at first appear more distant from women's health concerns can be shown in practice to be more proximate, or to be an essential component of exercise of a right more obviously connected to health. For example, the right to education is a basis of literacy, without which individuals cannot learn many precautionary strategies for the preservation of their health.

Several human rights, found in the various international and regional human rights treaties, can be applied to women's health interests.[5] For example, readers' literacy is of limited value if authors and publishers do not enjoy the right to impart information. Women's health is significantly aided by women's access to education and literacy, and on the right to impart to others the information they possess, for instance on matters of safe and effective control of infection and unwanted pregnancy.

The Committee on the Elimination of Discrimination Against Women (CEDAW), the body established by the Women's Convention to monitor compliance of States Parties with its terms, has paid specific attention to how women's subordinate and dependent status in many communities denies and compromises their opportunities for self-defence against HIV infection. CEDAW has directed attention to the need to prevent discrimination against women in national AIDS strategies, and has recommended that "programme[s] to combat AIDS should give special attention to the rights and needs of women and children, and to the factors relating to the reproductive role of women and their subordinate position in some societies which make them especially vulnerable to HIV infection."[6]

III. THE DUTY OF NONDIS CRIMINATION

Perhaps the most basic human right in social existence, individuals' right to nondiscrimination on such grounds as race and sex, has now been so universally endorsed and recognized as a minimum condition of civilized conduct as to have passed from the law based on acceptance of treaties to become international customary law, which binds all states without their explicit agreement. States are not legally free to claim a general exemption from this obligation on the ground that they have not subscribed to a particular international convention. It is sadly demonstrable that the practice of states falls short of full observance of this obligation, and equally demonstrable that the incomplete nature of the international legal order leaves states that violate this obligation free from systematic condemnation and sanction. The Race Convention has been widely adopted by states, and the Women's Convention was brought into legal effect with unusual speed and now has over 140 states parties. However, international entities, such as the Holy Sea and several

Islamic states, which claim religious inspiration and moral authority for their conduct, have declined to ratify the Women's Convention, or have limited their acceptance by such extensive reservations as to create doubts about whether they are member states in law.[7]

A. Sex Discrimination and Gender Discrimination

Women's liability to be excluded from equal rights with men, on grounds, for instance, of religious doctrines that exclude women from the exercise of equal spiritual influence with men within religious hierarchies, and women's exclusion from or subordinate representation within military structures that constitute governments or that are strongly influential on them, are illustrations of discrimination on grounds of both sex and gender.[8] Sex discrimination against women as such and negative gender stereotyping that limits the social roles of women are both sources of women's health disadvantage, and their undue vulnerability to HIV infection. Women's liability to suffer compromised health on grounds of gender is exposed by the broad description of "health" provided by the Constitution of the World Health Organization (WHO), which has been adopted by all countries that are members of the WHO. "Health" is explained to be "a state of complete physical, mental and social well-being and not merely the absence of disease or infirmity."[9] UN member states at the 1994 International Conference on Population and Development held in Cairo adopted the Programme of Action which built on this explanation to define reproductive health as:

> "a state of complete physical, mental and social well-being and not merely the absence of disease or infirmity, in all matters relating to the reproductive system and to its functions and processes. Reproductive health therefore implies that people are able to have a satisfying and safe sex life and that they have the capability to reproduce and the freedom to decide if, when and how often to do so. Implicit in this last condition are the right of men and women to be informed and to have access to safe, effective, affordable and acceptable methods of family planning of their choice, as well as other methods of their choice for regulation of fertility which are not against the law, and the right of access to appropriate health-care services that will enable women to go safely through pregnancy and childbirth and provide couples with the best chance of having a healthy infant".[10]

Many of the disadvantages that affect women's health arise from gender discrimination in their social circumstances, and from political, economic, spiritual and other sources of subordination that affect women's self-determination and their self esteem, creating frustration and perhaps depression reflected in a lack of mental and social well-being.

Sex is a matter of biological classification, but gender is a social construct applied by human societies through social culture and social psychology. Gender concepts influence social institutions including the family, individual role expectations and aspirations, and, for instance, the cultural senses of order, propriety and nature. For example, authority is seen as male gendered, credibly exercised by such male gendered institutions as governments, military administrations, religious, judicial and academic hierarchies and professional associations such as of physicians and lawyers. Male gendered characteristics are strength, decisiveness and willingness to stand against adversity and to struggle for ascendancy. Female gendered activities are subordinate and centre on service to others, particulary in families, such as through housekeeping, child-care and nursing the young, disabled elderly and sick. Female gendered characteristics are weakness, indecisiveness and submission.

Within the health care professions, nursing is female gendered, nurses being considered historically the compliant handmaidens of doctors and to constitute at most a subordinate profession. Nurses, who in many countries still wear the modest convent garb of nuns, were paid as meanly as others in lowly-esteemed service occupations, like domestic helpers and kitchen hands. Similarly, birth attendants and midwives are often still considered secondary health care providers to obstetricians, whose services, though delivered exclusively to women, are male gendered.

Actions that defy a prevailing social gender construction are frequently described as "unnatural", and explained as defying an order that is set independently of societies and cultures, for instance by authoritative (therefore male-gendered) interpretation of divine will. By these rationalizations, states claim that they are not responsible for the discrimination they practice on grounds of gender. They may point to legislation that prohibits discrimination on grounds of sex, and disclaim accountability for consequences that perpetuate the disadvantage that women suffer in practice. For this reason, the Women's Convention considered it necessary to reiterate the prohibition of discrimination on grounds of sex contained in the Universal Declaration and the Political and the Economic Covenants, observing that "despite these various instruments, extensive discrimination against women continues to exist".[11] The Convention also provides in Article 5(1) that states should "take appropriate measures to modify the social and cultural patterns of conduct to eliminate prejudices and customary and other practices based on the inferiority or superiority of either sex or on stereotyped roles for men and women".

B. Gender Discrimination and HIV Infection

Women's health is prejudiced by reference to their gender when in childhood girl children are fed from scarce food supplies only after boy children's appetites are satisfied. In many societies, girl children are considered a burden and detriment to their families, their births being at times publicly lamented and a source of condemnation and shame to their mothers. Health status is further compromised when girls become marriageable in early adolescence, at an age before that at which boys can marry, and when in marriage women have no control over the timing of sexual intercourse, their husbands' sexual activity outside marriage, or husbands' use of condoms to reduce sexually transmitted diseases including HIV infection. Women are frequently defenceless against the risk of HIV infection because of their subordinate and servile family and social status that the elimination of discrimination on grounds of both sex and gender should relieve. It is ominous that in many societies today, the population among which infection and AIDS are rising most rapidly is that of women of reproductive age.[12]

The Beijing Platform for Action explained that

> "HIV/AIDS and other sexually transmitted diseases, the transmission of which is sometimes a consequence of sexuial violence, are having a devastating effect on women's health, particularly the health of adolescent girls and young women. They often do not have the power to insist on safe and responsible sex practices and have little access to information and services for prevention and treatment. Women, who represent half of all adults newly infected with HIV/AIDS and other sexually transmitted diseases, have emphasized that social vulnerability and the unequal power relationships between women and men are obstacles to safe sex, in their efforts to control the spread of sexually transmitted diseases. The consequences of HIV/AIDS reach beyond women's health to their role as mothers and

caregivers and their contribution to the economic support of their families. The social, developmental and health consequences of HIV/AIDS and other sexually transmitted diseases need to be seen from a gender perspective".[13]

Gender discrimination can be found even within otherwise enlightened health care systems. "Mandatory" HIV testing is usually taken to mean that testing is required only if individuals want to avail themselves of a particular right, service or opportunity.[14] For instance, donors of blood for transfusion will be subject to mandatory testing, but do not have to volunteer to donate. Oppression of women occurs when testing is mandatory for receipt of medical services that women cannot conscientiously forego, particularly existing services associated with pregnancy, childbirth and care of newborn infants. Mandatory testing becomes coercive and discriminatory when hospitals' general practices that are gender-neutral on their face are applied to medical services that only women seek. Moreover, pregnancy and neonatal care arise not out of sickness, but out of women's conscientious concern for themselves and for the children they intend to bear.[15] The practice of universal precautions in delivery of these services reduces the need for HIV testing of women and infants.

Sex and gender discrimination continue to operate.in mod ern times to predispose women in many cultures to unduly high levels of HIV infection and AIDS.[16] A stereotype of young women is that they are sexually coy and passive, and that only "loose" girls prepare themselves for sexual activity. The pervasive difficulty that adolescents face in the quest for such birth control means as condoms, which may draw communal attention to them, is aggravated for adolescent girls, in that their reputations and value in marriage may be degraded if they compete for access to scarce supplies of condoms against the males destined to be their sexual partners. An obstetrician in Zimbabwe has observed that "adolescents have an impossible task to find condoms in the rural areas where 80-90 per cent of them live. Community-based distributors mainly responsible for contraceptive pills and condoms in such areas do not cater for unmarried individuals. A rural or small-town boy, let alone girl, could rarely obtain a condom without the whole community talking about it. This problem needs urgent attention since up to 30 per cent of 15-19-year-old pregnant girls are HIV positive.[17]

When women in late adolescence are uneducated and illiterate, they have few means of sustaining themselves outside their parents' homes except through marriage. The gendered conditions of access to economic opportunities even for the educated deprive women of means to enter all but the most modest forms of industry or commerce. Women's employment opportunities are limited, and then confined to service functions of a domestic character, usually paid at minimum industrial rates where minimum rates are legislated and actually enforced. Accordingly, many young women are denied opportunities for self-sustaining employment, except by sale of their sexuality in prostitution. Even afforded the more dignified title of sex workers, they may earn little, but remain exploitable and at high risk of HIV infection through inability to compel condom use by their possibly promiscuous clientele.

More traditional gender discrimination often compounds women's vulnerability to HIV infection and AIDS. Married at early ages to perhaps considerably older men, they face early widowhood under legal regimes that exclude or minimize widows' rights of land and property inheritance. As widows, they become burdens to their husbands' families and communities, but unable to rejoin birth families that were relieved to give them in marriage.[18] As their fathers' daughters, their inheritance, if any, will be secondary to that of their brothers.[19] In cultures where survival depends on land holding, subsistence farming and modest husbanding of cattle, women's inability in law and fact to hold land denies them means to support themselves and their families in widowhood; the sons they have borne may be supported by their deceased husbands' families, but they remain responsible for the survival and welfare of their daughters.[20] Again, prostituting themselves or daughters may be their only means to support themselves and their dependent families. Enforcement of laws of sexual and gender equality in such areas as inheritance, land tenure, education and training, equal employment opportunities, equal pay for work of equal value and, for instance, bank loans and other forms of commercial credit, though not immediately related to considerations of infection and disease, would afford women opportunities in life that would reduce their vulnerability to HIV infection derived from the lifestyle of selling their bodies to which sex and gender discrimination may commit them.

IV. OTHER INTERNATIONALLY PROTECTED HUMAN RIGHTS

A. The Rights fo Life and Survival

A measure of how far international human rights law must

develop to contain the spread of HIV infection and to protect women's fundamental interests more effectively is the narrow meaning that international practice has given to the right to life and survival. This right appears at the beginning of the Universal Declaration, the Political Covenant, the three regional human rights conventions, and, for instance, the Children's Convention. The tragic record of HIV infection and AIDS links infection closely to premature death and denial of the right to life. Present experience shows that the right has been applied, however, only to the issue of due process of law preceding a judicial sentence of capital punishment. Considerable scope, therefore, exists to enlarge this concept to create and enhance legal claims of AIDS sufferers to life-prolonging care, of HIV infected persons to treatment to postpone the onset of AIDS, and, for instance, of those at high risk of HIV infection to preventative care and education. Interests arising under different conventions may be tied together in resistance of HIV infection. For instance, women's means to protect their health through provisions of the Women's Convention would protect the children they conceive, deliver and rear, whose rights are expressed in the Children's Convention.

B. The Right to Health Care

The right to health care is addressed in the Economic Covenant, Article 12(1) of which recognizes "the right of everyone to the enjoyment of the highest attainable standard of physical and mental health". The Article further identifies some steps to be taken for this purpose, and indicates the several points of intersection between rights to health care and other rights that contribute to health protection and promotion. The Article demonstrates that health care includes the avoidance of HIV infection, but also that those who are HIV infected enjoy rights to the highest health status they can achieve, including maintenance of a symptom-free condition, reduction of symptoms in the shortest possible time when they occur, and experience of maximum health following the onset of AIDS, including the postponement and maximum treatment of mental deterioration associated with AIDS, such as clinical depression and AIDS-related dementia.

HIV infection compromises the immune system. Similarly, pregnancy suppresses a woman's immune system, since the placental, embryonic and fetal tissue is genetically distinct and would be at risk of rejection by the woman's normal immune reaction to alien tissues. Therefore, pregnancy can aggravate vulnerability to HIV infection and to opportunistic infections associated with AIDS, and HIV infection during pregnancy can aggravate the risk of maternal morbidity, and mortality. Danger to a woman's life from pregnancy provides an indication for medical termination of pregnancy. This is accommodated in even conservative abortion laws, which permit the procedure when there is danger to life or danger to enduring health. Legislation may expressly allow abortion on the basis of HIV infection, as in Guyana.[21]

The right to health care is afforded significant amplification in the Women's Convention. It is for each woman to determine whether she wants to undertake pregnancy when she knows she is HIV infected, and whether she wants to risk HIV infection through pregnancy, for instance by having the child of an HIV infected partner. The woman's right to health requires, however, that she can decide to reduce the chance of unwanted pregnancy through the practice of birth control. The Women's Convention therefore instructively provides in Article 12 that:

> "States Parties s0hall take all appropriate measures to eliminate discrimination against women in the field of health care in order to ensure, on a basis of equality of men and women, access to health care services, including those related to family planning."

Health care services related to family planning include information on the use of condoms, and access to them. Condom use reduces unwanted pregnancy and abortion, and is a means of reduction of sexually transmitted diseases, including HIV infection. It is fortuitous that condoms serve the goals both of family planning and of containment of the spread of HIV infection. Promotion of condom use is justified on both of these grounds, but persons and institutions that oppose the use of condoms as an illicit or unnatural form of fertility control deny human rights of both birth control and protection of health. States parties to international conventions that respect the right to health care compromise the integrity of their observance of human rights if they deny or obstruct access to condoms.

Provisions in human rights instruments on health care, including means of family planning, raise the pervasive jurisprudential question of whether rights recognized in established human rights conventions are negative rights or positive rights, or impose obligations that contain both negative and positive components.

Negative rights are so described because they impose only negative obligations on states, meaning obligations not to deny or obstruct individuals' actions taken in pursuit of their rights. Individuals are to be legally free to serve their own health and other interests as they see them, subject only to legal regulation concerning the safety and efficacy of the means they choose to employ. When those means invalves medical treatment, for instance, states can regulate the training and qualifications of practitioners entitled to provide such treatment.

Freedom of religion and conscience are individual rights, and include freedom from imposition of the religious and conscientious convictions of other persons, and of institutions and governments. States are not entitled to deny services of which individuals can avail themselves by invoking, for instance, religious or moral principles.[22] Individuals are free to offer, use or reject services on the basis of their own religious, moral, social, political or other convictions. Those acting in accordance with their convictions are not to be obstructed by police or other state officers on the basis of an asserted public morality or state religion. States are legally entitled to subscribe to a preferred moral vision and to a state religion, of course, but not to impose such a vision or religion by legal sanctions against nonconformity. There is an interaction between positive and negative duties in that, where states have laws or practices that deny or obstruct negative rights, their acceptance of international human rights conventions may require that they take positive steps to amend or repeal such laws and change such practices, but in general this will not convert such rights into positive rights.

The normal meaning of a positive right is that its enjoyment is dependent on a state's acceptance of an affirmative duty to apply its resources in a positive way to make available services and instruments for the purpose of providing an opportunity of which individuals may avail themselves for instance, the right to health care need only be a negative right is the means to supply themselves with the services and instruments, such as pharmaceutical products, that protect or enhance their health status, but would have to be a positive right for states to be obliged to make provision for those who lack resources for self-determination of their health status, and who can maintain or achieve a state of good health status, and who can maintain or achieve a state of good health only through services and related instruments, including drugs, that the state provides.

In many instances, health services that individuals cannot supply for themselves are not supplied by states, but are made available by international aid through agencies or foreign government programmes, or by initiatives of national nongovernmental organizations. If national governments have no obligation under international human rights conventions to provide for these health services, for instance by reaching agreements with international or national suppliers, the right to health care would not offer more than a negative right. That is, although such health services would not have to be made available through initiatives of government, an obligation would exist binding governments not to deny nationals access to such health services, and not to prevent or obstruct their delivery through, for example, provisions on importation of means unrelated to the safety and effectiveness of the particular health services, or on entry of specialized health personnel. Therefore, countries that are unable themselves to provide means to contain the spread of HIV infection should accommodate international and national initiatives for this purpose, and amend legislation that obstructs the effective delivery of such services. For instance, legislation restricting the importation of condoms or access to them by unmarried people on moral grounds would obstruct HIV containment programmes.

C. The Right to Liberty and Security of the Person

The right to liberty and security of the person has its legal expression in the Political Covenant rather than the Covenant that addresses social and cultural rights. This shows that liberty and security were viewed under the Universal Declaration primarily as political interests that are vulnerable to removal and limitation by the unlawful exercise of governmental power. In the context of HIV infection, rights to liberty and security may appear personal rather than political. However, governmental conduct may directly and indirectly affect the extent to which individuals may maintain their liberty and security against the risk of infection, and against inadequate health care services when they are infected. The right to liberty and security closely intersects the right to health care when governmental policies deny individuals the means to protect themselves against infection. For instance, if governments do not require HIV screening of blood donations that contribute to the national blood supply, patients who require transfusions will be denied security against HIV transmission if they could not store their own blood in anticipation nor obtain donations in advance from family members and others they know to present minimum risk.

Governmental denial of liberty and security against HIV

infection has more obvious political dimensions when governments fail to provide security against sexual violence and abuse. Women's vulnerability to rape in circumstances of military turmoil is well documented,[23] but they are also at risk in countries not in a general state of armed conflict when, for instance, police and prison authorities abuse women pending trial and after conviction.[24] Men who intend rape, whether for political purposes of ethnic dominance or as an act of gender superiority, will not restrain themselves for fear of spreading sexually transmitted diseases, and will not use condoms unless perhaps they fear suffering infection.

It is the responsibility of governments to compel restraints against sexual and other abuse on military, police, prison and, for example, refugee management personnel whose access to victims is based on governmen,tal power. States will be in breach of obligations of equality before the law under the Political Covenant if they fail to anticipate and prevent such abuse, to investigate accusations of abuse by acceptance of women's complaints and evidence in accordance with international standards of legal due process, and to punish abuse severely. For example, if the testimony of a woman is not afforded the same procedural weight as the testimony of a man, and if a woman confirming sexual relations with a man faces,undue obstacles in establishing that she did not consent, and she therefore becomes liable to prosecution for fornication, her rights to equality before the law and to security of the person are violated.[25] The outrage to human rights is compounded when the convicted woman has also been infected, and is then stigmatized and refused appropriate care in detention.

In many governmentally maintained institutions, such as prisons, mental hospitals and orphanages, including those in which there is no military or politically motivated action, residents or detainees who are believed to be HIV infected suffer discrimination and are denied health and other services, such as dental and sanitary care, considered to present caregivers with a risk of infection. As against this, however, residents and detainees in such institutions may themselves be denied protection against infection. Homosexual rape of prisoners and mental health detainees is a familiar phenomenon.[26] Further, consensual sexual activity is known to take place in single-sex institutions such as prisons. Institutional authorities frequently refuse to make condoms available, and classify them as contraband when brought in from outside, on the ground that such sexual activity is a violation of institutional rules.[27] Drug taking is also common in many prisons, and because needles are scarce they tend to be shared, aggravating the risk of transmission of HIV infection and, for instance, hepatitis. Prison authorities have refused to implement or permit needle exchange programmes in prisons on the same basis as they refuse to allow condom supplies. Such policies violate the rights of victims to security of the person. The moralistic response, that there would be no risk if people in institutions refrained from sexual and drug taking activities, fails to recognize sex as a natural part of life and the range of compulsive addictive behaviours.

A common expression of the right to liberty is the right to foreign travel, whether for purposes of business, employment or, for instance, recreation. The international human rights movement has not significantly weakened the sovereignty that states may exercise over whether non-nationals may enter their territory, except for obligations regarding refugees. An early international reaction to HIV infection and AIDS was to presume that infection originated outside of countries,[28] and that they could defend their populations by broader controls on entrants, including requiring evidence that those proposing more than brief visits were HIV-negative. Regulations were introduced by many countries that violated international travel agreements endorsed by WHO.[29] A few countries went further, in breach of the long standing provision of international law that countries cannot refuse return of their own nationals, and required nationals who had spent some time abroad, such as students, to present evidence that they were not HIV infected. Such requirements are perhaps more acceptable if their purpose is to provide appropriate care on return rather than to prevent return, but they might still deter persons from return who would suffer stigmatization if they are infected.

There is evidence that a significant percentage of foreign travellers are sexually active outside their countries, including businessmen who are incidentally "entertained" and men who travel on deliberately promoted "sex junkets" to countries where sex workers are a common feature of the entertainment industry. Compulsory HIV testing may be offensive, and futile when conducted on travellers' return within the incubation period following infection. Similarly, compulsory testing of immigrants at or after their arrival in a country may violate anti-discrimination principles. Nevertheless, human rights principles do not preclude states from making health clearance a condition of entry of visitors and immigrants. Barring individuals who present a serious risk of infection to a country's population because of HIV infection may not be different from barring them due to other infections, or on grounds of the costs their care would impose on nationally funded health services. Blanket prohibitions on entry may be less defensible, however, than case-by-case decisions taking account of such factors as individuals' life style and family circumstances.

D. The Right to Freedom from Torture or Ill-Treatment

The right to freedom from torture or ill-treatment, including freedom from inhuman and degrading treatment, is closely related to liberty and security of the person, and equally violated in breach of international human rights law when governments fail to exercise necessary discipline on their military, police, prison and similar personnel. The Inter-American Commission on Human Rights recognized the rape of women by military personnel in Haiti as torture, which would be aggravated were HIV infection to be transmitted to victims.[30] Torture tends to be understood as wilful cruelty inflicted in direct or indirect pursuit of a public or political purpose. The private conduct of an HIV infected person that recklessly or even deliberately risks the infection of another, for instance through unprotected sexual intercourse, would not constitute torture. However, if states do not have or employ means to restrain or to investigate, prosecute, convict and punish such conduct, their tolerance of this ill-treatment would constitute a violation of their obligations under the Political Covenant and, for instance, relevant regional human rights treaties.

States must equip themselves to discharge their international duties, and so be able to act diligently and in good faith to protect the human rights of residents against ill-treatment even when the immediate violation is by a private person not acting under the authority of the stave. Private persons are not directly bound by international human rights law, but must be amenable to preventive and punitive regulation by the laws of states, and to the competent enforcement of those laws. For instance, persons who prove positive on HIV testing should be subject to counselling by public health officers against the deliberate and negligent spread of infection.

Because torture arises from acts to promote the purposes of states in military, political and strategic spheres, not only is the concept itself male gendered, but victims of torture, primarily military, political and strategic adversaries of governments in the quest for power and authority, are also conceived of in male gendered terms. The image of the shackled and tormented victim of torture is essentially male. Male torture victims obviously exist, and their victimization through sexual and other cruelty is documented, but less visible have been the innumerable female victims of torture through which state agents have advanced their purposes.

Women face multiple vulnerabilities to sexual and other forms of torture. They are vulnerable to torture in their own right if they defy gendered expectations of their subordination and passivity, and become outspoken leaders in protests against political, social and other injustice. They are vulnerable if militia want to assert ethnic dominance, the ethnic inferiority of the populations to which women belong, and that particular populations should be "cleansed" from the territories in which they have settled.[31] Women are also vulnerable to torture for the instrumental purpose of menacing, punishing and humiliating their husbands, brothers, fathers and sons for their military, political and other activities.[32] Women's victimization is aggravated not only by risk of their suffering HIV infection but also when they are considered degraded within their own families and communities by even the involuntary loss of virginity, which is stigmatizing for women but not for men. Their rape is compounded by its consequences of rendering them unmarriageable in their own communities and unacceptable into any other that also practices gender discrimination in approving only virgin brides.

Women s vulnerability to ill-treatment in private sector employment can implicate international human rights conventions against ill-treatment, and perhaps indirectly contribute to infection. In many work environments, women become vulnerable to sexual harassment including intercourse they cannot resist because of their economic dependency on their employers. Beyond sexual abuse, they may be compelled to deal with others, such as through care giving, in unsafe ways that expose them to infection. Further, women who are or who may be HIV infected may be compelled to conceal infection and their health vulnerability, and perhaps forego necessary treatment, lest they may forfeit their employment. Enforcement of human rights laws against industrial and related ill-treatment would empower such women to preserve their health interests, employment and integrity.

E. The Right to Marry and Found a Family

The modern international human rights movement was triggered largely by state policies of extermination of ethnic and racial groups, including laws against their intermarriage and on compulsory sterilization. The human rights reaction is the emphasis on rights of marriage and family foundation expressed in all of the leading international, regional and specialized human rights conventions. Limitations on rights of marriage are permitted only on narrow grounds such as mental and physical immaturity, incest prohibitions and severe mental impairment. An unresolved jurisprudential issue is whether the human right to found a family is contingent on marriage, or whether the right to found a family can be separated from marriage in the same way that people unable or unwilling to have families are free to marry.

Some jurisdictions have reacted to HIV infection by mandating that an HIV test be made a condition of the grant of a licence to marry.[33] Such laws are not only offensive to human rights principles of non-discrimination on grounds of disability, but may be ineffective or dysfunctional if their purpose is to obstruct marriage by infected persons. Of course, this would also offend the right of freedom to marry. In many cultures, co-habitation and childbirth without marriage are commonplace, and policies for containment of HIV disease through control of marriage would be futile. Such legislation is equally futile to resist homosexual spread of HIV infection, since same-sex partners are almost invariably not permitted to marry each other.[34]

Denial of same-sex marriage may actually be counterproductive, since the spread of HIV infection would be limited by encouraging and facilitating HIV infected partners to remain with each other and not be sexually promiscuous. In many cultures too, a legislative supposition that heterosexual intimacy does not occur before marriage is naive. Cultures in which the supposition is justified, furthermore, may be suspect in their general respect for human rights, since they tend to be those in which unmarried women's human rights of self-determination in social conduct and association are most frequently violated in the enforcement of their chastity.

The justification that laws mandating pre-marital HIV testing are designed only to ensure that prospective marriage partners are adequately informed may be more defensible, but is patronizing in presuming that legislation has a role in enforcing the obligations of protection against HIV infection that partners in marriage owe to each other. The legislation would violate human rights against discrimination against HIV infected persons where it does not apply equally to other sexually transmitted diseases. Where the sexes are equal, women do not require legally mandated information or protection against risks of sexually transmitted diseases contracted through husbands, and men do not require such legislative protection against their wives. Such legislation indicates that countries are in violation of their human rights obligations to achieve equality of the sexes.

Legislation of this nature also indicates the risk of gender inequality if it reflects men's perceived needs of protection. It suggests that women are both inherently deceivers of men, and sources of uncleanliness and venereal infection. The cultural construction of women as potential vectors of disease is historically profound, denigrating women as liable to be unclean, sexually promiscuous and prone to prostitution. It is an obstacle to women's rights of marriage if they are required to demonstrate, for instance through evidence of chastity or non-infection, that they are fit to be wives and mothers.

The right to found a family is dependent on the capacity for procreation and on the potential of both mothers and children to survive pregnancy and childbirth. The capacity for procreation is normally a negative right, in that the duty of states is not to interfere with conception, pregnancy or adoption. However, infertility may require medical treatment, and, where such services exist, medically assisted reproduction, to afford infertile persons the opportunity to have children. The duty of states to provide medical treatment, including reproductive technologies, is not established as a positive right by inter-national human rights law. However, where such treatment is provided by a state, and where a state observes its negative duty to permit such services to be available, the state is bound by the human rights duty not to permit discrimination against people who are disabled due to HIV infection .

Observance of the duty not to permit discrimination that obstructs HIV infected people's right to found families can present a conscientious dilemma. It has been seen that HIV infection aggravates the dangers of pregnancy through further compromising biological immunity, and that pregnancy may be therapeutically contraindicated for an uninfected woman whose partner is HIV infected. Nevertheless, human rights principles indicate that counselling should be nondirective, and women should be permitted to exercise their right to found a family with informed autonomy. The knowledge that their children on birth will be at risk of succumbing to HIV infection, and that the women themselves may not long survive childbirth, are important matters that women will take into account. They vvill not necessarily be deterred, however, from initiating pregnancy, for instance where this risk does not overwhelm other risks they and their newborn infants would normally face. In any event, the choice must be exercised by them and not by their counsellors.

Pregnant women who are HIV infected have the same right to prenatal care, assistance in labour and postnatal care as uninfected women, and their children are entitled to the same standard of care as those of uninfected mothers. Different treatment is not necessarily discriminatory,[35] however, and care may appropriately be given by personnel and facilities that are able to apply universal precautions so as to minimize the risk of infection to assisting personnel and other recipients of health care.[36] Counselling should be offered to women on such matters as prenatal care, methods of delivery that may minimize the risk of HIV infection to a child, breast feeding, and management of a newborn child. Counselling should be offered in addition to women's partners. If they are HIV infected, they are parties to risks that women may face in bearing their children, and if women are infected, their partners are similarly involved in the risks of their pregnancy. Both partners have important decisions to make in exercise of their right to found a family.

F. The Right to Private and Family Life

The right to marry and found a family is an important component of the right to private and family life, but the latter right goes considerably further. The right to private life reinforces duties of confidentiality and privacy that arise in relations between health care providers and patients. Confidentiality is of special significance regarding HIV infection and AIDS because in many social environments these conditions are widely stigmatizing, and associated with lifestyles that result in social condemnation, marginalization and alienation. Legislation mandating reporting of HIV infection is consistent with human rights principles where public health authorities that receive reports are obliged to respect the confidentiality of their data, and to undertake public health protection without undue disclosure of identities of reported persons .

The right to private life may be compromised where public health legislation permits quarantine of infected persons. Since a detained person will not cease to present a risk of infection, detention and isolation may persist for some time. Public health authorities may not consider the public to be secure unless, for instance, infected persons' undertakings of behaviour modification or lifestyle change are credible or can be reliably policed. Historic instances exist of infected persons being kept in detention for over 26 years,[37] and the experience might be internationally replayable under the impact of the AIDS pandemic, subject to limitations and alternatives compelled by international human rights law. Legislation may be dysfunctional and in violation of human rights law, for instance, when it obstructs the wish of two HIV infected persons to establish a permanent household between themselves, and live a private life together that presents no danger to public health.[38] The European Court of Human Rights has found violatipn of the right to private life, for instance, in Irish legislation that criminalizes homosexual relations among consenting adults.[39] Partner notification requirements may also be dysfunctional if women are vulnerable to domestic violence and other forms of spousal abuse.[40]

The right of HIV infected persons to adopt children is usually contentious, but may be defended under rights both of nondiscrimination and of private and family life. The claim to the right may be resisted because of children's superior rights to safety and to placement where they would have a minimally interrupted upbringing. Children's rights may be consistently invoked in support of their adoption by parents' same-sex partners, however, for instance where the partners are involved in their care and would continue to discharge parental functions, for instance on death of the natural parent.

G. The Right to the Benefits of Scientific Progress

The Economic Covenant addresses the human right to the benefits of scientific progress, but the issue has a political or democratic aspect in that the Covenant anticipates scientific advances offering benefits to all persons without discrimination. Applied to HIV infected persons, the right includes the negative component that private initiatives to advance and apply evolving scientific knowledge for their benefit should not be impaired, and the positive component that states should ensure that the new knowledge that emerges from the initiatives they sponsor will be made available without discrimination on such grounds as sex, race and physical or mental disability. The negative right concerns tolerance, for example, of private pharmaceutical industry and other research under regulations that are neither prohibitive nor unduly restrictive, and under conditions of participants' free and informed consent that conform to international standards.[41] It also includes permitting research, for instance, to develop and test an HIV vaccine and to reinforce resistance to infection and postponement of the onset of AIDS.

It remains difficult, however, to contend that states or international agencies have a positive legal duty, as opposed to a moral duty, to sponsor AIDS research in priority to research into other infections, since states may have no legal obligation to sponsor health research at all or by any particular means. Those whose conditions are studied may in time enjoy benefits, but it is not discrimination against those whose disabilities are not investigated by state initiative that others are treated more favourably. Discrimination is denial of an entitlement, but where there is no entitlement thete is no discrimination when some receive benefits and others do not. States are free to pursue whatever health research agenda they find most promising and most suitable to their needs. Further, the science whose benefits must be made available is not limited to biomedical science but includes, for instance, social science. Similarly, the science may address preventative health care rather than curative treatment. Accordingly, states may discharge any positive obligations they bear under the Economic Covenant by pursuing programmes of preventive community health care to resist the spread of HIV infection rather than by sponsoring clinical studies to aid persons living with AIDS-related disorders.

The need for more successful research into HIV infection, its prevention, and in time, its cure is self-evident from rising statistics of infection. A special challenge is development of gender-sensitive studies that address women's special vulnerability to infection in the ordinary conduct of their lives. Sufficient knowledge exists to achieve behavioural change that would considerably reduce rates of infection, but the gendered functioning of many cultures and societies denies women sexual and reproductive self-determination. Women who have no real alternatives in life to early marriage, to partners they cannot require to be sexually abstinent outside marriage or to use condoms within marriage, are denied means of self-protection against HIV infection and unwanted pregnancy. They have a legitimate claim to research to develop effective female controlled means of resistance to sexually transmitted diseases and unwanted pregnancy.[42] A female condom has been developed, for instance, but women may be unable to overcome partners' hostility to their using it. The right to scientific progress may not afford the means to hold states to account for their inadequate research initiatives in this regard, but respect for human rights against sex and gender discrimination may condition greater sensitivity to women's special needs by both private and public sponsors of biomedical research.

Governments committed themselves through the Beijing Platform for Action to "support and expedite action-oriented research on affordable methods, controlled by women, to prevent HIV and other sexually transmitted diseases, on strategies empowering women to protect themselves from sexually transmitted diseases, including HIV/AIDS, and on methods of care, support and treatment of women, ensuring their involvement in all aspects of such research".[43]

H. The Rights to Information and Education

Information, literacy and the capacity to acquire, process and apply knowledge accurately are necessary tools for self-determination. Individuals must be able to understand particularly the modes of transmission of HIV infection, and strategies to avoid the risk of infection, to themselves and others, that they can apply effectively in the circumstances of their lives. It is commonly observed that knowledge is power, and information and its educated use empower individuals to exercise autonomy and responsibility. Accordingly, rights to information and to the achievement of understanding of uses of information underpin most if not all of the human rights considered above.

The European Court of Human Rights has found a human rights violation when a government attempted to limit information for fear that individuals would employ it for purposes the government disapproved.[44] The Court thereby recognized a limit on governmental means of censorship of information that individuals could use for self-determination, because such censorship violated individuals' human rights. The case concerned reproductive self-determination and access to abortion services, but the Court's decision is applicable to information relevant to HIV infection and management of AIDS.

International experience demonstrates how women may be denied the opportunity to protect their health, including against HIV infection, because of sex and gender discrimination in education. In many cultures, the schooling of girl children is not considered as important as the schooling of boy children; girls enrolled in schools may more easily be kept away to assist mothers in domestic work; and girls' education may be prematurely ended by early marriage. Moreover, some schools expel girls who become pregnant when boys who cause pregnancy face no similar sanction. In Botswana, such school policy on pregnant school girls was successively challenged as constituting sex discrimination under the Constitution of Botswana.[45]

Levels of literacy among girls are frequently lower than levels among boys, and states do not apply resources to encourage and facilitate families to keep their girl children in school.[46] A disincentive to families to invest in girls' education is the devaluation of women's education in employment, and the enduring concept that a woman's only proper destiny is caregiving in the home. Wider recognition of the high percentage of women who are heads of households, and of women's essential contributions to their families' economy, would lead to recognition of how necessary it is that women be informed and educated for the discharge of the functions even conservatively considered to define women's role.

Conservative resistance to the education of girls, and of other marginalized social underclasses, should not be underrated. Literacy and education permit individuals to develop sensitivities to their own circumstances, to gain awareness of the injustices and subordination to which they are subject, and to demand that they and their perceptions be taken seriously, be respected, be treated equally with others and be influential in future developments. The concept that individuals can shape their own destiny and defences, and escape controls exercised, for instance, by those who traditionally have defined natural and supernatural authority that governs individuals' destiny, challenges traditional power within societies.[47] Prohibition of information has long been the instrument of politically and othurrwise oppressive forces protective of their authority. Only in recent years, for instance, has the Roman Catholic Church discontinued its Index of Prohibited Books, which limited the literature that observant members of the Church could read in good conscience. Some Islamic authorities continue to consider the abandonment of faith by reception of different ways of thinking, namely apostasy, as properly punishable by death. Conservative forces are willing to tolerate HIV infection and death, perhaps seen as the divinely ordained wage of sin, rather than tolerate the challenge to their traditional values represented, for instance, by condom use to reduce sexually transmitted disease.

I. Associated Rights

Closely allied to rights to information and education are rights to communicate and apply the understandings that individuals have developed through information and its interpretation. The human rights to freedom of thought, conscience and religion, to political participation and to assembly and association, recognized in the Political Covenant and, for instance, the regional human rights conventions, both contribute to and depend on rights to information and education. Knowledge is power, and power is applied in political, social, spiritual and related ways. Political power can achieve and secure rights to information and education, but democratic political power frequently depends on rights to assembly, association and collective action.

Improvement in public health and health education in a community is frequently possible through collective and political initiatives, and initiatives can become effective through the application of historical, social and strategic understanding. Accordingly, although these associated rights are of immense democratic importance in themselves, they can be of decisive significance in health protection and promotion, regarding resistance to HIV infection and AIDS and to other dangers to life, only when applied interactively with each other. The indirect implication for health that each of these rights has in isolation becomes direct when they are used in combination.

V. DOMESTIC APPLICATION OF INTERNATIONAL HUMAN RIGHTS LAW

International law in post-medieval Western Europe was taught, for instance by Gentili, the professor who first taught the subject at Oxford University before the end of the 16th century, as The Law of Nature and Nations. As part of Natural Law, international law was an inherent component of all law, and all countries governed by law necessarily included international law as an element of their jurisprudence. Subsequent developments led to a distinction, however, in how domestic legal systems regarded international law. The Monist theory kept faith with history and considered international law to be directly applicable by domestic courts, although subject to domestic legislation that could direct courts differently. In contrast, the Dualist theory considered the international and domestic legal systems to be separate, the law of nations not being relevant within the domestic legal order.

In practice, few states applied either theory in a pure form, and modern states define the domestic significance of international law according to historical and political influences. The modern constitutions of some states, such as Germany, explicitly afford the principles of international law priority over national law where the two appear to be in conflict. Accordingly, international human rights law prevails within the domestic legal system over any contrary provisions within that system. Other states have achieved the same effect with regard to human rights principles, but not necessarily other provisions of international law. Countries in the English Common law tradition do not give domestic effect to international treaties unless they have been given the force of domestic law by explicit national legislation, but treat international customary law as part of domestic customary or Common law. In yet others, provisions of constitutional law permit the state's ratification of certain international treaties to be self-executing, meaning that they become directly applicable within the domestic legal system, while other international treaties do not have that effect but require explicit adoption by legislation. Where international law is not incorporated or adopted into domestic law, however, domestic courts of all countries will normally try to avoid inconsistencies in their interpretation of domestic law so as not to place their countries in breach of their international responsibilities if that result is avoidable.

States' domestic laws that are applied in ways that violate international human rights law may be exposed and condemned by international human rights tribunals, when states are subject to their jurisdiction under human rights conventions. Condemnation is possible even concerning matters that states claim to be of moral concern. For instance, the European Court of Human Rights has condemned criminalization of homosexual relations between consenting adults when the relevant national law was internally perceived as upholding moral values.[48] As the international jurisprudence on human rights evolves, such rights as those to non-discrimination on grounds for instance of sex or disability are being recognized to form part of international customary law, and therefore to be incorporated into many national legal systems, and not to be dependent on states' legislative adoption of a particular convention.

It may be anticipated that international human rights law relevant to HIV infection and its prevention will evolve to set international norms by which the humane character of countries' internal laws and practices will be assessed. Further, although individuals as such are not generally governed by international law, for instance concerning acts of domestic violence and those liable to spread HIV infection, countries themselves are responsible under international law to take appropriate preventive, remedial or punitive action when those subject to their jurisdiction violate principles of international human rights law. In more extreme cases, individuals may face direct legal accountability under international human rights law for war crimes and crimes against humanity. Accordingly, international human rights law concerning HIV infection will have considerable potential for both international and domestic enforcement.

Under Strategic Objective C.3 of the Beijing Platform for Action, governments agreed to undertake gender-sensitive initiatives that address sexually transmitted diseases, HIV/AIDS, and sexual and reproductive health issues that include reviewing and amending laws "that may contribute to women's susceptibility to HIV infection and other sexually transmitted diseases, including enacting legislation against those socio-cultural practices that contribute to it, and implement legislation, policies and practices to protect women, adolescents and young girls from discrimination related to HIV/AIDS".[49] Significant efforts are underway in several regions, including Asia,[50] to review laws and policies and enact new laws that facilitate the protection and promotion of reproductive health, including the prevention and treatment of HIV/AIDS. The challenge is to ensure that such efforts are accelerated and progress in a gender-sensitive manner.

REFERENCES

1. Henkin L, Pugh R.C., Schachter O., Smit H. Eds., *International Law: Cases and Materials.* St Paul, Minnesota: West Publishing Co. 2nd ed. 1987 at 107.
2. Brownlie I. *System of the Law of Nations, State Responsibility,* Part I. Oxford, UK: Oxford University Press 1983 at 81.
3. Taylor A.L. Women's health at a crossroad: global responses to HIV/AIDS. Health Matrix 1994;4:297-324.
4. Paragraph 97, Platform for Action adopted by the United Nations Fourth World Conference on Women: Equality, Development and Peace, Beijing, China, Advance Unedited Draft, 15 September 1995.
5. Cook R.J. Human rights and reproductive self-determination. *The American University Law Review* 1995; 44:975-1016 at 978.
6. General Recommendation No. 15: Avoidance of Discrimination Against Women in National Strategies for the Prevention and Control of Acquired Immunodeficiency Syndrome (AIDS), in Report of the Committee on the Elimination of Discrimination against Women, 9th Sess., UN Doc. A/45/38 (1990).
7. Cook R.J. Reservations to the Convention on the Elimination of All Forms of Discrimination against Women. *Virginia Journal of International Law* 1990;30: 645-716.
8. Cook R.J. Gender, health, and human rights. *Health and Human Rights* 1995;1(4): 153-168.
9. Constitution of the World Health Organization, signed July 22, 1946 and entered

into force on April 7, 1948, in *Basic Documents,* 39th ed. (Geneva: World Health Organization, 1993).

11. Preamble to the Women's Convention.
12. Mann J., Tarantola D.J.M., Netter T.W. The HIV Pandemic: Status and Trends. In: Mann J., Tarantola DJM, Netter T.W., eds. *AIDS in the World: A Global Report.* Cambridge: Harvard University Press, 1992: 11-108, 30.
13. Paragraph 99, Platform for Action adopted by the United Nations Fourth World Conference on Women: Equality, Development and Peace, Beijing, China, Advance Unedited Draft, 15 September 1995.
14. Dickens B.M. Health Care Practitioners and HIV: Rights, Duties and Liabilities. In Jayasuriya DC ed., *HIV Law, Ethics and Human Rights* - Text and Materials, New Delhi: UNDP, 1995.
15. Goldstein K.L. Balancing risks and rights: HIV testing regimes for pregnant women. *Cornell Journal of Law and Public Policy* 1995; 4: 609-637, and Post LF. Unblinded mandatory HIV screening of newborns: cure or coercion? *Cardozo Law Review* 1994; 16:169-227.
16. See generally, Marge Berer ed., *Women and HIV/AIDS: An International Resource Book,* London: Pandora, 1993.
17. Verkuyl DAA. Practising obstetrics and gynaecology in areas with a high prevalence of HIV infection. *Lancet* 1995; 346: 293 6 at 295.
18. Owen M. *The World of Widows.* London: Zed Press, forthcoming, 1996.
19. Halim A.M.A. Challenges to the application of international women's human rights in the Sudan. In Cook R.J. ed. *Human Rights of Women: National and International Perspectives.* Philadelphia, Penn: University of Pennsylvania Press, 1994: 397 421.
20. Butegwa F. Using the African Charter on Human and Peoples' Rights to secure women's access to land in Africa. In Cook R.J. ed. *Human Rights of Women: National and International Perspectives.* Philadelphia, Penn: University of Pennsylvania Press, 1994: 495-514.
21. Guyana Medical Termination of Pregnancy Act 1995.
22. *Open Door Counselling and Dublin Well Women Centre* v. *Ireland* 15 Eur. H.R. Rep. 244 (1992).
23. Swiss S., Giller J.E. Rape as a crime of war: a medical perspective. *JAMA* 1993;270:612-615.
24. Human Rights Watch, *Double Jeopardy: Police Abuce of Women in Pakistan,* New York: Human Rights Watch (1992).
25. Id at 35.
26. Meier R.F. *Crime and Society* Boston: Allyn and Bacon, 1989 at 414-5.
27. Correctional Services Canada, *HIV/AIDS in Prisons Final Report of the Expert Committee on AIDS and Prisons,* Ottawa: Minister of Supply and Services Canada, 1994.
28. Sabatier R. *Blaming Others: Prejudice, Race and Worldwide AIDS.* London: Panos, 1988.
29. Id. at 118.
30. OEA/Ser.L/V/II.88, February 9, 1995 at 12-13, 39-47, 93-97.
31. International Human Rights Law Group. No justice, no peace: accountability for rape and gendered-based violence in the former Yugoslavia. *Hastings Women's Law Journal* 1994;5:18-128.
32. Human Rights Watch. *Untold Terror: Violence Against Women in Peru's Armed Conflict.* New York: Human Rights Watch, 1992.
33. Closen M.L., Hermann D.H.J., Horne P.J. *et al., AIDS: Cases and Materials.* Houston, Texas: The John Marshall Publishing Com., 1989 at 406.

34. Hawaii's Supreme Court has recently held in *Baehr v. Lewin* (1993) 852 P. 2d 44 that Hawaii's marriage statute discriminated on the basis of gender in permitting only heterosexual marriage, and so violated the equal protection clause of the state constitution.
35. Vos v. *The Netherlands,* Communication No.218/1986, U.N. Doc. A/44/40 at 232 (1989) (U.N. Human Rights Committee).
36. Supra note 14.
37. Leavitt J. Gendered Expectations: Women and Early Twentieth Century Public Health. In Kerber L.K., Kessler-Harris A., Sklar K.K., eds. U.S. *History as Women's History.* North Carolina: University of North Carolina Press, 1995: 147-169.
38. See text above, following note 34.
39. *Norris v.* Ireland 142 Eur. Ct. H.R. (ser. A) (1989).
40. North R.L., Rothenberg K.H. Partner notification and the threat of domestic violence against women with HIV infection. *New England Journal of Medicine* 1993;329: 1194-96.
41. *International Ethical Guidelines for Biomedical Research Involving Human Subject,* Council for International Organizations of Medical Sciences (CIOMS), Geneva: CIOMS, 1993.
42. Potts M.The urgent need for a vaginal microbicide in the prevention of HIV transmission. *Am* J. *Public Health.* 1994; 84 :890-1.
43. Paragraph 109(o).
44. Supra note 22.
45. *Student Representative Council, Molepolole College of Education v. Attorney General of Botswana* Unreported, Civil Appeal No. 13 of 1994, Misca No. 396 of 1993. Judgment delivered on 31 January 1995; for discussion of the judgment see Quansah EK. Is the Right to Get Pregnant a Fundamental Human Right in Botswana? *Journal of African Law* 1995;39:97-102.
46. United Nations, *The World's Women 1995: Trends and Statistics.* New York: United Nations, 1995 at 92.
47. Seidel G. The competing discourses of HIV/AIDS in Sub-Saharan Africa: Discourses of rights and empowerment vs. discourses of control and exclusion. *Soc. Sci. Med.* 1993;36:175-194.
48. Supra note 39.
49. Paragraph 109(b) of the Beijing Platform.
50. Jayasuriya DC ed. *HIV Law and Law Reform: Asia and the Pacific,* New Delhi: UNDP, 1995.

22

Women, the HIV Epidemic and Human Rights: A Tragic Imperative

Ms. Julie Hamblin
Partner
Elsworth and Ebsworth
Sydney Australia

Ms. Elizabeth Reid
Director
HIV and Development Programme
UNDP, New York

INTRODUCTION

> "Like every other epidemic, AIDS develops in the cracks and crevasses of society's inequalities. We cannot face the epidemic if we try to hide the contradictions and conflicts which it exposes."—
>
> *Herbert Daniel, Brazil*

Women require special and urgent consideration in the response to the HIV epidemic. It may not be clear why, in the case of a virus that can infect a person regardless of sex, race or social status, we should single out women as one group for separate consideration. This seems to deny the universality of the threat of HIV infection.

However, the HIV virus is not random in its spread or in its impact. The epidemic is inextricably bound up with the social and cultural values and economic relations which underlie the interaction between individuals and within communities. In its impact, the spread of the virus is facilitated by social inequalities and, in turn, reflects and reinforces those inequalities. It differentiates not only in its medical manifestations but also in its disproportionate impact on those who are socially, sexually and economically vulnerable.

Women, because of their social and sexual subordination, are disproportionately affected by the epidemic. The dynamics of sexual relationships mean that many women are unable to protect themselves against sexually—transmitted HIV infection, the predominant mode of infection. Globally, it is estimated that 60 per cent of all cases of infection occur through vaginal intercourse. In sub-Saharan Africa, the estimate is 80 per cent.

As wives and sex workers, women are at risk of sexual transmission. As mothers, women must deal with the implications of HIV infection for unborn children. As mothers, aunts, sisters, grandmothers and daughters, women will have to care for the children orphaned by the epidemic. As carers, women bear the burden of caring for sick and dying partners, children, relatives and neighbours and attempting to hold the family unit together in the face of sickness and death. On all these counts, women are disproportionately affected by the epidemic.

An understanding of the factors that affect women is critical to any effective measures to contain the spread of HIV and to deal with its effects for both women and men. The vulnerability of women to HIV must be understood in the broader context of deeply embedded social and gender inequalities which lie at the heart of women's inability to deal effectively with the risks and needs created by the epidemic. Unless the interaction between HIV infection, cultural values and the rights and needs of women is recognised, the fundamental changes required to stem this epidemic will be unattainable.

THE EPIDEMIOLOGY OF HIV INFECTION AND AIDS IN WOMEN

In 1990, the World Health Organization estimated that there were between 8 and 10 million people worldwide infected with HIV. More than 3 million of these people are women.[1] Even more alarming is the rate at which infection among women has been increasing. The number of infected women rose sharply during the second half of the 1 980's and, in some areas of Africa, Latin America and the Caribbean, there was more than a fourfold increase over a period of between two and four years.[2, 3] It is estimated that during the next decade the prevalence of HIV infection among women will equal and, in some cases, overtake that of men.

The World Health Organization estimates that during the 1990's, the number of women and children dying of AIDS will rise to 3 million. In most central African cities and in some major cities in America and Western Europe, AIDS is already the leading cause of death for women between the ages of 20 and 40. In sub-Saharan Africa over the next few years, infant mortality is expected to increase by up to 30 per cent as a result of perinatal transmission of HIV.[1]

It is estimated that approximately 80 per cent of the total number of women and children currently infected with HIV are in sub-Saharan Africa. In this region, one in every twenty adult women is thought to be infected,[4] and women represent more than 50 per cent of the total number of AIDS cases.[1]

The majority of infected women are of child bearing age, opening the way for perinatal HIV transmission to these women's children on a large scale. UNDP has estimated that over 85 per cent of the cases of paediatric infection in Africa have resulted from perinatal transmission. For the Caribbean the estimate is 97.5 per cent.[5]

Even where the children do not themselves have HIV infection, the number of children orphaned by AIDS is increasing rapidly. World Health Organization has estimated that as many as 10 million children in sub-Saharan Africa will be orphaned by the epidemic by the end of the 1 990's.[1]

The primary HIV risk activity for women globally is sexual activity. Over 90 per cent of women currently infected with HIV have been infected as a result of transmission through vaginal intercourse. Efficacy of transmission is increased where women have poor general health and suffer from genital lesions, inflammation, secretions and scarification. Women are also at increased risk of being infected with HIV infection through contaminated blood and injections because of the high incidence of blood transfusions and injections associated with pregnancy, childbirth and post-pregnancy haemorrhage or treatment for anaemia caused by repeated pregnancies.[6]

The World Health Organization has admitted that its estimates of the levels of infection among women and children should be viewed as very conservative.[1] It is likely that underreporting of HIV infection and AIDS in parts of Africa, the Caribbean and Asia, where women make up a large proportion of the infected population, has helped to conceal the true levels of infection. However, even the estimates currently available leave no doubt as to the magnitude of the impact of the HIV epidemic on women.

THE STATUS OF WOMEN AND THE HIV EPIDEMIC

While the levels of HIV infection and AIDS among women

demonstrate clearly the magnitude of the problem, an understanding of HIV infection in women requires more than just an appreciation of the statistics. The social and cultural determinants of HIV infection in women are very different from those for men because they relate to the-role of women within relationships, families and communities which, in turn, determines the nature and patterns of sexual activity and other factors that place women at risk of HIV infection. An understanding of the epidemic must therefore include not only how women have been affected but also why they have been affected.

HIV infection is preventable. Given access to information and appropriate preventive measures and the means of implementing these measures, there need be no new cases of infection. But poverty, dependency and powerlessness strip a person of the ability to protect herself or himself against infection. It is therefore inevitable that, as the epidemic progresses, those people who have the power to protect themselves against infection will be in a position to do so while those people who do not will continue to be infected in ever-increasing numbers.

The link between powerlessness and the risk of exposure to HIV provides the key to understanding the source of women's vulnerability to HIV infection. It is the reason why HIV infection is increasingly a condition of all women, regardless of race, colour or economic status. In more developed countries, the full impact of these social and cultural dynamics was not apparent in the early years of the epidemic when the majority of reported cases was among homosexual men. With dramatic increases in infection levels in women in both the developed and the developing world, however, there has been a shift in the global demographics of HIV infection. This shift has forced a reassessment of the role of socio-economic factors in the spread of HIV in order to address the ways in which women are being affected by the epidemic.

The male orientation of the understanding of the epidemic to date is evident also in the way HIV-related illnesses and AIDS have been defined. The case definition of AIDS issued by the United States Centres for Disease Control and used worldwide focuses on the marker diseases that are characteristic of HIV- related illness in men and omits conditions that often signify the onset of HIV-related conditions and AIDS in women, including pelvic inflammatory disease, cervical cancer, vaginal candidiasis and conjunctivitis. This has had serious consequences for women, leaving many women undiagnosed or wrongly diagnosed, delaying diagnosis and treatment and denying women access to disability and other benefits and services because they have not been diagnosed with AIDS.[7]

The patterns of social and economic dependency that render women vulnerable to HIV infection are manifested in many different ways. First and foremost, they lead to women being deprived of the power to determine the basis upon which their sexual-relationships with men take place. For many women, sexual intercourse is not a question of choice but rather a question of survival. Cultural attitudes and norms leave no place for unmarried or childless women. A woman's fertility and her relationship to her husband will often be the source of her social identity. Moreover, for many women, marriage provides forms of economic and social support that would not be available to them if they were to remain single.[2, 8, 9]

Similar social constructs also dictate that a married woman has little or no power to negotiate the basis upon which her sexual relationship with her husband will take place. Once married, women are usually expected to remain faithful to their husbands but are unable to compel fidelity in return. In many parts of the world, multiple sexual relationships on the part of men are actively condoned or at least regarded as an acceptable practice. The tendency for men to have sexual relationships outside their marriage is reinforced by male migration and mobility common in many developing countries where men leave the village to obtain work elsewhere.[10]

Women have little alternative but to accept the risk that sexual intercourse with their husband entails. They usually have little or no means of support for themselves and their children other than by remaining within the marriage. Even if condoms were available to them at an affordable price, most women would not be able to ensure that their husbands used them.

Although it is almost invariably the husband who is the vector of HIV infection for wives, a married woman who is found to be infected with HIV will often be expelled from the family unit by the husband. The husband will then seek a new wife, often a younger woman who is believed to be uninfected and therefore safe and who, in turn, will be exposed to HIV. In some parts of Africa, there have been reports of increased rape of young girls, because they are believed to be free of HIV infection.'[11]

Prostitution is often the only means of support for deserted, separated, divorced or unmarried older women, highlighting once again the close link between economic need and exposure to HIV infection. The term "prostitution" is used in this paper to refer to a wide variety of ways in which women exchange sexual intercourse for cash or other forms of economic support, food, shelter or care.

There has been a serious distortion of the understanding of the way this epidemic has affected women because of the singling out of sex workers by epidemiologists, researchers and national HIV/AIDS programmes as a target or high risk group. The overwhelming majority of women are not sex workers and the largest group of women at high risk of infection are wives. Recent data from Mexico indicate that only 0.8 per cent of all reported AIDS cases have been among sex workers and 9 per cent among housewives.[12] Similar figures can be found in other countries, both developed and developing. In Senegal where the epidemic is still in its infancy (less than 2 per cent of the adult population infected), modes of transmission to women in one infectious diseases ward were 20 per cent acquired iatrogenically, 30 per cent occupationally (sex workers) and 50 per cent had no risk factor other than being a wife.[13] As the epidemic proceeds, the proportion of wives to all infected women increases and that of sex workers and iatrogenically acquired transmission decreases.

The targeting of sex workers encourages blame, stigma and discrimination not only against them but against all women. It allows others, both the men who infect sex workers and the wives of these men, to deny that they are at risk. However, it has brought some benefits to some sex workers. HIV prevention programmes which have provided counselling, support and services for these women and their children and which ensure women access to affordable, quality condoms have assisted women to adopt condom usage in their work.[2] In some cases, sex workers have been empowered through collective action and instituted condoms-only policies in their area of operation.

However, programmes of assistance and support to sex workers and-regular supplies of affordable, quality condoms are still rare. Furthermore, even where sex workers have adopted condoms in their work place, research shows an endemic failure to use them in their personal relations.[2] In this, sex workers are no different from the vast majority of women.

Women's access to the cash economy other than through prostitution, is often limited by land ownership or usage regulations, by their limited access to education, training, credit or employment, and through their culturally restricted mobility. The sale of sex is also something that women may engage in from time to time in order to support themselves and their families. For these women, sex work is not an occupation or even a chosen lifestyle, but a pragmatic measure to overcome transitory economic hardship. The risk of HIV transmission to which they are exposed has to be tragically balanced by them against need.

The economic dependency of women increases their risk of exposure to HIV infection in other ways. Lack of access to affordable health care, particularly treatment of sexually transmitted diseases and other conditions that increase susceptibility to HIV, means women are more likely to become infected as a result of sexual intercourse with an infected partner. Low levels of literacy among women means that they are less likely to have access to information about HIV prevention strategies. The social and geographic isolation of women further reduces their ability to protect themselves.[9]

Women are also in a markedly disadvantaged position with respect to confidentiality. The majority of HIV-infected women discover their HIV status during pregnancy or when one of their children becomes sick with AIDS. At this point, any confidentiality protection for the woman disappears as local knowledge of the child's illness leads to open assumptions about the HIV status of the mother. The child's father often refuses to be tested. The woman is frequently held responsible for having transmitted HIV to her children, even though it is usually the husband who introduced HIV to the family unit. The consequences of this lack of control over the disclosure of her HIV status can be blame, social alienation and repudiation by her husband.[2,14]

The inability of women to control the factors that place them at risk of HIV infection is compounded by the fact that many societies define the social and cultural identity of women primarily through their role as child- bearers and child rearers. HIV barrier preventive measures, such as the use of condoms, that inhibit women's ability to fulfil their reproductive role are not acceptable. The experience with family planning programmes in the past has highlighted the extent to which the cultural value placed upon reproduction has been an obstacle to change and has demonstrated that women rarely have control over the reproductive process.

The impact of the HIV epidemic on women is not confined to their own risk of being infected with HIV. As the primary carers, women bear the burden of caring for the sick, of holding the family unit together in the face of sickness and death and of coping with the emotional trauma of the dying. They must often forego productive activities or employment opportunities in order to fulfil their duties as care-givers. The psychological burdens and responsibilities carried by women in these circumstances are great and will be exacerbated where the women herself is infected with HIV and experiences anxiety about her own health and the future care of her children.[15]

These scenarios paint a grim picture of a cycle of dependency in which women are forced into activities that place them at risk of-HIV infection and where their ability to free themselves from their dependent role is further reduced by the day to day reality of coping with the consequences of the HIV epidemic. Unless the cycle can be broken, there is every risk that it will be perpetuated, leading to the deaths of increasing numbers of women and men. HIV infection and AIDS have become frightening manifestations of the underlying social and economic inequality of women. Measures to address this inequality must be central to efforts to contain the spread of HIV.

PREVENTION IN WOMEN

Given the greatly increased vulnerability of women to HIV infection because of their emotional, social, cultural and economic dependency, the task of preventing HIV transmission in women must be recognised as presenting very different challenges to that of preventing infection in men. It is necessary to consider not only whether proposed preventive strategies are inherently effective in reducing transmission risks but also whether the cultural environment is such that women are in a position to implement the preventive strategies. Knowing what has to be done in order to protect oneself from HIV is meaningless if one has no power to control the circumstances that give rise to the risk or in which prevention must occur.

HIV prevention efforts to date have failed to offer women effective and achievable ways of reducing their exposure to transmission risks. The prevention efforts have focused on three issues—a reduction in the number of sexual partners, monogamy or fidelity within relationships and safer sexual practices, in particular the use of condoms, that reduce the likelihood of HIV transmission when exposure occurs. These prevention measures are drawn from men's physique and lifestyle and should be directed at men. As means by which women can protect themselves from HIV, they are hopelessly inadequate.

As a prevention strategy, reducing the number of one's sexual partners is of no help to the many women who have sexual intercourse only with their husband or regular partner. Having only one sexual partner has been a tragic failure as a means of protection against HIV for wives. Even where a woman does have multiple sexual partners, she will often be powerless to change this behaviour because, for the reasons discussed above, her sexual relationships are too often born out of economic need and dependency. Unless these women are offered some other solution to the underlying problem, warnings about the risks involved in multiple sexual relationships, while increasing women's anxiety about HIV, will not in themselves lead to any actual reduction in the risk.[8,9,14]

Similarly, HIV prevention messages that emphasise the importance of monogamy within relationships are not of any practical relevance to most women. It is estimated that between 60 per cent and 80 per cent of HIV-infected women in Africa have had sexual intercourse with only their husband.[14] The problem is not that these women are not faithful to their husbands but that they are unable to compel faithfulness in their husbands in return. In a society where it is culturally acceptable for men to have sexual relationships outside marriage. but-not for women, women have fewer alternatives but to accept these cultural determinants. Their lack of choice is exacerbated once again by economic dependency which provides a powerful disincentive for a woman to leave a sexually unsafe marital relationship.

If one accepts that women are not able to avoid contact with HIV-infected sexual partners, the third prevention strategy which relates to safer sexual practices could still provide significant protection for women. Even here, however, it is evident that the inequality of women within relationships obstructs their ability to protect themselves against HIV. The only barrier method of preventing HIV transmission advocated at present is the male condom. It is an unfortunate biological reality that women must ask men to use condoms and not the other way around. If women have no power to negotiate the basis upon which their sexual relationships take place, they will equally have no power to compel the use of condoms by their male partners nor to negotiate abstinence. Moreover, the use of barrier protection to reduce HIV transmission presents difficulties for many women because of the desire and, in many cases, the cultural imperative to bear children.[9,14,16] Yet again, social and cultural inequality is translated into an increased risk of HIV infection.

HIV prevention measures advocated to date have offered women little or no protection from infection. By placing the lives of women in jeopardy in this way, the failure of HIV prevention programmes to address the needs of women can be seen as a fundamental abuse of human rights. This imbalance in the focus of

HIV prevention efforts must be redressed as a matter of urgency.

STRATEGIES FOR CHANGE

The Philosophical Issues

This epidemic calls for an affirmation of faith that the irrational will not prevail. Refusing to use a condom or to curtail or change sexual behaviour in the face of the fatality of infection is irrational. Traditionally, ideals of rationality and of morality have been drawn from male thought styles and moral consciousness.[17] The character traits traditionally associated with-femininity are considered to place ideals of rationality and the objectivity of truth, the male character traits, in jeopardy. Human excellence and virtues are considered to be exemplified in the range of activities and values associated with maleness.

However, this equating of human excellence with male character traits has been placed under attack by the epidemic. So many men seem reluctant to change their lifestyles that this would seem to indicate defects in the concept of masculinity and an impoverishment of male consciousness, especially moral consciousness. It can never be considered to be a virtue or rational to act repeatedly in a situation such as this to place one's own life and that of others in danger. In this case, there is no overriding defence such as patriotism or heroism which might justify such behaviour. Thus, a tension is created between ideals of rationality and moral consciousness on the one hand and cultural norms-of maleness on the other. Behaviour which has such devastating consequences not only for the self but for others, women and children in particular, undermines both.

The HIV epidemic thus carries within itself a cultural critique. Cultural ideals of masculinity and femininity in themselves have become responsible for a devastating toll in human lives, especially women's lives. Culturally created norms of masculinity place men at high risk of becoming infected through accepted male lifestyles. Culturally created norms of femininity place women and children at high risk of becoming infected through the same male lifestyles.

The same behaviour can place both men and women at risk of infection since the cultural norms of masculinity and femininity have operated in societies not as descriptive principles of classification but rather as expressions of values. Maleness and male paradigms of rationality are identified with superiority. The feminine becomes one with subjugation and oppression. This systemic sexual, social and economic subjugation denies to women one of the few effective preventive measures for them: the negotiation of safer sexual intercourse.

It is not just that women lack the power to act or the means to influence male behaviour obecause of these structural gender differences. Women have been stripped of voice and self-esteem. They feel powerless even to talk about safer sexual behaviour and practices with their husbands or regular sexual partners.

The epidemic thus provides an imperative for fundamental cultural and social change. But such changes may not occur in an acceptable time frame: the epidemic also imposes an imperative for urgent action. Approximately 1,500 - 1,700 women are becoming newly infected each day[18] and this number is increasing.

This creates a potential tension between prevention strategies for women directed towards lessening their subordination so that they can take greater control over their lives and prevention strategies that they can use immediately. Addressing strategies that are achievable in the short term without also addressing the inequalities that have given rise to the risk of infection creates the possibility that the impetus for more fundamental cultural and social change will be defused.[19] Is it possible to overcome the tension between the urgent need for immediate, practical interventions to protect women from HIV infection and the need to address the systemic inequalities that render women vulnerable in the first place?

The experience in recent times with family planning provides a relevant analogy. The pattern has been that women have increasingly taken responsibility for the consequences of sexual relationships, either through the use of contraceptives, overwhelmingly measures to be adopted by women rather than men, or through being the primary carers for children. However, while on one level this has increased women's control over the consequences of sexual activity, it is possible to question whether it has in fact reduced the sexual exploitation of women. It is certainly arguable that the availability of contraceptives for women has merely assisted the sexual exploitation of women since men need no longer be concerned that-intercourse will lead to unwanted pregnancies and paternal obligations.

With the HIV epidemic, we see the same philosophical dilemma played out but with vastly-increased stakes. Any effort to redress women's vulnerability to HIV must be recognised as being potentially a two-edged sword. On the one hand, there is an urgent need for HIV prevention measures that women can control because they are unable to compel condom use or monogamy on the part of their male partners. On the other hand, by encouraging women to be the initiators of HIV prevention measures within sexual relationships, there is a risk that we will further entrench the sexual exploitation of women by men who will, once again, be absolved of responsibility for the consequences of their sexual activity. Similarly, other measures aimed at reducing HIV infection risks for women, such as treatment of sexually-transmitted diseases, may only serve to obscure the fact that it is sexual subordination and not poor health that is the primary HIV risk factor for women. It must be clearly understood that the most effective prevention strategy for women is behaviour change in men.

It is critical that the need to reconcile this potential conflict between the long-term and the short-terrn goals for women be recognised when formulating strategies to respond to HIV/AIDS. Clearly, where there is the possibility of implementing immediate and effective measures to reduce women's risk of HIV exposure, it would be morally reprehensible to withhold these measures in the interests of furthering the long term objective of achieving the required cultural and social changes. However, the important point to bear in mind is that the two objectives need not necessarily be in conflict. Thus, the two goals of improving the status of women and protecting women against HIV are entirely consistent, as long as HIV/AIDS policy is properly informed by an understanding of the philosophical issues that underpin it.

It is important that these concerns guide HIV prevention efforts towards interventions that lead to the greater rather than the lesser empowerment of women. This could be done, for example, by interventions to assist women collectively to develop strategies to take greater control over sexual relationships or by increasing the role of community-based organisations in HIV prevention since these groups are more accessible to women. HIV/AIDS education programmes can focus on ways in which women can themselves exercise control rather than on interventions that require little active participation by women. Measures that address the legal and economic inequality of women can provide real and immediate prospects for reducing women's risk of infection because they give women autonomy, alternatives to dependent relationships. Initiatives such as these not only offer the best prospects for the effeetive containment of HIV both immediately and in the long term but also assist in addressing the fundamental structural inequalities that have denied women control over their lives.

Research and National Policy Strategies

HIV infection risks for women necessitate a re-thinking of HIV research strategies, both biomedical and social. Because women are often unable to control the basis upon which their sexual relationships take place, research efforts directed towards developing barrier protection methods that do not rely upon the co-operation of men have the potential to offer women immediate and effective protection against HIV infection.

The primary barrier protection currently available — the male condom — clearly does not meet this need and it is notable how little medical research has been devoted to HIV prevention methods that women can use. The proposed female condom has little appeal for women and has limited application where protection must be surreptitious. Little has been done to investigate whether other devices, such as a modified diaphragm, may also offer protection to women from HIV transmission. Diaphragms have been thought to be as effective as condoms in protecting women from gonorrhoea and other sexually transmitted diseases. There is still no form of chemical barrier protection, such as a virucide, available to women. These are all matters that should be an urgent priority of research.[16]

It is also important that research assist in accommodating the social and cultural factors that otherwise would prevent women from protecting themselves against HIV. This could be done, for example, by working to develop a virucide that does not at the same time prevent contraception. In this way, practical measures could be put in place to ensure that the desire or social imperative for women to have children does not also expose them to an increased risk of HIV infection.[8,16,19]

In addition to effective barrier protection, there are other interventions that can protect women against HIV infection. Foremost among these is effective treatment of sexually transmitted diseases and other genital conditions which increase the risk of HIV transmission. In relation to iatrogenically-acquired HIV, improved sterilisation procedures, blood screening, the use of blood substitutes and measures to decrease the likelihood that a woman will require a blood transfusion during childbirth could also be effective in reducing risk factors.[9]

The fact that these measures have not yet been given a high priority in HIV strategies indicates the extent to which those strategies have failed to place women at the centre of the analysis that is, to give adequate consideration to the concerns and needs of women in the development of prevention strategies.

Pregnant women are frequently advocated and used as sentinel groups for determining HIV infection rates in the general population. The need to find a proper balance among surveillance, prevention and other HIV programmes is noted here but will not be addressed.

For many, men and women, unauthorised delinked testing is considered to be an invasion of bodily integrity. The testing of pregnant women without consent and without disclosure to them of their results is justified by those responsible on the grounds of the public health need to monitor the spread of the virus. This might be a justification of this non-democratic policy if there were no other equally cost- effective way of monitoring spread. There are, however, studies indicating that data with acceptable degrees of confidence can be obtained if such testing is voluntary. If women are tested, they have a right to know the results. This is a general right but particularly applicable to women since too many decisions relating to their own life, to child bearing and to the future of their children might be made differently on the basis of this knowledge. Voluntary testing can both respect women's right to knowledge of their infection and provide the required epidemiological data.

Women are at the heart of this epidemic, not as transmitters of the virus, as they are so often depicted, but as bearers of its.consequences in families and communities.[20] It is, therefore, critical that their voices be heard and that they be actively involved in all policy discussions and in programme development at all levels. Women's experiences will be the primary source of information about social impact and knowledge of their foregone productive activities can provide insights into future socio-economic consequences. They will cushion the emotional trauma, social strain and economic disruption of the epidemic and so are of decisive importance to effective responses to the epidemic.

The International HIV Policy Framework

Just as HIV prevention strategies to date have neglected the rights and needs of women, so too has the response of the international community failed to recognise the source of women's vulnerability to HIV and the measures necessary to overcome this vulnerability.

Since 1987, the World Health Organisation, through its Global Programme on AIDS, has issued 18 consensus statements on specific issues surrounding the HIV epidemic. Only one of these statements — that dealing with the health of mothers and children — has dealt specifically with issues affecting women. However, it limits its attention to women's role as mothers and, even in this context, focuses more on the ramifications for families and children of HIV infection in women than on the consequences for women themselves.[21] Statements have been issued dealing with the issues of prostitution and sexually-transmitted diseases. However, any consideration of these issues will necessarily be inadequate for women if it fails to adopt a woman-centred analysis that identifies how the sexual and economic subordination of women is the primary reason why women must run the risk of exposure to HIV. None of the World Health Organisation statements has adopted such an analysis.

The Paris Declaration on Women, Children and AIDS issued on 30 November 1989 reinforces the view that women's issues in relation to HIV/AIDS are essentially those that also affect children.[22] It emphasises the importance of prevention and support programmes that are directed specifically at women but does not state why women require independent consideration and analysis in the context of HIV and, therefore, what must change if the factors that place women at risk are to be overcome.[23] Similarly, the World Health Assembly resolution adopted on 13 May—1988 on the Avoidance of Discrimination in relation to HIV-infected People and People with AIDS, while recognising that respect for the human rights of people with HIV is vital to the success of HIV prevention programmes, fails to deal with the broader discrimination and human rights issues that are critical to a proper understanding of why the risks faced by women as a result of the HIV epidemic are so grave.[24]

It is only in the last two years that there has been an emerging recognition within some areas of the international community of the inter-relationship between the status of wome n and women's risk of exposure to HIV. In July 1989, the Centre for Human Rights conducted an International Consultation on AIDS and Human Rights. The Report resulting from this consultation includes a statement that special attention should be given to the human rights of women. It notes that there are "certain factors relating to the reproductive role of women and their subordinate position in society which render them particularly vulnerable to infection."[25] Women's lack-of equal access to education, health, training, independent income, property and legal rights was acknowledged to affect both their access to knowledge about-HIV and their ability to protect themselves from infection. This theme was taken up by the Committee for the Elimination of Discrimination Against Women in its 9th session (1990) at which a recommendation was passed that stated, among other things, that national programmes to combat AIDS should give special attention to "the factors relating to the reproductive role of women and their subordinate position in some societies which make them especially vulnerable to HIV infection".[26]

The United Nations Development Programme has prepared a set of policy principles to assist and guide UNDP policy formulation relating to programming and personnel policies. These include the principle that "the power imbalances in interpersonal relationships and in society which create women's subordination must change if women are to be able to protect themselves from HIV infection and its consequences". Within the UNDP policy framework, priority has been given to:

> "measures to address women's needs for prevention, care, support and access to treatment, to reduce discrimination and trauma, to strengthen their ability to protect themselves from infection and to assist affected women to meet their child rearing, domestic and economic responsibilities."[27]

In November 1990, a World Health Organisation consultation on women was called to consider research priorities for women and HIV/AIDS. The meeting recognised the need to redress the neglect of gender specificity in existing research on HIV/AIDS and to focus on research that will contribute to the empowerment of women. Among the specific issues allocated research priority were the cultural factors that inhibit behaviour changes necessary to enable women to protect themselves against HIV, the impact of different contraceptive methods on HIV transmission to women, the diagnosis and treatment of sexually-transmitted diseases in women and the impact of geographical mobility on changing sexual patterns and HIV transmission risks for women.[28]

These initiatives are an important first step towards an international policy response to HIV/AIDS that will give proper weight to the rights and needs of women, but the urgency of the need for action must be communicated. We are now a decade into the epidemic and hundreds of thousands-of women have already died of AIDS. Millions more will die because of the inadequacy to date of the international response to the risk of HIV infection in women. Women's sense of urgency must be communicated to the international community.

Human Rights and the HIV Epidemic

Prevention strategies will only ever be effective in protecting women from the effects of HIV if they embrace a recognition and active promotion of the human rights of women. Human rights can and must be used pro-actively in this context. They do not merely provide the backdrop against which HIV/AIDS skategies should be planned, but rather are a powerful tool that can be actively used to enable women to protect themselves against HIV. The urgent and critical need to improve the social and economic status of-women and thereby to-overcome their vulnerability to HIV means that human rights considerations in this context must look beyond immediate concerns such as discrimination against people with HIV and access to health care to address the fundamentally unequal social and economic position of women.

The HIV epidemic has already launched a savage assault on the human rights of women. Foremost among these is the right to life which is being denied women who are forced, by reason of their subordination, to be exposed to HIV infection and who are powerless to adopt any measures to avert death from AIDS. The failure on the part of governments and the international community to take any adequate steps to enable women to protect themselves against HIV infection represents a profound denial of the value of the lives of women. Equally, women have been denied the right to health and even the right of access to health care, further increasing their vulnerability to HIV. They have been denied the right of access to education and to economic independence, both of which impact critically upon abuse of the human rights of women.

Women infected with HIV suffer further denials of human rights through being deprived of the right to bear children and the right of freedom of reproductive choice. Their right to privacy is stripped from them when their own HIV status becomes known because of the illness of their children, when they are denounced as being "responsible" for having transmitted HIV infection to an unborn child, or when they are rejected by their husbands because they are infected with HIV.

The right to freedom from discrimination has a powerful meaning for women who are blamed by men for the consequences of HIV infection. Women who are powerless to avoid the risk of exposure to HIV, whether through sexual contact with their husbands, prostitution or other means, are nonetheless blamed for having been a vector of HIV infection and suffer stigmatisation, rejection and expulsion from family and community structures. The failure to recognise the rights of these women to protection against discrimination, in addition to being morally indefensible, has further compounded the inability of women to protect themselves against the effects of HIV.

Women also have a right to knowledge—a right which has been transgressed in a number of ways in the course of the HIV epidemic. The denial of this right is linked directly to cultural assumptions about who best exercises rational deliberation, to women's lack of participation in decisions affecting their lives and to women's social subjugation. The recognition of women's right to knowledge is essential to their informed choice and action. A women who knows about patterns of infectivity in HIV infected people, for example, may be able to devise strategies to avoid sexual intercourse with her husband during periods when the infection risk is highest even though she may not be able to achieve long-term sexual abstinence. Similarly, it is a woman's right to know the facts about perinatal HIV transmission through breastfeeding so that she can make an informed choice about breastfeeding, weighing the risk of HIV transmission against other factors, such as the threat to the child's health of not breastfeeding.

The human rights abuses experienced by women as a result of the HIV epidemic and which continue to place women's lives at risk must be addressed at a fundamental structural level if the international community is to fulfil its moral, ethical and legal obligations to women. The changes required are far- reaching. They include changes to cultural values and expectations that deny women the power to control their own sexual relationships, changes to the law and culture that deny women the same economic rights and opportunities as men, and changes to the role of women within their communities in order to give recognition to women's individual identity and consciousness. These changes are the minimum that is require if human rights for women are to be a reality.

The nexus of women and the HIV epidemic provide a compelling demonstration of how the philosophical underpinnings of human rights are central to an effective policy response and have a direct and immediate impact upon policy outcomes. Thus, the urgent need to act to protect women against HIV demands that policy-makers move human rights concerns to the top of their political priority list. Unless this priority is recognised, efforts to contain the spread of HIV among women are bound to fail.

The Role of Law

The inescapable link between human rights and effective HIV/AIDS prevention for women points to the role of law in bringing about the changes necessary to enable women to protect themselves against HIV. The law has always been one of the principal mechanisms by which human rights have been given direct recognition both through international law and through domestic human rights codes and charters. A rights- focused analysis of the factors that render women vulnerable to HIV immediately demonstrates how human rights instruments can be used directly in HIV/AIDS strategies for women. In addition, the law can and should be used to promote and protect human rights indirectly by redressing structural inequalities and injustices in a way that actively seeks to bring about social change.

The Direct Role of Law

In its efforts to contain the spread of HIV, the international community has a responsibility to utilise fully the human rights protection afforded by existing international law. If used creatively and appropriately, international instruments offer wide scope to promote and reinforce the human rights of women that have been so seriously affected by the HIV epidemic. Among the instruments that could be used in this context are the United Nations Charter of 1945, the Universal Declaration of Human Rights, the International Covenant on Civil and Political Rights, and the International Covenant on Economic, Social and Cultural Rights. There are also number of regional treaties, such as the African Charter of Human Rights and People's Rights and the European Convention on Human Rights. These instruments explicitly recognise rights such as the right to life, the right to privacy and the right to bear children, which go to the heart of the HIV epidemic as it affects women.

More must be done to give formal legal effect to these international instruments through the domestic law of each country. This has been one area of notable neglect in international law, and one where immediate and tangible recognition of human rights could be implemented by the passage of appropriate domestic law enactments.

In countries where human rights codes and charters already exist as part of the domestic law, there is debate as to the extent to which these instruments are of practical effect in the context of the epidemic, either in preventing human rights abuses or in providing remedies in the event that discrimination or a breach of rights occurs. As with any legal remedy, issues of accessibility and cost may mean that legal protection that is available in theory is not available in practice. In developing countries, in particular, practical access to the legal system is likely to be non-existent for all but a very small number of people.

Nonetheless, the symbolic effect of explicit and legally-enforceable human rights protection should not be under-estimated. The experience in Canada, for example, where the Canadian Charter of Rights and Freedoms has been in force only since 1982 has shown that these legal instruments can have an effect upon the philosophical orientation of government policy, if only by introducing the language of human rights into the policy debate. It may be wrong to believe that human rights codes by themselves can provide adequate protection of individual rights, but equally it would be wrong to dismiss them as being entirely ineffectual.

The Indirect Role of Law

The notion of the law as an instrument of social and behavioural change has been the subject of a long and controversial jurisprudential debate. There are countless examples of how the law has been ineffectual in changing social behaviour either because it has been ignored or because it has been selectively enforced. The issues of rape and domestic violence are two such examples that are particularly relevant to women. Despite this experience, however, there is reason to believe that a creative use of the law, based on an appreciation of the complex social and cultural dynamics that are involved, may be able to bring about changes in social attitudes and practices that represent an abuse of rights.

What could this mean, in practical terms, for strategies to protect women from the effects of HIV? There is no universally applicable answer to this question for effective strategies must, by their nature, be culturally-specific. However, there are a number of areas where the role of law could usefully be explored.

First, there is the interaction between the law and economic dependency. In many developing countries, the law upholds the economic dependence of women through land ownership, marital property laws and credit regulations which deny women the right to independent ownership of property or through laws which prohibit women access to certain forms of paid employment or to financial credit.[29] Laws such as these effectively leave women only two means of economic support—marriage and prostitution. The removal of these legal barriers to economic independence may be a first step towards enabling women to control the circumstances that give rise to the HIV transmission risks. It could permit women access to the cash economy other than through prostitution which, in turn, could facilitate access to better health care, for example, for sexually transmitted diseases. Within the marital relationship, measures that reduce the economic dependence of the wife may also assist in increasing her power to negotiate over matters such as condom use and faithfulness on the part of her husband or partner.

Second, the law can be used to enhance the status of women within marriage or other sexual relationships. In many countries, for example, the absence of any criminal sanctions attaching to rape within marriage reinforces attitudes about the sexual subordination of women. By enacting laws that recognise the rights of women to make their own decisions about sexual relationships, the ability of women to protect themselves against the risks of HIV transmission within sexual relationships will also be increased. Similarly, cultural traditions embodied in law and which encourage or condone activities that may spread HIV can be the subject of legal reform. In such cases, changes to the law provide necessary support and reinforcement for other efforts to change cultural practices.

Third, the law can be used to express an appropriate policy response to activities, such as unprotected sexual intercourse, prostitution and injection drug use, that increase the risk of HIV transmission. Depending upon the context, the appropriate response will vary. For women whe are already isolated from access to information, prevention measures and support, laws that seek to criminalise or otherwise regulate the behaviour that places them at risk of HIV infection will only entrench the alienation they already experience. A legal regime that is coercive and unresponsive to the powerlessness of women will inevitably be ineffective. If women are unable to exercise control over the factors that force them to engage in prostitution, for example, punishment will certainly not act as a deterrent and may actively impede efforts to give these women access to appropriate education and support.

On the other hand, however, women's interests may be protected by laws that seek to change the behaviour of men. This has been shown to be possible in parts of southern Africa where the introduction of laws requiring men to pay maintenance for children they father has led to marked changes in men's sexual behaviour in that they have fathered fewer children. By attaching legal obligations to certain forms of behaviour, these patterns of behaviour have changed. For women whose risk of exposure to HIV results directly from patterns of sexual behaviour controlled by men, the law can be used constructively to confront and change the cultural values and behaviours that place women at risk.

Finally, the law can be used to provide positive incentives for measures that assist in containing HIV. For women, this may mean affirmative action programmes that require the participation of minimum numbers of women in the process of policy formulation, either in relation to HIV/AIDS specifically or more general matters, such as economic assistance and health care. Economic incentives can be legislated in the form of tax concessions or training programmes to encourage a greater participation by women in the workforce. Such initiatives, by enhancing the economic and social status of women, would contribute directly to the ability of women to protect themselves against HIV.

CONCLUSION

The HIV epidemic has taken the sexual, economic and cultural subordination of women and translated it into a death sentence for women. The virus has attacked the fundamental human rights of women, leaving them powerless to protect themselves against infection. The international response to the epidemic has compounded this abuse of rights by failing to recognise that the disadvantaged status of women is the cause of their vulnerability to HIV and by refusing to permit the rights and needs of women to play a part in shaping HIV strategies.

While millions of women are already condemned to die of AIDS, the lives of many more can be saved if immediate action is taken to address the human rights violations perpetrated on women by the HIV epidemic. Strategies that permit women to exercise control themselves over factors that place them at risk of HIV infection are critical. Mechanisms must be established to uphold human rights for women as a reality and to impose sanctions for abuses of rights. Laws must be put in place to change the structural factors that deny women equal status with men.

These changes require a fundamental reorientation of the values, beliefs and laws that shape the perception and role of women within relationships, families and societies. The challenge is great, but so too is the moral imperative that demands urgent action.

REFERENCES

1. Chin, James. Current and Future Dimensions of the HIV/AIDS Pandemic in Women and Children. Lancet 1990; 336:221-224.
2. Sabatier, Renee. Women and AIDS: Strategies for the Future. Proceedings of the meeting on Women and HIV/AIDS. CIDA, Ottawa, Canada, 1990.
3. Diaz, F.G. and Rodolfo N. Morales. HIV/AIDS in Mexico. AIDS Action. AHRTAG newsletter, issue 10, April 1990.
4. World Health Organization. The Global AIDS Situation Update. WHO, Geneva, 1990.
5. Narain, Dr. Jai. Caribbean, AIDS Action. AHRTAG newsletter, issue 10, April 1990.
6. United Nations Division for the Advancement of Women. Interrelationships Between the Status of Women and HIV- Epidemic: A Review of Published Literature. Paper prepared for the Expert Group Meeting on Women and HIV/AIDS and the Role of National Machinery for the Advancement of Women. Vienna, 24-28 September 1990.
7. Center for Women Policy Studies. Memorandum on Federal Women and AIDS Legislation. Washington, D.C., 6 March l991.
8. Carovano, Kathryn. More Than Mothers and Whores: Redefining the AIDS Prevention Needs of Women. International Journal of Health Services 1991; 21:131-142.
9. Panos Institute. Triple Jeopardy: Women and AIDS. Panos Publications Ltd., 1990.
10. Reid, Elizabeth. Young Women and the HIV Epidemic. Development Journal of SID, 1990: 1, February 1990.
11. Jochelson, Karen, Monyaola Mothibeli and Jean-Patrick Leger. Human Immunodeficiency Virus and Migrant Labour in South Africa. International Journal of Health Services 1991; 21:157-173.
12. Akeroyd, Anne. Socio-cultural Aspects of AIDS in Africa: Topics, Methods and Some Lacunae. Paper presented at the Conference on 'AIDS in Africa and the Caribbean: The Documentation of an Epidemic'. Columbia University, New York, 5 November 1990.
13. Uhlig, Mark. Prostitutes Join Mexico AIDS Fight. New York Times, 10 April 1991.
14. Personal communication, Dr. A.M. Coll Seck, Dakar, Senegal.
15. Reid, Elizabeth. Placing Women at the Centre of the Analysis. Proceedings of the meeting on Women and HIV/AIDS. CIDA, Ottawa, Canada, 1990.
16. Hankins, Catherine. Psychological and Social Consequences of HIV Infection in Mothers and Children. Proceedings of the International Conference on the Implications of AIDS for Mothers and Children, Paris, 27-30 November 1989.
17. Stein, Zena. HIV Prevention: The Need for Methods Women Can Use. American Journal of Public Health; 1990:460-462.
18. Lloyd, Genevieve. The Man of Reason: 'Male' and 'Female' in Western Philosophy. Methuen, London, 1984.
19. This figure is derived from WHO estimates of 4,000 new infections each day.
20. Hankins, Catherine. Women and AIDS: Strategies for the Future. Proceedings of the meeting on Women and HIV/AIDS. CIDA, Ottawa, Canada, 1990.
21. Bailey, Michael. Report of the Fifth International Conference on AIDS in Africa. Save the Children Fund, United Kingdom, 1990.
22. World Health Organization, Global Programme on AIDS. Statement on health of mothers and children in the context of HIV/AIDS, Geneva, November 1989.

23. Paris Declaration on Women, Children and AIDS, 30 November 1989.
24. Reid, Elizabeth. UNDP Statement. Proceedings of the International Conference on the Implications of AIDS for Mothers and Children, Paris, 27-30 November 1989.
25. World Health Assembly Resolution on the Avoidance of Discrimination in relation to HIV-infected People and People with AIDS, Geneva, 13 May 1988.
26. Centre for Human Rights. Report of an International Consultation on AIDS and Human Rights. Geneva, 26-29 July 1989.
27. Committee for the Elimination of Discrimination Against Women. General Recommendation No. 15 on the Avoidance of Discrimination Against Women in National Strategies for the Prevention and Control of Acquired Immunodeficiency Syndrome (AIDS). Report ofthe 9th Session (1990).
28. United Nations Development Programme, Policy Framework for UNDP's Response to the HIV/AIDS Epidemic, May 1990.
29. World Health Organization, Global Programme on AIDS. Report of the Meeting on Research Priorities Relating to Women and HIV/AIDS, Geneva, 19-20 November 1990.

23

Prevention and Control of Sexually Transmitted Diseases Including AIDS: Some Public Health, Legal and Ethical Issues

Dr. D.N. Jayakuru
Director
STD/AIDS Control Programme, Sri Lanka

Notification

Why Some Diseases are Made Notifiable?

Notification allows immediate public health measures to be instituted to prevent their spread. While STDs are no longer notifiable, AIDS requires to be notified. However, since public health preventive measures are not instituted in the case of AIDS, it is doubtful why AIDS cases need to be notified.

What Actions Follow Notification?

- Confirmatory test
- Counselling of patient and immediate family
- Provision of social support
- Partner notification
- Provision of medical follow-up
- Activation of domiciliary care service
- Information collection for interventions

While notification is beneficial to both the patient and the health authorities, the present system jeopardizes confidentiality. Notification procedures, therefore, need to be modified.

Testing

When testing for STDs other than HIV, consent is implied. Tests are performed as and when indicated by the disease condition.

Testing for HIV Infection

The nature of the testing can be:

- Voluntary confidential
- Voluntary anonymous
- Unlinked anonymous
- Mandatory

The two problems facing HIV infection testing are: (a) informed consent is not always feasible, and (b) laboratories are inadequately equipped.

Circumstances Under which Testing is Carried Out

• Surveillance	Unlinked anonymous
• Client's request	Voluntary confidential Voluntary anonymous
• Clinician's request	Voluntary confidential Mandatory ? (Unconscious) (Dementia)
• Request from court	Voluntary confidential Rape Soliciting
• Visa requirements	Voluntary confidential
• Requirement for domiciliary residence	Voluntary confidential
• Insurance requirement	Voluntary confidential
• Accidental exposure	Voluntary confidential
• Surveys	Unlinked anonymous seroprevalence in groups engaging in 'at risk' activities

Partner Notification

This is carried out in the case of certain STDs and HIV/AIDS. Partners may be notified in one of the following ways:

1. Patient is requested to bring/send his/her partner/s.
2. Patient requests Health Care Worker (HCW) to trace, contact and treat.
3. HCW takes the responsibility for tracing contact.

Among the issues partner notification raises are: (a) how much can be told to the partner? and (b) can the HCW be liable?

Confidentiality

This is maintained only while the patient is HIV positive. Confidentiality gets breached during hospitalization and also in the event of: (a) domiciliary care, (b) social support, and (c) death.

Condoms and Sex Workers

The inability of sex workers to refrain from having multiple partners makes it crucial that they use condoms. However, they face the following problems:

1. Arrest of individuals carrying condoms.
2. Assault of sex workers coming to collect condoms.
3. Arrest of persons for having condoms on the premises.

Police raids and arrests impede easy accessibility to condoms.

Refusal to Provide Care by Institutions and HCWs

Patients suffering from HIV infection may be denied treatment in the following ways:

1. Discharged from hospital.
2. Transferred to an infectious diseases hospital.
3. Refused surgery/delivery.

In a few cases the patients may refuse medication.

Some Problems Encountered by HIV/AIDS Patients

- Ejection from places of residence.
- Refusal to be treated by health care providers—both individuals and institutions.
- Rejection by the family.
- Rejection of the patient and his family by the community.
- Targeting of HIV infected persons by irresponsible media sources.

Some Issues of Concern

- Infectious disease control procedures not in place to any satisfactory degree.
- Insufficient attention with regard to the disposal of needles and contaminated hospital waste.
- Haphazard testing for the HIV antibody by some non-governmental organizations.
- Refusal to be hospitalized by PLWAs—where there is a need for isolation.

24

Information and Education Laws

Mr. Michael Alexander
Legal Policy Analyst
Australian Federation of AIDS Organisations, Australia

1. INTRODUCTION

HIV/AIDS programmes have two primary objectives: the prevention of HIV transmission, and minimization of the personal and social impact of HIV. The provision of information and education is central to both of these objects. Therefore, it is apparent that the laws regulating information and education will have a significant impact on the success or otherwise of HIV/AIDS programmes.

The task of law-makers and lawyers is to create a legal environment which enhances the work of HIV/AIDS educators, rather than (as is often the case) block or interfere or counteract it.

Prevention of HIV transmission depends on individuals changing their behaviour. At the most basic level, people need to be informed about the virus, about how it is transmitted, and how they can protect themselves. Since HIV is most commonly transmitted through sexual intercourse or shared needles, explicit information is required about these activities—activities which are not openly discussed in many societies. Information is necessary, but in itself is not sufficient to bring about behavioural change. HIV is transmitted primarily through behaviour which is private, secret, often hidden, and in many places illegal. Individual decisions and actions in the areas of sexuality and drug use do not necessarily follow the rules of logic or rationality, however much we0 would like them to. They are areas of human behaviour which are subject to strong emotions and passions, often illogical and sometimes dangerous.

The experience of HIV educators (and of people working in other areas of health promotion such as anti-smoking campaigns) is that people need more than just information, even explicit information. Just as people continue to smoke even though the evidence of adverse health consequences is clear, people continue to engage in unsafe sex and needle sharing, even when they have full access to information about HIV transmission. HIV educators face the following complex tasks:

- Provide explicit information about the virus and how it is spread.
- Provide explicit information about how individuals can protect themselves.
- Persuade the individual that HIV constitutes a real risk for him or her; i.e., challenge the common perception that it is a disease of the other (e.g., foreigners, adults or homosexuals).
- Empower people to take action to protect themselves.

In terms of prevention, information and education must be supplemented by other programmes, for example ensuring that the blood supply is safe, and making sure that condoms and safe injecting equipment are readily available.

Information and education are also important to the second major aspect of HIV/AIDS programmes—minimizing the social and personal impact of HIV infection. People with HIV, or people who think they may be at risk of acquiring HIV, must not be frightened of presenting themselves for testing or treatment. If people fear stigmatization or discrimination, they will be dissuaded from coming forward. This has implications not only for the health of the individual, but also for HIV prevention, as people who do not know their status are more likely to transmit the virus to others. Fear campaigns, or education campaigns which (often unintentionally) demonize people with HIV, can thus be counterproductive, not only for people with HIV and society generally, but also for HIV prevention.

2. THE RIGHT TO INFORMATION—INTERNATIONAL LAWS

The International Covenant on Civil and Political Rights recognizes in Article 19 the right to information as a universal human right:

1. Everyone shall have the right to hold opinions without interference.
2. Everyone shall have the right to freedom of expression; this right shall include freedom to seek, receive and impart information and ideas of all kinds, regardless of frontiers, either orally, in writing or in print, in the form of art, or through any other media of his choice.
3. The exercise of the rights provided for in paragraph 2 of this article carries with it special duties and responsibilities. It may therefore be subject to certain restrictions, but these shall only be such as are provided by law and are necessary:
   (a) For respect of the rights or reputations of others.
   (b) For the protection of national security or of public order (order public), or of public health or morals.

Also relevant to HIV/AIDS information and education are Article 21 (the right of peaceful assembly) and Article 22 (the right to freedom of association).

3. THE RIGHT TO INFORMATION—NATIONAL LAWS

Some countries have laws, often contained in their Constitution or Bill of Rights, which assert general rights to information, freedom of expression, or freedom of speech. For example:

- The Constitution of the Philippines explicitly provides for the right of the people to information on matters of public concern, as well as ancillary rights of freedom of speech, freedom of expression, and freedom of the press;[1]
- In Papua New Guinea, section 46 of the Constitution guarantees freedom of expression, which is defined to include freedom to hold and communicate opinions and information, and specifically guarantees freedom of the press and mass media[2];
- Article 9(1)(a) of the Constitution of India guarantees the right to freedom of speech and expression to all persons[3].

Many other countries have similar constitutional guarantees. Their enforceability varies between countries, depending on the structure of the constitution and the legal system generally. However such guarantees are invariably subject to exceptions, sometimes explicitly stated or implicit in judicial interpretation. Exceptions commonly relate to such issues as defamation, national security, morality or obscenity.

4. DECISION-MAKING ABOUT AIDS EDUCATION PROGRAMMES

HIV/AIDS information may be conveyed in a variety of ways, including posters, printed pamphlets, performances, movies, videos, radio, television, telephone, computer games and networks, lectures, group discussions, and individual counselling. A large wide range of different laws are likely to apply to these various situations.

However the law is only one among several factors that determine what can be portrayed or discussed in these various situations. The content of AIDS information and education materials and programmes depends on a wide range of factors, starting with the nature of the target group. How is the target group at risk? What information do they need to change their behaviour? What is the best way of getting through to them? What is their level of literacy or general education? What will offend or shock them? Is it a good idea for people to be offended or shocked—will this galvanize them into action or will it merely prompt them to switch off or ignore the message? The content is also determined by the values and social attitudes of the person or organization designing or propagating the information, and those who have control or influence over the means of propagation. Will the television station be prepared to telecast educational programmes? Will commercial advertisers object to unpleasant subjects being portrayed alongside the advertisements for their products? Who decides whether a film or video can be shown, and in particular whether it can be shown to children? Will printers object to printing the pamphlet? Will the school principal permit an open discussion? Will the local council allow the poster to be displayed? Will religious bodies support or oppose the proposed material or programme? Will funding bodies object? These are some of the complex questions that AIDS educators confront regularly, in addition to the potential problems posed by the law.

Lawyers must look far and wide to identify the many different laws which impact HIV/AIDS prevention and education. Depending on the political and legal system, such laws may be national, state or provincial, or local government laws. Religious and customary law is also significant in some countries. The relevant laws and regulations existing in many countries include:

- Obscenity laws.
- Laws about advertising or promotion of condoms.
- Laws prohibiting advertisement of false cures or treatment.
- Laws regulating the licensing and content of television and radio.

- Laws regulating the classification, distribution and exhibition of films and videos.
- Laws regulating the printing and distribution of printed materials.
- Customs laws regulating the importation of films, videos and printed materials.
- Laws regulating advertising;
- Local government laws regulating aspects such as advertising in public transport, public toilets, or on billboards.
- Laws against promotion or assistance of criminalized activities (e.g., prostitution, adultery, sex outside marriage, under-age sex, homosexuality, injecting drug use).
- Laws about school education.
- Laws about prisons.
- Laws against vilification of certain social groups.
- Religious or customary laws.
- Laws affecting the status of women.
- Laws about the use of national or minority languages.
- Laws about dealing with or assisting illegal immigrants.
- Laws restricting the ability to form community based organizations, either generally or for particular groups (e.g., sex workers, injecting drug users, homosexuals).
- Laws restricting the use of government funding.

Some of these laws are very prescriptive and clear; whereas many others are likely to give wide scope for administrative or judicial discretion. Several of these laws overlap with each other. Others tend to place restrictions on HIV/AIDS education and information; however some of them may be used to overcome or challenge restrictions.

4.1. Obscenity Laws

Most countries have laws prohibiting obscene or pornographic materials or actions. What is considered obscene varies considerably from one place to another, and from time to time depending on the prevailing social and moral values.

As an example, Section 292 of the Indian Penal Code makes it an offence to sell, hire, distribute, exhibit and circulate obscene books, pamphlets, paper writings, drawings, paintings, representations, figures or any other objects. Exceptions are made if the publication is for scientific, literary, higher learning, or bona fide religious purposes or that which is sculpted, painted, depicted or represented on ancient monuments or temples. Section 293 of the Code makes the sale of obscene products to young people punishable, and Section 294 of the Code makes it an offence to commission an obscene act and/or sing or recite or utter an obscene song, ballad or words in or near a public place.

In India, obscene is defined as that which is lascivious or appeals to the carnal interest or tends to deprave or corrupt those to whom it is addressed.

This definition, as in most countries, is very subjective and open to a broad interpretation. This particular law came into the Indian Penal Code during British colonial rule, and similar provisions appear in the laws of many countries in the region. It is clear that such a view of obscenity has not always been a part of India's values, as demonstrated by the reference to ancient temple carvings, which explicitly portray a range of sexual couplings which would be considered obscene if produced today.

A Malaysian lawyer has written, in relation to a similar provision in the Malaysian Penal Code, prosecution would be unlikely if materials carrying information on HIV/AIDS are genuinely educational in nature.[4] This comment confirms the wide discretion possessed by authorities in the area of obscenity.

When obscenity is assessed by reference to community standards, the question which arises is, which community? In every society there is likely to be a wide range of standards, and different communities are likely to be offended by different things. This is a real issue for HIV/AIDS educators, who need to target programmes at particular groups within society. Are sex workers, for example, likely to be depraved or corrupted by exposure to sexually explicit language or depictions of sexual conduct? Gay men are not likely to be shocked or depraved by depiction or discussion of homosexual conduct, whereas some non-homosexual people may be disgusted by any mention of homosexuality. Young people are most at risk of contracting HIV -should educational material targeted at them be judged by the standards of older people, who may be more conservative? Some religious leaders would argue that chastity and fidelity are the only ways to counter HIV/AIDS, and are opposed to condom use in any circumstances; they may contend that any suggestion of condom use, even in the context of HIV/AIDS, is likely to deprave and corrupt.

4.2. Laws about Advertising or Promotion of Condoms

Condom promotion is a central part of HIV prevention programmes. However, some countries have laws banning or restricting the advertisement or promotion of condoms. In many countries, though, such restrictions have never existed, or have been removed to be consistent with family planning and HIV/AIDS programmes.

In Australia, for example, the state government of Victoria prohibited the advertising of condoms in the Police Offences (Contraceptives) Act 1935. Apart from issues of morality or propriety, this law was supported by arguments that the Australian race would die out if contraceptives were widely used, that young people should not be able to indulge themselves without any responsibility, and that wealthier (i.e.,better) people were limiting the size of their families through condom use.[5] Until recently, condoms could not be openly displayed or advertised in Australia. Since the onset of the HIV/ AIDS epidemic, laws and practices have changed radically, and condoms are now openly sold in such places as supermarkets and are advertised in the press, on television, and on the sides of buses.

In Myanmar, condoms were banned until 1992 and are still not widely available or promoted.[6] In Cambodia, a 1992 survey by the Ministry of Public Health found that 77 per cent of the population said they didn't know what a condom is and don't know about their use in protecting against HIV/AIDS.[7]

In Vietnam, a man who hosted a condom party at a Ho Chi Minh City hotel was jailed in 1993 for degrading national culture. A year later it was reported that the HIV epidemic had led the Vietnamese government to break with the past, and officially sanctioned pamphlets had been issued warning: "If you don't have a condom, don't get drunk.[8]

In Malaysia, condom advertisements are not allowed in the electronic media, but are permitted in the print media, with the proviso that the advertisements are in the context of HIV prevention.

In Papua New Guinea, whilst there is no bar to condom promotion as such, there have been problems with condom packaging and instructions for use. In 1991 a line of condoms sold under the brand name Protector was marketed in Papua New Guinea, with an instruction insert in Pidgin, the national language. The condoms were a great success. But conservative Christian forces complained to the National Censorship Board, which found the insert to be pornographic because the line drawings implied the presence of a sexual partner while the man was putting the condom on. All stores selling the condoms were ordered to remove the inserts, until the drawings were altered to remove the visible legs of the sexual partner[9]. A similar problem exists in Fiji with pictorial depictions of condom use in instruction inserts (Personal communication: Fiji AIDS Task Force, 1995).

In Japan, on the other hand, legal and social barriers to condom promotion are minimal:

> ... distribution is widespread, supermarkets everywhere carry stocks, conveniently placed next to women's sanitary goods, as it is Japanese women who are the main condom buyers. Vending machines are also common, although there are initial problems with children mistaking them for bubblegum machines (which probably put a lot of Japanese children off bubblegum for life). In Japan, distribution is so widespread that women even sell condoms door-to-door. One brand was actually packaged to look like an encyclopedia... Furthermore packaging is as attractive and tempting as possible. Leading Japanese commercial artists are employed to promote condoms in the same way as any other household items, novelty packaging, accessories and gimmicks are all part of the incentive to buy. You can buy condom packs disguised as cigarette boxes or as packs of cosmetics; some condoms even have musical movements activated when the packet is opened.[10]

4.3. Laws Prohibiting Advertisement of False Cures or Treatment

Advertisement of false cures and treatment for HIV/AIDS is obviously counter-productive to HIV education. Such cures or treatment may be promoted simply as a money-making scam, or because of genuinely misguided belief on the part of the promoter. In either case, gullible people may be persuaded to part with their money and put their health at risk.

For example in Papua New Guinea Section 140 of the Public Health Act makes it an offence to publish statements promoting the sale of any medicine, instrument or appliance for the alleviation or cure of venereal diseases, complaints or infirmities arising from or relating to sexual intercourse, diseases affecting generative functions, etc. The provision does not apply to publications in relation to medical research, and publications sent to medical practitioners or pharmacists for the purpose of their businesses, or advertisements approved by the Commissioner for Venereal Diseases. Such a provision will appear in the laws of other countries. However, many people (including people with HIV/AIDS), have strong beliefs in traditional and herbal remedies. It is difficult for the law to strike a balance between protection of people from fraud, and allowing for genuine belief in the efficacy of traditional and herbal remedies.

In Thailand there was an uproar in early 1994 when the owner of the Living with Nature Club in Chiang Mai was arrested and charged with distributi.ng herbal water without a license and defrauding the population. Over 1,000 people with HIV were members of the club. Angered by the arrest, a group of people with HIV got together to protest. The group swore they were not victims of deception, and received support from non government organizations. They sent representatives to see the Prime Minister asking the government to reconsider its action and show compassion for the people depending on the man's herbal medicines to treat their condition. As a compromise, the Public Health Ministry allowed association members to continue preparing their herbal treatments, but they were not allowed to advertise it.[11]

4.4. Laws Regulating Licensing and Content of Television and Radio

Regulatory systems for television and radio vary widely between countries. Many countries in the Asia - Pacific region exercise very tight control over radio and television broadcasting. Some exercise a government monopoly on broadcasting, not permitting any competition to government owned stations. In other countries, there is a mix of government and commercial operators, with decision-making about content and censorship powers sometimes being delegated to the broadcasters themselves.

Generally speaking, censorship (including self-censorship) of sexual content in the electronic media is stricter than for other forms of media, because of its accessibility to all age groups throughout the region, who have the necessary equipment. At the same time, because of their extensive reach, television and radio are attractive and important for HIV/AIDS information and education campaigns.

In Australia, where the attitudes towards sexuality are relatively liberal, the Department of Health has run several major AIDS campaigns on television. However television advertisements are the subject of self-regulation by a non-government body, the Federation of Australian Commercial Television Stations (FACTS), which the Department of Health regularly consults before launching its campaigns:

> In 1989, following discussions with FACTS at the script development stage, the Department of Health decided not to accept a proposal to include homosexual couples in the 'Beds' television commercial, which had originally only been planned for heterosexual couples... FACTS had advised that it may have difficulty giving the advertisement clearance, and even if it did, some member stations would probably refuse to broadcast it. Some stations, such as the regional television station in North Queensland, declined to even screen the final version of the commercial showing heterosexual couples only.[12]

> An international AIDS journal has reported the following incident in Pakistan:

> "As a report about AIDS in Poland begins on BBC's 'Health File', the scrambler in Pakistan Television Corporation's control room rushes into action, distorting the picture and muffling the sound. It is almost a reflex action on the part of the official on duty because the government's censorship policies do not prohibit AIDS-related news or features. But the practice is common in many Muslim countries. 'If they are talking of AIDS, sex can't be far behind', says a TV official in Pakistan."[13]

Media regulation laws are not only about censorship - they also have the capacity to be used to the advantage of HIV/AIDS educators. For example, an expert committee in Australia has recommended that the government should require television and radio broadcasters to provide free time for community service announcements which would include HIV/AIDS and other government health promotion campaigns, and that announcements should be screened at a variety of times including prime time. The committee noted that the Australian Minister for Communications already had the power to direct broadcasters to broadcast information of 'national interest', and that this should be broadened to include 'community interests' enabling the minister to direct that broadcasters carry information relating to serious threats to health, including HIV/AIDS.[14] This recommendation has not yet been implemented.

4.5. Laws Regulating Classification, Distribution and Exhibition of Film and Video

All countries have legally established systems for the censorship and classification of films and videos. Films are often censored or classified on the basis of sexual or violent content, and also for political reasons.

In India, for example, before being exhibited all films must have a certificate under the Cinematograph Act, 1952. The Act states that a film shall not be certified if, in the opinion of the authority, the film or any part of it is against the interest of the sovereignty and integrity of India, the security of the state, friendly relations with foreign states, public order, decency or morality, or involves defamation or contempt of court, or is likely to incite the commission of an offence. Guidelines have been framed by the central government, including a guideline stating that visuals or words depicting women in ignoble servility to man or glorifying such servility as a praiseworthy quality shall not be permitted. Moreover, the authority is to ensure that the film is examined in the light of contemporary standards of the country and the people to which the film relates.[15]

In Australia, films are generally classified by the Commonwealth Office of Film and Literature Classification. This office has stated that its general principles applied to film and video classification are as follows:[16]

- Adults should be free to see what they wish provided there is sufficient protection for young people, and those people who do not wish to see certain material should not have it thrust upon them.
- The classification should reflect what a reasonable adult person would consider within the acceptable limits of community standards for that age group.
- The closest attention is paid to the portrayal of violence and, in particular, sexual violence.
- Certain classes of activity, such as sexual child abuse, bestiality, and the incitement to or encouragement of crime or violence are refused classification.

Most Australian state governments accept the determinations of the Office of Film and Literature Classification for the purposes of their own state laws, but some states reserve the right to override the decision in certain circumstances.

4.6. Laws Regulating the Printing and Distribution of Printed Materials

These laws cover such important purveyors of HIV/AIDS information as newspapers, magazines, books, pamphlets and posters. Some countries maintain a tight control over the publishing of newspapers and magazines by requiring licensing or registration, as well as monitoring content. Other countries allow a free press, but there are invariably a range of laws determining the content, and in some cases, how the publications may be distributed.

In Australia, the Office of Film and Literature Classification also classifies printed matter in most states and territories. It is a voluntary scheme; materials are only classified if they are presented for classification or if a complaint is lodged. They may be classified into one of four categories:

- Unrestricted.
- Restricted Category 1 (restricted to persons over 18 years and must be displayed in a sealed wrapper).
- Restricted Category 2 (restricted to persons aged over 18 and displayed for sale only in restricted premises).
- Refused Classification.

In the state of Queensland, Category 1 and Category 2 material is banned, while other states operate their own classification systems.

The office has shown some flexibility in classifying HIV/AIDS education material. For example the office was asked to classify a very explicit pamphlet 'Six Tips for Hard Cocks', produced by the AIDS Council of NSW for gay men, demonstrating the proper use of condoms. The pamphlet was given an Unrestricted classification, based on an undertaking that it would be distributed to only adults in places such as gay bars. This was an important recognition of the need for explicit, targeted information in HIV/AIDS education, and that material which might be considered offensive to some parts of the community should be permitted distribution to targeted groups.

4.7. Customs Laws Regulating Importation of Films, Videos and Printed Materials

The customs laws of countries often judge imported materials by criteria different to those applied to locally produced materials. This has implications for HIV/AIDS educators who wish to import AIDS materials from overseas. HIV/AIDS educators often get ideas from each other, and use or emulate successful campaigns and materials from other countries. At international conferences and study tours, information and materials are often exchanged. It is important that educators should not have to keep reinventing the wheel. Educators returning to some home countries may have to bear in mind the possibility that their newly acquired material may be examined and possibly confiscated by the customs authorities, and that they may even be subject to prosecution for attempting to import sexually explicit material, or material which is explicit about injecting drug use.

In Australia, the Customs (Prohibited Imports) Regulations apply to films, slides, video tapes, video discs, and any other form of recording from which a visual image can be produced, books, papers, magazines, films or other written or pictorial matter. Regulation 4A(4) says that importation of the following goods is prohibited unless permission is obtained from the Attorney-General:

- Pictures of child pornography, or of bestiality, likely to cause offence to a reasonable adult.
- Pictorial representation of acts of considerable violence or cruelty or of sexual violence against non-consenting persons.
- Publications and films that promote or incite crime, violence or drug abuse.

If films or videos are for public exhibition, they must first be registered. It can be seen that there is duplication and potential conflict with the domestic process for approval and classification.[17]

4.8. Laws Regulating Advertising

Advertising is one of the important media for HIV/AIDS education, and often has its own system of regulation.

In Australia, for example, advertising is self-regulated by the media industry, where most decisions are made by an Advertising Standards Council. This body has often ruled against health promotion advertisements, including anti-smoking and HIV/AIDS campaigns, on the grounds of taste and decency.

For example:

> In September 1990 the Advertising Standards Council banned the Victorian AIDS Council's poster showing two men kissing with the headline "When you say Yes, Say Yes to Safe Sex". The ban came in response to a complaint by a coalition of church and community groups in Bendigo, who claimed that the advertisement breached several clauses of the Media Council Codes, including that it was

> misleading and deceptive and would cause serious offence to a significant section of the community. Although the Council noted that it was the type of advocacy advertisement where it has traditionally allowed wide latitude to advertisers, it concluded that the material 'went way beyond the bounds of advocacy and acceptability to community standards'. The Council said it appeared that the advertisement was 'less concerned with the prevention of AIDS and more concerned with encouraging homosexuality' and was likely to cause serious offence to a significant section of the community.[18]

One of the difficulties caused by such a system of self-regulation is that there is no right of appeal against such a decision.

4.9. Local Government Laws

Regulation of advertising in such places as public transport, publis toilets or billboards is often the responsibility of local governments Powers may be found in local government legislation or planning and environment legislation. There is the potential for local authori ties to use this power to censor HIV/AIDS information and education material.

For example, in the Australian state of NSW, the Local Government Act, 1919, gives councils the power to regulate advertisements and structures used or to be used for the display of advertisements. This power has occasionally led to problems for HIV educators:

> In late 1991, problems arose for the AIDS Council of New South Wales and the Wollongong and Shellharbour Council over the wording of a stencil to be used in council toilets as part of a 'Beat' programme. The original stencil said: 'Always use a condom when having anal or vaginal sex'. The Councils objected to the explicitness of the message and asked that it be replaced with 'Always use a condom when having casual sex'. Wollongong Council eventually agreed to use the stencil in its original form, but Shellharbour Council has refused to use it.[19]

In the Australian context, it has been recommended that local councils should not use their legislative powers to impede HIV related health promotion campaigns[20].

In the United States, the Massachusetts Bay Transportation Authority refused in 1993 to place condom advertisements in its trolleys and subways. The advertisements, prepared by the AIDS

Action Committee of Massachusetts, displayed a large colour picture of a condom wrapped in a package, and messages stating that condoms are an effective means of preventing the transmission of HIV. The advertisements used humour and suggestive language to overcome adolescents' and men's reluctance to use condoms. The AIDS Action Committee successfully used, claiming violation of the First Amendment (freedom of speech) and the Fourteenth Amendment (due process) of the US Constitution. The US District Court, upheld on appeal by the US 1st Circuit Court of Appeals, found in favour of the AIDS Action Committee. The court pointed out that at the same time as the Authority was refusing to run the condom ads, it was displaying sexually suggestive posters for a Hollywood movie featuring the bare, crossed legs of a woman. The court said that if the authority was displaying commercial ads which were overtly sexual, it could not block public service ads of a more modest nature without violating the First Amendment protection of freedom of speech. The court added that both sets of ads fall well within the heartland of speech that we, as a secure society, should be willing to tolerate in the marketplace of ideas.[21]

It is inappropriate for local authorities to impede HIV/AIDS programmes designed and promoted at a national or state level. It must be remembered, though, that attitudes in local authorities vary enormously, and that local authorities may be able to use their powers to the benefit of HIV/AIDS programmes, even if there is indifference or hostility to such programmes at higher levels of government.

4.10. Laws Against Promotion or Assistance of criminalized Activities

If self-injection with a prohibited drug is a criminal offence, is it lawful to tell someone, or to demonstrate to someone, how to inject safely? This is a major problem for HIV educators in every country. In China, the National People's Congress passed a resolution in 1990 that a penal sentence is to be given to those who cajole, abet, deceive and/or coerce others to take or inject narcotic drugs[22]. One approach to HIV education with injecting drug users is to say that the only way to protect yourself against HIV is to stop using drugs. This is a method which has demonstrably failed, and has led to high rates of HIV infection amongst injecting drug users in places where it has been the sole strategy. In order to minimize infection, there is a need to be realistic and to say, in effect we accept that you are going to use drugs and this is how to do it safely. Such a message is not, in terms of the Chinese law, cajoling, deceiving or coercing, but it may be seen as abetting or assisting.

Similar questions arise in other areas of HIV/AIDS education:

- If prostitution is illegal, is it lawful to talk to sex workers about strategies and sexual practices which aim to assist them in protecting themselves or their clients from HIV infection? Is this aiding or abeffing acts of prostitution?
- If homosexual acts are illegal, is it;lawful to talk about how to do them safely? Can programmes specifically targeted at gay men be seen as promoting homosexuality?
- It lawful to talk to young people below the age of consent about specific sexual practices?

4.11. Laws About School Education

Young people approaching or entering sexual maturity are most at risk of contracting HIV. The school system is a crucial point for children and young people to be exposed to information about HIV/AIDS and how to protect themselves. Sex education has long been a controversial issue in most countries, and HIV/AIDS gives added urgency to the resolution of this issue.

In the Philippines, a strong Catholic nation, debate has taken place in the legislature on the question of HIV education in schools. Some legislation has supported the need for HIV education. However:

> ...legislative counter reactions can also be seen in Senate Resolution No. 314 which, while recognizing the necessity of teaching HIV prevention and control and integrating it into the High School curriculum, opposes the Department of Education Culture and Sports programme of integrating into the First and Second Year High School's 'Physical Education Health and Music' Programme the promotion and use of condoms, on the ground that such plans promote promiscuity among tonnages who should be taught moral values and standards instead.[23]

In the American state of Alabama, a bill passed through the legislature in 1992 which stipulates that any sex education programme in Alabama public schools should include, at a minimum:

- That abstinence from sexual intercourse is the only completely effective protection against pregnancy and STDs, including AIDS when transmitted sexually.
- An emphasis on the importance of self-control and ethical

conduct pertaining to sexual behaviour.

- An emphasis in a factual manner and from a public health perspective, that homosexuality is not a lifestyle acceptable to the general public and that homosexual conduct is a criminal offence under the laws of the state.[24]

A familiar argument in this context is that sex education will increase sexual activity and might thus lead to more, not less, transmission of HIV. Dr Michael Merson, formerly Director of the World Health Organization's Global Programme on AIDS, argues the contrary view:

> Research has shown that, contrary to popular belief, children who receive sex education do not become sexually active earlier than others. Quite the opposite: such youngsters delay their sexual experimentation, and when they do engage in intercourse they are more likely to take the right precautions, including contraception.[25]

In many countries where there is extensive sex education and HIV education in schools, it remains a matter of dispute whether condoms should be promoted or made available in schools. For example, there has been extensive litigation on this issue in New York City[26]. In Thailand, the long-time condom promoter (and former Cabinet Minister) Mechai Viravaidya has no doubts about what is needed in school education:

> Condom Man was last seen valiantly striding from bar to bar in Bangkok, talking with bar girls and patrons alike, always making sure to distribute his trusty condoms. Our plan ... is to take Condom Man beyond the bars and have him reach a broader base. In fact, we plan to send him to where his popularity will be the highest and most effective: to school-age children. We have yet to secure the permission of the Thai Ministry of Education for this somewhat radical departure from traditional education, but I am confident that when Condom Man himself lands in the Minister's office, permission will be granted.[27]

4.12. Laws About Prisons

Prisons are environments which are potential hothouses of HIV transmission, because of the high level (in many countries) of injecting drug use, and the high level (in most countries) of sexual activity between men, both consensual and non-consensual. HIV infection is not contained within the prison; prisoners are eventually released and return to their families and regular lives, which may lead to further infections in the community. Prison laws and regulations must provide for HIV education and information, and provide prisoners with the means to protect themselves from the virus.

Prisons present a very clear example of the near futility of providing information and education without giving access to condoms and safe injecting equipment.

4.13. Laws Against Vilification of Certain Social Groups

As noted above, stigmatization or discrimination against people with HIV/AIDS or affected communities will be counter-productive for HIV information and education programmes.

Bearing this fact in mind, the Australian state of NSW has passed laws against the vilification of people on the basis of their race, their sexual preference, or the fact that they have, or are thought to have HIV. Under Section 49ZXB of the state's Anti-Discrimination Act:

> It is unlawful for a person, by a public act, to incite hatred towards, serious contempt for, or severe ridicule of a person or group of persons on the ground that the person is or members of the group are HIV/AIDS infected or thought to be HIV/ AIDS infected (whether or not actually HIV/AIDS infected).

The Act also creates a criminal offence of serious HIV/AIDS vilification, where the above acts occur by means which include:

- Threatening serious harm towards, or to wards any property of, the person or group of persons.
- Inciting others to threaten physical harm towards, or towards any property of, the person or group of persons.

The offence is punishable by a fine of up to $5,000 or imprisonment for six months or both.

Anti-vilification measures send an important message from governments and complement and assist HIV education campaigns.

4.14. Religious or Customary Laws

Some countries recognize religious or customary laws alongside their formal legal system. A good example of the impact these laws can have on HIV education programmes comes from Papua New Guinea:

> As part of the public awareness campaign already instituted

in the country, a man living with HIV from the Highlands area volunteered his services in various outreach programmes. He did an excellent job, travelling around villages all over the remote and rugged Highlands area, explaining demonstrating, counselling. A video was made in which he starred in his role as an outreach worker. Shortly afterwards he died. The video has had to be suppressed. The subject is dead, and a dead person has passed into the spirit world and it is vital that his privacy be respected. If the video were to be released for public showing, his angry relatives would object and ask for compensation for the infringement of sacred taboos.[28]

In some aboriginal communities in Australia, tribal elders have banned photos of male and female genitalia showing STD symptoms, even for same sex audiences[29].

In Malaysia, the Islamic Syariah Law applies to Muslims. As premarital sex is prohibited under Islamic law, condoms cannot be given to unmarried persons in any official programmmes, since this would suggest that the authorities are condoning premarital sex.

Much of the content of HIV/AIDS educational and information programmes is not, of course, customary in most cultures. The advent of HIV/AIDS has meant that customs and cultures have had to change and adapt in order to minimize the harm to their communities. This is not to argue against the need for cultural appropriateness, or to doubt the validity of customary or religious laws. However, if the effect of customary law is to set customs in concrete or to create a perception that customary laws are unchangeable, this create problems for HIV/AIDS programmes. HIV/AIDS educators need to bear in mind that all cultures evolve and change over time; none are static. In Uganda health workers believed that it was wrong to tell people that they have HIV because it is not customary to talk about death, dying or related issues. Despite this, a Ugandan NGO conducted surveys that found that people actually wanted to know if they were positive or negative, and they are now mobilizing support services and informing people of their HIV status, despite the supposed cultural in appropriateness.[30]

4.15. Laws Affecting the Status of Women

In many countries women are likely to be more difficult to reach with HIV/AIDS information and education programmes because of the laws and customs which subordinate and disempower them. An Indian woman lawyer has written that:

> Women are the subordinate sex, relegated to second-class status, kept uneducated, dependent, isolated and confined within the four walls of their homes. They are often denied access to education, health, independent income and property rights. All these factors combine to increase women's vulnerability and obstruct any effective prevention campaign.[31]

Even if women can be reached by education campaigns, how can they act to protect themselves against HIV (e.g., by insisting on condom use) in societies where the law strips them of rights or power in sexual negotiation, and most other aspects of life?

4.16. Laws About the Use of National or Minority Languages

In some countries there are laws or legal systems which require the use of national languages in certain contexts (e.g., education) and restrict the use of minority languages. Such legal requirements pose a number of problems for AIDS educators in reaching minority, indigenous populations, since material dealing with such sensitive and personal issues as sexual behaviour and drug use is often best presented in everyday, colloquial language. If HIV/AIDS education material is only presented in a language other than the person's mother tongue, the problems are:

- The material does not reach people who are not literate or influent in the official language.
- Even if people understand the words, will they understand the message?
- There may be a tendency for minority groups to see HIV as not applicable to them if it is not in their own language. It may be seen as a disease of the national majority group, rather than their own minority group.

These considerations apply not only to indigenous minorities, but also to immigrants. With uneven economic development, there is a huge influx of immigrant workers from one country to another country, often working in lowly paid jobs, poorly educated or illiterate even in their own languages. In Malaysia, for example, there are over 1 million migrant workers in a population of 18 million, many of them from the neighbouring countries of Thailand and Indonesia. Despite their large numbers, there is very little HIV/AIDS education targeted at them in their own languages.

Article 26 (equality before the law) and Article 27 (rights of ethnic religious and linguistic minorities) of the International Covenant on Civil and Political Rights have particular relevance to these situations.

Many countries in the Asia Pacific region have within them a wide variety of spoken and written languages. Reaching all these people is enough of a challenge to HIV/AIDS educators, without the additional burden of legal or bureaucratic restrictions on use of languages.

4.17. Laws About Dealing with or Assisting Illegal Immigrants

In many parts of the Asia Pacific region there are large illegal population movements from country to country, caused by wars, political repression or instability, economic opportunities and other factors. It is estimated for example, that there are about one million Burmese living illegally in Thailand.

Thai law makes it illegal to assist or harbour illegal immigrants, and most other countries have similar laws. Large numbers of women and girls are trafficked from neighbouring countries into the Thai sex industry, primarily from Burma, but also from China and Laos. Many of these illegal immigrants come from rural farming communities and have little education, and little or no knowledge of HIV/ AIDS. There is an obvious and pressing need for HIV education among these women, yet there is virtually no material about HIV written in Burmese available in Thailand, and virtually no programmes are targeted at them. The problem for non-government organizations is that if they work with illegal immigrants, they are likely to be breaking the law.[32]

In every country illegal immigrants try to remain invisible; they do not wish to identify themselves for fear of arrest and deportation. While this fact provides a considerable challenge to HIV educators, they do not, however, need the additional challenge of fearing arrest themselves merely for trying to work with these most marginalized communities.

4.18. Laws Restricting the Ability to Form Community Based Organizations

Whilst governments have a vitally important role in the fight against HIV/AIDS, community based organizations also have a central role to play. Governments cannot do everything. They are subject to financial and logistical constraints. But more significantly, governments cannot hope to muster the same commitment or recognition or support as a community based organization fighting to protect its own community.

In Australia, North America and parts of Europe, where the impact of HIV initially fell largely on gay men, organizations formed by the gay communities took much of the responsibility for responding to the epidemic. The same phenomenon was observed in developing countries as diverse as Mexico, Zambia and Thailand[33]. These organizations were able to formulate strategies to inform and educate their own communities in a way which governments either could not, or were unwilling to do so. It is now recognized that the best way to reach injecting drug users is to empower organizations of injecting drug users to do so, and the most effective way of speaking to sex workers is to utilize sex worker organizations. The same principle applies to other groups and communities: both communities of interest and geographical communities. Women's organizations, youth groups, and organizations of ethnic and linguistic minorities all have a role to play. Large scale information campaigns, such as those run by governments, must be supplemented by peer education programmes which are more accessible to the individual.

This principle was recognized in the 1986 Ottawa Charter for Health Promotion, which states that:

> Health promotion works through concrete and effective community action in setting priorities, making decisions, planning strategies and implementing them to achieve better health. At the heart of this process is the empowerment of communities, their ownership and control of their own endeavours and destinies.[34]

As noted above, the rights of peaceful assembly and freedom of association are human rights recognized in the International Covenant on Civil and Political Rights. Despite this, some countries have laws which restrict the rights of people to organize themselves into groups. In some authoritarian countries there is a general prohibition on non-government organizations. In other countries there are considerable deterrents. Dennis Altman observes:

> Knowing that one requires government registration to establish a group is a powerful deterrent from organizing, say, a sex workers' association in Indonesia or even a 'general' AIDS organization in Kuwait.[35]

4.19. Laws Restricting the Use of Government or other Funding

Non-government organizations working on HIV/AIDS education

often rely on funding from governments, and this often comes with strict conditions on what it can be used for. Often, if a government is funding a non-government organization to produce education material, the government reserves the right of final approval of the material, and also maintains copyright over material produced.

Material produced using government funding is more susceptible to protest from conservative elements of society than is material produced using money from other sources. For example, a Safe Sex Diary produced by the Family Planning Association using Australian government funding had to be withdrawn from distribution after the Prime Minister had his attention drawn to it by a State Premier[36]. This was not done through any formal legal process of censorship, but through the naked power of the government as the funding body, pursuant to the funding conditions.

Similar restrictions may be imposed by other organizations providing funding, such as development aid agencies or religious bodies.

5. CONCLUSION

In the introduction it was stated that the task of law-makers and lawyers is to create a legal environment which enhances the work of HIV/AIDS educators, rather than interfere with it. This brief (and very incomplete) survey shows that, in all countries there is a great deal of work to be done before we achieve this important goal.

REFERENCES

1. See discussion in Jimenez C. Information Law, Privacy and HIV/AIDS in the Philippines. In: Glick RA (ed.,) *Law Ethics and HIV.* New Delhi: UNDP, 1993: 27-39, 29.
2. See Stewart C. Existing Law on HIV/AIDS in Papua New Guinea. In Glick, *op cit.,* 133-150, 141.
3. See discussion in Grover A. HIV/AIDS—related law in India. In Glick: *op cit.,* 111-131, 118.
4. Siraj M. The HIV Epidemic in Malaysia. In Glick: *op cit.,* 97-110, 103.
5. The Communications Law Centre. *HIV/AIDS and the Media—Broadcasting, Censorship and Privacy Law.* Canberra: Department of Health, Housing and Community Services, 1992. Discussion paper for Intergovernmental Committee on AIDS Legal Working Party. 18.
6. Asia Watch/ Women's Rights Project. *A Modern Form of Slavery: Trafficking of Burmese Women and Girls into Brothels in Thailand.* New York: Human Rights Watch, 1993. 141.
7. Peace, at a Price. *Campaign* 1992 Sep: 9.
8. Murdoch L. Vietnam starts fight against lethal new foe. *The Sydney Morning Herald.* 1994 March 7, 12.
9. Jenkins C. Condom Backlash hits Papua New Guinea, *World AIDS* 1993: 29 Sept:1; Stewart C, Kase P. Law, Custom and the HIV/AIDS Epidemic in Papua New Guinea. In Glick: *op cit* 63-76, 64.

10. Parisot J. *Johnny Come Lately.* London: Journeyman, 1985: 52-53. Quoted in Jayasuriya D.C. *AIDS* and *Condoms.* Nawala Sri Lanka: Institute of Comparative Health Policy and Law, 1989: 24-25.
11. New Life Friends. *Thai-Australia Northern AIDS Prevention and Care Programme Newsletter* 1994: (July- Aug.); Suwanna Asavaroengchai "AIDS: For many, hope lies in herbal medicine" *Bangkok Post* 1994: February 17.
12. The Communications Law Centre. *HIV/AIDS and the Media - Broadcasting, Censorship and Privacy Law.* Canberra: Department of Health, Housing, Community Services, 1992. Discussion paper for Intergovernmental Committee on AIDS Legal Working party, 11.
13. Hanif M. AIDS and Islam, *World AIDS* 1995 (Mar):6-10, 9.
14. *The Final Report of the Intergovernmental Committee on AIDS.* Canberra: Department of Health Housing and Community Services, 1992: 78-79.
15. Grover A. *op cit.,* 119.
16 *Office of Film and Literature Classification and Films Board of Review: Report of Activities (1990-91).* Canberra, 1991, pars 2,13-14.
17. Godwin J., Hamblin J. Patterson D., Buchanan D., *Australian HIV/AIDS Legal Guide,* 2nd ed, Sydney, The Federation Press, 1993, 366-67.
18. The Communications Law Centre *op cit.,* 10-11.
19. The Communications Law Centre *op cit.,* 1l.
20. *The Final Report of the Intergovernmental Committee on AIDS op cit.,* 79.
21. *AIDS Action Committee of Massachusetts Inc v. Massachusetts Bay Transportation Authority et al.,* 1st Cir 94-1116. Decided 9 November 1994. Summarised in Court enjoins Boston Transit Agency from Banning Racy Condom Posters. *AIDS Policy* s *Law* 1994 December 2, 6-7.
22. Wang Yan & Zhao Ning. A Brief Introduction to the Legislation of China Governing the Prevention and Control of AIDS. In Glick *op cit.,* 183-90, 189.
23. Jimenez C. *op cit.,* 32.
24. Alabama Senate OKs Compromise Deleting Question on Condoms. *AIDS Policy* and *Law* 1992 April 2: 2-3.
25. Quoted in *The Hidden Cost of AIDS: The Challenge of HIV and Development.* London: The Panos Institute, 1992: 129.
26. *Alfonso v. Fernandez,* NY Sup Ct AppDiv, 2nd Dept, No. 92-06950, 30 December 1993. NYC Board of Education Votes Not to Appeal Court Mandated Opt-Out on Condom Distribution. *AIDS Policy* and *Law.* 1994 January 21:1.
27. Mechai Viravaidya Confronting a Culture at Risk: A Curbside View of AIDS Education and Prevention in Thailand. Paper delivered at 1st Conference on AIDS in Asia and the Pacific, Canberra, 5-8 August 1990, 6.
28. Stewart C. and Kase P. *op cit.,* 64.
29. Brady M. *Vaccinating with Videos: A Preliminary Assessment of HIV/AIDS Media Strategies for Aboriginal and Torres Strait Islander People.* Canberra, Department of Human Services and Health, 1994, 36.
30. Goodgame R.W. AIDS in Uganda - Clinical and Social Features, *New England Journal of Medicine* 1990, 323, (6) 383-89. Cited in Brady *op cit.,* 36.
31. Ayappa G.D. Women and HIV/AIDS: An Indian Scenario. In Glick *op cit.,* 55-61, 57.
32. Asia Watch/Women's Rights Project. *op cit.,* 120-123, 144-146.
33. Altman D. *Power and Community: Organisational and Cultural Responses to AIDS.* London: Taylor and Francis, 1994, 3.
34. The Ottawa Charter for Health Promotion was adopted at the first International Conference on Health Promotion in Ottawa in November 1986.
35. Altman, D. *op cit.,* 158.
36. Boyd M. Fact and Fantasy File, *National AIDS Bulletin* 1992, 6(2), 23-24.

25

Health Care Practitioners and HIV: Rights, Duties and Liabilities

Prof. Bernard M. Dickens
Faculty of Law, University of Toranto
Toranto, Canada

1. INTRODUCTION

This framework of the legal rights, duties and liabilities of health care practitioners concerning the risk of HIV infection and AIDS is based on perceptions that have evolved in the Common law jurisprudence of a developed country. The jurisprudence and legal institutions of other legal systems, including those based on Civil law, Roman-Dutch law, and religious law, may require the principles addressed here to be applied somewhat differently. Similarly, the chapter may reflect circumstances of health care professional licensure, discipline, supply and funding that differ among countries. It certainly reflects experiences of legislation, litigation in courts and access to lawyers' services that depart from experiences in other settings.[1] Its aim is to focus on issues that are likely to arise in different legal and health care cultures, and to identify a number of key legal questions that are likely to be asked, rather than to present uniform answers. It is hoped that the parts that are not relevant to any particular jurisdiction are balanced by parts that are, and that the discussion will contribute to understanding through comparisons and contrasts that readers can make with the legal and health care systems with which they are most familiar.[2]

2. HEALTH CARE PRACTITIONERS

In conventional western analysis, the primary health care practitioners are physicians, including specialists in such areas, for instance, as virology and urology, and general practitioners, who may include family practitioners in areas where family practice is not considered a speciality. Nurses are an obvious parallel cadre of health care practitioners, and, evolving from their historical role as handmaidens to physicians, public health nurses and nurse practitioners are achieving status in some areas as independent professionals in health care. They enjoy powers to prescribe medications derived from the right to make clinical diagnoses. Similarly, midwives are emerging from the supervision of physicians and the nursing profession in some areas to be recognized as professionals who practise under independent licensure. Psychiatric and other social workers, lacking any basis in medical sciences as such, are also health care practitioners, in that their services contribute to patients' and families' health in the sense in which the World Health Organization characterizes health, namely as "a state of complete physical, mental and social well-being and not merely the absence of disease or infirmity."[3]

Traditional healers and, for instance, birth attendants significantly practice health care in many areas. They often serve where western-recognized practitioners are not found, but also practise as alternative health professionals where the latter are available, sometimes practising with them as mutually respectful colleagues. A legal distinction remains, however, between academically qualified, professionally licensed health care practitioners such as physicians and nurses, and practitioners who have received no training that complied with widely recognized standards, who accept allegiance to no enforceable code of ethical practice, and whom the law would not hold to higher standards of knowledge, proficiency and care than are expected of a layperson. The legal rights, duties and liabilities of those who deliver health care services differ, depending on their status and the expectations they reasonably create of the availability and calibre of the services they offer.

Where HIV infection is concerned, important health care services may be performed, neglected or repudiated by professionals who are not health care practitioners. School teachers have abilities to inform pupils of dangers of infectious diseases in general, including their modes of transmission, and HIV and other sexually transmitted diseases in particular. Ministers of religion may also provide preventive health care information, not just in moralistic condemnation of sex outside marriage but for instance by reinforcing the moral imperative of practising safer sex, in marriage and outside, where risk of HIV infection arises. Similarly, industrial personnel and related staff training officers dealing, for instance, with adolescent and slightly older recruits to a workforce coming from rural areas may inform and alert newcomers to the dangers of HIV infection, particularly from sexual interactions and drug use. Such practitioners fall outside the analysis of this chapter, although the ethics of their actions in promoting, failing to promote and obstructing promotion of HIV prevention programmes are amenable to evaluation comparable to that applied to health care professionals.

Health care practitioners who are not routinely exposed to high risk may face unusual dangers from HIV infection. Dentists, for instance, may be exposed to patients' blood, and if their equipment is not appropriately sterilized they may transmit infection between one patient and another. Laboratory technicians, clinic waste disposal personnel and staff who clean operating theatres following surgery who are not exposed to patients as such are in contact with their body fluids that may be a source of infection, to themselves or to others their employing institutions have legal responsibilities to protect.

Accordingly, there are few if any health care practitioners whom the risk of HIV transmission does not affect, in discharge of their professional or work-related activities, or in protection of their personal health or of that of their family members. Self-interest and the interests of others dependent on them require them to maintain vigilance and skill, and to be aware of evolving knowledge and experience of HIV spread and prevention.

3. THE DUTY OF DUE AWARENESS

The legal duty to maintain professional awareness in good repair[4] has a direct and an indirect component. The direct component concerns those to whom health care professionals owe legally enforceable duties of care, notably their patients and patients' family members but also their colleagues and staff members. Duties to the former, who lack means of self-protection against unknown risks, are somewhat greater than duties to the latter, who may be expected to take due precautions and therefore may contribute to any injury they suffer. The indirect component concerns professional responsibility to maintain educational and technical fitness to practise as a condition of continuing or renewed licensure, and liability to licensing authorities' disciplinary charges of misconduct and unprofessional behaviour arising from lack or misapplication of relevant knowledge of HIV infection and prevention.

Even where professional licensing authorities impose no obligation on licensees to attend at continuing professional education courses as a condition of licensure, professionals are expected by the courts and by their own professional associations to keep abreast of the literature and evolving perceptions and standards of performance in their field. For instance, the Australian Medical Association's June 1991 policy on AIDS provides that "medical practitioners have an ethical and professional obligation to inform themselves about all conditions they care for and to behave in a scientifically responsible manner" (Art.1.2) and that "Both this tradition and this obligation must be maintained throughout the AIDS epidemic" (Art.1 .3).[5]

Where professionals charge fees for services, an implied term of the fee-for-service contract is that professionals maintain the standards of awareness and proficiency that induce patients to place their health care in such professionals' hands. Like fee-for-service practitioners, salaried health care professionals and others with no contractual links to the patients they treat are bound by the law of torts or delict, since the duty of care that must be observed under the law of negligence is set by courts as a matter of policy and of keeping faith with popular expectations.

How widely professionals should inform themselves of matter pertinent to their practise, and how promptly they should incorporate new understanding and awareness into their clinical or public health care practise, are more complex matters. Not every new perception is sound and scientifically established, and not every prevailing practice that a study shows ineffective or countertherapeutic need be abandoned. There is a legal doctrine that a practice supported by a "responsible body" or "respected minority" of practitioners of a health care profession satisfies the standard of care set in negligence law.[6] The responsible or respected minority rule permits maintenance of a conventional therapy that most practitioners have discontinued for persuasive reasons, and also, at the other end of the evolutionary spectrum, adoption of a promising new procedure not incorporated into general patient care. Accordingly, prevailing understanding, for instance, of the safety of a procedure, need not yield instantly to reasoned criticism based, for instance, on the evident liability to transmit HIV infection. Equally, a reasonable belief that a new practice is effective to resist viral transmission may be held in preference to a management of proven efficacy, even though subsequent evidence and clinical experience may discredit the innovation. It is ultimately for the courts to determine if a practice, whether old or new, majority or minority, satisfies legal standards of competence, and ineffective or harmful practices will quickly be found unsatisfactory.[7]

Awareness is central to clinical diagnosis of HIV infection, public health care concerning, for instance, safety of the blood supply for transfusion, and to implementation of clinical and community health protection practices. Unawareness that, by good fortune, does not result in HIV infection to a patient or compromise community health will usually escape legal liability in a direct sense. Liability for negligence requires proof that failure to meet the legal standard of care caused calculable injury. Liability for breach of contract could arise without proof of resulting injury, but an award of damages is usually related to material loss and calculable pain and suffering. However, indirect legal liability may arise when a health professional's licensing authority finds a degree of unawareness that constitutes professional misconduct or unfitness to practise. The mandate of governmental licensing authorities is usually protection of the public, and such authorities are not limited to acting *ex post facto.* They are empowered and ethically bound to take preventive action in reasonable anticipation of the individual or community health disaster that a practitioner's lack of due awareness threatens.

Popular political, religious and other obstacles to awareness of the risks of HIV infection are not usually amenable to correction by the legal system. Health professionals' standards of practice are legally monitored at the clinical level by litigation and at the level of public protection by professional regulatory authorities appointed under legislation and acting according to due process of law, and they are thereby held to higher standards than non-professionals. Beyond the risks implicit in their own practices, they are legally required to be aware both of risks implicit in patients' known and reasonably interpretable circumstances and lifestyles, and of the incidence of HIV infection among categories of the populations they treat. Practice based on crude mischaracterization of AIDS and HIV infection as disorders of only homosexual and bisexual men, commercial sex workers and people who use drugs by injection, will fail to satisfy legal standards where viral infection is significant among the heterosexual population, and the epidemic is prevalent among women of adolescent or older reproductive age. Not every country or region produces accurate data of HIV prevalence from reliable screening programmes, but global, national and regional data exist that provide a basis of relevant awareness. The law requires professionally competent responses to the knowledge that exists, and incorporation of that knowledge into practice, even if that knowledge subsequently proves imprecise, inaccurate or inadequate.

4. THE DUTY TO DIAGNOSE

HIV infection is diagnosable by laboratory detection of properties of body tissue samples, particularly antibodies to the human immunodeficiency virus, but AIDS itself is not a disease. It is a syndrome that explains various manifestations of individuals suffering compromised immune systems due to viral infection. Suspicion of a patient's suffering from AIDS can be confirmed or refuted by testing for HIV infection, but a health care professional may be legally obliged to recognize a patient's symptoms as possibly being AIDS related. Some conditions may be strongly indicative of severe HIV related disease, but other conditions such as unexplained wasting of body tissues should serve to put health care professionals on notice that a patient may be infected with HIV. The frequent linking in the literature of such conditions as Kaposi's sarcoma and *Pneumocystis carinii* pneumonia with HIV infection, particularly when such conditions are recurrent, should also alert health care professionals to the need to consider the HIV diagnosis. Whether pulmonary or extra-pulmonary tuberculosis, invasive cervical cancer or, for instance, cytomegalovirus retinitis should sound the same alarm will depend on its general prevalence in the patient's community or relevant subpopulation, and whether a diagnosis of HIV infection can reasonably be discounted. A high incidence of familial cervical cancer, for instance, may explain a woman's condition sufficiently to make HIV infection a less probable diagnosis.

The legal duty of competent diagnosis is primarily owed to the patient, but the relationship between physicians and patients, and courts may find between other health care professionals and their patients or clients, is legally considered special. The law recognizes that, in such a special relationship, a duty is owed to whoever the health professional actually foresees, or reasonably should foresee, would be liable to be injured by his or her act or omission. Accordingly, if a professional should perceive that a patient may be

HIV infected and is liable to infect another person such as a sexual partner, the professional owes a legal duty to both the patient and also the partner at risk of infection to offer the patient diagnosis, due counselling and advice. If the patient declines diagnosis and related services,[8] the health professional's duty to the partner may be satisfied, but the professional may nevertheless have a power, if not a duty itself, to warn the partner of the suspected risk (see 8, below). No duty may arise, however, when a woman patient who has been adequately informed takes the risk of transmitting HIV infection to a child *in utero*, if the only preventive means is non-conception or abortion, because of general legal policies not to punish voluntary conception and not to compel advice or performance of abortion. Others to whom health care professionals owe duties are those at risk of infection through professionals' use of unsterilized or inadequately sterilized equipment, and those who may foreseeably be exposed, perhaps inadvertently, to patients' body fluids when they could be a source of HIV infection.

Health care practitioners have different degrees of familiarity with those they treat. Some are aware of patients' family histories, personal characteristics and lifestyles, while others have only a transitory and superficial interaction with them. General or family practitioners of medicine may have a depth of personal knowledge of patients that specialist consultants do not achieve, and, for instance, hospital emergency room personnel may know nothing beyond the immediately presenting conditions of those for whose care they suddenly become responsible. In many cases, however, professionals can ask questions of patients, and interpret the significance of their answers. This is important in diagnosis of HIV infection because, when a clinical diagnosis is unavailable, or negative, a social or lifestyle diagnosis may be relevant. During the incubation period following infection, a patient may prove negative when tested for viral antibodies, but nevertheless be capable of transmitting the infection to others. The risk of transmission may be perceived by a health care professional who has knowledge of a patient's lifestyle.

Epidemiological data disclose the risks of HIV infection in many segments of societies, including for instance adolescent girls from rural areas who take employment in large cities and are subject to sexual inducements and depredations by more worldly men. Similarly, married men may have sexual encounters when on business or other travel,[9] and acquire HIV and other sexually-transmitted infections they spread to their wives. Accordingly, a health care professional should be aware of the different ways in which HIV can be acquired and transmitted, and seek information from patients that may indicate HIV infection as a possible diagnosis of the conditions they present.

5. "UNIVERSAL PRECAUTIONS" AND DUE CARE

Because many patients may have to be treated before a diagnosis of HIV infection can be made, and infected patients in the early stages of incubation may not have developed the antibodies that tests detect and therefore provide a negative test result although they may transmit infection, health care practitioners cannot await an HIV positive test result before they take appropriate precautions against infection. These are often described as "universal precautions". They are "universal" in the sense that they need to be taken regarding every patient and every other person to whose body fluids a health professional may become exposed. They are not necessarily uniform, however, but may be calibrated to the degree of risk of exposure. The risk of a surgical patient's spurting blood, for instance, requires more precaution than moving a sealed sample container. The former involves use of eye protection as well as protective cover of exposed facial and other skin, while the latter requires little if anything more than routine gloves and use, if available, of shatter-proof containers that open without spilling contents.

Hospital emergency room personnel and health care professionals who go to treat trauma patients where accidents occur should ideally be educated, trained, equipped and mandated to exercise universal precautions, but many professionals will be exposed to the risk of infection in circumstances that are less than fully secure against risk of HIV infection. For instance, women giving birth and newborn babies infected *in utero* may present irreducible minimum risks of viral transmission to health care and related attendants. The goal of professionals' self-protection must always be to minimize infection risk without prejudicing patients' care. Similarly, employers of health care practitioners often have legal obligations, as terms of contracts of employment and/or under occupational health and safety legislation, to provide employees with a safe work environment and with secure conditions of employment. Education, training and equipment may have to be made available as part of this obligation, although staff who refuse or fail to accept them may alone assume the risk of suffering infection.

In many instances, courts will have to decide whether the precautionary services available to practitioners satisfy legal standards of care. The ways in which inadequate resources are allocated and priorized among limitless demands of, for instance, patient care, community preventive education programmes, institutional, clinical and out-patient services, staff training and provision of staff equipment may be called into question. Courts are often disposed to defer to governmental or other public agencies on the level of protective services that should be available in order to determine legal standards of care owed to staff, so that what level of precautions should be provided to health care practitioners will be influenced by what public authorities actually provide. If this is woefully inadequate, however, or where courts are prepared to require public agencies to reallocate budgets as judges indicate, courts may be prescriptive in establishing the extent to which health care practitioners must be facilitated to take universal precautions. At a minimum, courts may expect guidelines to contain the spread of hepatitis from patients to health facility staff to be observed and enforced.

Precautions are also necessary for protection of patients, health facility employees who do not attend patients directly, and others at risk of so-called "nosocomial" or institutionally spread HIV infection, such as through use of unsterilized or inadequately sterilized equipment. Improper sterilization of medical apparatus and instruments presents obvious dangers of spread of HIV infection, and equally obvious areas of potential legal liability for negligence. More problematic is infection through contamination of the supply of blood for transfusion, since no system can guarantee safety from infection. Absence of any effective screening of donors may create legal liability, but when a system exists, no liability will arise for its unavoidable imperfections.

The problem of multiple use of single-use or "disposable" medical devices is becoming commonplace as health care practitioners and institutions, even in relatively wealthy areas, cannot afford to use costly or scarce devices on only a single patient when the devices remain physically capable of re-use, particularly following sterilization.[10] The use of devices in ways that contradict or depart from their manufacturers' instructions raises legal questions, particularly under the laws of liability for negligence and of product liability.[11] Due care must be taken, for example, against excessive dilution of solvents employed in sterilization, operator error in the sterilization process and damage to the safe and effective use of devices caused for instance by solvents, and surface scratching of materials that causes crevices in which contaminated debris may lodge.[12] Courts may be called on to set the standard of care that governs reuse of devices that manufacturers and suppliers describe as designed or intended for single use, when reuse may spread HIV infection from one patient to another. When scarcity of essential devices compels reuse, however, health care practitioners and facilities may invoke the law of necessity to excuse their risk-taking in use of the only means available to them to treat patients in emergency. Outside cases of emergency, the law of consent may require that prospective patients for whose care reuse of devices supplied for single use is proposed be so informed, so that they can exercise choice regarding the convenience, immediacy and risk of the care they accept.

6. THE DUTY TO TREAT

In many countries, health care practitioners in general have not proven better informed or more enlightened than members of the lay public about the sources and spread of HIV infection, and have shared the dysfunctional misperceptions and negative stereotypes that prevail among the general population. One result has been a refusal by some practitioners to treat those they know are HIV infected, or who they think, for instance from their lifestyle, may be HIV infected. A refusal by health care practitioners to render care to people in need of their services on the ground that such people may be sick seems perverse, and a negation of the conscientious commitment to their calling that health care practitioners often profess and that justifies public esteem. Disregard of the ethical duty to treat the sick gives rise to legal liability in different circumstances. Practitioners employed in a contractual relationship with a health care facility, for instance, may violate terms of their contracts by failure or refusal to render care to those eligible to receive it from them, provided that facilities have observed reciprocal duties to provide an adequately safe work environment. It is clear from the nature of their functions that health care facilities cannot provide those they engage with work settings free from the risk of infection, and the undertaking of minimization of risk is not an assurance of its elimination.[13]

The legal claims of those wrongly refused health care depend on their circumstances. A tendency exists, not least among health care practitioners, to describe those eligible to receive treatment as "patients", but an important legal difference is drawn between those who are patients in law and those who are seeking to become patients. Where a diagnostic or therapeutic relationship exists between a health care practitioner and a person, that person is a patient, and a refusal or failure to render due care exposes the practitioner to legal liability for negligence, abandonment and/or breach of contract. Similar liabilities may arise where the patient's legal relationship is not with one or more particular practitioners but with a particular hospital or other health care facility. Patients cannot demand every or any particular treatment even when the costs of treatment can be met, since practitioners and facilities may exercise judgment about what treatment is indicated by patients' circumstances and what treatment is contraindicated in patients' best interests or would be futile. Nevertheless, they are legally obliged to offer care that is indicated, and to refer patients elsewhere for indicated care that they lack the specialization to provide. The standard of care that patients are entitled to be offered is ultimately determinable by a court, as an implied term of the contract of care and/or as an element of the law of negligence.[14] Some courts are reinforcing patients' rights to due care by invoking the concept of fiduciary duty,[15] which binds health care practitioners to conscientious duties to keep faith with the reasonable expectations of persons in need whom they have agreed to assist through their superior knowledge.

Where no prior relationship exists between a person who wants to become a patient and a particular health care practitioner or facility, no duty binds the practitioner or facility to enter such a relationship. Some facilities may in emergency treat persons they do not admit as patients, and must then conform to a legally determined standard of care, but the legal status of facility outpatients differs among jurisdictions and must be studied in detail to determine whether or not they are patients like those legally admitted as such. Some health facilities and practitioners have legally binding funding or other agreements with governmental or other public or private agencies, including religious and charitable foundations, that require them to admit designated people, such as residents of specified areas or people in evident need of emergency treatment, as patients. Refusal or failure to treat such eligible people will violate those agreements, but it is a matter of law in each jurisdiction whether such third party beneficiaries of agreements acquire legal rights to enforce them and to sue upon their breach.

Many licensing authorities of health care practitioners and

professional associations, health care facilities and health service funding agencies impose obligations of non-discrimination that preclude practitioners and facilities from declining to accept and treat persons on the bases, among others, of any physical or mental disability they may have. Further, jurisdictions at municipal, state or provincial and federal or central levels of government may have legally enforceable human rights codes that prohibit discrimination on grounds not only of race, sex and religion, but also of physical or mental disability. These are inspired by international human rights treaties that give legal force to the United Nations' Universal Declaration of Human Rights of 1948.[16] For instance, the International Covenant on Economic, Social and Cultural Rights recognizes rights to the highest attainable standard of physical and mental health and to the benefits of scientific progress on the basis of non-discrimination, and the International Covenant on Civil and Political Rights apparently includes rights to non-discrimination on the basis, for instance, of sexual orientation. Similarly, the Convention on the Rights of the Child recognizes children's rights to health care.

Practitioners and facilities that decline to accept people as patients on the grounds of their actual or presumed HIV infection may be in breach of laws that give effect to countries' domestic implementation of these international commitments. Action may be initiated by persons denied services, but alternatively they may complain to police or other public authorities, which may consider the matter to transcend a private wrong between the person and practitioner or facility, but to affect the public interest. Public prosecutors may feel obliged to become involved, and in some jurisdictions actions may be taken, for civil or criminal remedies, by an officer as high as an Attorney General or Minister of Justice. At stake is not just the denied right to due health services of the person requesting care, but the integrity of the country's commitment to principles of non-discrimination against disabled persons, and the seriousness of its commitment to its international human rights duties. Indeed, a state's failure to act against private acts of discrimination may represent a violation of the country's obligation under international law to give effect to its human rights obligations.[17] Even when no legislation or public law enforcement authorities give effect to human rights principles of non-discrimination, however, private law may be invoked. Health care practitioners who are members of professional associations whose ethical codes require non-discrimination, and/or who are licensed to practise subject to their observance of a code of professional practice, may face expulsion and loss or suspension of licensure, and may violate contractual obligations of employment that require their compliance with ethical codes and rules of licensure. Thus, both public law and rivate law may be applied against discriminatory conduct. .

The legal measures outlined above that might enforce the duty to treat persons who are HIV infected supposes that refusal to treat due to HIV infection amounts in law to discrimination on grounds of physical or mental disability. AIDS-related dementia affects many persons in advanced stages of sickness, but, at the other end of the spectrum of infection, many people who are HIV infected are asymptomatic and functioning well. They may require medical care, however, for conditions not related to infection, or indeed to illness; they might, for instance, break limbs in accidents or be pregnant and preparing for childbirth. The legal issue is whether denial of services to them on account of their HIV status is illegal discrimination on a ground of disability, when they are neither mentally not pathologically impaired.

An influential decision of the United States Supreme Court was given in the *Arline* case.[18] This did not directly concern AIDS or HIV positivity, and actually reserved whether it was applicable to HIV infection, but is widely considered relevant.[19] The Court held that if others refused to work or otherwise deal with a person on account of that person's infectious or other medical condition, even when the person was mentally and physically capable of discharging routine functions, they were discriminating on grounds of disability. The person affected was not able to function, because the interactions with others on which normal ability to function depends was denied by those others. The person was not medically disabled, but disabled from functioning in social, employment, economic or other ways that anti-discrimination legislation also addresses and prohibits. Thus, health care practitioners who refuse or fail to accept or treat a person as a patient on the ground of the person being HIV infected, even when the person shows no symptoms, disable that person, and face liability for discrimination on grounds of the disability that person suffers that they have caused.

It does not follow, however, that HIV infected persons can therefore legally demand any health service from any practitioner or facility. Practitioners are entitled and often legally obliged by licensing authorities to decline to act beyond their trained skills, but must refer applicants for care to practitioners or facilities able to give it There is no duty to treat beyond the ability to treat, but rather a duty not so to treat. Further, when a person who is HIV infected or who is responsibly considered liable to be infected seeks health care from a practitioner or facility capable of giving it, a refusal would be legally justifiable, and consistent with human rights and antidiscrimination law, if an accessible alternative centre had been established to give care to such persons. A practitioner or facility may refer to an alternative regional source of care available to the HIV infected person where the regional resource has personnel trained, equipped and experienced to treat such patients.

A local facility or practitioner may justifiably refuse to deliver treatment that is offered elsewhere that is as convenient to the person seeking care, or that presents no significantly greater inconvenience, when, for instance, the agency first approached is the principal health resource for a sizeable population but lacks the means, such as sterilization equipment or operatives, to protect other patients against spread of HIV infection. Treatment is not discriminatory in law simply because it is available in specially designated facilities, provided that there is no substantive disadvantage or stigma attached to receiving care there. Accordingly, the duty to treat HIV infected persons is discharged by referring them to accessible facilities that are best suited to provide care, including appropriate counselling. Specialized facilities may attract practitioners specially sympathetic to those with HIV infection. Facilities that do not accept such persons but refer them to specialized alternative facilities may attract practitioners fearful of suffering infection or averse to those whose behaviour presents high risk of infection, but the law is not effective to address the bias and prejudice that health care practitioners feel, but at best only the discrimination they exhibit.

In routine medical management of patients, therapeutic treatment is usually distinguishable from research, and although therapeutic innovation often has an experimental aspect, it is usually considered to be a category of treatment. However, since no cures exist for AIDS or HIV infection, infected persons may demand that they be given unproven medical and other products in the hope that improved care and even a cure will be achieved.[20] It has been observed regarding management of HIV infected patients that "experimentation and research come to look more and more like treatment."[21] The duty of health care professionals to undertake research is ethical rather than legal. Professionals may incur research duties to institutions that employ them, but they owe no legal duty to patients for whose care they are responsible to propose research on them. Any research that is undertaken, even at patients' insistence, must conform to requirements of ethical approval by institutional review boards,[22] and the law on research subjects' consent. Further, research outcomes must be carefully monitored, on both legal and ethical grounds, to assess their implications for treatment.[23] This is an element of health care practitioners' legal duty to be aware of scientific developments in their field.

Underlying the duty to treat is the capacity to treat. Those bound by the duty must employ resources reasonably available to them for this purpose, but management of HIV infection and AIDS in many regions of the world is beset by unavailability of indicated means. The cost of such drugs as AZT, which can for instance significantly reduce the risk of a mother transmitting HIV to her baby, may be beyond the means of national health services and individual patients to pay.[24] The law does not require that the impossible be accomplished, and unless indicated treatments are reasonably available there is no legal duty to employ them or to disclose them as options that patients may want to pursue by their own means and expenditures. Indeed, tantalizing desperate patients by giving information that means of relief exist to which they have no real possibility of access may be adverse to their well-being, and inimical to their care. Information that impresses patients with their powerlessness, isolation, poverty or subjection to misfortunes they cannot restrain or escape may justifiably be omitted from discussions about their care.

7. THE DUTY TO COUNSEL

Counselling of patients regarding HIV infection and testing cannot be adequately undertaken by health care practitioners whose own understanding of the infection, its transmission and epidemiology is inadequate. Practitioners who are competent to counsel should be able to offer counselling regarding whether HIV testing is indicated because of a patient's symptoms or high risk behaviour or experience, regarding the implications of a positive and a negative test result, and the medical, social, moral, and perhaps legal implications of a patient declining an indicated test. Counselling on the appropriateness of taking an HIV test is in some ways the most difficult because of mixed social messages about HIV infection and AIDS. As awareness grows of the risks of infection and rising statistics of HIV infection and AIDS-related deaths, patients can be panicked into believing they should be tested, including patients whose behaviour places them in a low risk category for infection. As against this, since the virus does not survive long in air and is transmissible primarily through intimate exchanges of body fluids, particularly in sexual relations, needle-sharing injection of drugs and transfusion of unscreened or contaminated blood, the virus is not casually spread. People who engage in high risk behaviour may accordingly feel justified in believing in their immunity, particularly when they recognize no symptoms of infection. Counsellors, therefore, face the double challenge of comforting the inappropriately troubled, and troubling the inappropriately comfortable.

A patient whose HIV test proves negative must be questioned about earlier conduct, and counselled about the incubation period during which negative results will be shown in tests on recently infected persons who are capable of transmitting the virus to partners. That is, patients must be counselled that a negative test result must be interpreted in the context of preceding and subsequent behaviours before it can be taken to show the absence of infection. If a health care practitioner does not adequate]y counsel a patient whose test is negative but who later infects another due to a belief that there was no need, for instance, to take sexual precautions, the practitioner is at risk of legal liability, particularly if that other was induced to rely on the practitioner's implied assurance that the patient was not HIV-infected.

More extensive counselling must be offered when a patient's test produces a positive result.[25] Initial discussion with a patient who accepts counselling concerns whether the result may be a false positive, but once this possibility is minimized, a patient must be counselled as if truly HIV infected. Counselling must be offered that addresses strategies to remain symptom free, how to receive treatment for opportunistic infections to delay the onset of AIDS, how to live with AIDS and postpone its more debilitating effects, and how to maintain morale and maximize functional capacity through progressive stages of disability. No less important is counselling on protection of others the patient may infect,"[26] including reproductive counselling and counselling of risks of transmitting infection to a child *in utero* or in childbirth. Pregnancy itself reduces the immune response, and when this is already compromised by HIV infection, susceptibility to infection may be aggravated. Nevertheless, counselling should conform to professional standards, and be non-directive regarding patients' responses and decisions.

Protection of intimate partners may be proposed through joint counselling, but patients' assumption of responsibility for partners' protection is legally problematic, since a failure of such protection resulting in partners' infection may implicate health care practitioners. Patients may be unwilling to disclose to health care practitioners who all of their sexual or drug-sharing partners have been, for instance when they prefer to keep their bisexuality secret. Further, patients who regard their positive test result as a death sentence may grieve, and early stages of grieving include anger and denial.[27] Patients who deny the implication of the test result may angrily deny the advice given in counselling and behave as if they are not infected, so endangering sexual partners and others. Counterproductive counselling of patients raises legal issues if it results in third parties being infected.

Legislation in many jurisdictions proposes containment of the spread of contagious and infectious diseases, including sexually transmitted diseases, by mandating that health care practitioners who learn of such disorders must notify a public health officer.[28] The officer will attempt to detain an infected person or otherwise reduce risk of spread of infection, learn identities of the person's associates at risk and undertake partner notification and contact tracing, as far as possible,[29] to warn partners and contacts that they may have been exposed to infection. This legislation represents the coercive or policing power of the state to protect public safety and welfare,[30] and is not dependent on infected persons' consent. Whatever its practical effect may be, its legal effect is to protect the health care practitioner whose HIV infected patient does not comply with advice given in counselling aimed at protection of third parties against infection by a patient. The practitioner's report to the designated public health officer may discharge any duties owed to patients' partners at risk of infection .

Whether legislation mandates reporting of patients a health care practitioner finds not to have AIDS but believes may be HIV infected when they decline to be tested depends upon its particular wording. However, when reporting is not mandatory, practitioners usually have a legitimate discretion to report any person they believe reasonably and in good faith may be a danger to public health by being a potential source of infection to others. Under these conditions, there will be no illegal violation of the patient's confidentiality if the belief of infectivity is correct, nor actionable defamation if it is incorrect because disclosure will be covered by the law of qualified privilege. Practitioners themselves do not need to know a person's HIV status in giving treatment, since they should take universal precautions, including in treating persons who test HIV negative. Whether practitioners can legally withdraw from treatment of patients who decline to be HIV tested depends on the law of contract and abandonment, and on antidiscrimination law, but proposed withdrawal requires the practitioner to offer counselling on both the patient's protection of others and on how to maintain his or her health and secure appropriate services from other practitioners.

Counselling should also address differences between compulsory, mandatory, routine and voluntary HIV testing, where relevant to a patient's conduct. The terms are not always used consistently, but compulsory testing is usually taken to mean involuntary testing compelled by legislative or judicial authority, such as testing of persons convicted or accused of sexual assault,[31] perhaps in violation of human rights principles such as the presumption of innocence. Mandatory testing makes submission to testing a condition of exercise of otherwise voluntary choices. For instance, patients who seek treatment for HIV infection may reasonably be expected to permit testing to establish that they are infected, plaintiffs who sue defendants they claim infected them may be required to provide evidence that they are actually HIV infected, and persons who want to serve as donors of blood, sperm or organs must expect that the donated materials will be tested for protection of potential recipients. Patients do not have to take treatment, plaintiffs do not have to sue and persons do not have to donate, but if they want to proceed with their plans to be patients, plaintiffs or donors it is mandated that they submit to relevant tests, and have test results made appropriately available.[32]

Routine testing is based on implied consent. When a patient gives a blood or other tissue sample to be tested, it is in the context of a particular diagnosis or circumstance, such as monitoring of therapy. The patient knows the overall purpose of testing, but not necessarily each of the individual characteristics or properties of the sample it will be tested to detect. Some centres and health care practitioners believe that samples should routinely be tested for HIV infection, such as by detection of antibodies to the virus, and that patients need not specifically be asked to consent to this, or be explicitly informed that this test will be performed. Other authorities find this highly objectionable, and forbid HIV testing without explicit consent.[33]

Patients should be counselled that what is presented to them as routine testing may include an HIV test, however, and that they may take an initiative to ask about this test and to object to it if they wish. An ethical view that prevails in many health care settings to which courts of law may be sympathetic is that an HIV test is not just a test like many others, because of the severe stigmatization and prejudice that may follow if the test proves positive. Accordingly, an HIV test should be performed only following a person's adequately informed and freely given consent. Courts may determine in each case whether an HIV test may legitimately be included in routine testing on the basis of implied consent, but if the sample was taken for any legal purpose its taking does not become an assault simply because a test to which no legal consent was given is conducted. That is, illegal testing of the sample for HIV antibodies is not an assault on the patient provided that the sample was taken for another, legitimate purpose. A patient will, therefore, have to seek a legal remedy on other grounds such as breach of privacy or confidentiality, if such grounds are available.

8. CONFIDENTIALITY AND THE DUTY TO WARN

The stigmatization and prejudice often directed against persons with HIV infection provide reasons why HIV infected patients' confidentiality should be preserved. The implied terms of a contract, the law of negligence, the law on breach of fiduciary duty and, in some jurisdictions, the law on privacy may reinforce the duty of confidentiality. The countervailing consideration, however, is that timely disclosure of a risk of HIV infection may prevent it, preserve a person's health and prolong a life. Health care practitioners may accordingly confrortt the dilemma of preserving a patient's confidentiality but appearing complicit in an innocent persons' suffering and premature death, or of prioritizing the welfare of a non-patient over that of a patient by betraying the patient s trust. The dilemma of a health care practitioner is aggravated when the person at risk of HIV infection is also the practitioner's patient, such as a patient's spouse, other family member or companion for whose welfare the practitioner is also responsible.[34]

The legal dilemma of preservation of confidentiality is eased, if only in an analytical sense, by an observation of the Supreme Court of California in 1976 that has achieved considerable currency. In the much discussed *Tarasoff* case,[35] where health care practitioners were held civilly liable for not giving appropriate warning to an identified person at risk of a grave danger they correctly anticipated would be caused by a patient, the Court identified the special nature of the therapist-patient relation, held that this imposed a duty towards the person at risk to protect from foreseen harm, and observed that "the protective privilege [of confidentiality] ends where the public peril begins".[36] Disclosure was thereby analysed not to be a breach of confidentiality, because what the Court described as "the privilege" of confidentiality did not extend so far as to preclude disclosure where an individual was considered to be in grave peril. This confirms that, while confidentiality is an important value in the relation between a health care practitioner and a patient, it is not the only value, nor necessarily the highest. The Court prioritized a duty to warn of anticipated grave peril, limiting the scope of confidentiality. Because confidentiality is not necessarily absolute, courts may give added force to antidiscrimination legislation.

The legal duty under the *Tarasoff* principle is not to make accurate predictions of risk, but only to act appropriately in light of the prediction actually made, so that a competently reached assessment that thére is no or little risk will be an excusable error if it proves incorrect.[37] In *Tarasoff*, the potential victim was identifiable, and the predicted menace was great. The same may be the case when a patient who is HIV infected has a heterosexual or same-sex partner. Where local legislation requires the reporting of identities of HIV infected persons to a public health officer, a health care practitioner should inform the patient of the reporting duty and of prospective contact tracing, but in any event should counsel the patient about risk of transmission to the partner. Unless the practitioner is assured that the partner is or will be appropriately notified of the risk and afforded protection, for instance by the patient and/or the local public health officer, the practitioner may have to be proactive.

The practitioner may, for instance;, ask the patient to have the identified partner contact the practitioner, inform the patient that the practitioner will directly contact the partner or, for instance if the practitioner is not a physician but knows a physician responsible for the partner's health care, contact that physician. If the patient discloses no identifiable partner at risk, the practitioner has no duty of investigation, but may discharge legal duties to unidentified others by informing an appropriate pubic health officer of the patient's HIV status. Whether such officers act under legislative authority or not, they are legally obliged to afford due confidentiality to the identities of persons of whose health status they learn, and are usually expected not to disclose identities of their informants.

If local jurisprudence does not accept the Tares off rationale that confidentiality does not negate duties to warn, but recognizes instead the priority in principle of confidentiality, a practitioner who feels morally obliged to notify an identified person at apparent risk of infection may invoke the legal principle of necessity to protect human life.[38] In law, there are mandatory, justifiable, excusable and capable disclosures. Mandatory disclosure arises, for instance, under public health legislation and the Tarasoff principle, and justified disclosure would arise with patients' consent and if patients fail to object when adequately notified of intended future disclosures. The law on necessity provides that, although it does not justify unauthorized disclosure, which is therefore unlawful, it may excuse from capability a person who discounts other legal duties when a considerably more significant value is at stake. The law regarding the confidentiality of HIV status protects patients against social stigmatization and prejudice in pursuit of many interests, but a court may find that protection of an unaware person against avoidable HIV infection and its consequences to health and life is a more significant value. The intention to provide such protection may accordingly be held excusable so as to exempt a health care practitioner from punishment or culpability for the unlawful act of unauthorized disclosure.

Lawyers may find it difficult to advise health care practitioners to act in reliance on necessity, however, because a court may not accept the priority of the claimed necessity, and in any event the conduct would be unlawful, even if considered not punishable or culpable by a court of law. A professional disciplinary authority may be able to impose sanctions for professional misconduct for behaviour that is unlawful, even when a court finds it excusable.[39] Accordingly lawyers may advise health care practitioners about their legal obligations of confidentiality, and that if they choose to violate them in order to warn others of the risk of infection that patients present, the breach of confidentiality may be found excusable and so not punishable or compensable. However, lawyers are unlikely positively to advise health care practitioners to act unlawfully and to hope that courts will excuse them. Courts may not, and even if they do, professional disciplinary authorities may not. Further, legal professional disciplinary authorities usually will not permit lawyers to give advice that the law may be broken, even if courts find particular breaches to be excusable. Necessity may offer an *ex post* facto defence, but not a prospective basis of legal advice to disregard the law of confidentiality, where the *Tarasoff* principle does not limit the legal scope of confidentiality in the face of public peril .

When a patient requests a health care practitioner to send a copy of the patient's medical record to a third party, the practitioner is obliged to do so. Even though the record may be contained on materials owned and possessed by a health care facility or the practitioner, courts increasingly recognize that the information itself belongs to the patient[40] and that the practitioner, as trustee of the information, must supply it and give copies of it according to the patient's directions. Nevertheless, since patients often do not know the full contents of their medical records or appreciate the way information contained there may be understood and used by others, health care practitioners are legally bound to offer patients counselling about foreseeable consequences of their compliance with patients' requests to disclose confidential medical information.

Patients seeking, for instance, employment or insurance may not appreciate that their medical records may include information that motivates prospective employers or insurers not to accept them, and to give honest or contrived reasons for refusal influenced by local anti-discrimination laws. Health care professionals cannot advise or be parties to deception of those with whom their patients may interact, but must ensure that patients are afforded means to exercise adequately informed consent in releasing their confidential health information to others. When patients' information needs to be shared with other health care practitioners, however, practitioners are entitled and usually bound to make disclosure to them of information relevant to serve the patients' interests. Even when patients are unaware of such sharing of information, it is a part of legitimate practice to advance patients' interests to which they impliedly consent, and no breach of confidentiality arises. Recipients of such shared information owe patients the same duties of confidentiality as the practitioners who make it available.

Testing of identifiable patients raises confidentiality concerns, but testing is different from screening. Population screening studies are epidemiological surveys to determine, for instance, the prevalence of HIV infection in a target group.[41] The group is composed, of course, of individuals, but data are gathered to learn not about the individuals as such but about the incidence of infection in the group as a whole. Screening studies may use personally identifying health records or, for instance, unlinked anonymous data, gathered from individual records or from aggregated data sources. Legal concerns about individual confidentiality are occasionally invoked to prevent or regulate screening studies designed to establish HIV prevalence in a given population, but this appears a misapplication of clinical values to the detriment of public health systems. Individuals' health is endangered where public health authorities lack information of the incidence of diseases, and therefore cannot take effective preventive or remedial action or develop and locate treatment resources appropriately. Those who conduct HIV prevalence screening programmes may on occasion learn personally identified health information, but they are usually legally obliged to observe confidentiality. Often, however, no individual confidences are violated by screening studies. Some are authorized by public health legislation that explicitly supersedes or limits individual confidentiality.[42] Since such studies are directed to the welfare of individuals as a public health measure, they may be taken to have consent given at a communal or macroethical level,[43] and not to violate the ordinary legal obligations to preserve confidentiality of individual health information.

Death certificates are frequently public documents. In law, duties such as of confidentiality are not usually owed to people following their deaths, but forms of certification can implicate the HIV status of living persons such as companions and family members of those who have died, including their young children. Where death is certified as AIDS-related, no confidence of the deceased is legally violated, but interests of living persons may be endangered. Local law governs how explicit and comprehensive death certification must be, but unless legislation or regulations expressly provide otherwise, physicians have a discretion to certify death as due only to its immediately precipitating causes, such as carcinoma, pneumonia or tuberculosis, or to add that the causes were AIDS related .

9. THE HIV INFECTED HEALTH CARE PRACTITIONER

The danger of patients being exposed to health care practitioners' HIV infected body fluids has appeared so low that some have claimed the problem to be non-existent.[44] However, surgeons or dentists may cut themselves through their protective gloves, particularly in undertaking procedures in which they do not have sight of their hands, and they may then bleed into patients' bodies before it is surgically or otherwise appropriate for them to remove their hands. There are few if any proven instances of an HIV infected health care practitioner infecting a patient,[45] but were a practitioner to do so, a court would probably assess liability by strict criteria because the practitioner would be held to a higher standard of care than a layperson. This is not to say that HIV infected health care personnel cannot practise as such; indeed, they may be peculiarly suited and perhaps willing to attend certain HIV infected patients. In countries where HIV infection is endemic and health care practitioners scarce, there may be no alternative to infected practitioners remaining in practice. They would be expected, however, to maintain a high level of vigilance and care to protect patients against any threat they might pose. If an HIV vaccine is developed and practitioners decide to take it for protective purposes, their HIV status will become positive because they will develop antibodies to the virus, but they will pose little, if any, risk to patients.

Infected practitioners might be expected to remove themselves from all but the irreducible minimum risk of exposing patients to their body fluids. For instance, HIV positive surgeons might limit their practice to external procedures, and forego undertaking any in which they wouid not have full sight of their hands at all times. They might also be expected, for instance, not to work in emergency or trauma centres. They might be required to explain to health facility department or unit heads why they are unsuited to certain styles of practice. All infected health care practitioners should seek specialist advice and monitoring on their professional practice, because compromised immune systems might leave them particularly susceptible to contract infections from patients, and to spread such infections other than HIV itself. Their stamina might also decline, although they might well become incapable of practice some time before becoming susceptible to AIDS-related dementia.

Health care practitioners who diagnose or otherwise learn of a colleague's HIV infection have a duty to inform appropriate institutional, or licensing authorities if they believe that advice to protect patients is not being followed and that the colleague's fitness to practise may be impaired. Due warning protects both patients and the colleague from catastrophe, and may facilitate the colleague's appropriate care. Those who learn of a colleague's HIV infection must observe confidentiality in the ordinary way, but selective disclosure to protect patients and also the colleague would not constitute a breach of confidentiality, since colleagues are expected to monitor and ensure each other's professional capacity to practise. It must be remembered that, where legislation requires that a designated public health officer be notified that a patient has been diagnosed with AIDS or HIV infection, the duty to notify applies no less to patients who are health care practitioners than to others. Several health care professions have specified practitioners' duties to protect patients on suspicion of their own HIV infection in ethical codes, and it has been seen that ethical codes may be legally enforced through licensing authorities' and others' disciplinary powers to contain professional misconduct. As against this, a practitioner's dismissal from employment or denial of the right to practise on account of HIV infection alone raises legal issues under antidiscrimination laws, including whether non-infection is a *bona* fide employment requirement for the tasks the practitioner seeks to undertake.

Local law will determine whether HIV infected practitioners must inform patients of their status before undertaking invasive or other procedures on them.[46] If patients inquire about practitioners' HIV status, they must be answered honestly. In principle, however, there seems to be no requirement to volunteer disclosure in view of the relatively low risk of practitioners infecting patients, and of analogies with the more easily infectious conditions practitioners might transmit to patients that they are not required to disclose. Information that patients are usually entitled to receive centres on what is material to the choices they have to make,[47] and risks that are so low as to be almost insignificant do not have to be disclosed, unless patients show that they consider them significant by asking about them.

Some patients in the United States who were treated by health care practitioners they did not know were HIV infected were not infected themselves, but nevertheless brought legal proceedings claiming that, once they learned of their practitioners' HIV status, they became fearful of the risk of infection and had to undergo invasive testing to determine their own HIV status.[48] The basis of the claims was deliberate or negligent infliction of emotional distress. It will have to be seen whether such "AIDS phobia" claims will become influential in a country's jurisprudence. Fearing liability, health facilities may bar surgeons, dentists, and possibly other health care practitioners from performing certain and perhaps any procedures on patients who have not given prior consent to receive services from practitioners who may be HIV infected. Alternatively, facilities may outline the protective measures they take, and say that persons unwilling to receive care under those measures should not become patients there. Neither strategy would cover emergency care, however, which may justify the exclusion of HIV infected practitioners from delivering such care except when life is in immediate danger and no alternative practitioners are available. A counter-argument, however, is that the universal precautions that health care practitioners take to protect themselves against HIV infection from patients also protect patients against infection spread by practitioners and that their exclusion from routine emergency services would be unlawful discrimination on grounds of their HIV-based disability. Health care practitioners remain members of the general community protected by human rights laws against discrimination.

NOTE

[Ed.: The text of the Statement issued by the General Medical Council of the United Kingdom on 'Guidance on Ethical Aspects of HIV Infection and AIDS' is reproduced in Annexure E].

REFERENCES

1. See generally Fluss S.S., Zeegers D. "AIDS, HIV and health care workers: some international legislative perspectives" *Maryland Law Review* 1989; 48: 77-92.
2. See Jayasuriya D.C. (ed.) *HIV Law and Law Reform: Asia and the Pacific* (New Delhi: UNDP Regional Project, 1995).
3. Constitution of the World Health Organization, in *Basic Documents,* 39th ed. Geneva, World Health Organization, 1992. The Constitution entered into force on 7 April, 1948.
4. D. Giesen, *International Medical Malpractice Law* Tubingen: JCB Mohr (Paul Siebeck); Dordrecht: Martinus Nijhoff, 1988, 112 *et* seq.
5. Godwin, J. *et al. Australian HIV/AIDS Legal Guide* (Sydney: Federation Press, 2nd ed. 1993) 167.
6. Kennedy I., Grubb A., 2nd ed. *Medical Law: Text with Materials* London: Butterworths 1994 at 450 *et. seq.*
7. See Giesen D., note 4 above at 117 *et seq.*
8. Temmerman M., Ndinya-Achola J., Ambani J. *et al.* The right not to know HIV-test results. *Lancet* 1995; 345: 969-70, and Green J., Kentish J. *ibid.* 1508.
9. See Von Reyn C.F. Mann J.M. and Chin J., International travel and HIV infection, *Bulletin World Health Organization.* 1990; 68: 251-59, and Canada Communicable Disease Report, Statement on travellers and sexually transmitted diseases, *Canadian Medical Association Journal* 1995; 152:1826–8.
10. Canadian Hospital Association, "The Reuse of Disposables: A Discussion Paper", Ottawa: CHA Press, 1994.
11. See Giesen D., note 4 above, at 115.
12. See for instance Bentolila P., Jacob R. and Roberge F., "Effects of reuse on the physical characteristics of angiographic catheters", *Journal of Medical Engineering and Technology* 1990; 14: 254-259.
13. See Verkuyl D.A.A., "Practising obstetrics and gynaecology in areas with a high prevalence of HIV infection", *Lancet* 1995; 346: 293-96.
14. See Giesen D., note 4 above.
15. See for instance *McInerney v. MacDonald* (1992), 93 D.L.R. (4th) 415 (Sup. Ct. Canada).
16. See R.J. Cook "Human Rights HIV Infection and Women", in Jayasuriya D.C. (ed.) HIV *Law, Ethics and Human Rights: Text and Materials* (New Delhi, UNDP Regional Project, 1995).

17. See R.J. Cook, "State responsibility for violations of women's human rights", *Harvard Human Rights J.* 1994; 7; 125-75.
18. *School Board of Nassau County* v. *Arline* (1987), 480 U.S. 273 (U.S. Sup. Ct.).
19. The *Arline* judgment was applied to AIDS in *Chalk* v. *United States District Court* (1988), 840 F.2d 701 (9th Cir.) and *Baxter* v. *City of Belleville* (1989), 720 F. Supp. 720 (S.D. Illinois).
20. For instance, on a controversial proposal for a transplantation of a baboon's bone marrow into a patient with advanced HIV infection, see Thompson C., No cheers for baboon tó AIDS patient xenotransplant, Lancet 1995; 346:369-70.
21. Gostin L.O. Preface: Hospitals, health care professionals, and persons with AIDS. In Gostin L.O. ed., *AIDS and the Health Care System.* New Haven and London: Yale University Press, 1990: 3-12 at 9.
22. See Council for International Organizations of Medical Sciences, International Ethical Guidelines for Biomedical Research Involving Human Subjects. Geneva, CIOMS, 1993.
23. See for instance Lowe D. HIV study raises ethical concerns for the treatment of pregnant women. *Berkeley Women's Law Journal* 1995; 10: 176-182.
24. Cohen, J., "Bringing AZT to poor countries," *Science* 1995; 269:62426.
25. Counselling must be offered, but see Temmerman M., Ndinya Achola J., Ambani J., note 8 above.
26. See *Pitman Estate* v. *Bain* (1994), 112 D.L.R. (4th) 257 (Ont. Ct. (Gen. Div.).
27. Kubler-Ross E., *On Death and Dying* New York: Macmillan, 1969, at 34-43 (denial of death is the first major stage in the psychology of dying).
28. See Fluss S.S., Zeegers D., note 1 above at 82.
29. But see North R.L., Rothenberg K.H. Partner notification and the threat of domestic violence against women with HIV infection. *New England Journal of Medicine* 1993; 329: 1194-96.
30. *Jacobsen* v. *Massachusetts* (1905), 197 U.S. 11 (U.S. Sup. Ct.).
31. See Stevenson C.M. Note [HIV Testing of Sex Offenders]. *Journal of Contemporary Health Law and Policy* 1994; 11: 281-315.
32. Mandatory testing for women seeking care in pregnancy may amount to unlawful coercion to submit to testing if the alternatives are to forego care, to the detriment of a woman and a child she delivers, or voluntary termination of pregnancy; see Goldstein K.L. Balancing risks and rights; HIV testing regimes for pregnant women. *Cornell Journal of Law and Public Policy* 1995; 4: 609-637. See also Post L.J. Unblinded mandatory HIV screening of newborns: care or coercion? *Cardozo Law Review* 1994; 16: 169-227.
33. See Fluss S.S., Zeegers D., note 1 above at 84-7.
34. Bayer R., Toomey K.E. HIV prevention and the two faces of partner notification. *American Journal of Public Health* 1992; 82: 1158-63.
35. *Tarasiff v. Regents of the University of California,* (1976) 551 P. 2d. 334 (Calif. Sup. Ct.).
36. *Ibid.,* at 347.
37. See *Whitehouse v. Jordan,* [1980] 1 All E.R. 650 (C.A.), affirmed at [1981] 1 All E.R. 267 (House of Lords).
38. See *R. v Bourne,* [1939] 1 K.B. 687 (Cent. Crim. Ct.) and *Perka* v. *The Queen* (1984), 14 C.C.C. (3d) 385 (Sup. Ct. Canada).
39. For instance following the decision of the Dutch Supreme Court to impose no sentence for unlawful euthanasia committed by medically assisted suicide in the *Chabot* case of 21 June 1994 Nederlandse Jurisprudentie (1994) 656,

the Amsterdam Medical Disciplinary Board found a violation of professional standards; see M. Milo "The Chabot cases", (editorial), 2 *Maastricht J. of European and Comparative Law,* 1995; 2: 1-3.

40. See *McInerney* v. *MacDonald,* note 15 above.
41. See Last J.M. Epidemiology and ethics in Bankowski Z., Bryant J.H., and Lat J.M. (eds.) *Ethics and Epidemiology: International Guidelines,* Geneva, Council for International Organizations of Medical Sciences, 1991, 14-28.
42. See *Jacobsen* v. *Massachusetts,* note 30 above, on police powers exercised for protection of the public.
43. Gostin L. Macro-ethical principles for the conduct of research on human subjects: population-based research and ethics. In: Bankowski Z., Bryant J.H. and Last J.M., eds., note 41 above at 29-46.
44. See DiMaggio S.L., "State regulations and the HIV-positive health care professional: a response to a problem that does not exists", American Journal of Law and Medicine 1993; 19: 497-522.
45. In case in Florida, five patients of an HIV infected dentist were found to be infected, but investigations and sterilization and infection control procedures, such as would prevent transmission of infection from other patients, rather than from patients' exposure to the dentist's infection; see *ibid.* 498.
46. Some early decisions in the U.S. seemed sympathetic to practitioners' duty to make prior disclosure of their HIV status, but this is contrary to the principle of informed consent that only material risks need to be disclosed; see DeVille K.A., "Nothing to fear but fear itself: HIV-infected physicians and the law of informed consent", J. *Law, Medicine and Ethics,* 1994; 22: 163-175, and Logan M.K., "Who's afraid of whom? Courts require HIV-infected doctors to obtain informed consent of patients", *DePaul Law Review.* 1995; 44: 483-511.
47. See *Canterbury v. Spence* (1972), 464 F.2d 722 (U.S.C.A., Dist. Of Columbia Cir.), *Rogers* v. *Whitaker* (1992), 109 A.L.R. 625 (H.C. Aust.) and generally D. Giesen, note 4 above, at 252 *et seq.*
48. See note 43 above.

26

HIV and Insurance

Prof. Joseph M. Kelly
Buffalo State College
State University of New York, U.S.A.

Insurance is an important necessity, especially in a free market, industrialized society. To HIV seropositive individuals, insurance is crucial, not only in order to obtain medical care, but also to pay one's debts after death and provide for spouses and children. This chapter compares the problem of insurance related to the HIV seropositive primarily in the United States, Europe, and certain African and Asian countries. Hopefully, by comparing different systems one may learn to resolve the HIV seropositive insurance issue better in one's own country.

The insurance industry in the United States is essentially a risk allocation contract where the policy holder "transfers certain risks of loss to another, the insurer, for a monetary consideration."[1] "It is axiomatic that insurance does not cover known losses. Insurance covers the risk of loss."[2] The industry is usually heavily regulated only by the state[3] unless a particular aspect of insurance is pre-empted by federal law.

A. HEALTH INSURANCE

1. U.S.

Because of the high risk of private health insurance, it is essential that employees, especially those with HIV, belong to some workplace health plan. While many states have protected HIV seropositive employees from insurance workplace discrimination, it was unpredictable that the Employee Retirement Income Security Act of 1974 (ERISA), a law designed to protect employee benefits, could be judicially interpreted to virtually eliminate HIV seropositive insurance protection. Whether the Americans with Disabilities Act (ADA) will restore such protection is still uncertain, although the federal administrative agency enforcing the ADA has clearly indicated that discrimination based on HIV is not only a violation of the ADA, but will result in financial penalties against the entity responsible for such discrimination.

Within the United States, private health insurance costs are extremely expensive. Approximately 83 per cent of all private health insurance is provided through the workplace,[4] with the employer often paying a major portion of premiums. It is undisputed that the more employees in a business, the more likely the company will have a health plan. For example, 90 per cent of the firms with twenty-five to forty-nine employees have a health plan compared to 54 per cent of those with five to nine workers and 26 per cent of firms with under four employees.[5]

2. Self-funding

In the United States, lifetime medical costs for HIV are estimated at $119,000.[6] Due to cost and other barriers for health insurance, HIV seropositive persons have sought work at those companies that have large group insurance policies[7]—these companies present fewer obstacles to obtain health insurance. Some employers have concluded that economic necessity should mandate a reduction for HIV benefits, a measure which would result in violation of many state anti-discrimination laws.

Rarely, very rarely, do corporations exclude HIV seropositive coverage because of HIV problems resulting from "personal lifestyle decisions". Circle K Corporation, the second largest operator of convenience stores in the United States, excluded HIV coverage for claims of gays and drug users, but not for claims resulting from blood transfusions. Public pressure forced Circle K to drop its HIV exclusion.[8] Galaxy Carpet Mill (Ga.) imposed a lifetime $10,000 cap' on health benefits on "voluntarily contracted HIV" and other sexually transmitted diseases. As in Circle K, the cap was dropped as a result of public pressure.[9]

Increasingly, however, companies are turning to self-funded insurance programmes[10] regulated by ERISA[11], which preempted state regulations. In fact, by 1995, "over 65 per cent of (US) workers who are provided health benefits ... are in self-insured plans.[12]

This federal law was passed long before HIV was an issue, and its purpose was partly to protect employees' pensions and health benefits granted by an employer. While ERISA created substantive regulations covering pension plans, it did not create the same for welfare plans.[13] It has come under judicial criticism, especially when applied to health care plans and HIV.[14]

Judicial decisions under ERISA have often been unfavourable to persons with AIDS (PWA). In *Phelps v. Field Real Estate Co.*,[15] plaintiff, hired in 1985, learned he was HIV seropositive in 1986, but did not disclose his condition. In 1988, he informed his employer that he had a fatal disease which he had kept secret out of fear of losing his job and health insurance. In 1989, after being terminated for poor work performance and for company reorganization, the plaintiff filed an ERISA complaint, alleging that his termination was the result of fear of catastrophic benefit cost increase. The Court of Appeals affirmed the trial court decision for the defendant because the latter did not base any part of its termination decision on saving benefit costs. The plaintiff was further'more unable to show that it was more probable than not that his medical condition motivated his employer to terminate his employment.

Under ERISA, there is no specification as to what the standard of review should be concerning the determination by an administrator in self-funded plans. In *Kennedy v. System One Holdings,*[16] the HIV seropositive former employee claimed that he was misled by the employer and plan administrator as to the allowed time to recover long-term disability benefits under the company welfare plan. Cane factor in granting the defendant summary judgment was that courts will defer to the plan administrator's factual determination unless there is an abuse of discretion.

Courts will generally defer to the decision of an insurance plan administrator concerning benefits and will uphold his decision as long as it is not arbitrary and capricious. In *Florence Nightingale Nursing Service v. Blue Cross* s *Blue Shield of America,*[17] the patient's employer provided medical benefits through a plan administered by the defendant. The plan provided reasonable charges only for medically necessary privateduty nursing. During the first month, the provider billed the defendant for at-home intravenous care for an HIV seropositive patient. During the second month, the defendant was billed for at-home care notwithstanding that the patient was no longer receiving IV treatment. Blue Cross paid less than half the cost of the first month and nothing for the second month since it said that the patient's family could have provided post-IV treatment care.

The court declined to defer to the claims administrator's expertise since Blue Cross had in this matter a potential conflict of interest, given that it had to follow the sponsoring employer's emphasis upon containing costs. The court then examined the matter de novo and concluded that medical costs were reasonable by comparing them to other home nursing services that cared for HIV seropositive patients, and because HIV seropositive patients were a special case. The trial court opined that "recruit(ing) nurses for treating AIDS victims must be like recruiting kamikaze pilots. It takes a special breed."[18]

When many employers in self-insurance plans realized that they, instead of the insurer, had to pay medical costs, they then introduced caps on HIV payments for all employees, while leaving intact medical benefits for other illnesses. In two instances, federal appellate courts upheld employer caps on HIV in self-funded plans.

In *McGann v. H and H Music Co.,*[19] the company changed from a group insurance plan to a self-insurance plan and reduced lifetime maximum health benefits from $1 million to $5,000 only for HIV. This had disastrous consequences for plaintiff McGann, who had been diagnosed HIV seropositive seven months (December 1987) before the policy changed. When McGann sued, alleging a violation of Section 510[20] of ERISA, the court granted the defendant summary judgment because the plaintiff had not shown discriminatory intent on the employer's part, notwithstanding the plaintiff being the only affected employee. H & H Music had also reserved the right to modify the plan which prevented the defendant from successfully alleging interference with any vested right. In dicta, the Court of Appeals stated that there would have been no ERISA violations "even though the employer's decision ... may stem from some 'prejudice' against AIDS or its victims generally. ..."[21]

A similar result was reached in *Owens v. Storehouse, Inc.,*[22] where the employer, in order to obtain stop-loss insurance, switched to a self-insurance plan that reduced lifetime benefits from $1 million to $25,000. *Owens,* in following *McGann,* concluded that ERISA pre-empted state law and that "absent evidence of retaliation or interference with the attainment of an entitled right ..., ERISA provides no right to perpetual health insurance with immutable terms." As in *McGann,* the plaintiff furthermore failed to show that his former employer intentionally interfered with any vested right of the plaintiff.[23]

3. The Americans with Disabilities Act

The Americans with Disabilities Act[24] (ADA) of 1990 extended certain anti-discrimination provisions of the 1964 Civil Rights Act to disabled persons. In 1991, a protected individual pursuant to a graduated damages provision could obtain a maximum award of $300,000. The ADA became effective for all employers with 25 or more employees on 25 July, 1992, and for employers with 15 to 24 employees on 26 July, 1994.[25] While the ADA does not mention HIV, its congressional history[26] and court decisions have concluded that even asymptomatic HIV seropositive has protection under the ADA.[27] The Equal Employment Opportunity Commission (EEOC) is the federal administrative agency responsible for the enforcement of much of the ADA, and its regulations are generally given significant deference by federal courts. Should the EEOC determine that an employer's HIV benefits policy is in violation of the ADA, it may obtain relief only through litigation in a federal court if settlement attempts fail.

The ADA requires an employer to make reasonable accommodations and prohibits discrimination against "a qualified individual with a disability" unless such accommodations would create undue hardship. Concerning insurance programmes, the ADA prohibits an employer from using insurance risk classifications "as a subterfuge to evade (the statutes) purposes."[28] The employer may neither ask about medical conditions nor require a blood test prior to offering employment. After an offer is accepted, an employer may reject an applicant for employment only if the physical examination demonstrates it is physically impossible for the applicant to work.

The "plain language" of the ADA "provides no express guidance" whether HIV is included. Therefore, "substantial deference" is given to the interpretation of its provisions by the EEOC.[29] The EEOC has issued "guidelines"[30] which would make caps on HIV reimbursement all but impossible for an employer to defend. When various companies enacted caps concerning HIV reimbursement, the EEOC issued determination letters claiming that such caps were in violation of the ADA.

According to the EPA-guidelines,[31] if there is a disability based distinction, then the burden of proof shifts to the employer to show that the distinction is not a subterfuge to evade the ADA. The employer may rebut this subterfuge allegation by showing disparate treatment is either based on sound actuarial data, accepted standards for fiscal soundness (underwriting risks), or to prevent a drastic reduction in coverage for other employees.

The ADA does not protect gay employees, but does protect an employee fired for reasons of HIV. In *Doe v. Cooper Investments,*[32] a terminated employee alleged he was fired two weeks after he disclosed that he was HIV seropositive. The judge ordered the employer either to obtain continuing insurance for the employee or to absorb his medical expenses. In Arizona, a gay HIV seropositive employee was fired shortly after filing an insurance claim for HIV illness. The company alleged it was the employee's poor work performance, and the judge informed the jury that if the dismissal was based "solely" on the plaintiff's sexual orientation, it should find for the defendant.[33]

4. Caps

There have been various attempts by companies to set caps on AIDS-related illnesses, but they generally have been withdrawn after objection by the EEOC. The following examples are typical: In *Mason Tenders District Council Welfare Fund v. Donaghey,*[34] a self-insured labour management health trust fund (the construction union fund) in 1991 had cut off medical benefits for Donaghey and three other HIV seropositive workers. When the EEOC concluded that *Mason Tenders* had violated the ADA, the fund then sought a declaratory judgment claiming that the fund was only covered by ERISA and not the ADA because it did not employ Donaghey and the other claimants.[35]

The fund was most adamant about not conceding or settling until a federal judge denied the fund's motion for summary judgment and also insisted that at a subsequent trial the fund would have to show an actuarial basis for HIV cap.[36] In September 1994, the US Attorney filed a RICO (racketeering) complaint, claiming that organized crime controlled the fund and had skimmed "benefit funds", including that which excluded HIV coverage. It was difficult for the fund to argue lack of money for HIV coverage while simultaneously defending charges that organized crime had pilfered its funds.

In *Estate of Kadinger v. IBEW, Local 110,*[37] a consent decree was entered between the EEOC and the plaintiff with the union and its benefit reimbursement plan. In 1987, the plan imposed a $50,000 lifetime cap for HIV costs while maintaining a $500,000 cap for other illnesses. Kadinger was diagnosed HIV seropositive after the implementation of the cap, but before the ADA became effective. In the consent decree, the fund agreed to remove the cap retroactive to 26 July, 1992 and pay $100,000 to Kadinger's estate, which would reimburse Kadinger's hospital costs and pay $2,500 to the Minnesota AIDS project.

In other settlements, the EEOC[38] reached an agreement with Connecticut Refining Company to eliminate a $10,000 cap for HIV while retaining a $1 million cap for other illnesses. In February 1992, the company instituted this cap retroactive to November 1991 when Collimore, the plaintiff, was diagnosed with HIV, but left intact the $1 million cap for other illnesses. In February 1993, the EEOC concluded that the defendant had violated the ADA. In March 1994, the parties signed a conciliation agreement whereby the defendant eliminated the $10,000 cap retroactive to 26 July, 1992, and agreed to pay $35,000 to Collimore for pain and suffering.

It is essential to emphasize that the settlements were made with no admission of liability and often only in order to avoid protracted litigation. In *Anderson v. Gus Mayer Boston Store of Delaware,* the plaintiff alleged that the employer changed its group health insurance carrier because of the plaintiff's HIV seropositive condition and that it knew the new carrier would reject the plaintiff; and therefore, this would result in lower premiums. The EEOC determined that the defendant had violated the ADA and made what defendants considered to be "a gun to the head 'offer of conciliation' requiring the defendant to pay $100,000."[39]

5. Jurisdiction

It appears that self-funded plans are jurisdictionally subject to the ADA. In Carparts Distri. Ctr. v. Automotive Wholesaler's,[40] the Court concluded that the ADA did cover a self-funded medical reimbursement plan. The plaintiff, who also was the sole shareholder of Carparts Inc., had enrolled in 1987 in the plan of Automotive Wholesale Association of New England, Inc., which sponsored a self-funded health benefit plan. The plaintiff was diagnosed HIV seropositive in 1986, but a lifetime cap of $25,000 for HIV was established effective from 1991, which left $1 million for other illnesses. The District Court concluded that the defendant was neither an employer nor a public accommodation within the meaning of the ADA. The Court reversed by concluding that the plan had the authority to determine the level of benefits and this was an "employer" subject to Title I of the ADA, and that the plaintiff might have a possibility of showing that the defendant is a public accommodation, and, therefore, subject to Title III of the ADA.

6. If No Insurance Workplace Coverage

While two-thirds of US employees are covered by an employment insurance plan, the remainder must either obtain a private plan or do without one. In 1991, it was estimated that 29 per cent of those with HIV had private health insurance. Forty per cent were covered by Medicaid, 2 per cent by Medicare, and 29 per cent had no health insurance.[41]

Private medical plans regulated entirely by states predictably will exclude pre-existing conditions, but often courts will interpret state statutes liberally in favour of the insured. In *Gonzales v. Associates Life Ins. Co.,*[42] the Court of Appeals overturned the summary judgment in favour of the defendant. The plaintiff, who sought reimbursement from the medical policy for HIV, was denied coverage because of the AIDS/ARC conditions limitation. The appellate court concluded that the AIDS exclusion clause was not disclosed in a conspicuous manner as required by Florida statute. While the AIDS exclusion was clearly legible and not buried in fine print, it was unenforceable.

Approximately 27 states have established risk pools which require insurers to share in underwriting policies for persons otherwise uninsurable. Generally, the state will form an association of all health insurance companies doing business within that state. One company would then be selected to administer the plan pursuant to guidelines on premiums, deductibles, and other matters. The plan would often provide for prescription costs and skilled nursing care.[43] The premiums, however, are generally 125 to 200 per cent higher than non-risk policies and exclude pre-existing conditions.[44] Very few states have established subsidies for indigent persons.

Should an HIV seropositive person lose his job, he would have a right to convert his health plan to private coverage pursuant to the Consolidated Omnibus Budget Reconciliation Act (COBRA).[45] COBRA, which is an amendment to ERISA, mandates that employers of at least 20 employees allow terminated employees, except for gross misconduct, to pay privately for group insurance plans up to 18 months.[46] This is especially significant for an HIV seropositive employee because COBRA, unlike a new insurance policy, may not exclude pre existing conditions.

While COBRA limits premiums to 102 per cent of the cost of insurance, the payment may be very difficult for a PWA. The Ryan White Care Act (The Comprehensive AIDS Resources Emergency Act) allows states to use federal funds to help PWA continue private health insurance coverage.[47] COBRA also may not protect a former employee from a cap on health benefits. In *Gonzales v. Garner Fast Foods Inc.*,[48] plaintiff was terminated once the employer discovered his HIV seropositive status when he submitted a medical claim through the company's self-funded health programme. Although the plaintiff exercised his COBRA rights, the company, six months later (October 1991), enacted an HIV cap of $40,000, down from $1 million lifetime. The judge granted the defendant's motion to dismiss because the cap was enacted before July 26, 1992, the effective date of the ADA.

Should an HIV seropositive worker lose his job and benefits, he will be forced to seek financial help, but only at the point of bankruptcy will he be eligible for Medicaid.[49] As explained by Congressman Waxman, Medicaid is often the last resort:

> "AIDS has shown that Medicaid is shallow and inadequate. Many middle-class Americans are learning the hard way that, in most states, you can qualify only if you are totally disabled and have less that $1,500 to your name.
>
> AIDS has shown that we can produce medical miracles for the rich and plain neglect for the poor. AIDS drugs and treatments are priced for kings, while Medicaid is only for people who have been made paupers."[50]

Even Medicaid coverage will not eliminate the problem of a PWA. In one documented instance, an HIV seropositive, young male without health insurance needed relief from collection efforts by a hospital for unpaid medical bills. His employment insurance was soon due to end, Medicaid did not fully cover his prescription costs, and he was barely able to pay his rent. The AIDS Law Project referred him to the local Consumer Bankruptcy Assistance Project.[51]

7. Health Insurance Outside the United States

In most other countries, obtaining medical insurance is not as crucial to an HIV seropositive person because it is often obtained either at work or through a national health service. Within Australia, "Medicare" pays for HIV medical treatment.[52] Health insurance is not an issue relevant to HIV in Britain "because of the free availability of medical treatment of high quality under the National Health Service (NHS)."[53] British law, however, has not been an impediment to those employers who utilize pre-employment HIV testing, and a HIV seropositive employee may not have protection against termination within the first two years of employment.[54]

Throughout Europe, the asymptomatic HIV seropositive employee has no duty to disclose and, generally, "when questioned has the right to remain silent or to lie." Sweden is an exception since the employer has both the right to test and ta refuse employment to those with HIV. The harshness of this policy is mitigated somewhat by the Swedish Social Security Scheme which will cover those HIV seropositive persons who are prevented from working. Should a worker become unable to work through HIV or any other illness, Belgian law would pay a guaranteed wage. In France, the person will be entitled to receive social security. In Germany employers will provide payment followed by public health insurance.[55]

Switzerland[56] has no national health service. Medical care is paid through private insurance plans which generally require the insured to pay 10 per cent of all medical costs. "In the case of HIV and AIDS, this can amount to extremely high sums of money. For people without health insurance, the situation is obviously graver still." There is also discrimination, not only in insurance, but also in many pension funds which mandate that applicants not test HIV seropositive. Without joining a pension scheme, "it is practically impossible to get a job."[57] Life insurance requires a HIV negative result, which is especially important in Switzerland since loans to professionals to set up a business practice "are often given only in conjunction with an insurance policy in favour of the lender in the amount of the loan."[58]

In many European countries, health insurance is organized by an employer for employees and should an HIV seropositive person not be covered, then an employer might not want to employ an uncovered worker. French law prohibits HIV exclusion and Belgian practice is to not exclude HIV-persons from group insurance.[59] Within South Africa, insurers have expressed concern that in "several instances" an employer will offer work to an HIV seropositive person in order to have the person "benefit from the company's group life and/or benefit scheme." This is because the group plan would not "require evidence of HIV status" and also allows conversion to life insurance when the HIV seropositive worker leaves employment.[60] Within the United States, testing is rarely used in group health policies.[61] In Uganda, insurers will not insure HIV "in the same way as if the illness were alcohol or drug related." Employees in Uganda are more concerned with the employer-paid group insurance policy that provides a death payment for HIV or some other illness.[62]

Canada has a National Health Service which provides free medical care.[63] Discrimination against HIV seropositive persons is prohibited. As early as 1987, an employer in a collective bargaining agreement could not order an employee "to remain off work even where the employer is prepared to maintain full pay and benefits" since such action could be "demeaning and corrosive to morale."[64] Generally, HIV discrimination law is provincial and the matter is heard by a provincial administrative body such as a Board of Inquiry. There has been litigation when an employee was denied long-term disability benefits pursuant to the following clause: "If an employee has incurred medical expenses, or received care or treatment by a Physician during the 90-day period prior to the date his insurance becomes effective, no Income Benefit shall be payable for any disability resulting from the same or related cause until" the employee was not treated by a physician for 90 days or had been insured for 12 months. The Board of Inquiry[65] concluded that the above exclusionary clause did not offend the Ontario Human Rights Code partly because it was standard insurance practice for employers with less than 100 employees. The Code[66] allowed distinctions that are reasonable and bona fide which would otherwise substantially increase an insurer's risk. But the court stressed the need to inform better all employees as to benefits and "to institute a review of all its contracts to make sure that the spirit of human rights legislation is observed, and especially it is requested to review its P(re) E(xisting) C(onditions) clauses. It will file a report of its review with the Superintendent of Insurance within eighteen months. The OHRC in turn is asked to monitor the effectuation of this order."

Public health insurance will range from coverage of all workers in France, to two different public funds in The Netherlands, to complicated German procedures. Unlike the United States, worker's compensation or invalidity insurance schemes have nowhere "excluded HIV/AIDS sufferers." When there is hardship, it is "more as a result of administrative delays in receiving benefits than as a result of substantive limitations on the nature or extent of those benefits."[67]

B. LIFE INSURANCE

1. U.S.

Unlike medical insurance and HIV, which is a serious concern only in a few countries besides the US, gays and certain other groups everywhere have concerns over obtaining life insurance. Throughout much of the world, the issues are—(i) at what amount and under what conditions should mandatory HIV testing be required of applicants; and (ii) what questions may be asked of applicants which would protect the interest of the insurers, but not be unduly intrusive into an applicant's privacy. There is some concern that inexpensive saliva tests might also be used by insurance companies, especially in developing countries.[68]

Insurers must develop categories for risk of loss and one of the basic categories is health and often, unfortunately, lifestyles.[69] Tied to lifestyles, some insurance companies also utilize factors such as an applicant's residence or occupation. Understandably, insurance companies are reluctant to underwrite huge policies for HIV seropositive applicants and are unwilling to cover persons with full blown AIDS. In order to test for HIV, companies have utilized blood tests which have been approved in all 50 states and the District of Columbia.[70] It would be financially prohibitive, however, for insurers to require testing for every application, and therefore, many insurers require testing only for a policy of over $100,000.[71] States occasionally have stringent requirements about informed consent, confidentiality, mandatory counselling, and disclosure of HIV tests.

AIDS exclusion clauses in life insurance policies are very rare. Life insurance policies are also unique in that state law generally limits the time for an insurer to contest a misrepresentation upto two years. Understandably, insurers, when faced with an expensive payment, "have a strong financial incentive to allege misrepresentation" or failure to disclose the material facts.[72] "Thus, in the case of a life insurance contract, the maxim 'fraud vitiates a contract' must be changed to 'fraud vitiates a contract, except for a life insurance contract which was issued more than two years ago.'"[73]

Since an insurance agreement is basically an adhesion contract and because insurance companies are held to a good faith standard, courts will "resolve any uncertainty in favour of the insured."[74] The following HIV issues in insurance contracts are illustrative of litigation results. In *Northern Life Insurance Co. v. Ippolito Real Estate Partnership,*[75] a person with haemophilia took out six life insurance policies for business purposes. After Ippolito died of HIV, Northern Life sought, through a declaratory judgment, to rescind the policies because the deceased had omitted material information on the amendment to the application. The deceased, after signing the first five policies, but prior to approval by the company, had experienced weight loss and sinusitis and did not disclose that he had twice seen a physician. The appellate court approved the trial court's decision for the deceased and concluded that as a matter of law there had been no material misrepresentation. The insurance company was granted summary judgment on the sixth policy because Ippolito had verified he had not "suffered any ... sickness or consulted or (had) been attended by a physician," when he earlier had been diagnosed with an HIV related illnesses. Thus, the court believed Ippolito intended to deceive and his answers "contained misrepresentations material to Northern Life's risks." In *New England Mutual Life Insurance Company v. Iohnson* (executor),[76] an insurance company attempted to rescind a $50,000 policy because the insured misrepresented his relationship with his beneficiary lover, by only disclosing him as a business partner. The judge criticized the company for having "searched through its files in an attempt to determine a way to escape its obligations" and concluded its actions were on a "bogus basis." The court further assessed the company with over $127,000 in attorney fees because if the deceased person's "illness was not one associated with homosexuality, no attempt to rescind the policy would have been made."

There is no obligation, generally, on the part of the insured to disclose his or her HIV status unless required surer. In *Waxse v. Reserve Life Ins. Co.*[77] the company was unsuccessful in attempting to rescind the health policy because the insurer failed to disclose his HIV seropositive status. An opposite result was reached in *Sapp v. Paul Revere Life Insurance Co.,*[78] Occasionally, an insurance company will litigate rather than pay a $10,000 policy. In *Hebert v. Magnolia Life Ins. Co.,*[79] an HIV seropositive applicant, diagnosed with HIV m 1990, purchased a $10,000 policy in 1991 and died in 1993. He answered "no" on an application question whether he had any medical examination in the last five years or whether he had any consultation/treatment which had been completed. The court concluded that the applicant had made statements which were intended to deceive and which materially affected the insurer's risks. Both factors were necessary under Louisiana law for an insurer to escape liability.

2. British Isles

Other countries, of course, also refuse to grant policies to HIV applicants and require blood tests if the policy is large and ask questions concerning HIV for smaller policies. In Britain,[80] there was concern that individuals might be denied life insurance because they have had an HIV test or belonged to high-risk groups Furthermore, it was "standard procedure" to test for HIV unmarried males who need life insurance in order to obtain large mortgages. Unlike in the United States, mortgages in Great Britain often mandate life insurance.[82]

In February 1987, a representative from an AIDS advocacy group informed the House of Commons Social Services Committee that individuals were denied life "insurance if they want to take out a joint mortgage with another man." Life insurance was also necessary for a self-employed person as security for an overdraft in business.[83]

While there was no set amount of insurance that triggered a mandatory test, Midland Bank required tests for a male desiring £150,000 or a female desiring £250,000 policies, as well as all intravenous drug users and gays.[84] Other firms generally tested for all policies over £40,000 for single males and £150,000 for everyone else.[85] The general reaction of the insurance companies to HIV was to increase premiums up to 150 per cent for single males.[86]

During the early 1990s there were occasional attempts in Parliament to get the government to obtain assurances from life insurance companies to eliminate offensive/irrelevant questions on applications. One MP asked whether life insurance companies "will no longer ask questions of (applicants) that have the effect of putting people off taking the HIV test."[87] The government responded that it was meeting with insurance representatives on this issue and conducting a study The result of this study by the Association of British Insurers and the Department of Health had concluded that possibly tens of thousands had put off taking an HIV test because of these questions. A government representative found this result to be "worrying. "[88]

By 1994, the Association of British Insurers (ABI) concluded that because HIV claims since 1987 (c. £50 million) were much lower than expected,[89] it recommended that the question "Have you ever had an AIDS blood test?" be replaced with "Have you ever tested positive for HIV/AIDS or Hepatitis B or C or have you been tested/treated for other sexually transmitted diseases or are you awaiting the result of such a test?"[90] It is still uncertain as to whether the test question issue is resolved. By the end of 1994, only one-third of the 105 insurance companies had changed the application wording.[91] Appllcants who are seronegative gay males still might have to pay higher premiums or accept an AIDS exclusion clause "in the early years of the policy."[92]

Within the Republic of Ireland, insurance companies have "no immediate plans" to follow the British example. The Irish Insurance Federation spokesperson said, however, that if the applicant had a negative HIV test, additional information would be sought only if the requested policy were "say over £I 100,000".[93]

3. Africa

In Egypt,[94] there is no need for HIV testing, although applicants must pass a certain number of medical examinations. An HIV seropositive person who does not disclose his or her condition will make the insurance contract a nullity. Sub-Saharan Africa has approximately 2 per cent of the world's population, but 60 per cent of the world's HIV seropositive persons.[95] Predictably, sub-Saharan Africans have difficulty in obtaining life insurance without testing.

In Zimbabwe, the government rejected requests of insurance companies to test applicants for all policies over Z$50,000 (US$6,250) instead of the present limit of Z$100,000 (US$12,500).[96] The Minister of Health of Zimbabwe declined to endorse the testing measure "since he is a strong supporter of the Geneva Convention banning (HIV) discrimination." The argument of the insurance company is that HIV accounts for 60 to 70 per cent of death claims during the first five years of the policy, and that one million of a ten and one-half million population is HIV seropositive.[97] In 1993, 42 per cent (1,428) of all claims were HIV related, but between January and June 1994, only 111 of 2,888 tested applicants were HIV positive.[98] Presently, applicants, in order to avoid being tested, obtain endowment policies "which provide insurance coverage for up to 25 years of a person's life."[99] It has been suggested that restrictions on HIV testing might "put an end to life assurance as a welfare option" in Zimbabwe as it did in Malawi."[100]

In South Africa, testing for HIV was set by the Life Office Association at R200,000.[101] As HIV increased, insurers utilized AIDS exclusion clauses for those applicants unwilling to be tested. One South African company, Southern Life, has initiated a policy called "Exclusive Life Insurance," which requires all policy holders to be tested every five years. If the insured is HIV seropositive, the policy amount is reduced to 10 per cent unless the HIV "can be proved to be blood transfusion, rape, health procedures or other 'non-blameworthy' factors."[102] At the workplace, insurance companies, at the employer's request, engage in pre-employment testing for HIV since "job applicants are still not covered by any of the legislation enforcing fair employment practices."[103] Medical plans including "employer operated schemes" have arbitrarily limited HIV claims. "Pension funds and provident funds have been curtailed to exclude" HIV.[104]

Within South Africa, HIV has increased 10 times since 1990 to nearly 8 per cent of the black population. The mine workers, virtually all black, have been especially hard hit by HIV. Consequently, the life insurance underwriter for the 350,000 National Union of Mine Workers wants to raise premiums by over one-third or reduce benefits for HIV.[105] In Swaziland, the Swaziland Royal Insurance Corporation, as of 1 July, 1995, would mandate HIV screening for all life insurance policies over Rand 25,000. "Applicants have to prove they do not have the virus in order to qualify for a life policy on normal terms."[106] In Uganda, HIV testing is utilized "for sums insured as low as $4,000."[107]

4. Asia

According to the WHO, over one million Asians are HIV seropositive,[108] with insurance issues being most controversial in Japan, Thailand, Singapore and Australia/New Zealand. Life insurers in Japan,[109] are contemplating mandatory HIV tests for large life insurance policies. A physician group serving as advisors to life insurance companies had earlier concluded that life insurance applicants should be tested for HIV.[110] This increase is also necessary because the industry is experiencing lower yields and also because policy-holders might be unwilling to pay increased premiums for higher HIV coverage. One major reservation to mandatory tests is the fear of "how well applicant's privacy could be protected,[111] no matter how strictly they guard test results," and whether HIV human rights might be violated by rejection. Should firms introduce questionnaires concerning HIV, which is regarded as more controversial than testing, they would only have two years to set aside applications for false statements.

In Thailand, instead of stressing more testing, the National AIDS Prevention and Control Administrative Committee has proposed to the Prime Minister that a regulation prohibit compulsory

HIV testing by insurance companies.[112] In addition to the usual arguments, viz., inadequate counselling, failure to keep results confidential, the Committee stressed that many HIV seropositive persons "do not suffer from any serious infections, if they receive the right medical treatment." The Committee instead urged that HIV seropositive persons be allowed to obtain insurance at a higher premium.[113]

Presently,[114] insurers can refuse payment within one year of a policy in a group scheme if an insured intentionally failed to disclose his or her HIV status. Applicants in high-risk provinces must take HIV blood and saliva tests for any policy, and the remainder of the country must take a test for a policy over B750,000. Thai insurers have argued unsuccessfully that no benefits be paid to an HIV seropositive person if he or she develops HIV within five years, or alternatively, have unsuccessfully attempted to develop a sliding timescale for payments.

In Singapore,[115] certain occupations have been listed as "highrisk" groups which require mandatory tests for insurance. A Prudential Assurance spokesperson specifically listed "male hairstylists, fashion designers and dancers [as tending] to be effeminate. 'We want to make sure they are not homosexuals."' While Prudential indicated it might insure some groups if they tested seronegative, other insurers said they would not accept any risk group members as policy-holders. While testing is usually required only for policies of S$500,000 and above, it is mandatory for risk groups. Any misstatement concerning a lifestyle would result in the contract being invalidated. Insurers have considered genetic testing impracticable.[116]

5. Australia and New Zealand

Australian insurance law is federal,[117] and state anti-discrimination agencies are precluded from dealing with insurance complaints. The Insurance Code of Practice now prohibits an insurance company from basing its decision solely on an applicant's lifestyle. Nor may any prior negative tests be utilized, which should eliminate the fear of individuals voluntarily taking HIV tests.[118] National Mutual,[119] one of Australia's largest insurers, has also agreed to drop a clause that excluded HIV seropositive persons from receiving payments in group life insurance. Previously, a person would be excluded from receiving moneys if HIV were contracted within two years of the policy date.

This action by National Mutual was based on an independent

study that the HIV spread in Australia "had not been as wide as insurers expected."[120] The Trowbridge Report, an independent study commissioned by the federal government concluded that "there was no statistical evidence to support exclusion clauses (by life insurance companies and superannuation funds) purely on the basis that applicants had the AIDS virus."[121]

It is still uncertain whether the Disability Act and Trowbridge Report would alleviate fears by gay spokemen that it is "almost impossible" for gays to purchase life insurance.[122] Australia does have, since 1988, a Code of Practice on Underwriting in Relation to AIDS, whose guidelines state that no decision will be based on sexual orientation or on a negative HIV result. In reality, "there is growing concern that there is a-slightly less than zealous adherence to the guidelines and principles."[123]

In New Zealand, life insurance claims for HIV did not suggest thathHIV applicants were deliberately purchasing life insurance. In 1989, the industry adopted a voluntary code for HIV guidelines concerning testing and counselling which asked specific questions about sexual practices rather than lifestyle. The head of New Zealand's insurance industry stated "AIDS and HIV exclusions may also be used, especially in group life insurance, disability insurance, mortgage repayment insurance, and direct marketed policies, while non-guaranteed premium rates may become more common."[124] The New Zealand Human Rights Act of 1993 permits discrimination insurance for HIV or gay status only if the discrimination is based on actuarial data, or if that is unavailable, the discrimination is based on either reputable actuarial opinion or medical data.[125]

6. Europe

In the Netherlands, insurers as of 1993, pursuant to a Code of Conduct with the government, may not ask life insurance applicants whether they have had HIV tests, but only whether they have had an HIV seropositive result from such a test. Tests for life insurance may be given only for a policy over $f.200,000. If the policy is under that, the applicants are asked "Have you got AIDS?" and "Have HIV antibodies been found in your blood (are you seropositive)?"[126] Legislation would have been enacted had not the above agreement been reached. In Belgium, any policy over BF5 million requires an HIV test.[127]

In Denmark, the National Insurers Association consulted gay groups before issuing guidelines. Testing for HIV is required for policies over DKK 2M; for policies over DKK 1M, a certificate of health is required from the family physician. For cheaper policies, an applicant is asked about test information.[128] Seronegativity is also required for an annual disability annuity of DKK 200,000. In Norway,[129] all life insurance applicants "must confirm that they have not undergone a blood test which shows that they are HIV seropositive." Germany has not had mandatory testing, but insurers are beginning to ask applicants to disclose HIV test results.[130] Applicants seeking a DM250,000 policy must undergo a medical examination. The company may require an HIV test.[131]

France[132] regulates its insurance industry and the issue of HIV pursuant to an agreement between the Minister of Economics, the Minister of Health, and the insurance industry. The insurer may test for seropositivity. If the applicant consents prior to the examination, the test is part of a full medical examination by a physician and the HIV results are given to a physician. The agreement also contains provisions for counselling and confidentiality. The Code of Conduct prohibits "questions concerning the intimate nature of private life, and, in particular, the sex life of the person applying for cover."

Testing is generally required only for policies over FF1 million. Yet, testing itself is not seen as controversial because "one in four men and women had taken the test". This ratio rises to just over one in two of all people between 25 to 34 [133] A more serious problem is the requirement of a life insurance contract to insure real property loans. Until 1991, PWA were effectively excluded from such insurance. Pursuant to a 1991 agreement, HIV seropositive persons may receive loans up to FF1 million for up to 10 years at a 4 to 6 per cent price increase. [134]

In Sweden,[135] life insurance companies may test and do test gays or those who have multiple partners. All applicants must inform a physician about their entire sexual history. Should an applicant provide false information and subsequently die from AIDS, the beneficiaries would receive nothing. In Italy, applicants for policies over LIT 300 million are required to take an HIV test. An applicant for a lesser amount may be required to be tested if from the application "it appears to be necessary to obtain more information as to the risk."[136]

7. Canada

Within Canada, the Canadian Life and Health Insurance Association utilized guidelines in 1987 that prohibited even indirect questions concerning the applicants "sexual orientation" or on past seronegative test results.[137] The Canadian Life and Health Insurance

Association Incorporation[138] (the Canadian trade association for about 100 companies) has decided that applicants would be tested only for policies over C$100,000. Testing for smaller policies would occur only if there was a history of promiscuity, e.g., sexually transmitted diseases.

C. OTHER MATTERS

1. Policies Against Contracting HIV

Insurance companies throughout the world have developed policies in case the insured contracts HIV. In Canada,[139] an applicant can pay C$4 and receive a $100,000 policy if the applicant becomes HIV seropositive during a trip. The insured must take two tests—one, 14 days after returning, which should be seronegative; and the other, 180 to 210 days after returning, which should be seropositive.

In Italy,[140] an insurance policy has been offered that will cover the applicant if he accidentally contracts HIV. The policy will be available to health care professionals, police personnel, and members of volunteer groups and later will be extended to dentists. In South Africa, SANA (the South African Nurses Association) has encouraged short-term insurance policies for nurses who may contract HIV through work. Applicants would not have to take a blood test or a medical examination and need only sign a "declaration of health."[141]

In Great Britain, a "critical insurance policy, pays a lump sum for cancer, heart attacks, and strokes, but generally excludes HIV. Some companies will cover HIV if it is contracted through blood transfusion or from medical occupation".[142] Australian insurers have provided coverage for police, medical providers and others who contract HIV through employment. The insured would receive $200,000 or twice one's annual salary, whichever is lower.[143]

Within the United States, various insurers will provide HIV insurance to health care workers who contract HIV in the course of employment. One insurer will provide, through its HIV carrier protection plan, up to $250,000. The insured must take a test and report any workplace incident within 24 hours and then take a blood test within five days.[144] A labour contract provision has provided special disability insurance of $100,000 to a nurse who acquires HIV through employment.[145] The American Medical Association also offers a nationwide plan of a lump sum insurance amount of up to $500,000 to a physician who contracts HIV.[146]

2. Death Futures

Some entities have offered to purchase life insurance policies of PWA through a Life Insurance Buyout The purchaser becomes the irrevocable beneficiary, and the PWA gets remuneration that can be used for medicine, vacations or any other purpose. The purchaser will also continue to pay premiums until the death of the insured. The amount often depends upon how much time the HIV seropositive person has left.[147] The buyout can range from 30 per cent to 80 per cent. There are concerns whether the proceeds are taxable by the IRS or whether the payment would result in a loss of Supplemental Security Insurance/Medicaid benefits.[148]

Two 26-year-old Americans have auctioned their policies in London. The first policy, paying $75,498 is expected to sell for $60,000, and the insured has a life expectancy between 1.5 to 2 years. The second policy worth $100,000 should sell for $90,000 since the insured has only 13 months to live.[149] The purchaser must insure that the policy is unencumbered (i.e., not committed to mortgage repayment), that the insurance company has a proven history of stability, and that the insured is neither under any duress nor suffering from lack of capacity.[150]

A new business has formed to deal with these "death futures." Life Partners, Inc., for example, "is one of the biggest of about 30 companies that invest in policies on their own or match buyers and sellers for fees or (3 to 5 per cent) commissions."[151] In February 1995, Dignity Partners, Inc., which had purchased policies from HIV seropositive persons, "closed a $35 million deal" with Ironwood Capital Partners, Ltd.[152]

For historical reasons, the British industry is "far less regulated than it is in the United States."[153] Within Great Britain, one might attempt to "surrender" a life insurance policy and one's success in obtaining moneys paid will increase if the policy has been in effect for over five years. An HIV seropositive person might obtain more money should he or she auction it or sell it to a company specializing in purchasing a policy from !'people with life threatening conditions."[154] An HIV seropositive person might be able to get the trustees of an occupational pension plan to pay immediately a lump sum on the condition that he or she has less than 12 months to live.[155] Parliamentary attempts to eliminate the requirement of "obtaining a medical certificate stating he will unquestionably die within 12 months" have been unsuccessful.[156]

3. Insurance of Coverage of Tort Actions of HIV

Insurance may cover an HIV seropositive person's negligent actions, but not those that are intentional. For example, in *Christian v. Estate of Rock Hudson,*[157] the jury concluded that Hudson's lover should be awarded $21.75 million because Hudson had not informed him of his HIV seropositive status while continuing intimacy. The amount was reduced by the trial judge to $5.5 million.[158]

One month after the jury award, Hudson's homeowners' insurance company filed a request for a declaration that it had no obligation to indemnify or defend Hudson's estate because the policy was inapplicable to damage "which is expected or intended by the insured." The 9th Circuit, interpreting what the California Court would do, concluded that for Hudson to engage in unprotected sex for eight months after realizing he was HIV seropositive was an inherently harmful act which was exacerbated "by the seriousness and deadliness of AIDS." Since Hudson had intentionally misrepresented that he did not have HIV, the insurance company had no obligation to his estate under a homeowners' insurance policy.[159] In Germany, an insurance policy will generally pay out if the insured is responsible for infecting another, as long as the insured is not grossly negligent or intentional in acting to transmit HIV. Italian insurance companies also would accept liability.[160]

4. Blood Transfusions

Blood transfusion liability and HIV is an issue that is beyond the scope of this section which is concerned only with the liability of the insurance coverage of a defendant. Nevertheless, some preliminary comments are necessary. In the United States, HIV seropositive blood transfusion recipients and persons with haemophilia have generally been unsuccessful either in litigation or in obtaining a settlement with blood product defendants or their insurance companies. There are many reasons for the plaintiffs' lack of success: unlike Canada, plaintiffs may sue neither in product liability nor implied warranty; plaintiffs' difficulty in proving negligence is exacerbated by utilization of a professional rather than an ordinary standard of care; there are also statute of limitation problems and often an inability to discover a donor's identity as well as the huge expenses of discovery. When plaintiffs do succeed at trial, the reward is often reversed on appeal or a new trial is mandated.

It seemed that a class settlement may have resolved the issue of allegations against manufacturers of blood products by HIV infected persons with haemophilia. In fact, a tentative settlement of $140—$160 millio[161] had been reached. Suddenly and unexpectedly, a federal judge granted partial class certification to the litigants.[162] The chair of the committee representing the persons with haemophilia then denounced the offer as "absurdly low."[163]

The court of appeals,[164] however, reversed the class certification partly because it doubted that there was constitutional authority for one trial under "a law that is merely an amalgam, or averaging of the nonidentical laws of 51 jurisdictions." The effect of this reversal would necessitate hundreds of separate cases and comprehensive costly discovery, subject to the laws of many jurisdictions. This is a terrible burden for attorneys operating on contingency fees and for clients who are responsible for court costs.

For insurance companies, such a settlement could have been a nightmare. Some of the defendants were "in litigation and negotiations" with insurers. One defendant, Baxter, sued in California, "seeking to force hundreds of liability insurers to defend and indemnify it against claims by (HIV) hemophiliacs." Insurers such as Zurich American insisted it "provided no coverage for this sort of claim against Baxter. Therefore, we will not contribute to the reported settlement."[165]

Insurance companies generally pay the defendant's litigation costs and often all or part of settlement or unfavourable verdicts. In the United States, however, only in rare instances they are directly involved in litigation, e.g., when a state law prohibits a charitable hospital[166] from being sued which necessitates it being substituted by the insurance company, or when the widow of an HIV seropositive person, who contracted HIV from a blood transfusion before 1982, sued her homeowner's insurance policy which would pay the balance of the mortgage in case of accidental death.[167]

It would seem that there must be a better approach than the adversarial system in blood bank litigation. One author has suggested the establishment of a strict liability "compensatory system similar to the National Vaccine Injury Compensation Programme. This would provide swift, certain compensation to HIV transfusion victims while they are still alive." Insurance companies would benefit because an occasional "multimillion dollar judgment (has) begun to trickle through their defenses."[168]

In Germany, a Parliamentary AIDS Investigating Committee concluded that about 60 per cent of Germany's over 2,300 HIV seropositive persons with haemophilia would not have become HIV seropositive between 1983 and 1987 had blood supply companies applied known screening procedures.[169] The German Red Cross, for example, utilized untested blood products through 1987 because "to acquire the required testing equipment was too expensive."[170]

Compensation or indemnification of victims has not been as difficult in Germany because of a peculiarity of industry/ insurance payments. In 1978, about 130 German insurers and reinsurers, as well as pharmaceutical companies, created a "pharma-pool" to compensate injured parties in strict or product liability claims against pharmacy companies.[171] By the end of 1994, the pool paid over DM120 million to over 1,250 HIV seropositive persons with haemophilia infected by blood products.[172] The settlements ranged from DM20,000 to DM500,000.[173] The insurance industry insisted that they did not require proof that a specific product caused HIV, "proof that most of the hemophiliacs would have had difficulty in supplying." The payment was made for loss of earnings and other material damages, but not pain and suffering since German law provides compensation only for proven negligence.[174]

The German government, created, in 1994, created a new fund (DM700 million) to compensate those HIV seropositive persons with haemophilia who have not received DM200,000 or more in settlement. Besides the federal government, the states and drug industry have indicted a willingness to contribute.[175] German insurers had refused to contribute partly because they claim to have already paid an average of DM60,000 per claimant.[176] The government has threatened the companies with legislation that would force contributions, especially since the fund is grown to DM400 million and earns DM30 million p.a. in interest.[177]

France, unlike Germany, has an insurance industry that had been quasi-public. Furthermore, the actions of the French National Transfusion Centre to release possibly HIV tainted blood for transfusion resulted in about 7,000 HIV infections, 1,200 of whom were persons with haemophilia. This has resulted in criminal prosecution, as well as serious questions of liability.

The French Insurance Companies Federation objected to a governmental proposal of compensation through a "special tax on damage insurance policies"[178] which would raise approximately FF10 to FF14 billion.[179] Eventually, a compromise was reached whereby insurance companies agreed to pay FF1.2 billion and the government agreed to replenish the fund after exhaustion. The trade body for the French insurance industry accepted the compromise "for the sake of national solidarity".[180] Victims who accepted compensation the amount of which was based according to circumstances, waived the right to further litigation.[181] The state-owned UAP and Assurances Generales de France agreed to pay, respectively, FF109 million and FF68 million. Group AXA, a major private insurer, paid FF85 million. Perhaps this compromise was induced by the fear of insurers that awards for HIV seropositive transfusion to about 400 plaintiffs averaged between FF1.5 million and 2.5 million. [182]

In some countries, litigation has been a viable alternative for HIV seropositive persons with haemophilia. In the Netherlands, an individual became HIV seropositive when injected with an unclean needle used on an AIDS patient. The insurer accepted liability and paid $86 000 as compensation and an additional $57,000 for pain and suffering. When the victim rejected the $57,000 and demanded $400,000, the Supreme Court awarded him $170,000 for pain, "the highest amount awarded in The Netherlands."[183]

In some countries is is difficult to sue a hospital for negligence concerning HIV seropositive transfusions. In Romania, the parents/ guardians of children with HIV have begun litigation against a government and medical system which "had benefitted from a quasi-immunity under a half century of communism." They are suing for $162, 000. "Equally novel is the attempt to cite individual doctors for malpractice. 'Professional responsibility is a reality when it is linked with a system of professional insurance, which does not exist yet in Romania." [184]

Within Australia[185] the vast majority of litigated cases have been lost by HIV seropositive persons with haemophilia because of the difficulty of proof. Fortunately for victims, almost all Australian states have settled claims. In one case litlgation costs totalled $15 million after an 87-day trial, with a payment of $87,000. In Victoria, federal state and insurance companies concluded a group settlement with 112 HIV seroposltive persons whe medically acquired HIV.

Great Britain and Canada have essentially settled all blood transfusion claims by creating a governmental fund. In Canada, unlike Great Britain, insurance companies have agreed to make substantial payments in the settlement with persons with haemophilia on the condition that the recipients sign a release or waiver of litigation. The insurance payments will benefit primarily spouses and children of HIV seropositive persons with haemophilia and blood transfusion recipients. Perhaps one major reason[186] for the settlement is that the judiciary has twice ruled against class action litigation by Canadians infected with HIV through transfusion or plasma.[187]

CONCLUSION

Insurance companies are, of course, in business to make a profit. All countries, however, impose a specially high standard by insurers. For insurers to simply refuse to insure people with different lifestyles is not only unfair, but irrational. Concerning individuals with HIV, governmental subsidy of insurance for PWA would be ideal because many people who are asymptomatic have many long years ahead of them. In most countries, such a suggestion would be considered unrealistic. Certainly for society to do nothing means that HIV seropositive individuals are forced to rely totally on charity or on programmes such as Medicaid in the United States. By not offering HIV seropositive persons early medical care, society will pay much more through programmes such as Medicaid.

REFERENCES

1. Ruth E. Kim & Kimball R. McMullin. AIDS and the insurance industry: an evolving resolution of conflicting interests and rights. 7 St. Louis u. Pub. L. Rev. 155, 155 (1988).
2. Sapp v. Paul Revere Life Ins. Co., 1994 U.S. App. LEXIS 15219 (9th cir). The court granted the insurance company summary judgment when an HIV seropositive person had not disclosed his pre-existing HIV seropositive status even though he had not been asked about HIV on the life insurance application.
3. The McCarran—Ferguson Regulation Act, 15 U.S.C. 1011-1015, et.seq. (1988).
4. Jonathan Gruber and Brigitte Madrian. Health insurance and job mobility: the effects of public policy on job outlook. *Indus. S. Lab. Rel. Rev.*, 1994; WL 2812315:4. Employee-sponsored health plans insure 65 per cent of all Americans under the age of 65. Comparahve Labour Law 1993; 14 (spring): 339. Sen. Jim Jeffords (R. VT) states that 92 per cent of persons covered by private health insurance are part of a group. *Speech at National Health Council.* 8 August. 1995.
5. *Technical Report. National Commission on AIDS,* at 17 (August 1991).
6. Fred. J. Hellinger. The lifetime cost of treating a person with HIV, *JAMA* 1993; 270:474. Group health insurance claims for HIV were estimated at $446 million for 1994, $483.9 million for 1993, and $525.2 million for 1992. Steven Brostoff, "AIDS Related Group Health Claims Drop for 2nd Year," *National Underwriter Life* and *Health Financial Services Edition,* 1995 August 14:3 (1).
7. Testing for HIV in group policies is rare. Some states prohibit testing in group health plans by statue; *see* Mark Scherzer. *Private insurance.* In:Scott Burris *et al.*, eds., *AIDS Law today: A new guide for the public.* 2d ed. 1993:419. Workers might also have the option of selecting Blue Cross or HMO plans. These topics are outside the scope of this chapter. New Jersey is presently considering allowing insurers to test for group health and life insurance, which insurers have already been doing covertly. Eugene Kiely, *Officials Ignoring AIDS Test Criticism, The Record,* 1995 October 5:A3.
8. Harold Jaffe. The medical facts about AIDS. In: *AIDS and the Courts* 8, (Clark C. Abt & Kathleen M. Hardy eds., 1990); *Business Insurance* 22 February 1993.

9. Michael Bradford. *Cap on AIDS claims dropped: firm revises benefit policy. Business Insurance 1990* February 19:2.
10. Between 1986 and 1991, self-insured medical plans increased from 46 per cent to 68 per cent. Even small firms (less than 100 employees) are utilizing self-insurance (1988, 8 per cent, 1991, 22 per cent). Edward Felsenthal. *Self-insurance of health plans benefits firms. Wall Street Journal* 1992. November 11,:B1. The plan is administered by a fiduciary which requires a high standard of care.
11. The Employee Retirement Income Security Act of 1974, 29 U.S.C. 1001-1461 (1988).
12. Elaina Goldstein. *ERISA: a key to market-based health reform. (Active Voice* 1995).
13. Neville M., Bilimoria. No relief in sight: the impact of the Americans with Disabilities Act on AIDS discrimination in employee medical plans. *Detroit College of L.Rev.* 1994 Fall: 1062. Yet, in Rucker v. Pacific FM Inc., 806 F. Supp. 1453 (N.D. Cal. 1992), the Court denied the defendant summary judgment when the defendant cancelled a medical benefit plan without informing the HIV seropositive plaintiff. The court concluded that the defendant might have intentionally concealed the termination of the plan. The court further denied that ERISA permitted the defendant 210 days after termination to notify the plaintiff.
14. In *Florence Nightingale Nursing Service v. Blue Cross and Blue Shield of America,* 832 F. Supp. 1456 at 1457 (N.D. Ala. 1993), the court opined that while "A hyperbolic wag is reputed to have said that ERISA stands for 'Everything Ridiculous Imagined Since Adam' .... this court is willing to believe that ERISA has lurking somewhere within it a redeeming feature. However, this is not the case in which to find it."
15. 1991 F. 2d 645 (lOth Cir. 1993). The decision is critized by Mark Isley, Tenth Circuit Survey: health law survey." 71 *Denver University Law Review* 1994:981, 993, 996.
16. 835 F.Supp. 947 at 949 (S.D. Tex. 1993).
17. 41 F. 3d 1476 (11 Cir. 1995), *aff'd* 832 F. Supp. 1456 (N.D. Ala, 1993), *cert. den.* 115 S.Ct. 2002 (May 22, 1995); see also *AIDS Policy* and *The Law,* March 10, 1995 at 3; Nikki M., Constantine. Insurance administrator ordered to pay court determined charges. *J. of L. Med.* and *Ethics,* 1994 Spring:89. In *Bradley v. Empire Blue Cross and Blue Shield,* 149 Misc. 2d 20 (N. Y. Sup.Ct. 1990), Blue cross was ordered to pay the claim of an HIV seropositive person for a bone marrow transplant which the insurer claimed was experimental and therefore outside policy coverage. Although, the plaintiff obtained a preliminary injunction during the eight weeks of litigation, the plaintiff developed other medical problems which precluded the above treatment; *see* Scherzer, *supra* n7 at 404.
18. *Florence Nightingale, supra* nl4 at 1465.
19. 742 F. Supp. 392 (S. D. Tex. 1990), 946 F.2d 401 (5th Cir. 1991), *cert.den.sub.nom., Greenburg v. H* and *H Music Co.,* 113 S.Ct. 482 (1992).
20. Section 510, in relevant part, provides: "It shall be unlawful any person to discharge,... or discriminate against a participant or beneficiary for exercising any right to which is entitled under the provisions of an employee benefit plan,... or for the purpose of interfering with the attainment of any right to which such participant may become entitled under the plan. .." or for the purpose of interfering with the attainment of any right to which such participant may become entitled under the plan..." 29 U.S.C. 1140 (1988).

21 *McGann*, 946 F.2d at 408. Had the company retained its group insurance plan, it might have been subject to any state anti discrimination measure. *McGann* has been criticized by experts, e.g., "the reasoning of the McGann case borders on the ludicrous," Scherzer, *supra* n7 at 425.

22. 773 F.Supp. 416 (N.D. Ga. 1991), *aff'd*, 984 F.2d 394 (11th Cir. 1993). The company also capped benefits in certain other areas, e.g., nicotine dependence $500; see also *Westhoven v. Lincoln Foodservice Products*, 616 N.E. 2d 778 (Ind. App. 1993), where an appellate state court concluded that because of ERISA pre emption, a state administrative agency erred in holding that state fair employment law prohibited AIDS benefit caps. At that the, approximately 20 states would have prohibited such insurer discrimination against PWA; *see* Scherzer, *supra* n7: 425, 432.

23. *Owens*, 984 F.2d at 400. For an excellent criticism of the reasoning in both *McGann* and *Owens, see* Samuel A. Marcosson. Who is 'us' and who is 'them'—common threads and the discriminatory cut-off of health care benefits for AIDS under ERISA and the Americans with Disabilities Act. *American University of Law Review;* 1990, 44(2): 361-432.

24. 42 U.S.C. 12101-12213 (Supp. 1995).

25. According to the EEOC, the ADA's expansion covers approximately 86 per cent of the United States workers. Daniel J. Murphy. *Sorting out ADA's enforcement. Investor's Business Daily* 1994 August 18:1.

26. *Newman v. GHS Osteopathic, Inc.*, 1995 U.S. App. LEXIS 17186 (3rd Cir.)

27. There is some authority that suggests in dicta that asymptomatic HIV seropositive is not protected. In *Ennis v. National Assoc. of Bus. and Educ. Radio Inc.*, 53 F.3d 55 (4th Cir. 1995), the Court of Appeals upheld the summary judgement against the plaintiff who alleged that she was discharged because her employer did not want to cover her HIV-seropositive son which would have a "possibly catastrophic impact ... on defendant insurance rates." The Court concluded that the plaintiff did not perform her job adequately, but suggested that the asymptomatic son would not be considered disabled under the ADA. Other federal decisions have concluded that discrimination against an asymptomatic HIV seropositive person is protected by the ADA. *Doe v. Kohn Nast*, 866 F. Supp.190 (E.D.Pa. 1994). The matter was settled out-of-court. *Daily Labour Report* (BNA) 1994 D-8. November 2.

28. 42 U.S.C. 12201(c), Murphy, *supra* n25.

29. *Newman v. GHS Osteopathic, Inc.*, 1995 U.S. App.LEXIS 17186 (3rd Cir.).

30. Equal Employment Opportunity Commission. Interim Enforcement Guidance on the Application of the Americans with Disabilities Act of 1990 to Disability-Based Distinctions in Employer Provided Health Insurance (8 June 1993) (hereinafter EEOC Guidelines). These guidelines are intended to be followed until the EEOC issues final regulations after considering public comments, see example 2 at 8 which specifically invalidates an HIV cap of $5,000 in self-insured plans while all other illnesses are capped at $100,000.

31. EEOC regulations prohibit discrimination in "fringe benefits available by virtue of employment, whether or not administered by the covered entity," 29 C.F.R. 1630.4(f).

32. Following the issuance of this temporary judicial order, the parties settled the case with a payment of $50,000 to the plaintiff *(Doe.* v. *Cooper Investsments*~ WL 336658 DC Col.) (1991).

33. John Douglas. HIV disease and disparate impact under the Americans with Disabilities Act: a federal prohibition of discrimination on the basis of sexual orientation? *Berkeley lournal of Employment and Labour Law* 1995; 1691) 288.

34. *Mason Tenders v. Donaghey,* 1993 U.S. Dist. LEXIS 17032.
35. Karen Donovan. Health fund held subject to ADA in AIDS exemption. *NAT.L.J.,* December 6: 17. The matter was subsequently settled out of court. *AIDS Policy* and *the Law,* 1995 Feburary 15:9.
36. *Mason Tenders, supra* n34.
37. *Estate of Kadinger v. IBEW, Local 110,* 1993 U.S. Dist. LEXIS 18982.
38. BNA Health-Care Daily, 1994 March 11. EEOC, *Connecticute* employer *reach agreement to drop AIDS benefit ceiling from health plan.* Collimore had rejected a settlement offer which would have reinstated benefits. "I wanted to send a signal to people like me that if this is happening to them, they can fight it and they can win." Trial. 1994 June:7; similar results were reached with Allied Services Division Welfare Fund (IL), September 1993, settlement $100,000 (cap $1 million to $5,000 for HIV); Truck Drivers & Helpers Local Union No. 355 (MD), August 1994, settlement $85,000; Tarrant Distributors Inc. (IX), September 1994, settlement $20,000 to the American Foundation for AIDS Research $40,000 in medical bills ($1 million cap to $10,000 lifetime for HIV); and Labourers District Council Building and Construction Health and Welfare Fund (PA), January 1995, settlement $42,500 (cap $100,000 to $10,000 for HIV); *AIDS Policy and the* Law 1995:4. In the consent decree, the $42,500 was to be paid to the AIDS Law Project of Pennsylvania on behalf of John Doe and the other deceased plaintiff. Plaintiff. Plaintiff's medical bills of $1,209 would eb paid. The cap was approved effective 5 January 1995. Consent decree on file with author. EEOC v. Lee Data ($1 million $ 100,000; $5, 000 paid to estate of the deceased for emotional distress.
39. *AIDS Policy & the Law,* 1994:2-3, Civil No. 94 CV232, (E.D. Tex. 1994); *see* defendant's reply to plaintiff's summary Judgment Motion, June 20, 1995 at 9. This may be the first case actually litigated on HIV caps and the ADA; by July 1995 both parties had filed summary Judgment Motions. For information on the EEOC, settlements, and pending litigation regarding HIV and insurance, see *AIDS Policy and Law* 1995 Sept. 8:6-9.
40. 37F. 3d 12 (1st Cir. 1994) *vacating* 826 F. Supp. 538. The appellate court relied on EEOP interpretative guidelines.
41. National Commission on A IDS, *supra* n5; Steven Eisenstat. *Capping health insurance benefits for AIDS: an analysis of disability based distinctions under the Americans with Disabilities Act, Journal of Law and Politics* 1993; X(1):41, suggests 44 per cent of HIV patients have private insurance coverage; T. Diaz, et al., *Health* insurance coverage among persons with AIDS: results from a multistate *surveillance project* (June 1994): 1015-18, states that as a result of a survey in 11 states and cities, overall, 25 per cent of HIV seropositive persons had no insurance, 55 per cent had public insurance, and 20 per cent had private insurance.
42. 641 So. 2d 895 (Fla. App. 1994).
43. Kimberly A. Ackourey, Comment: Insuring Americans with Disabilities: How far can Congress go to protect traditional practices? *40 Emory L.J.* 1183 at 1188 (Fall 1991). In South Carolina, a federal judge has approved the exclusion of HIV from the state risk pool and said the ADA was inapplicable to a quasi-public state pool. *Post and Courier* 1995 Aug. 27:A21.
44. *See* Lawrence Bartlett, *Financing health care for persons with AIDS: balancing public and private responsibilities.* Lawrence O Gostin, ed 1990. In: AIDS and the Health Care System., 216-17. Aaron K. Trippler, *Comprehensive Health Insurance for High Risk Individuals: A State by State Analysis 4,* (4th ed. 1990); Sally Squires. *State-sponsored health plans attract uninsured.* Washington Post 1991 Mar. 26:5 (Health Supplement).

45. 26 U.S C. 162. et. seq
46. If the employee leaves work due to a disability that qualifies him for Social Security Disability Insurance, his COBRA coverage would be for 29 months after which he would be eligible for Medicare.
47. According to Sen. Edward Kennedy, Florida, Minnesota and Wisconsin saved nearly $10,000 for each, PWA by using, the Ryan White Act moneys to help PWA continue private health care insurance coverage. *On Senate consideration of the Ryan White 'care' Reauthorization Act of 1995. Congress Press Releases* 1995 July 21. "Forty per cent of HIV-infected individuals in Riverside and San Bernardino County (California)... are receiving services through the Ryan White CARE because they have no health insurance whatsoever." *Floor remarks of Sen. Barbara Boxer.* Congress Press Releases 1995 July 26. In Minnesota, to qualify for the programme the person "must have an HIV-related disease and must have either lost his job or consider it likely to lose his job within the next three months. The applicant must also have a gross income that does not exceed 300 per cent of federal poverty guidelines and may not have more than $25,000 in assets, including his homestead." The programme also requires an applicant to be covered by his former employer's group insurance plan. *Minnesota okays program allowing state to pay insurance premium. AIDS Policy & the Law* 1990 Nov. 14 7
48. 855 F. Supp. 371 (N.D. Ga. 1994); EEOC Guidelines at 8 state the ADA has a retroactive effect even before July 1990. The matter is now on appeal before the 11th Circuit (NO. 95-8533).
49. Lisa M. Tonery. AIDS: *a crisis in health care financing.* 40 *Fed'N Ins. & Corp Couns. Q.* 1990; 133:146 1990. Approximately 40 per cent of all individuals with HIV receive health coverage through Medicaid, a federal entitlement programmed paid for by the federal, state and local governments.
50. Henry A. Waxman. Introduction to symposium on AIDS. 49 *Ohio State Law Journal* 1989; 877, 878. HIV seropositive people are eight times more likely to have lost health insurance than HIV negative people. Michael T. Isbell. *Health Care Reform Lessons from the HIV Epidemic.* Lambda Legal Defense and Education Fund, 1993:69.
51. 1994 ABI JNL LEXIS 2740 at 9 (Sep. 1994). Worker's compensation will not be of use to an HIV seropositive worker unless the HIV was acquired on the job. In Colorado, an HIV seropositive worker, who filed a worker's compensation claim based on becoming HIV through job-related bleeding, had his claim opposed by the state insurance authority which alleged he became HIV seropositive because of sex. AIDS *Policy & the Law* 1995: July 28. 3. In Pennsylvania, a claimant alleged workrelated injury in a worker's compensation claim, but was ordered to release his medical records to determine whether he was HIV Seropositive.
52. David Hirsch. *Sida et droit en Australia.* CNRS, *Droit Et Sida.* J. Foyer and L Khiaiat ed. In: 1994:93.
53. Peter Roth. *AIDS and insurance: some very British questions.* In David FitzSimons, Vanessa Hardy and Keith Tolley, Eds. *The Economic and Social Impact of AIDS in Europe.* Cassell, 1995 (hereinafter *Economic and Social Impact).*
54. B. Napier. *AIDS, discrimination and employment law.* 18 Industrial law Journal 1989; 18:84, 86. (1989). Within the first two years of employment, a worker is protected from unfair dismissal only on grounds of race or sex.
55. Anne-Sophie Rieben Schizas. *Employment, the law and HIV: An overview of European legislation.* In: FitzSimons, Hardy and Tolley, eds. Economic and Social Impact. 304-7. *Supra* n53.

56. Jacqueline De Puy. *Living with HIV/AIDS in Switzerland: exclusion or solidarity.* Id.:250.
57. Id.: 243. Testing in Switzerland for group insurance has been criticized by R. Charbonney in Aide Suisse contre le Sida, Zurich. *La selection des personnes seropositive pour le Sida operee par les assurances collectives (maladie et prvoyance professionnelle) en Suisse*, Schweiz. Med. Wschr. 1991; 1212-6; 12:6.
58. Comparative Study on Discrimination Against Persons with HIV or AIDS. Lausanne: Swiss Institute of Comparative Law and Strasbourg: Council of Europe, 1993:97.
59. *Ibid.* 95-96.
60. 5(5) AIDS Analysis Africa Journal (Southern Africa Edition), Feburary 1995:1. There is no HIV testing for group insurance. Life insurance at the workplace is negotiated between the insurance company and the employer. There is no HIV test for a basic policy. Letter to the author from Morna Cornell, September 18, 1995, The AIDS Consortium.
61. Scherzer, supra n7 at 419; certain states statutorily bar testing for group health policies.
62. John Carruthers. The impact of AIDS on the insurance industry with particular reference to Uganda. AIDS Analysis, 1995.
63. An HIV seropositive plaintiff had no cause of action pursuant to the Canadian Charter of Rights and Freedoms when the province of British Columbia put AZT on the Pharmacare Programme, which in effect, required HIV seropositive persons to pay for it. *Brown v. B.C. (Min. of Health)*, 42B. C.L.R. (2d) 294 (1990).
64. *Pacific Western Airlines v. Canadiart Airline flight Attendant Association*, 28 L.A.C. (3d) 291 (1987).
65. *Thonrton* v. *North American Life Insurance Co.* (No. 5), 17 C.H.R.R.D/481, 483-3, 495 (1992). The result was moot because the complainant had returned to work, became eligible for long-term disability, and then was fired and successfully sued the company, see Joseph Hall. Man with AIDS gets job back plus $ 35,000 in settlement. *Toronto Star*, 1992, March 20:A2. The decision was upheld by the Ontario Court General Division No. 720/92 unreported, 1995, March 31.
66. Sect. 24(25)(3)(a).
67. *Comparative Study on Discrimination, supra* n57 *at* 88. There are, of course, anomalies. In France, it is beneficial to HIV prinsoners, especially if they are not French nationals, to remain in prison because "treatment is fully covered by the Social Security's health insurance branch." British Medical Journal 1995:February 4.
68. New AIDS test using saliva unveiled. *Agence France Presse*, 1993: December 16.
69. Joyce N. Hoffman & Elizabeth Z. Kincaid. AIDS: the challenge to life and health insurers' Freedom of contract, *Drakel Law Review* 1987; 35:709. For example, Midland National Life Insurance required HIV testing for applicants wishing to purchase $100,000 or more coverage if they lived in ten three digit zip code areas. The New Jersey Insurance Department concluded that testing on the basis of lifestyle violated New Jersey law. New Jersey Charges Insurer with Zip Code Readlining. *AIDS Policy and the Law* at 4 (1990).
70. New York, Massachusetts and the District of Columbia had attempted to prohibit blood testing of applicants for HIV. *Health Ins. Ass'n of America v. Carcoran*, 551 N.Y.S. 2d 615 (N. Y. App. Div. 1990) (holding that use of HIV test results was a valid underwriting practice under New York law), Aff'd. 565

N. E. 2d 1264 (N. Y. 1990); *Life Ins: Ass'n of Mass. v. Commissioner of Ins.*, 530 N. e. 2d 168 (1988). The District of Columbia has also rejected its HIV testing prohibition; see Lawrence Bartlett, supra n43 at 215.

71. Peter Pockley. Insurers inconsistent over HIV. *British Medical Journal* 1993:Jun. 5, 1495, et. seq. According to the Director of Consumer Issues at Aetna Insurance, "There's virtually no testing of people who get group life insurance coverage through their jobs, their unions, or groups such as university alumni associations. Only if someone request coverage for five or ten times their annual salary may they be asked to take an HIV test. "
72. Scherze, supra n7 at 421.
73. Muriel Crawford, *et. at.*, Insurance & Employee Benefits. In: Donald Herman and William Schurgin, Challaghan, eds. *Legal Aspects of AIDS* 1990) at 13:21. This is somewhat of an oversimplification of the law. This might be inapplicable to a disability policy. In *Harrison v. Conn Life Ins. Co.*, 771 F. Supp.1053 (n. d. Cal. 1991), the incontestability clause was two years, but inapplicable to "any period of disability related to a misrepresentation (such as HIV) in your application." British Columbia's Insurance Act Section 135 (2) allows an insurance policy to be set aside after two years only for fraud, but not misrepresentation. In *Fioretti* v. *Massachusetts General Life Insurance* Co. 11th Cir. 1995, the Court of Appeals concluded that the "incontestability clause" in the insurance contract which barred the company from voiding the policy was inapplicable. The courst viewed the case as a "conflict of laws" issue and applied New Jersey common law which allowed an insurance company to rescind the policy even for an "innocent misrepresentation." *AIDS Polcy* and *Law* 1995 August 11:2.
74. *Northern Life Insurance Co v. Ippolito Real Estate Partnership,* 601 N. E. 2d 773 (Ist Dist. Ill. 1992), 624 N.E. 2d 1266 at 1274 (Ist Dist. Ill. 1993).
75. Id., 601 N. E. 2d at 776.
76. Junda Woo. Judge rules against insurer in AIDS case, *Wall Street Journal* 1992 July 24:B6.
77. 809 P. 2d (kan. 1991). Kansas is among the minority of states that require fraudulent intent for rescission.
78. 1994 U.s. App. LEXIS, *supra* n2.
79. 651 So. (2d 468 (La. App. 1995).
80. Il House of Commons Social Services Committee (3rd Report), 18 March 1987 at 261. See, for example, the testimony of Mr. R. F. C. Zamboni, Chairman, Life Insurance Council at 1128, "We have always focused on high risk groups. It is clearly established that homosexuals are high risk. We now ask this question because we have to assess what the risks are in every case. We are not turning people down just because they are homosexual but there is usually a medical related factor that comes in" Dr. M. A. Reynolds, Chairman, Medical Affairs Committee at 1130, "We are asking a question: have you received medical advice, treatment or had a blood test in connection with AIDS or an AIDS-related condition? We are searching out the high risk areas which are the very ones the Government have indicated in the campaign, the DHSS, and the blood transfusion centres." The Social Services Committee recommended in 1989 that questions about past HIV tests should not be asked by life insurance companies. Social Services Committee, 7th Report (1988-89), AIDS, HC 202.
81. Comment of the Association of British Insurers. Peter Victor. Single men face AIDS test on mortgages. *The Independent,* 1995 January 8. An endowment mortgage requires life insurance as will a mortgage where the lender required a mortgage protection policy. *The Insurance Leaflet, Advice on Insurance,*

Pensions, and Mortgages for People Affected by HIV or AIDS. Terrence Higgins Trust. 1995:9 (hereinafter *Insurance Leaflet)*.

82. According to the Director of Public Policy of the AIDS Action Foundation in Washington, "life insurance is not a condition of getting a mortgage in the U.S. although it is often purchased in connection with a mortgage." *British Medical Journal* 1993 January 5, *supra* n 69.
83. Il at 112, par 479, supra n80.
84. Jason Bennetoo, Healthy wrongly diagnosed with HIV. *The Independent* 1993 Sept. 19:9.
85. Spencer Leigh. UK: special report: speical risk: striking a balance on AIDS Question. *Money Marketing,* 1993 Feburary 4.
86. Roth at 285, *supra* n53; Policy exclusion for death from HIV was disfavoured for two reasons: (i) HIV often will not appear on death certificates, and (ii) mortgage companies would not accept such an exclusion, Id.
87. Written Question by Frank Field to Virginia Bottomley, Secretary of State for Health, 200 Parl. Deb., H.C. (6th ser.) (W.A.) 444, 11 December 1991 and 182 Parl. Deb., H.C. (6th ser.) (W.A.) 363, 11 December 1990.
88. *British Medical Journal,* 1993 June 5.
89. Debbie Harrison. Finance and the family: questions of life and AIDS—an HIV test may still signify high risk in spite of a new ruling, *Financial Times* 1994 July 30:7.
90. Lorne Burke. UK: a consumer's view—motorcycle insurance, *Money Marketing* 1994 August 4. "a more relevant question to identify high-risk individuals would: 'do you ride a motorcycle?' There is more chance of a young man in the 18-25 age group being killed in a motoring or motorcycle accident than contracting AIDS."'
91. Peter Victor, *The Independent, supra* n81. Perhpas the insurance industry was influenced somewhat by the threat of legislation since "A Private Members' Bill was due to be introduced into the House of Lords in the autumn by Lady Gardner of Parkes that would have stopped insurers asking about negative test results or counselling. This Bill is now being dropped." UK: dramatic switch on HIV questions. *Post Magazine* 1994 July 28.
92. *The insurance Leaflet, supra* n79 at 4; states "(i)f you are a single man, you will almost always recieve a supplemental questionnaire," Id.: 6. Persons who travel to the USA, Africa or Thailand are often required to be tested, Id.; see also Peter Victor. Single men face AIDS test for mortgages, *The Independent* 1995 January 8, *supra* n81. Andrew Verity, Term Policies Taking on a New Look, *Money Marketing* 1995 August 31:12.
93. Siobhan Creaton. Insurers consider HIV stance, *Irish Times* 1994 July 28:15.
94. Foutouh El Chazli. Le sida au regard du droit Egyptien. *Droit et Sida:* 161-62, *supra* n52.
95. Lynne Duke. South Africans face spiraling epidemic of AIDS: after apartheid, a plague/one in five Blacks at risk by the year 2000, *International Herald Tribune* 1995 July 26.
96. Zimbabwe rejects blanket AIDS tests for insurance. *Reuters World Service* 1994 November 1. See also Glen Williams and Sunanda Ray. AIDS in Africa: signs of hope from the workplace. at 353, *Economic and Social Impact of AIDS in Europe,* supra n53.
97. *AIDS Analysis Africa* 1994; 4(6):1.
98. AIDS and Life Assurance Claims in Zimbabwe, 2(4) *SAf AIDS News,* 1994 December 12.
99. Itai Masuku. Big AIDS shock on Insurance Claims, *Business Herald 1994*

June 2:1. The cost of an HIV test is at least $130 and the premium average is $500; therefore, the testing would have to be on a random basis. *Ibid.*

100. *Ibid*. 5(5):1.
101. *Ibid.*
102. Life Insurance Dilemmas, 1(3) ZIA Net AIDS News 1993 September 8.
103. 5(6) AIDS Analysis 1993 Apr/May:6. Until recently, there had been little litigation on HIV because a complainant did not have the anonymity. The AIDS Law Project has recently obtained a ruling that allowed anonymity "which is a major breakthrouh." Letter to the author from Morna Cornell, The AIDS Consortium 1995 September 18.
104. 5(6) *AIDS Analysis,* 1995 Apr/May 6.
105. Lynne Duke, South Africans face spiraling epidemic of AIDS: after apartheid, a plague/one in five Balcks at risk by the year 2000, *Int'l Herald Tribune* 1995 July 26. The new South African Constitution prohibits discrimination based on disability, such as HIV. The AIDS Law Project of the Univerity of Witwatersrand has challenged the policy and the matter should be litigated in September 1995, Id.
106. Swazi insurance firm starts screening for AIDS. *Reuters World Service* 1995 July 27. The health industry estimates 80,000 of the 900,000 population is HIV seropositive, World Corporate Ins. Rpt., *Financial Times* 1995 August 11.
107. *AIDS Analysis,* supra n62.
108. Luisetta Reuter. Hong Kig firms lag in AIDS battle, *Financial Post* 1994 May 21:54.
109. Hirotaka Terai. Insurers fear being hit by AIDS; and mull screening applicants. *Daily Yomiuri* 1993 August 24:8.
110. Doctors suggest AIDS tests for insurance applicants, *Japan Economic Newswire* 1993 Mar. 31.
111. Terai, *supra* n104. As of August 1994, only four persons in Japan had publicly admitted being HIV seropositive. Andrew Pollack. Japan facing up to its AIDS cases. *New York Times,* 1994 August 7:18.
112. Thailand: AIDS prevention panel to draft regulations for insurance firms, *Bangkok Post* 1995 May 14.
113. Thailand: longer period likely in which to dispute payouts, Ibid. 1995 March 20; *Financial Times Limited World Policy Guide* 1994 August.
114. *Financial Times Limited World Policy Guide* 1994 August.
115. Yohanna Abdullah. Companies cutting risk of insuring AIDS victims. *Straits Times* 1992 June 28:1.
116. Tan Hsueh Yun. Insurers here hesitant to ask clients to undergo genetic tests. *Ibid.* 1993 November 15:23.
117. The Disability Discrimination Act of 1992 covers superannuation and insurance companies, but allows an exception when "discrimination is based on actuarial or statistical data which justifies the discrimination."
118. Justice Michael Kirby. HIV and Law-a paradoxical relationship of mutual interest. IUVDT World STD/AIDS Congress, Signapore, 22 March 1995. David Hairsh. Sida et droit en Australie. *Droit et Sida,* supra n51:93.
119. David Adams. Australia: victims of AIDS gain in insurance reform. *The Age* 1994 (Melborne) October 24. By January 1995, AMP and Life Reinsurance of Australia, along with National Mutual, had dropped HIV exclusion claims for death and disability benefits. Gays were infuriated, however, when they heard that the Health Employees Superannuation Trust Australia would screen all new workers and those testing HIV seropositive would no longer get death or

disability benefits resulting from HIV. Australia: Gay Super Furore, *Ibid.* 1995 March 8. The federal government backed HIV/AIDS Implementation Working Group has been involved in extensive negotiations with the Life Insurance Federation of Australia to reach a solution to the problems caused by the AIDS exclusion clause.

120. *Ibid.* October 24, 1994.

121. Karen Middleton. Australia: insurance bar over AIDS under attack, *The Age (Melbourne)*, December 2, 1993. The Trowbridge Report has been used as authority in litigation by an HIV seropositive former teacher whose disability benefits were rejected by a medium-sized insurance firm. The firm said that if it had known that the teacher had participated in homosexual acts, it "never would have accepted him for the fund." Paul Robinson, Australia: Challenge to AIDS Bias in Insurance, *Sunday Age* (Molbourne) 1993 December 5.

122. *British Medical Journal* 1993 June 5, supra n69; Hirsch, supra n51 at 93.

123. Will Adler. A legal perspective on insurance industry reactions to AIDS. *Law Society Journal* 1992; May: 64. In 1992, the federal Disability Discrimination Act prohibited insurance discrimination based on disability lmless it were based on grounds of statistical/ actuarial data or reasonableness: Secs. 4, 24, 46.

124. New Zealand: AIDS insurance payouts total $1.5M, *New Zealand Herald* 1989 November 23; and New Zealand: payouts of $3.5 million on AIDS patients. *Ibid.* 1992 Jun. 24.

125. Secs. 21(1)(h)(vii), (m) and 44, 48. Compliance is monitored by the New Zealand Human Rights Commission.

126. *British Medical Journal* 1993 June 5. supra n69. Minister of Justice, Dept. of Civil Law Legislation, Ref. 307430.93/6; *Comparative Study on Discrimination, supra* n58 at 97.

127. *Ibid.* :96.

128. British Medical Journal, supra n71. Letter to author, September 4, 1995 by Henrik Stenbjerre, Esq.

129. Per Sandberg. HIV and life insurance: costs and ethics of nondiscrimination. *Economic and Social Impact of AIDS in Europe:* 293, supra n52. The author argues that with the Euroepan Union, all HIV positive persons should be allowed "small life insurance policies" without disclosure of HIV and that "a no-question policy is absolutely feasible economically." *Ibid.*" 300.

130. *Comparative Study on Discrimination, supra* n58 at 96-97.

131. Letter from Verband der Lebenvericherungs Unternehmen E.V. to Terrence Higgens Trust, November 30, 1992.

132. Adoption in France of a Convention on the insurability of seropositive persons and on the confidentiality of the handling of medical information by insurance companies. International Digest of Health Legislation 1992; 43(1).

133. British Medical Journal 1993 June 5, *supra* n71, "over 90 per cent of people would agree to an HIV test if it were free."

134. Comparative Study on Discrimination, *supra* n58 at 97.

135. Ake Saldeen and Lotta Westerhall. Reflexions sur le sida et droit suedois, *Droit et Sida,* supra n 52 at 402ff; and Benny Henriksson. Social Democracy or Societal Control. A Critical Analysis of Swedish AIDS Policy, *Institute for Social Policy* 1988; *Comparative Study on Discrimination,* supra n58 at 97.

136. Decree of the Minister of Indistry and Handicrafts of 23 November 1990, *Ibid.*:97.

137. NAIC Model Regulation Service, Medical/Lifestyle Questions on Applications and Underwriting Guidelines Affecting AIDS and ARC. 1988.

138. *British Medical Journal* 1993 June 5, supra n71 Testing for HIV in life insurance

policies had been common only in C$50,000. *Toronoto Star* 1993 January 10.

139. AIDS cover for travellers, *Financial Times Limited World Policy Guide 1993* October.
140. Italy: Reale Mutua provides cover against risk of contracting AIDS, *Italia Oggi* 1995 March 31.
141. Cas St. Leger. Questions over AIDS insurance plan for SA nurses, *Sunday Times* 1994 September 11:15.
142. Helen Pridham. As state pay-outs shrink, more people are insuring their health. critically important. *The Herald* (Glasgow) 1995 August 12:20.
143. Steve Lewis. Australia: cover against catching AIDS now on market, *Australian Financial Review* 1989 October 17.
144. Maginnis & Associates announces new insurance for health care workers exposed to HIV. *Business Wire* 1992 June 1.
145. Massachusetts Hospital Insurers for HIV Infection of Nurses, *Reuters North American Wire* 1992 April 29.
146. AMA offers HIV insurance for U.S. doctors, *Reuter Lib. Rpt.* 1992 February 12.
147. Gracian Mack. Insurance for the living. *Black Enterprise* 25 (12); 1995 July: 100-2. "If the doctors determine that you're going to live for three years, you might get 50 per cent of the policy's value. If you've only got about six months, you'd probably get 80 per cent." For an excellent analysis of the subject, see Jennifer Berner. Beating the grim reaper, or just confusing him? Examining the harmful effects of viatical settlement regulation. *Journal of Marshall Law Review* 1994; 27:581-616.
148. Allan H. Terl. Life insurance buyouts (allowing AIDS carriers to "sell" policies to third party, which in turn gives carrier cast value of policy in exchange for future benefits upon death), *Human Rights* 1993; Spring:7.
149. Jon Ashworth. AIDS victims put life policies up for sale, *Sunday Times* 1994 August 6. Prudential Insurance of America will pay about 95 per cent of a policy's face value for an insured who has less than six months to live. Greg Steinmez. New companies are forming to buy policies of AIDS patients, *Wall Street Journal* 1992 July 31:4.
150. Duncan Hughes. Money-go-round: a new trade in life cover, *Daily Telegraph* 1992 June 20:23.
151. Leslie Scism and Jeffrey Taylor. SEC questions insurance deals for the dying, *Wall Street Journal* 1994 August 18.B1.
152. Cecile Gutscher, New Class of Investment Cashes in on Terminally Ill, *Ariz. Republic* 1995 April 23:E7. In August 1994, the SEC filed suit against Living Partners. Inc., because the policies were unregulated investment contract securities. Lois Caliri, Gambling on death: life policies for sale, *Central Pennsylvania Business Journal* 1995 August 4:1. In August 1995, a federal judge issued a preliminary injunction ordering Life Partners to transfer $100 million to an independent third party pending resolution of the case, but the judge also observed that the SEC had failed to produce even a dissatisfied party; *SEC v. Life Ptnrs.*, 1995 U.S. Dist. Lexis 12657 (D.C.).
153. Iskandar Hamwi, Past and Present Dangers in Living Policy Values. *Journal of the American Society of CLU and CHFC* 1994; 48(6).
154. *Insurance Leaflet,* supra n81:10.
155. *Ibid.*
156. Written Question by Lord Kilmarnock, 559 Parl. Deb., (H.L.) (5th ser.) 30 November 1994, WA 38-39.
157. *Christian v. Sheft,* (Cal. Super Ct. Feburary 17, 1989).
158. Jury award is sharply cut in Hudson AIDS suit. *New York Times* 1989 Apr.

22:7 Hudson's lover settled for an undisclosed amount while the appeals were pending *Press Association Newsfile* 1993.

159. *Aetna Cas.* and *Sur Co v Sheft*, 989 F. 2d 1105 at 1108, (9th Cir. 1993).
160. *Comparative Study on Discrimination*, supra n58:100.
161. Thomas M. Burton and G. Pascal Zachary. Baxter and Rhone Poulenc Rorer to settle hemophiliac AIDS *suits, Wall Street Journal* 1994 August 3.B7.
162. *Wadleigh v Rhone-Poulence Rorer, Inc.*, 157 F.R.D. 410 (N.D. Ill. 1994).
163. Burton and Zachary. Hemophiliacs quit settlement of suit on clotting agents, *Wall Street Journal* 1994 August 10:B6.
164. *Matter of Rhone-Poulenc Rorer, Inc.*, 51 F. 3d 1293 at 1302 (7th Cir. 1995).
165. *Business Insurance* 1994 August 8.
166. *Kirekendall v. Harbour Ins. Co.*, 698 F. Supp. 768 (W.D. Ark. 1988).
167. *Cheney v. Beel Nat'l Life Ins.*, 520 A. 2d 402 (Md. App. 1987).
168. See Keith M. Garza. Administrative no-fault recovery for transfusion-related HIV infection. Defence Counsel Journal 1993; 60:384 (discussing the compensation of HIV transfusion victims without a showing of the provider's fault). Most authorities agree that there has been a significant decrease in blood bank litigation; see blood products: tainted blood suits going, going, gone?, *AIDS Policy* and *the La7a* 1994 May 27:5.
169. Don Lewis Kirk. Germany, blood screening faulted in report, *Business Insurance* 1994 November 24.
170. *Insurance Research Literature* 1993 August 1.
171. Kirk. supra n169.
172. *Ibid*, Germany *Lloyds Product Liability International* 1994 December 31.
173. Argument over humanitarian fund. *World Insurance Report* 1993 November 19.; *Lloyds Insura1tce International* 1993 December 1.
174. *World Insurance Report* supra n165
175. *Agence France Presse* 1995 January 21
176. Kirk. supra n169.
177. *Ibid.*
178. Ian Davidson. France sets aside billions for AIDS victims. *Financtal Times* 1991 November 28:2.
179. William Dawkins. French Insurers Step In With AIDS Cash. *Financial Times* 1991 December:14.
180. *Ibid. Business Insurance* 1992 November. 2.
181. *Ibid.*
182. *Ibid.*; see also Caroline Bettai. Responsables et coupables, une affaire de sang, *Editions du Seuil* 1993, and Andre Picard, France makes ar. example of misdeeds, *Globe and Mail* 1993 September 7:A4.
183. *Insurance Research Literature* 1993 August 1.
184. *Agence France Flresse* 1995 January 27.
185. *The Age* (Melborr.e) 1991 December 26. Ex gratia payments for medically acquired HIV have been made through the Mark Fitzpatrick Trust Fund established by the Federal Government through a $13.2 million seed grant and also by the New South Wales Government which set up a seed grand of 516 million for all HIV seropositive persons.
186. Lisa Priest. Insurers may join tained blood deal. *Toronoto Star* 1993 September 10: A3; Andre Picard. Terms of deal over blood draws protest, *Globe and Mail* 1993 December 7:A5. In Great Britain, local governments were self-funded, and therefore, insurance was irrelevant.
187. *Sutherland et al. v. Canadian Red Cross Society, et al.*, (Ont. Feburary 1994); *Mr. "X" v. The Canadian Red Cross Soceity and the Attorney General of Quebec*, (August 10, 1992).

HIV/AIDS AND LAW, ETHICS AND HUMAN RIGHTS

INTERNATIONAL ENCYCLOPAEDIA OF AIDS - 4

HIV/AIDS AND LAW, ETHICS AND HUMAN RIGHTS

PART - II

Editor

Dr. Digumarti Bhaskara Rao

M.Sc., M.A., M.A., M.Ed., Ph.D.

Dean, Faculty of Education

Member, Academic Senate

Ex-Chairman, Board of Studies in Education

Member, Research Advisory Committee

Acharya Nagarjuna University

D-43, S.V.N. Colony

Guntur - 522 006 (India)

DPH

DISCOVERY PUBLISHING HOUSE PVT. LTD

NEW DELHI-110 002

First Published - 2000

Reprinted - 2015

ISBN: 978-81-7141-526-7 (Set)

HIV/AIDS and Law, Ethics and Human Rights

Published by:

DISCOVERY PUBLISHING HOUSE PVT. LTD.

4383/4B, Ansari Road, Darya Ganj

New Delhi-110 002 (India)

Phone: +91-11-23279245, 43596064-65

Fax: +91-11-23253475

E-mail: discoverypublishinghouse@gmail.com

sales@discoverypublishinggroup.com

web: www.discoverypublishinggroup.com

Printed at:

Infinity Imaging Systems

Delhi

Preface

The HIV/AIDS is a new phenomenon in the human society. HIV destroys the immune system of human individuals, producing a defenselessness fatal state known as AIDS. The World Health Organisation has estimated that already one in every two hundred and fifty adults in the world is infected with Human Immunodeficiency Virus and according to WHO's projections a total of forty million men women and children worldwide will have been infected with HIV by the turn of this twentieth century. Visualising the devastating effects of the HIV/AIDS epidemic within our life times and beyond is difficult. Probably, no other disease in recent times has had the impact on human society generated by HIV/AIDS.

The HIV/AIDS epidemic has brought into focus many health related ethical, legal and human rights issues. This epidemic requires immediate and effective responses in new programming areas: attitudinal and behavioural changes, community-based care and support initiatives, and the maintenance of human development in the face of increasing rates of illness and deaths. At this point, education enters the scene as it can alter the HIV/AIDS situation since it brings change in the behaviour of the people.

This *'International Encyclopaedia of AIDS'* presents the worldwide information about HIV/AIDS, issues and challenges, reports and reviews, ethics laws and human rights, and educational activities and programmes to keep the policy makers, planners, professionals, activists, researchers, educationists, teachers and students well informed of the epidemic.

Dr. Digumarti Bhaskara Rao,
26 January 1999
The Republic Day of India

Acknowledgement

I am thankful to the World Health Organisation and its associated offices for using their material namely School Health Education to prevent AIDS and STD: A Resource Package for Curriculum Planners-Handbook for Curriculum Planners. Student's Activities, Teachers' Guide, Global Programme on AIDS-HIV Prevention and Care: Teaching Modules for Nurses and Midwives, Global Programme on AIDS–Community HIV Prevention Handbook; STD care Management-workbooks 1-7, Facing the Challenge of HIV/ AIDS STDs: A Gender-based Response; HIV/AIDS and STD surveillance Data Management and Use-Report, Bangkok, 1995; Carrying out HIV Sentinal Surveillance–A Guide for Programme Managers, AIDS Prevention and Care in the workplace: Enhancing the Role of Private Sector; HIV Testing Policies and Guidelines; Carrying out HIV Sentinel surveillance; AIDS Prevention; Understanding and Living with AIDS; AIDS: A Modern Epidemic; HIV/AIDS in South-East Asia: IXth meeting of the National Programme Managers, New Delhi, 1993; Information, Education and Communication: A Guide for AIDS Programme Managers, Handbook on AIDS Home Care; HIV/AIDS in South-East Asia: A Pictorial Summary; etc.

I am thankful to the United Nations Development Programme, UNDP's HIV and Development Programme, and UNDP's Regional Projects on HIV and Development for using their material namely Economic Implications of AIDS in Asia; Socio Economic Implications of the Epidemic; NGOs Working with Sex workers; NGO Responses to HIV/AIDS in Asia-Case Studies; HIV in the Workplace: Dealing with the Issues-Role Plays, Development and the HIV Epidemic, Law Ethics and HIV; HIV Law and Law Reform; Issue Papers; Study Papers; Working Papers; etc.

I am thankful to the Health and Nutrition Centre, Republic of

Philippines for using its material namely sourcebook on HIV/AIDS Prevention Education for Tertiary Educational Institutions.

I am thankful to the Curriculum Development Programme, Ministry of Education, Government of Thailand for using its material namely Institutional Modules for AIDS Education.

I am thankful to US Department of Health and Human Services; Whitman-Walker Clinic, Inc., USA; East-West Centre, USA; National AIDS Control Organisation, Government of India; Academy of Culture Communication Education Science and Service, Guntur, United Nations and its agencies for using their material.

I am grateful to Bhaskar Bhattacharji; V. Alexeev, Geeta Sethi, Elizabeth Reid, Mina Mauerstein-Bail, A. A. Trinidad, Palomi Cuchi, D. Pushpa Latha for their kind co-operation.

Dr. Digumarti Bhaskara Rao,
Secretary
ACCESS
D-43, S.V. N. Colony,
Guntur-522 006

Contents

27

The Australian Legal Response to HIV

Michael Alexander
Australian Federation of AIDS Organisation
Australia

INTRODUCTION

In Australia, as in many countries, initial legal responses to HIV were knee jerk ones. Governments moved to require doctors to report names and addresses of people with AIDS to the states to stop people belonging to risk groups from donating blood, and to criminalize sexual conduct of people with AIDS. These moves provoked immediate reactions from the newly formed community based AIDS organizations, mostly made up of gay men mobilizing to combat the threat of AIDS to their communities in New South Wales, the largest state and the epicentre of HIV infection in Australia. Many people taking HIV tests gave their name as Neville Wran (the then state premier).

These measures also sparked off an intense debate, and many of then were revoked. Since that time Australia's legal response to HIV has more often (but not always) followed the path of consultation in line with the pattern followed in relation to other aspects of the epidemic. This is characterized by a partnership between the government, health professionals, and organizations representing people affected by HIV/AIDS.

Australia's Federal System

Australia's federal system, with eight state and territory governments responsible for most of the relevant areas of law, creates obvious difficulties for a co-ordinated national response. Unfortunately the virus does not recognize state boundaries. States and territories have governments of different political complexions and with different ideas on appropriate responses to HIV.

The federal government has taken the responsibility for the legal response to HIV. It has at its disposal certain tools (mostly involving funding) to persuade the states and territories to follow its lead. However, ultimately, the federal government has no power to make the states and territories comply with its policies.

Government Responses

The federal government has established a number of mechanisms to examine the legal changes necessary to prevent HIV transmission and to minimize the personal and social impact of HIV.

In 1989 a National AIDS Strategy was released, putting in place a three year plan with detailed measures to be implemented during that period. It covered all aspects of the response to HIV/AIDS, including the need for legislative reform. These measures had the broad support of all state and territory governments, and community based AIDs organizations.

The law reform recommendations of the national Strategy were largely based on an earlier report of a Panel on Discrimination, and other legal issues, which held public hearings in capital cities. Recommendations were made in the areas of public health laws, immigration, legal standards for condoms. prostitution laws, laws on homosexuality, drug laws, laws affecting procedures on death, censorship and media law, confidentiality and privacy, prisons, insurance and superannuation.

However, the National Strategy did not make detailed recommendations on most of these issues. Instead, it recommended the establishment of a Legal Working Party (LWP) comprising representatives of federal and state Attorneys-General and Health Departments to review these areas of law, and to make more detailed recommendations.

It also recommended the establishment of a Privacy and HIV/AIDS Working Party to formulate guidelines for government departments handling HIV related information.

Significantly, the national Strategy also recognized the need for legal advice and advocacy services for people with HIV, and for the first time provided funding to the Australian Federation of AIDS Organizations (AFAO) to employ a solicitor. It also acknowledged the need for lawyers and other HIV workers to be better aware of the existing laws relating to HIV/AIDS, and provided funding to AFAO to produce the first edition of the *Australian HIV/AIDS Legal Guide.*

The Legal Working Party

The Legal Working Party was set up in 1990 under the Intergovernmental Committee of AIDS (IGCA). It produced a series of nine discussion papers with possible options for reform, and public comment was sought. They received over 300 submissions from various organizations and individuals. People making submissions ranged from government departments to church bodies, unions, academics, legal groups and AIDS organizations.

In November 1992 the Legal Working Party produced its final report, containing a series of detailed recommendations for reform. The recommendations are in general very progressive, remarkably so in view of the fact they were drafted by a committee of bureaucrats. Whilst not agreeing with every recommendation, AFAO and other community based AIDS organizations have in general embraced the report and have adopted it as a desirable agenda for reform.

Members of the Legal Working party were at pains to emphasize that their task was to produce a broad prescription for legislative action, rather than attempt to find the lowest common denominator based on the current position in each state and territory. They saw their job as producing logical solutions to problems, rather than pragmatic compromises. They emphasized that adoption of the recommendations by a particular jurisdiction did not commit that government to immediate reform in all areas.

Some of the recommendations were controversial. They are too numerous to be comprehensively listed here, but include the following:

- Removing criminal penalties for homosexual conduct in private between consenting adults.
- Adoption of consistent ages of consent for homosexual and heterosexual activity.
- Legal recognition for partners in non-traditional domestic relationships, including homosexual as well as heterosexual *de facto* arrangements.

Removing criminal penalties for sex industry work.
Repeal of offence relating to possession of needles and syringes.
Repeal of drug self-administration offence.
Non-custodial offence for minor drug offence.
Repeal of legislative barriers restricting distribution, promotion, advertising or sale of condoms.
All jurisdiction to adopt anti-discrimination legislation covering disability (including HIV/AIDS) and sexuality.
Public health legislation to require notification of HIV and AIDS only in coded, non-identifiable form.

Implementation has been painfully slow. While the majority of the recommendations are to be implemented at the state and territory levels, most governments appear to have taken precious little interest in them. Worse than being inactive, some states have introduced new laws which are contrary to certain LWP recommendations. Queensland, for example, has passed a new prostitution law which is highly restrictive and virtually makes all sex work illegal. Tasmania has obstinately refused to decriminalize homosexual acts (all other states and territories have now done so). The situation for gay men in that state has changed only by virtue of an individual complaint to the UN Human Rights Committee, followed by controversial federal legislation implementing the sexual privacy aspect of the International Covenant on Civil and Political Rights.

NSW set up its own committee to produce a substantial report on how recommendations should be implemented at the state level. However, there has been little legislative change.

At the federal level, the Ministers for Justice and Human Services and Health have established an HIV/AIDS Implementation Working Group to oversee reforms. The Working Group is compiling a status report on the implementation of the various recommendations in each state and territory, which is to be raised at various ministerial meetings, and directly with the state and governments.

The Implementation Working Group is also working on a number of areas of federal responsibility which are outstanding-notably issue involving insurance and superannuation privacy and media regulation.

Discrimination Initiatives

In 1991 the NSW government asked the state's Anti-Discrimination Board to conduct an inquiry into HIV and AIDS related discrimination. The inquiry heard evidence and received and produced a report in 1992 entitled Discrimination-the other Epidemic. The report found that HIV discrimination was pervasive and extensive, and documented many instances of discrimination.

This very significant and conclusive documentation of the extent of HIV related discrimination led to a number of further initiatives. The federal Department of Human Services and Health has subsequently media campaign on HIV discrimination, and funded a number of community based projects aimed at reducing instances of discrimination.

Community Based Organizations

Community based AIDS organizations in Australia recognized the significance of the law in the fight against HIV/AIDS at a very early state and have consistently pressed for, liaised with and responded to the various government activities outlined previously. Much of this activity has been driven by legal working groups.

The primary focus of activity has been the AIDS Council of NSW (ACON) in Sydney. Since the mid-eighties ACON has had an active group of volunteer lawyers and other interested people involved in its legal working group. This group has been at the forefront of the push for law reform in numerous areas of law. It has also produced a number of publications on HIV law and conducted other educations activities for people with HIV/AIDS affected communities, lawyers, and general community.

Agitation by the ACON Legal Working Group led to the establishment and funding of the AFAO Legal Project has had at least one (and sometimes more than one) paid staff member working on legal policy issues, education and legal cases. The paid staff members have always relied to a very heavy extent on the volunteers of the ACON legal Working Group, and the other legal working groups which have since sprung up in some of the other states and territories. AFAO itself now has a national Legal Working Group, drawing together people from around the country to advise it one legal policy issues. This group has recently drafted a Legal Strategic Plan for AFAO, nominating priority areas for law reform.

In addition to legal policy issues, legal working groups and the AFAO Legal Project have attempted to meet the HIV legal education needs of people with HIV, affected communities, lawyers, other service providers, and the general public. Their publications include the following:

HIV/AIDS and *Your Rights,* a pamphlet on HIV legal issues for people with HIV/AIDS and affected communities, now in its fourth edition.

Australian HIV/AIDS Legal Guide, a book of over 500 pages containing a detailed exposition of the relevant law in each state and territory of Australia, now in its second edition.

Planning Ahead for People with HIV/AIDS, a series of pamphlets dealing with wills, powers of attorney, advance treatment directives, and superannuation.

A Guide to HIV/AIDS Confidentiality and the Law.

Applying for Permanent Residence in Australia, an information sheet for people with HIV/AIDS and their advisers.

HIV/AIDS Legal Link, a quarterly newsletter on HIV related law and policy.

Most of these publications have been funded by the federal Department of Human Services and Health.

The legal working group in Sydney provides a regular forum for various HIV related legal issues, and sends legal speakers to activities organized by other groups.

Arising out of work of the legal working groups, specialist HIV/AIDS legal centres (HALCs) have been established in Sydney and Melbourne to provide legal advice and representation for people with HIV/AIDS. The centre in Sydney employs a full-time lawyer who works with a larger roster of volunteer lawyers and law students to meet the heavy demand for specialist, well-informed legal services. The centre in Melbourne receives no funding, and is dependant on volunteers. There is also a specialist legal service in Brisbane, based at the Queensland AIDS Council, where a lawyer from the Legal Aid Office attends on a regular basis.

Each of these centres is connected to an extensive network of people working in the field such as doctors, hospital social workers and other service providers who refer clients needing specialist legal advice. These service providers themselves also tend to rely heavily on the HIV/AIDS legal centres for legal and ethical advice which arise in the course of their work.

A significant aspect of legal casework is that it informs the legal policy and education work of community based AIDS organizations. Because they daily confront the legal problems of the people with HIV/AIDS, HALCs have an excellent picture of which legal issues are involved, what laws need to be changed, and of the education and information needs yet to be met.

Several government inquiries and working parties on various legal issues have relied substantially on material from the casework database of HALC to inform them of the nature and extent of the problems confronting people with HIV.

Coalitions

AIDS organizations involved in legal issues recognize the need to work in coalition with other non-government organizations. For example, the HIV/AIDS legal centres are a part of a network of community legal centres around Australia, which are generally concerned with social justice issues. HALC workers and volunteers regularly run workshops at community legal centre conferences to build knowledge about HIV legal issues.

Other networks in which AIDS organizations are involved include:

Human rights organizations. AFAO is a member of the Australian Forum of Human Rights Organizations, and participates in its regular consultations with the Department of Foreign Affairs and Trade.

Other disability organizations. AFAO is a member of the National Coalition for the Development of Disability Standards, and participates in, regular consultations between the Federal Disability Commissioner and national disability peak bodies.

Other health advocacy organizations.

There are also networks and coalitions which come together to deal with specific issues. For example, when working on prison law reform issues relating to HIV/AIDS, it makes sense to join people and organizations working on other aspects of prison reform. Sometimes these networks do not exist when they are needed and have to be set up. For example, AIDS organizations have been at the forefront of community efforts in Australia in grappling with the complex laws relating to superannuation. It was the initiative of AIDS organizations that to a Superannuation Consumer Coalition been established in Sydney, comprising a broad range of consumer and legal organizations with an interest in the general area of superannuation.

Successes and Failures

From the point of view of community organizations, law reforms rarely go as far as we would like them to. In most areas we would like to see further reform. Whilst conceding that in many areas Australia has fairly enlightened laws and policies in place, acknowledgement of success is almost always qualified by some reservations.

Successes

Discrimination laws: The federal government, and all the states and territories (except Tasmania) now have discrimination laws which make discrimination against all people with HIV unlawful. In NSW it is also unlawful to vilify people with HIV/AIDS. This is a powerful symbol for and a potential weapon in the hands of people with HIV/AIDS. Unfortunately, though, complaint and investigation mechanisms are often very slow, and this constitutes a disincentive for people with HIV. There are also continuing problems with the reliance of the system on individual complaints to take on systematic probes, e.g., the ongoing discriminatory policies of the Cornmonwealth Employment Service and the Australian Defence Force, which are in clear breach of the Disability Discrimination Act.

> *Needle and syringe exchanges*: One of the most important and successful aspects of Australia's response to HIV has been the early acceptance by governments of the need for harm minimization policies to prevent HIV transmission amongst injecting drug users. Needle exchanges are funded by governments in every state and territory to try to ensure that if people use drugs, they use clean needles and syringes. It is no longer against law to possess needles for the purpose of injecting illegal drugs, and exchanges generally operate with the support of police services. There are still a number of legal problems with needle exchanges, and many drug law reform issues are still to be tackled. However, it must be acknowledged that Australia's needle and syringe exchange programme has meant that there is a much lower rate of HIV infection amongst injecting drug users than in most other comparable developed countries, which have generally been slower to adopt this form of harm minimization.

Decriminalization of homosexuality: Homosexual activities have now been effectively decriminalized throughout Australia. However ages of consent in many states are inconsistent, and there is a higher age of consent in many places for male homosexual sex as compared with heterosexual sex.

Media discussion censorship: Since the advent of HIV/AIDS, there is now much more open discussion and depiction of sexual activities, and advertising and availability of condoms. However problems still occur from time to time, as evidenced by the recent banning of AIDS education swap cards produced by the Queensland AIDS Council.

Immigration: People with HIV/AIDS who are married to or in permanent relationships with Australian citizens and permanent residents are now eligible for grant of permanent residence in Australia, as are the children of Australians and refugees. This is a significant advance over all applicants for permanent residence are tested for HIV, and other classes of applicant (e.g., business migrants, other relatives of Australians) are not eligible for residence.

Superannuation: After a long battle, HIV exclusion clauses for death and disability benefits have now been removed from most superannuation funds.

Failures

Prostitution: Prostitution laws vary considerably from one state to another, and no state has fully implemented the recommendations of the IGCA Legal Working Party.

Prisons: Some states carry out mandatory testing of prisoners, and several still segregate prisoners with HIV from the general prison population. Condoms are not supplied to prisoners with HIV from the general prison population. Condoms are not supplied to prisoners except in the ACT, and needle and syringe exchanges are not available in prisons in any state.

Voluntary euthanasia: Many people with HIV/AIDS who become very ill choose to die when their lives become unbearable, but need assistance to do so. Assisting a person to die was illegal in every state and territory at the time of writing. AIDS organizations in several states are undertaking a major law reform push in this area in 1995.

Conclusion

Australia has done very well in documenting HIV related legal issues and in producing detailed reports and discussion papers. The AIDS community sector has been active in the legal area, but there is still no great deal of knowledge or expertise about HIV in the mainstream legal profession. After an early and quite limited bout of enthusiasm for law reform, the attitudes of the state and territory governments towards legal issues have become quite complacent.

Good work has been done in setting the agenda for law reform. We know what we need to do. Our governments now need to muster the political will to actually implement it.

28

An Introduction to the Legislation of China Governing the Prevention and Control of HIV/AIDS

Wang Yan
Bureau of Legislation
The State Council China

Zhao Ning
Policy and Law Unit,
Ministry of Public Health, China

INTRODUCTION

The worldwide prevalence of AIDS has become a serious issue of global concern. In recent years, there has been a rapid increase of AIDS in the Asian-Pacific region, particularly in those adjoining countries to China, such as India, Thailand, Japan and Nepal, etc., where, some two million people are estimated to be infected with HIV. The rapid spread of HIV in the Asian Pacific region constitutes a threat to the continental part of China.

China is a country of low HIV prevalence. However, the increase of HIV/ AIDS cases detected in the country can not be overlooked. Since the first AIDS case detected from among a foreign tourist group in this country in 1985, there have been reported 261 AIDS cases and 969 HIV infections by the end of November 1992. Out of the 30 provinces/municipalities/ autonomous regions of the country (not including Taiwan Province), HIV infections have been detected in 18 provinces and autonomous regions.

With the implementation of China's policies of reforms and

opening to the outside world, China's communication with foreign countries has been increasing in political, economic and cultural areas, etc. Correspondingly, there are more opportunities and routes for HIV to be transmitted into the ,country. China is a developing country with a large population of which 80 per cent is rural based. If there is a rampant prevalence of HIV/AIDS in the country, it would have an inestimable bearing on the economic development of this country and the world as a whole. It is to this end that China's government has assigned a high priority to the prevention and control of HIV/AIDS by formulating a national comprehensive programme comprising of therapeutic, administrative and economic measures, and by formulating a plan of action for its implementation. The state legislative bodies have, at the same time, promulgated relevant laws, legislations and regulations for its prevention and control with the hope to ensure, by mandatory force of the state, the implementation of relevant laws and regulations. The legislative activities are the most important link for the prevention and control of HIV/AIDS of the country. A brief introduction in this aspect is hereunder given.

AIMS

China is a populous country with high population density. Historically, the rampant prevalence of certain infectious diseases, i.e., plague and smallpox, etc., had brought about a heavy death toll. Hence, "putting prevention first" for the protection of health of the broad masses of people has been the consistent foundation of China's policy in health services, as well as in the prevention and control of HIV/AIDS. HIV/AIDS is a disease both with a medical and social nature. It has been, therefore, specified in the legislation that HIV/AIDS patients are subject to respect and protection under the precondition of ensuring the interests of the great majority of the population.

MAIN CONTENTS

China's legislation governing the prevention and control of HIV/AIDS covers the following contents, *inter alia,* quarantine services at the border, civil law governing marriage and family, and criminal law. A brief description of relevant aspects and its background are given hereunder.

A. General Public Health

As an infectious disease HIV occupies an important place in the state legislation governing the control of infectious diseases. "The Law Governing the Control of Infectious Diseases in the People's Republic of China" adopted by the National People's Congress in February of 1989 and the procedure for its implementation as approved by the State Council in October of 1991 are of prime importance to the prevention and control of infectious diseases of the state. Aspects related to the control of HIV include:

(i) It has been specified in the epidemiological reporting system that, whenever an AIDS case is detected, a report must be made to local health authorities within 6 hours from city/ township and within 12 hours from rural areas.

(ii) Measures for the control of pathogen transmission include: establishment of strict managerial and operation procedures in medical health institutions to prevent iatrogenic infection; strict management is applied to the storage, delivery and transportation of virus strains of infectious diseases (management of HIV virus is subject to that applicable to infectious diseases:) and establishment of strict hygienic managerial requirements for the disposal of water and solid wastse contaminated by HIV.

B. Specific Legislations Governing the Prevention and Control of AIDS

Since the detection of the first AIDS case in 1985 in this country, surveillance centres on AIDS have heen set up by health authorities in most of the provinces/municipalities/autonomous regions and the prefectures under its jurisdiction. In order to strengthen its activities, the State Council approved and promulgated, in 1987, "Certain Regulations Relating to the Surveillance and Management of AIDS" as jointly submitted by nine clepartments concerned, including the Ministry of Public Health, the Ministry of Foreign Affairs, and the National Tourism Administration. This is the first legislation specifically formulated for the prevention and control of HIV/AIDS with the following main contents:

(a) Target persons for surveillance are specified;

(b) Serological tests are to be given, upon their entry into this country, to those foreigners applying for residence and /or for a stay longer than one year, and appropriate measures are to be taken by health departments if HIV is detected;

(c) Chinese citizens, having resided.and/or having stayed outside the country for a period longer than one year, are subject to physical examination by health departments concerned within a certain period of time after their return; and

(d) Strict management is applied to blood and blood products as a possible transmission route of HIV.

C. The Management of Blood and Blood Products

Blood and its products are known as an important route through which HIV is transmitted. Health authorities under the State Council have, since the detection of the first AIDS case in China, formulated a series of regulations and notifications including, *inter alia*:

(a) Notification on the Restriction of Import of Blood Products made of VIII factor Products;

(b) Notification on the Strengthening of Management of Imported Blood Products;

(c) Regulations for the Necessary Requirements and Test for Acceptance of Manufacturing Units of Blood Products;

(d) Notification for the Use of Disposable Syringes, Needles, Tubes for Infusion and Blood Transfusion;

(e) Basic Requirements for Blood Banks; and

(f) Managerial Procedure for the Collection and Supply of Blood and its Storage.

D. Quarantine Services at the Border

With the increase of communication with the outside world, the transmission of infectious diseases across borders has constituted an important component of health services of this country. The distribution of the infected population in China is mainly of the following four groups, i.e., drug injectors, venereal disease patients, returnees from abroad either for visiting friends/relatives or for labour assignment. It can thus be seen that two out of the four are those of the returnee groups. Hence, the quarantine services at the border stand at the forefront in the prevention of HIV transmission into the country.

Since the implementation of the "Frontier Health and Quarantine Law of the People's Republic of China" adopted by the National People's Congress in December of 1986 and its plan of action for implementation approved by the State Council in February of 1989, more than 50,000 cases of infectious diseases have heen detected, and of the total, more than 120 are of HIV cases.

According to the Frontier Health and Quarantine Law of the People's Rcpublic of China, the health and quarantine authorities of this country have heen authorised to undertake necessary health and quarantine measures to all incoming and outgoing passengers, transportation facilities, as well as packages, cargoes and postal parcels that could possibly transmit infectious diseases, including HIV.

The Frontier Health and Quarantine Law of the People's Republic of China and its plan of action for implementation specifies the following systems for the prevention of HIV/AIDS:

Epidemiological Reporting System

Whenever an AIDS case is detected, a prompt report shall be made to the health and quarantine authorities. A system of mutual notification shall be established between the health departments and health and quarantine authorities .

Surveillance System of Infectious Diseases

All incoming and outgoing passengers are subject to surveillance for infectious diseases. They are required to fill in the health declaration form and to produce health certificates and other relevant documents. The health and quarantine authorities shall issue a " FOR YOUR HEALTH" card for medical care to those infected passengers and put them under observation.

Control System

The health and quarantine authorities shall apply medical control measures, i.e., isolation of the infected passengers for observation, and shall refuse the entry of any AIDS patient.

E. Women's Rights and Interests, Marriage and Family Life, and Maternal and childrent's Health

HIV brings about grave suffering to anyone infected. Due to their specific status, women suffer the worst and encounter more difficulties. To them being vulnerable in their status, the prevention and treatment of HIV infection cannot be seen merely from a medical point of view, but as an issue that is closely associated with their status in their family and society as a whole. It is to this end that the state has formulated legislation to ensure women's rights and interests and to protect the health of women and children .

Legislation of this country for the protection of women's rights and interests, of women's and children's health, and for the prevention of HIV infection include, *inter alia*:

(i) The state ensures women's equal rights and interests to that of men in political, economic, cultural, social aspects, as well as in family life. This aspect has manifested itself to the full in the Constitution Law, the Law for the Protection of Women's Rights and Interests, the Marriage Law, and the Civil Law of this country.

(ii) The state has established a series of systems to ensure the health of women and children. The Ministry of Public Health has formulated "The Routine Regulations for Health" specifying the establishment of pre-marital health care, health care in the period of pregnancy and delivery, defining duties and responsibilities of health-care providers and its work performance requirements (including the dissemination of knowledge relating to sexology and pre-natal health care), and provision of physical examination and medical treatment.

Prevention of HIV Infection

Sexual behaviour is the most important causative factor for HIV infection of women, while venereal diseases constitute an important factor for women's vulnerability. Hence, the control of venereal diseases is an important link to prevent women from being infected. The state and departments concerned have issued a number of laws and documents in this aspect mainly of the following:

(a) regulations concerning the registration for marriage;

(b) regulations concerning the management of venereal diseases;

(c) provisional regulations governing the surveillance of venereal diseases; and

(d) diagnostic standards of venereal diseases and its treatments.

F. Criminal Legislation

Criminal sanction is the most severe measure the state adopts against unlawful practice. In order to ensure effectively the implementation of the systems and measures established for the prevention and control of HIV/ AIDS, and to curb and crack down the malfeasance and criminal acts that cause the spread of HIV,

Article 178 of "The Criminal Law of the People's Republic of China" stipulates that those in violation of the "Frontier Health and Quarantine Law of the People's Republic of China" are subject to a fixed term imprisonment up to three years and/or detention. Corresponding penal articles are stipulated also in the "Frontier Health and Quarantine Law of the People's Republic of China" and the "Law Governing the Prevention and Control of Infectious Diseases of the People's Republic of China."

Of the 969 HIV carriers, 585 are Chinese nationals, of which 537 are drug injectors residing in the border areas of Yunnan Province. Hence, IV drug users constitute the main threat of the spread of HIV in this country. A resolution was thus reached in December of 1990 by the National People's Congress that penal sentence is to be given to those who cajole, abet, deceive and/or coerce others to take or inject narcotic drugs. Education, compulsive means and/or administrative sanction are to be given to those who take and/or inject the drugs.

Venereal diseases were eradicated as early as the 1960s in this country. However, they have since re-occurred in some large cities and have been rising rapidly in the number of patients and spreading gradually to rural areas. The accumulated number of cases in the period covering 1984-1990 reached 370,000. Venereal diseases also constitute a causative factor to the spreading of HIV. Hence, their control constitutes a link of key importance to the control of HIV transmission. The National People's Congress adopted, in 1991, a resolution to strictly forbid prostitution. A test for venereal diseases and their treatment through compulsive means are to be given to prostitutes, and administrative punishment or penal sanction is to be given depending on the seriousiess of the wrong-doing.

SUMMARY

The number of HIV/AIDS cases in China and its socio-economic impact to the continental part of the country is not yet significant. However, with the increase of its prevalence, more socio-economic problems can be foreseen, i.e., the increase of economic expenditure (the expenses for surveillance and treatment of HIV patients, for eradicating drug addiction and for health education, etc.); the decrease of socio-productivity as the result of increases in the number of HIV carriers; and the protection of people with HIV and AIDS patients (their employment and medical care), etc.

The legislation relating to the prevention and treatment of HIV/AIDS of this country is still at its initial stage and with certain limitations. The established standards are incomprehensive, mainly concentrated on measures for its prevention and treatment. More exploration, investigation and proofing are needed in a number of aspects in the legislation. It is imperative, therefore, to sum-up the experiences both of the positive and negative sides of other countries, and to further emphasise that preventive measures are far more important than remedial measures.

Of prime importance for the formulation of corresponding policies and legal measures is the better understanding of the specific features of HIV/ AIDS, and by approaching it from medical, social, economic and legal points of view. Based on this understanding, the authors are of the opinion that the following measures need to be taken in order to further strengthen and improve the legal and other related measures for the prevention and control of HIV/AIDS:

1. Strengthening of health education to help cultivate a heathy life-style. Health education shall not he limited only to the dissemination of medical/health knowledge, but should also include subjects relating to psychology, sociology, ethics ancl to legal matters, which shall be gradually integrated into the education programme of the country.
2. Revising legislation relating to the rights and obligations of people with HIV and AIDS. In particular, the social status and basic rights and obligations of HIV/AIDS patients are to be defined further in order to alleviate social discrimination of HIV/AIDS patients, and the fear of people with HIV among the society and community.
3. Managerial procedures shall be intensified over the main causative factors for the spreading of HIV such as blood and iatrogenic infection.
4. Legislation relating to maternal health and delivery are to be perfected; a series of health-care systems are to be defined for women from their pre-marital stage until after they give birth to a baby, as well as for infants with an aim to reduce the suffering and adverse effects of HIV infection in women.

29

The HIV/AIDS Situation in the Cook Islands

Mr. Tingika Elikana
Sergeant of Police
Police National Head Quarters
Rarotonga

Ms. Tamarua Herman
Health Educator
Division of Public Health
Rarotonga

Introduction

The Cook Islands consist of 15 islands, scattered over more than 2 million sq km of the south-west Pacific Ocean.

It has a total population of 18,552, of which 10,198 live in Rarotonga, the seat of the local government.

In 1988 the Ministry of Health, assisted by WHO, launched an AIDS prevention programme to limit the spread of HIV and reduce the impact of the infection on individuals and society. A Short-Term Plan was developed for this year followed by a Medium-Term Plan (MTP) for 1990-1994. In April—May 1994, a programme review was carried out to assess the AIDS prevention programme activities.

Nature and Extent of HIV/AIDS Problems

Current Situation

To date, the Cook Islands has reported no HIV infections. There have been a couple of cases in the past when visiting tourists have revealed their HIV status to health workers while receiving medical care in Rarotonga.

HIV Antibody Test

HIV antibody tests have been conducted since 1987. HIV screening has been carried out for blood donors, antenatal cases, STD patients and some out-patients on request at the Rarotonga Hospital the only medical institution with facilities for HIV testing in the country.

Most tests have been on donated blood and samples drawn in antenatal clinics. No specific HIV serosurveillance studies for highrisk groups have been conducted.

Geographical Factors

Although geographical isolation from the rest of the world may have protected the island from HIV transmission, Cook Islands has close contacts with New Zealand, Australia and other countries with higher prevalence. Lifestyles and traditional values especially among your Cook Islanders have undergone rapid changes in recent years.

Since a substantial number of Cook Islanders live overseas, it is likely that those infected with HIV may return to spend the remaining years of their lives in their home islands.

Strategies and Interventions to Prevent HIV Intection

Prevention of Sexual Transmission of HIV

There are three major activity areas in the provision of information, education and communication:

1. Awareness raising and education of the general public;
2. Promotion of safe/safer sexual behaviour among potential high risk people; and
3. Education of school-going youth.

Condoms Procurement and Distribution

Condoms are available free of charge from government pharmacies. They can also be purchased from two private chemists in Rarotonga. A pamphlet entitled 'How to Use Condoms', has been developed and translated to Maori language; it is given with the condoms.

Prevention of HIV Transmission Through Blood

1. The need for blood transfusion is reduced by early

intervention, e.g., maternal anemia is detected through antenatal services.

2. Safe blood supply for transfusion is promoted by the rational and efficient use of blood.
3. Donor recruitment and selection is carried out by the laboratory staff with the assistance of Red Cross Society. Blood donors are mostly family members of the patient. In case of an emergency a small number of blood units are stored in the blood bank donated by the Red Cross.
4. Blood and blood products are routinely screened and tested for HIV, Hepatitis B and VDRL. To maintain confidentiality of the HIV test results a coding system is used. However the recording of the results by the blood system is not satisfactory as the code is entered with the name of the patient and the book is accessible to anybody in the laboratory. It is recommended that HIV test coding should be done by the requesting medical officer to ensure confidentiality.

Promotion of Safe Drug Use Behaviour

There have been no reports of injecting drug use in the country.

Promotion of Sterile Conditions

No specific guidelines for HIV infection control have been developed for health care settings. However, health workers appear to follow universal precautions. Disposable devices are used and equipment is properly disposed. Regular supplies of equipment such as gloves, gowns and instruments are a problem, especially in the outer islands.

Tattooing and other traditional customs do not seem to be of significant importance.

Prevention of Perinatal Transmission

Routine antenatal services include HIV testing. However no preor post-test counselling is provided.

Personal and Social Impact of HIV Infection

The provision of access to health care services for HIV infected persons is being promoted by awareness raising among health workers. This has been a priority area of the AIDS programme. Training workshops on all related issues have been organized for health workers.

Home or community care for HIV infected persons has been discussed at various community AIDS education workshops. However, without a single case of HIV infection, it may be difficult to deal with the issues realistically.

Legal Impact of HIWAIDS

There is no HIV/AIDS-related legislation in the country as yet.

30

HIV/AIDS in Cambodia

Dr. Tia Phalla
National AIDS Committee
Combodia

Situation in Cambodia Regarding HIV and AIDS

As of January 1995, more than 1,000 people in the Kingdom of Cambodia have been reported as HIV infected. The first cases of AIDS in Cambodia were diagnosed in 1994. Two of the patients have since died.

HIV infections were first seen in Cambodia in 1991 among volunteer blood donors, when three donors tested positive for antibodies to HIV. Since then, each year there has been a sharp increase in the numbers infected in this group. In 1994 alone, 401 donors were reported to be HIV positive. This rapid increase in infected cases is also evident among other groups such as commercial sex workers.

Based on the available data it is estimated that at least 6,000 people in Cambodia may be HIV seropositive. However, this is considered to be a conservative estimate.

Contributing Factors

The situation in Cambodia is characterized by large shifts in populations, porous borders, socio-economic disruption and limited public services. These factors have resulted in an increase in the sexually transmitted diseases which are seen as an indicator of

HIV transmission. According to Dr. Michael Merson, Executive Director of the Global Programme on AIDS, a comparison of HIV trends among blood donors suggests that Phnom Penh is likely to experience an even larger epidemic than Chiang Mai, the worst-affected city in Thailand.

The available data suggest that risk behaviour can be characterized as primarily sexual. With economic liberalization, the influx of foreign businessmen, expanding tourism, increase in the number of relief and development personnel and United Nations Peace-Keeping Forces (UNTAC), the commercial sex trade has grown rapidly since 1991. In one commercial sex area alone in Phnom Penh, it is estimated that there are some 1,000-2,000 workers. There are many other such readily identifiable smaller areas in Phnom Penh, in addition to the less obvious locations such as bars, dance halls and massage parlours. Further, there are large numbers of 'indirect' sex workers such as hotel workers, beer and cigarette promotion staff and peddlers who do not work in commercial sex establishments. Outside Phnom Penh the pattern is repeated with commercial sex work growing in economic centres, most notably in the western provinces and in the ports of Sihanoukville and Koh Kong.

While missions to Cambodia by the United Nations International Drug Control Programme and the WHO Programme on Substance Abuse have found no firm evidence of a serious drug problem, they have expressed concern over the potential for such a problem given the proximity of Cambodia to opium producing countries and development trends that could increase drug abuse in the future (urban migration and a limited urban infrastructure and job market to absorb increases in the population).

The preference for injections as a mode of treatment of illness in Cambodia should be noted as a potentially significant route for the transmission of HIV. The use of injections for treatment exceeds the availability of sterile needles and syringes necessitating re-use without sterilization between patients. Also lack of barrier protection places health personnel at risk of infection.

The National Blood Transfusion Centre began screening volunteer blood donors for antibodies to HIV in 1991. Provincial transfusion centres have now been established in nine provinces, but unscreened blood is still being used in certain parts of the country.

Comprehensive National Plan for AIDS Prevention and Control in Cambodia

Overall Objectives

1. To reduce HIV transmission.
2. To reduce the morbidity and mortality associated with HIV infection

The National Plan represents a nationwide effort to prevent and control HIV/AIDS. It addresses programme strategies and specific target areas of implementation for reducing HIV transmission and associated morbidity and mortality. Recommended by the World Health Organization's Global Programme on AIDS to all countries with national AIDS programmes, the strategies have been adapted to the special needs of Cambodia. The Plan, which comes at an appropriate time, can be utilized to mobilize the large number of intergovernmental organizations present throughout Cambodia. There is good potential for a far-reaching and well-co-ordinated control programme.

The Plan concentrates on the following assessed needs for the period 1993-1998:

1. Prevention of sexual transmission.
2. Prevention of transmission through blood.
3. Prevention of perinatal transmission.
4. Surveillance for HIV/AIDS and STDs.
5. Socio-economic impact studies and research.
6. The care and management of HIV infected individuals.

Factors Affecting Programme Implementation

Given that the primary mode of HIV transmission is sexual, prevention and control efforts often require that issues concerning sex be addressed. Cultural and societal norms, however, inhibit open discussion on sexual matters among the population.

In Cambodia, this reluctance can limit the implementation of programme strategies critical to HIV transmission prevention and control such as condom promotion, education campaigns for the general public and specific target groups, including commercial sex workers, and the care and management of sexually transmitted diseases.

Issues about HIV Law

While there is no law or bill yet to protect the rights of HIV infected people, health education materials have been used to dispel the fears, prejudices and misconceptions among the general public. The message of compassion for the infected and of the sense of responsibility of the non-infected have been often stressed on TV, radio and other media. A recently established STD clinic in the centre of a red-light area provides free STD care and health Education information to Commercial Sex Workers (CSWs) -this project was meant to send a signal to the public that CSWs should not be marginalized.

Moreover, the training at central and provincial level for health care workers is designed to make them understand that mandatory testing prior to the provision of medical services is not useful; health care workers should, instead, follow the universal precautionary guidelines to protect themselves from contracting HIV infection. National blood transfusion centres, while seeking blood donors, observe strict confidentiality concerning the identity of individuals found to be HIV positive and arrange for their counselling at the National STD Centre.

Thus, besides legal measures, health education can play an important role in protecting the rights of HIV infected people and in preventing the spread of infection to the non-infected.

Furthermore, since 1993 the Kingdom of Cambodia has adopted a new Constitution which enshrines respect for human rights as defined in the Universal Declaration of Human Rights, as well as the conventions on human rights and the rights of women and children. Thus, future laws regarding HIV to be adopted by the national bodies cannot be in contravention of the national constitution which is the supreme law of the land.

31

HIV Law: The European Scene

Sev S. Fluss
Advisor on Health Legislation to Director
Division of Publishing, Language and Public Services
World Health Organisation, Geneva

1. Introduction and Historical Perspectives

In keeping with its traditional function of compiling, processing, and disseminating information on all aspects of health legislation, WHO's Health Legislation Unit in Geneva has been carefully monitoring all significant regional, national, and subnational developments in the field of HIV/AIDS legislation in Europe. This chapter briefly describes the major legislative and regulatory developments that have occurred during the period 1983-1995. As one reviews the complex legislative scene in late 1995, it is salutary to bear in mind that legislative activity on HIV/AIDS in Europe commenced in the spring of 1983 (less than two years after the first cases of AIDS were described in Mortality and Morbidity Weekly Report). It was on 8 March 1983 that regulations were issued in Sweden by the National Board of Health and Welfare which declared it to be a matter of urgency "to survey suspected and confirmed cases [of AIDS] in order to provide the information needed to determine whether preventive measures are required." (Only one other jurisdiction, the Canadian Province of British Columbia, is known to have introduced earlier provisions on reporting/notification [on 31 January 1983]).

No less noteworthy is the fact that France appears to have been the first jurisdiction to draw attention to what was then described as "the possible transmission of AIDS through blood transfusions." The particular circular was issued by the Directorate-General of Health on 20 June 1983; three days later, on 23 June, the Committee of Ministers of the Council of Europe issued a recommendation (R [83] 8) on the blood safety issue. Governments of the Member States of the Council of Europe were recommended to, *inter alia,* provide all blood donors with information on AIDS, so that "those in risk groups will refrain from donating." It is significant that on 20 January 1984, the European Parliament (an European Community institution) adopted a resolution on "an emergency Community programme of research into and measures to combat AIDS disease"; this included a call on what was then known as the Commission of the European Communities (now the European Commission) to translate the Council of Europe's non-binding recommendations on blood safety into "binding Community law."

Another significant event in this sphere in 1983 was the adoption on 3 November, by the Parliamentary Assembly of the Council of Europe, of Resolution 812(1983) on AIDS. While the term "human rights" does not actually appear in the text of the Resolution, one of the preambular paragraphs reaffirms the Assembly's "unshakeable attachment to the principle that each individual is entitled to have his privacy respected and to self-determination in sexual matters." The Assembly recalled a Recommendation and Resolution, both adopted in 1981, that addressed the issue of discrimination against homosexuals, and expressed its concern at the "inaccuracy in the information circulated on AIDs by some of the media, whose sole concern is sensational news." It emphasized that "campaigns of this kind establish a link between AIDS and homosexuality, so spreading anti-homosexual reactions." This particular text, which appears to have received relatively little attention at the time, was of course the precursor to many subsequent developments, culminating in the Declaration adopted by the Paris AIDS Summit on 1 December 1994.

As early as 16 March 1983, the Federal Ministry for Health and Environmental Protection of Austria issued a Decree containing a series of precautionary recommendations addressed to health and laboratory personnel (corresponding provisions were introduced in Greece by a Circular of 14 July 1983).

WHO has been monitoring the literature on the legal/ethical aspects of the pandemic and, rather surprisingly perhaps, only one book devoted to these issues appears to have been published in Europe during the period 1983-1986.[1]

There have, of course, been many other milestones in the development of HIV/AIDS legislation. Thus, it appears that Austria was the first Europe country to enact (on 16 May 1986) a fairly comprehensive statute on AIDS. Known as the AIDS Law (and amended by laws promulgated in 1989 and 1993), it includes provisions on the following aspects:

- Notification of AIDS cases and deaths from AIDS
- Preservation of confidentiality
- Prohibition on AIDS-infected persons engaging in prostitution
- Screening of prostitutes
- Counselling of seropositive persons
- Approval of diagnostic kits
- Promotion of epidemiological studies on AIDS
- Preparation of a plan of information dissemination
- Funding of institutions and associations concerned with counselling and care in the AIDS context

Provisions on diverse aspects of AIDS research also appeared at an early stage. Thus, as early as 15 October 1983, a Notice was issued in Germany aimed at the promotion of research and development projects concerning AIDS. In what is now Slovakia, a reference laboratory for AIDS was established by a Directive dated 17 January 1984; its tasks included research on AIDS and the coordination of testing for infection.

One of the first European countries to introduce mandatory screening was Austria, as mentioned above. More comprehensive provisions that could be described as "coercive" appeared in the German Land of Bavaria in May-June 1987. The first provisions in Europe concerning HIV in the immigration context appeared to have been introduced by a Notice of 19 May 1987 of the Bavarian Ministry of the Interior, and indeed the same Ministry subsequently issued provisions requiring applicants for posts in the civil service and the judiciary in Bavaria to be tested for HIV infection. Later that year, the Ministry of Health of what was then the USSR issued regulations requiring the following to be tested:

- Blood and tissue donors.
- Nationals returning from assignments abroad of more than one month's duration.
- Aliens intending to reside in the country for more than three months.

- Persons belonging to "high-risk" groups, i.e., recipients of multiple blood transfusions, drug-dependent persons, homosexuals, and prostitutes.
- Contacts of AIDS patients or carriers of the virus identified in epidemiological investigations.

A number of European countries established what are known as "alternative testing sites" at a relatively early stage, notably in response to certain provisions contained in a Council of Europe Recommendation (R [85] 12) of 13 September 1985. What might have been a trend towards the introduction of mandatory testing programmes was to some extent pre-empted by a series of international recommendations, formulated both by WHO and by other European institutions. Thus, an European Community text, dated 15 May 1987, set forth the basis of community policy on various aspects of AIDS. One of the preambular paragraphs emphasized "the inefficacy, in terms of prevention, of recourse to any policy for systematic, obligatory screening, particularly during health controls at frontiers."

Few countries were as early as Norway in developing an integrated programme for the control of AIDS. Thus, a Circular dated 2 July 1985 issued by the Director-General of Health Services addressed the following aspects, *inter alia:*

- Objectives and basic principles.
- Epidemiological surveillance.
- Measures to prevent the spread of infection.
- Ethical issues.

Norway was one of the countries that first addressed the issue of transmission of AIDS in the dental context (a Circular of 7 February 1986 concluded that there was no risk of transmission of the disease from one dental patient to another in the dental care provided under normal conditions of hygiene); particularly comprehensive measures for the control of HIV infection in dental services, and in laboratories, were introduced in December 1986. That country also appears to have been one of the first to have recognized AIDS and HIV infection as "occupational injuries" in the case of health professionals and others engaged in professional activities involving exposure to a risk of HIV infection.

As early as 1987, France and Belgium introduced legislation waiving certain restrictions on the advertising of condoms, as well as provisions designed to facilitate access to clean syringes and needles. In the same year, France established mandatory standards for condoms.

As regards institutional mechanisms, a National Commission for the Co-ordination and Monitoring of Programmes for the Prevention of AIDS was established in Spain in June 1987, by a Decision of the Council of Ministers. A National AIDS Control Commission was established in Italy by a Ministerial Decree issued in January 1987. The first provisions concerning the prescribing of zidovudine (formerly known as AZT) appeared in Austria, the Netherlands and Span in the course of 1987.

One of the European countries to classify infection by what was then known as HTLV-III as a sexually transmitted disease was Iceland (by a Law dated 7 April 1986).

Denmark may well have been the first country (in 1987) that established compensation mechanisms for persons with haemophilia and blood transfusion recipients infected with HIV as a result of treatment in hospitals.

The United Kingdom appears to have been one of the first countries to enact legislation (in 1988) concerning access to HIV-testing kits.

Particularly comprehensive legislation has been enacted in Sweden on diverse forms of potential HIV transmission in the hospital/laboratory context; as an example, detailed provisions were issued in April 1987 designed to prevent the transmission of HIV through infected wastes.

The above are, of course, only examples of some of the forms that early and relatively early legislation on HIV/AIDS took in Europe.[2]

2. Sorne Features of the Current Configuration of HIV/AIDS Legislation in Europe

Space constraints render it impessible to provide more than a necessarily incomplete and non-comprehensive panorama of the legislative situation as it exists in mid-1995. Moreover, a relatively comprehensive overview is in preparation by Cattorini *et al.*, (1995)[3]; in recent years, the literature has been enriched by numerous publications containing information on a country by-country or topic-by-topic basis (Kirp & Bayer[4]; Swiss Institute of Comparative Laws[5]; Foyer & Khaiat[6]; Manuel & San Marco[7]; and Feuillet-Le Mintier[8]).

It must be recognized that the legislative responses to HIV/AIDS from country to country have shown major differences, both quantitatively and qualitatively. The reasons are multiple; one self-evident reason is the fact that measures that require legislative (or regulatory) intervention in one country may be introduced elsewhere without resorting to primary or secondary/subsidiary legislation. This is true for the 15 Member States of the Brussels-based European Union as it is for the 34 Member States of the Strasbourg-based Council of Europe. Perhaps the best illustration of this point is the fact that, at least one country that is a Member State of both institutions, namely Ireland, has so far not introduced legislation of any nature on HIV/AIDS. Legislative intervention in the Netherlands appears to have been limited to three Decrees, all issued in 1987.

The reason why some countries have tended to enact or issue a substantial amount of "hard law" (i.e., statute law and implementing regulations or the equivalent) and others have preferred to rely on "soft law" (i.e., guidelines, circulars, or the equivalent) are grounded in the legal, administrative, social and political traditions and contexts.

This section of the chapter will provide brief comments on some of the legislative provisions introduced during the last few years in selected European countries. These are cited for illustrative purposes only and no attempt is made to elucidate the background to or genesis of particular instruments. Nor is information provided on how the legislation is being implemented in practice, although such information is clearly significant and relevant.

Albania: There are specific provisions on AIDS in Law No. 7761 of 19 October 1993 on the control of communicable diseases. Thus, provision is made for the establishment of a national commission to address issues in the prevention and control of AIDS. Provisions on blood safety require all blood donors to be tested for HIV infection on each occasion when they donate blood. A Resolution of the Council of Ministers, dated 13 March 1995, provides for the free supply of medicaments to persons suffering from AIDS (and undergoing treatment on an out patient basis).

Andorra: An interministerial Commission on the AIDS Prevention and Control Programme was established by a Decree of 23 June 1994; its remit focuses primarily on activities in the field of health education and prevention.

Austria: An Ordinance of 1994 deals in detail with quality control and quality assurance within the context of the diagnosis of HIV infection and on the modalities for carrying out HIV tests; an earlier Ordinance of the same year addressed the issue of evidence of the presence of HIV infection and indicator diseases for AIDS. On the subject of notification, a 1993 Decree pointed out that seropositivity, alone, is not subject to notification.

Belgium: There have been several noteworthy items of

legislation in recent years. For example, provisions requiring testing for HIV-1 and HIV-2 are included in the Law of 5 July 1994 on blood and blood derivatives. An interesting development, at the institutional level, was the establishment (by an April 1991 Decree) of the AIDS Prevention Agency and the Scientific and Ethical Council on AIDS Prevention for the French Community.

Bulgaria: The conditions and procedures governing-testing for HIV infection were established by an Order issued by the Minister of Health on 2 April 1992. Provisions on mandatory testing covered:

1. All blood units obtained from donations.
2. Tissue and organ donors.
3. Sperm donors.
4. Milk donors.
5. Children born from HIV-infected mothers.
6. Foreign nationals and stateless persons spending more than one month in Bulgaria for purposes of study or for professional reasons, and immigrants, irrespective of the length of their stay.

Also included are provisions on voluntary testing (under conditions of strict confidentiality). Health personnel providing care to pregnant women are required to inform them of the risks incurred by the offspring of HIV-infected mothers and to advise them to undergo testing (and, specifically, to have blood withdrawn for the purpose). An order issued two months later, i.e., July 1992, established requirements for the testing of blood products for HIV-1 and HIV-2.

Croatia: A Law promulgated in September 1992 on the control of communicable diseases includes provisions requiring (a) the notification/reporting of cases of AIDS as well as cases of seropositivity for HIV, and (b) all health establishments to test blood, organ, and semen donors for HIV infection.

Dcnmark: The procedures for notlfying (a) AIDS cases and (b) seropositivity for HIV were most recently defined by an Order of December 1993. In April of that year, a Law was enacted providing for the payment of compensation to HIV positive minors, persons contaminated as a result of blood transfusions, etc., (this Law was given retroactive effect from 3 June 1987). Two items of subsidiary legislation (a Circular and Guidelines) were issued in September 1994; these set forth the detailed modalities for the testing of donated blood for HIV-1 and HIV-2.

Estonia: Two items of HIV/AIDS legislation have so far been reported to WHO. The first is the Penal Code of May 1992, which includes a Section (119-2) entitled "Infection by the AIDS virus." The other is a Decree, also issued in May 1992, which established an AIDS Prevention Programme in the Republic.

France: There is perhaps no country in Europe that has witnessed as much legislative activity relating to HIV/AIDS as France. Only a small selection—not necessarily representative—is cited below:

- International co-ordination of AIDS control was addressed in a May 1994 Decree.
- Measures to avert any risk of HIV-1 or HIV-2 infection are included in a Decree of February 1992 (amended in May 1994) designed to prevent the transmission of infectious diseases in the use of human organs, tissues and cells.
- A Circular issued in August 1994 deals with the establishments of an experimental programme for "therapeutic accommodation" for persons suffering from AIDS.
- AIDS control is stated to be an essential requirement of public health—with absolute priority being given to prevention—in another Circular issued in August 1994.
- A whole series of recent legislative texts have addressed the issue of transfusion safety, including the institutional, organizational and administrative aspects.

Germany: There has been little Federal legislation on HIV/AIDS, and legislation at the Land level (other than in Bavaria) has also been limited. The October 1983 Notice referred to above was followed by only two instruments, viz. 1985 Guidelines of the Federal Health Office on the detection of anti-LAV/HTLV-III antibodies in blood, and a Laboratory Notification Ordinance of December 1987 (providing for the anonymous reporting of positive confirmatory tests to the Central AIDS Infection Registry of the above-mentioned Office).

An important recent development was the promulgation, on 24 July 1995, of a law on humanitarian assistance for persons who have become HIV infected through blood products (the HIV Assistance Law). This establishes a foundation known as the "Humanitarian Assistance for Persons who have become HIV-infected as a result of Blood Products". The endowment of the foundation is currently DM 250 million.

Iltaly: Only a small number of the many significant items of HIV/AIDS legislation enacted or issued in recent years can be cited here. They include Decrees of September 1991 and October 1992 of the President of the Republic, which address the issue of the setting up of services for the domiciliary treatment of persons affected by AIDS and associated pathological conditions; a Law enacted in February 1992 which stipulates compensation arrangements for persons who have become HIV infected as a result of the administration of blood or blood products; a series of legal instruments issued in 1992 and 1993 on HIV/AIDS in prisons; a December 1992 Decree requiring all donated blood and plasma units to be tested for HIV-2; and an April 1994 Decree of the President of the Republic adopting the "AIDS Project-Objective for 1994-1996" (which places emphasis on prevention, care, training, co-ordination and research).

Russian Federation: A Federal Law on the Prevention of HIV infection was enacted on 30 March 1995. Particularly detailed provision on "Guarantees by the State" are contained in Section 4. Thus, the following are guaranteed:

- Regular dissemination of information to the population, notably through the mass media, on available means for the prevention of HIV infection.
- Epidemiological surveillance on the spread of HIV infection in the territory of the Russian Federation.
- Development of means for the prophylaxis, diagnosis and treatment of HIV infection; and the control of the safety of medical preparations, biological fluids, and tissues used for diagnostic, therapeutic and scientific purposes.
- Availability of medical testing for the detection of HIV infection (referred to hereinafter as "medical testing"), including anonymous testing, accompanied by counselling before and after testing, and the assurance of the safety of such medical testing both for persons being tested and for persons carrying out the test.
- Free provision of all forms of qualified and specialist medical care to HIV-infected persons who are citizens of the Russian Federation; the free supply of medicaments to such persons within the framework of out-patient or in-patient care; and free transport for such persons to and from the place of treatment within the confines of the Russian Federation.
- Development of scientific research on the problems of HIV infection.
- The inclusion, in the teaching programmes of education establishments, of thematic problems as part of moral and sexual education.

- Social and housing assistance to HIV-infected persons who are citizens of the Russian Federation; and arrangements for such persons to receive training, professional retraining, and work adjustments.
- Training of specialists for carrying out measures for preventing the spread of HIV infection.
- Development of international co-operation and regular exchange of information within the framework of international programmes for preventing the spread of HIV infection.

A Chapter in the Law devoted to "Medical care for HIV infected persons" includes general provisions on testing, followed by specific provisions on voluntary testing, mandatory testing, conditions for the entry of aliens, the consequences of detection of HIV infection, the right to a second medical test, certain rights of HIV-infected persons, and the development of a programme for the prevention, diagnosis, and treatment of HIV infection. Another Chapter deals with "Social protection of HIV-infected persons and members of their families", while the penultimate Chapter addresses the "Social protection of persons exposed to a risk of HIV infection in the performance of their professional duties."

Spain: A Crown Decree of April 1993 laid down that the National Commission for the Co-ordination and Monitoring of AIDS Prevention Programmes serves as the agency responsible for co-ordinating the programmes for HIV/AIDS prevention and control undertaken by the Public Administrations. A Crown Decree-Law issued in May of the same year established a programme of social assistance to persons infected by HIV as a consequence of procedures carried out within the public health system (including HIV-infected persons with haemophilia and blood-transfusion recipients who were treated before compulsory testing for HIV infection was instituted). A special commission—Commission on Assistance to Persons Affected by HIV—was established by a July 1993 Order.

Switzerland: Two fairly recent items of Federal legislation are noteworthy. The first, an Ordinance of February 1993, requires the authorization of the Federal Office of Public Health for the marketing of *in vitro* diagnostic kits, including those intended for the diagnosis of HIV infection. The second, the Ordinance on HIV studies of June 1993, establishes detailed standards and criteria for carrying out epidemiological studies on HIV.

Ukraine: An extensive Law on the Prevention of AIDS and the

Social Protection of the Population was enacted in December 1991. It establishes mandatory testing for *inter alia,* persons engaging in prostitution, and self-injecting drug-dependent persons (as well as aliens under certain conditions). There are provisions intended to safeguard confidentiality. Successive Chapters deal with: (a) the obligations of HIV-infected persons and all persons subject to "medical testing for AIVS; (b) social protection of HIV-infected persons, persons suffering from AIDS, and members of their families; (c) social protection of members of the "medical professions" at risk of being infected with HIV; and (d) liability for violating the legislation on the control of AIDS (this Chapter includes criminal law provisions, reflected in amendments to the Penal Code introduced by another Law promulgated on the same date).

Council of Europe: Two recent Recommendations adopted by the Committee of Ministers should be mentioned. One of these, Recommendation R (93) 6 of 18 October 1993, addresses "prison and criminological aspects of the control of transmissible diseases including AIDS and related health problems in prison [sic]." Details of the principles and policies to be followed in the prison and criminological contexts are formulated in a lengthy appendix. The other, Recommendation R (94) 10 of 10 October 1994, addresses the issue of "early pharmacological intervention against HIV infection." One of the criteria for such intervention is stated to be "full protection of a person's privacy, as well as full respect for a person's free choice."

3. Conclusions

Writing a decade ago, a distinguished former US Assistant Secretary for Health, Edward Brandt (1985), referred to the need for the scientific community to "study this [AIDS] epidemic and the total societal response to it."[9] Legislation is clearly one of these responses and this chapter has sought to demonstrate how the European countries and intergovernmental institutions have addressed the complex and interrelated issues that have arisen over the years. The international context has been, and continues to be, critically important and the various measures and instruments adopted by WHO, and by other entities within the United Nations system, have influenced the current, and constantly evolving, configuration of HIV/AIDS legislation in Europe.

It is highly likely that over the next few years, the human rights and social dimensions of AIDS will play an increasing role in the legislative responses to AIDS by European jurisdictions. It is clear that WHO and the various United Nations bodies that have considered AIDS and AIDS-related issues, have been placing increasing emphasis on these dimensions. It is noteworthy that resolution 1995/44, adopted on 3 March 1995 by the Commission on Human Rights, included a call upon all states:

> "... to take all the necessary steps, including appropriate and speedy redressal of procedures and the introduction of protective legislation and appropriate education to combat discrimination, prejudice and stigma, to ensure the full enjoyment of civil, political, economic, social and cultural rights by people living with HIV/AIDS, their families and associates, and people presumed to be at risk of infection, with particular attention to women children and vulnerable groups, and to address such concerns within their activities in the context of the United Nations Year for Tolerance, 1995."

More specifically, the Commission called upon all States to:

> "... ensure, where necessary, that their laws, policies and practices, including those introduced in the context of HIV/ AIDS, respect human rights standard, including the right to privacy and integrity of people living with HIV/ AIDS, prohibit HIV/AIDS-related discrimination and do not have the effect of inhibiting programmes for the prevention of HIV/AIDS and for the care of persons infected with HIV/AIDS."

In a recent address to the Forty-seventh Session of the Sub-Commission on Prevention of Discrimination and Protection of Minorities of the Commission on Human Rights (Geneva, 31 July—25 August 1995), Peter Piot, Executive Director of the Joint United Nations Programme on HIV/AIDS, stated that:

> "A key part of the multisectoral response is the human rights response. UNAIDS will be a strong advocate for the respect of human rights in the context of HIV/AIDS and will incorporate human rights concerns in all its activities. Furthermore, we intend to develop a partnership between the public health community and the human rights community, and to help ensure that human rights concerns are part of the national response to HIV/ AIDS in every country."

He went on to add that:

> "... the epidemic has forced us to reconsider what 'public health' means in the context of transmissible diseases and

what it means as a valid limitation on human rights. Many of the drastic measures that have historically been directed against sick people in the name of public health are clearly not appropriate or useful in the context of HIV/ AIDS. Only now are these measures being challenged on the basis of human rights. Thus, there is a need to clarify the meaning of the public health limitation on human rights and to subject it to the human rights scrutiny it deserves."

Just 17 years ago, the Lancet published an editorial that contained the following affirmation: "Public-health legislation and related measures have probably done more than all the advances of scientific medicine to promote the well-being of the community in Britain and in most other countriesl.[10]

To what extent has legislation on HIV/AIDS in Europe helped to stem and contain the spread of HIV/AIDS since 1983? The time is, perhaps, not yet ripe to give an authoritative response to this crucial question. What is clear is that many in Europe and elsewhere, will have much to contribute in the years to come in determining what role legislation has played for example in protecting the blood supply and in combating discrimination. It is clear that at least in some countries, the political dilemmas described recently by Rita Sussmuth, a former Minister of Health of the Federal Republic of Germany (1986-88) and currently President of Bundestag, are still on the agenda. In a special issue of the UNESCO Courier (June 1995) devoted to AIDS, Sussmuth poses the following question: Can the epidemic be contained more effectively by coercion or by a liberal policy based on education and individual responsibility?

It is clear that there is an international consensus, indeed a powerful consensus, that the second of these alternatives is the optimal one at this juncture and for the foreseeable future. In other words, most would be in agreement with the affirmation by Porter that "History says no to the policeman's response to AIDS.[11]"

REFERENCES

1. W Eberback. *Rechtsprobleme der HTLV-III Infektion (AIDS).* Berlin (West): Springer-Verlag, 1986.
2. Many of the important items of legislation on the control of HIV/AIDs referred to in this article have been reported in the WHO quarterly journal, the *International Digest of Health Legislation.* The reader is also referred to *Legislative Responses to AIDS.* Dordrecht and Boston: Martinus Nijhoff, 1989. Furthermore, reference should be made to the regularly updated listing, produced by WHO, entitled "Tabular information on legal instruments dealing with HIV infection and AIDS" (the current version of this document, WHO/ GPS/HLE/94.1, was produced in July 1994).

3. Cattorini P. *et al. Comparison and Analysis of European Legislation on AIDS from the Ethical and Legal Standpoint.* Milan: International Research Centre on Ethical, Legal and Forensic-Medical Questions Related to AIDS and Scientific Institute H. San Raffaele. In preparation.
4. Kirp DL. Bayer R., eds. *AIDS in the Industrialized Democracies: Passions, Politics, and Policies.* New Brunswick, NJ: Rutgers University Press, 1992.
5. Swiss Institute of Comparative Law. *Comparative Study on Discrimination Against Persons with HIV or AIDS.* Strasbourg:Council of Europe, 1993.
6. Foyer J., Khaiat L., eds. *Droit et Sida: Comparaison internationale.* Paris: CNRS Editions, 1994.
7. Manuel C., San Marco J-L, eds. *Sida: Les Enjeux Ethiques.* Paris: Doin Editeurs, 1994.
8. Feuillet-le Mintier B., ed. *Le SIDA: Aspects Juridiques.* Paris: Economica, 1995.
9. Brandt EN. Implications of the Acquired Immunodeficiency Syndrome for health policy.—*Annals of Internal Medicine* 1985; 103:771 -3.
10. Anonymous. [Editorial] *The Lancet* 1978; 2:354-5.
11. Porter R. *British Medical Journal* 1986; 293:1589-90.

32

National HIV/AIDS Programme in Fiji Islands

Dr. Salik R. Govind
Acting Director
Primary and Prevantive Health Services
Fiji

BACKGROUND

The Ministry of Health established the National HIV/AIDS Programme in 1988 in collaboration with the WHO Global Programme on AIDS. A Short-term Plan of Action (STP) with the following objectives was implemented successfully in 1989:

1. To prevent HIV transmission.
2. To reduce the morbidity and mortality associated with HIV infection.

The STP was followed by a Medium-term Plan of Activities (MTP) with the following broader objectives:

1. To prevent the further spread of HIV.
2. To reduce the morbidity and mortality associated with HIV.
3. To reduce the social and economic impact of HIV.
4. To stimulate applied research on the social, epidemiological and clinical aspects of the disease.

The MTP covered the period 1990-1995, with funds provided by WHO. Currently, a draft MTP II is being finalized to continue the HIV/AIDS programme upto the year 2000.

EPIDEMIOLOGY

The first case of HIV was reported in 1989 in a woman who had undergone a blood transfusion during her pregnancy some five years earlier. Since then HIV cases have continued to rise. The current total number of cases diagnosed stands at twenty-eight. The majority of the cases (78 per cent) falls within the 20-40 years age group, with males being more commonly infected (M:F=3.6:1). Hetrosexual tr'ansmission has been the most predominant mode of spread (64.2 per cent), followed by homosexual transmission. Perinatal, blood transfusion and IVDU transmission have also been noted.

PROGRAMME MANAGEMENT

The Ministry of Health, through its Primary and Preventive Division, is responsible for the overall implementation of the HIV/AIDS programme. A National Advisory Committee on AIDS with a membership drawn from multiple sectors, governmental and non-governmental, deals with policy formulation and preparation of guidelines on HIV/AIDS activities. A National Programme Coordinator within the Ministry of Health is responsible for the day to day administration of the programme.

PROGRAMME STRATEGIES

To achieve the objectives of both the short- and medium-term plans of activities, the following strategies are being implemented:

Epidemiological surveillance.
Prevention of sexual transmission.
Prevention of transmission through blood and blood products.
Prevention of perinatal transmission.
Case management and reduction of impact.

LEGAL ASPECTS

1. Fiji, as a member of the World Health Organization, has adopted the resolution (WHA 41.24) of the World Health Assembly on the avoidance of discrimination in relation to HIV infected people and people with AIDS.
2. HIV is a notifiable disease, as are other sexually transmitted diseases, under the Public Health Act.
3. Confidentiality regarding patient information and medical records of HIV/AIDS cases are treated in the same way as in other cases under the Hospitals Act.

33

Discrimination Against Persons with HIV/AIDS: Hong Kong's Experience

Ms. Lin-Oi-Chu
Hong Kong AIDS Foundation
Hong Kong

Prevalence of HIV Infection in Hong Kong

In Hong Kong, since the first AIDS case was known 10 years ago, a cumulative total of 520 persons were reported to have been infected with HIV as at the end of December 1994. The government estimates that there are currently 4,000-7,000 people with HIV in Hong Kong. Assuming a straight line increase in this number at the rate of 25 per cent per annum, which has been the average in the past few years, by the year 2000 15,000—27,000 people, or 0.25 per cent - 0.45 per cent of Hong Kong's population will be infected with HIV. The majority of this part of the community are, and for many years will remain, asymptomatic and belong to the young and middle age groups, who are socially and economically active.

Discrimination Faced by People with HIV/AIDS in Hong Kong

People with HIV/AIDS have been subjected to serious, unjustified discrimination in Hong Kong. Not only people with AIDS but HIV positive people who have not yet developed AIDS are often unfairly treated. Following are some of the major areas in which people with HIV/AIDS in Hong Kong are discriminated against:

Medical and Health Care

Many private hospitals and medical and dental practitioners openly or are known to refuse to treat patients who are PWHIV/AIDS. Even in public hospitals there have been instances of the staff refusing to give injections to AIDS patients. The health authorities have publicly announced that the clinical management of AIDS patients requires no major special equipment and that universal blood precautions are adequate for the prevention of HIV transmission in health care settings. There is, therefore, no ground for hospitals or health care workers to reject patients with HIV/AIDS.

Social Services

Most home help service agencies refuse to provide their services to PWHIV/AIDS, even when the service required is only meal delivery or escorting the patient to the clinic or hospital. It has also been reported that some drug rehabilitation service agencies would administer HIV antibody tests on potentiai clients before admission, possibly to screen out those who are HIV positive.

Education

There have been instances in which HIV positive school children were required or requested by the school authorities to discontinue education in the school. While in the last reported incident the Director of Education announced that schools which reject HIV positive students would face sanctions, the findings of a subsequent survey showed that 37 per cent of the secondary school principals and 41 per cent of the teachers thought that infected children should be kept in special schools. A small percentage of the principals and teachers felt that infected children should not attend any school at all.

Work

A major reason why most PWHIV/AIDS want to keep their HIV status strictly confidential is the fear of loss of opportunity to work. There have been incidents of PWHIV/AIDS being dismissed from employment or requested to leave partnerships. A survey conducted in 1992 among a group of executives showed that 21 per cent of the respondents would either resign from the company, if they had a PWHIV/AIDS colleague at their workplace, or ask for a transfer of the positive colleague or themselves.

Accommodation

Loss of living accommodation is another major concern of PWHIV/ AIDS if their HIV status becomes known to others. In a case known to the Hong Kong AIDS Foundation, a landlord who suspected his tenant of having AIDS requested the latter to move out. In another case a relative of a PWHIV/AIDS reportedly threatened, in a family dispute, to disclose the latter's HIV status to a public housing authority, in the erroneous belief that the authority terminates the tenancy of PWHIV/AIDS.

Funeral Service

PWHIV/AIDS face discrimination even after death—most major funeral parlours refuse to provide services for people who have died of AIDS.

Thus, PWHIV/AIDS in Hong Kong face discrimination or threats of discrimination in many major aspects of their daily life. With the number of infected persons steadily increasing, positive measures are needed to deal with the injustice.

Legal Remedies Being Considered in Hong Kong to Deal with Discrimination

Equal Opportunities Bill

The Hong Kong AIDS Foundation has strongly emphasized that HIV/ AIDS aspects should be covered by the Equal Opportunities Bill. Specifically, the AIDS Foundation has urged the establishment of an Equal Opportunities Commission which should be charged with the responsibility to not only handle and adjudicate complaints of discrimination, but also take positive steps to promote the elimination of discrimination in the community. The significance of protecting the identity of the complainant in processing any complaints of discrimination has also been stressed. However, the AIDS Foundation advocates treatment of PWHIV/AIDS on the same basis as people with other disabilities and prefers inclusion of HIV infection in the definition of disability, as is the case in the present bill, rather than specifically mentioning it in separate legislation.

Disability Discrimination Legislation

The Hong Kong Government has announced its intention to enact disability discrimination legislation in 1994-95 and has set into motion the consultative procedure. . At these consultations, the Hong Kong AIDS Foundation and other AIDS related organizations have raised the following points concerning HIV/AIDS:

1. Confidentiality of the complainants.
2. Blood screening—it should be regarded as discriminatory despite that it may be required for all employees or applicants.
3. Difficulty in proving discriminatory dismissal.
4. Prisoners' rights—their rights to lodge a complaint and the power of the proposed Equal Opportunities Commission to investigate complaints relating to correctional institutions.
5. Funeral services, where discrimination is against the deceased.
6. Discrimination based on suspected disability.

34

HIV/AIDS-related Law in India

Anand Grover
Attorney Bombay
India

India has the second largest population in the world of approximately 844.3 million persons, out of which 627.1 million (74.3 per cent) reside in the rural areas and 217.2 million (25.7 per cent) reside in the urban areas. The decedal rate of growth recorded in the 1991 census was 23.6 per cent.

The vast majority of the working population is engaged in agriculture and allied activities (68.8 per cent). Mining and manufacturing account for 13.5 per cent and services for about 17.7 per cent of the working population.

The overall literacy on an all-India basis is 52.1 per cent,63.9 per cent for males and 39.4 per cent for females. The vast majority of children, over 90 per cent, attend primary eelucation.

India is a multi-lingual, multi-ethnic, multi-religious and a multi-cultural nation. Though a large number of people are Hindi speaking (39.9 per cent), there are over 16 different recognised languages and 250 regional dialects. The largest religious group, the Hindus, constitute the vast majority (82.6 per cent). The other religious groups form a substantial minority—Muslims 11.4 per cent, Christians 2.4 per cent, Sikhs 2.0 per cent, Buddhists 0.7 per cent and Jains 0.5 per cent. The historically oppressed castes and tribes recognised by the Constitution as Scheduled Castes and Scheduled Tribes form 23.6 per cent of the population.

India is divided administratively into 22 States (based on

language) and a Union territories which are controlled by the Central Government. Each State and Union territory is divided into districts, totalling 434 districts in the country.

FUNDAMENTAL RIGHTS

India is a sovereign, socialist and secular democratic republic. It is governed by a written Constitution, the longest in the world.

The most important chapter in the Constitution is Chapter III, the fundamental rights chapter. These rights include, among others, Equality before Law (Article 14), Prohibition of Discrimination on grounds of religion, race, caste, sex or place of birth (Article 15), Equality of opportunity in matters of public employment (Article 16), Protection of certain rights regarding freedom of speech, etc. (Article 19), Protection in respect of conviction for offences (Article 20), Protection of life and personal liberty (Article 21), Protection against arrest and detention in certain cases (Article 22), Freedom of conscience and free profession, practice and propagation of religion (Article 25), and Protection of interests of minorities (Article 29).

There are various sources of law in India: the Constitution, customary law, common law, statutory law and rules and regulations framed under various statutes.

PERSONAL LAW

Customary law varies in different parts of the country, even amongst the same religious group. Historically, this was superseded to an extent by religious laws. Thus, with the establishment of the Moghul empire in India, Muslims came to be governed by Muslim Law and Hindus by Hindu Law. This was not confined to personal relations but was also extended to the field of contractual relations and crime. The British, through their policital rule, left some spheres of law untouched, but legislated on certain other spheres. Thus we had the Indian Penal Code,1860, the Transfer of Property Act, 1860, the Indian Contract Act,1872, the Indian Evidence Act,1872, and the Code of Civil Procedure,1908. All these laws were to facilitate trade and commerce for the exploitation of the resources in India. However, laws relating to marriage, divorce, succession, guardianship, custody, etc., known as family law or personal law, remained untouched. There are different personal laws for different religions. After independence, Hindu law was substantially codified and "secularised," as was the Parsi law, though much later. All other religious groups continue to be governed by their "non-secular" personal laws.

THE HIV/AIDS EPIDEMIC IN INDIA

The first HIV positive person was identified in 1986 in Madras. From the surveillance carried out, the HIV prevalence rate was 1.3 per cent in 1990 amongst those screened. High prevalence rates were found in sex workers in Bombay (27 per cent), sex workers forced out of Bombay to Tamil Nadu (over 70 per cent) and amongst IV drug users in Imphal in Manipur State (over 43 per cent).

The first AIDS case was reported in May, 1986. Until December 1991, 104 AIDS cases had been reported. It is estimated that there were about 400,000 HIV positive persons in India in 1990. The projection for the year 2000 is 5 million.

A. PUBLIC HEALTH

1. Notification

There is only one law which provides for the notification of AIDS (Section 51, Goa Public Health Act). In addition, local Municipal laws require every medical practitioner who treats or becomes cognisant of the existence of any dangerous disease to give information of the same to the Executive Health Officer (Section 421, Bombay Municipal Corporation Act). Section 2 of the Epidemic Diseases Act also confers powers on an officer of the State Government, in case of threat of an outbreak of a dangerous epidemic disease, when ordinary provisions of law are insufficient to tackle the disease, to take such measures including prescribing temporary regulations to be observed by the public or any class of persons that may be deemed necessary to prevent the outbreak and/or spread of any such epidemic diseases.

2. Testing, Counselling, Consent

The Goa Public Health Act provides that no person, including a foreigner, shall refuse the collection of blood for investigation of HIV or other communicable/infectious diseases if the Health Officer has reasonable grounds to suspect that such person is infected with HIV or other infectious diseases (Section 53, (1) (vi) Goa Public Health Act). Though other statutes do not empower testing for HIV specifically, the Epidemic Diseases Act confers the power to frame regulations for such a purpose (Section 2, Epidemic Diseases Act). These powers are amenable to challenge under Articles 14 and 21 of the Constitution and remain untested. In states of India where there is no specific statute, consent will be required before any testing can be done.

There is no statutory provision regarding consent for testing. A combined application of the doctrine of unconscionable contracts, Article 14 (Equality clause) and Article 21 of the Constitution (no person shall be deprived of his or her liberty except by procedure established by law) may help in developing the argument that consent has to be informed and supported by counselling services.

3. Confidentially

There is no specific statute providing for medical confidentiality in India. Section 126 of the Evidence Act protects from disclosure, professional communications hetween lawyers and their clients. No such provision exists in the case of doctors. However, the common law doctrine would apply, under which because of the relationship between doctor and patient, the patient reposes confidence in the doctor and passes on all personal and confidential communication to the doctor; the law protects it from disclosure to third parties.

4. Prevention Measures

Preventive measures are contained in local municipal laws, local public health laws as well as in the Epidemic Diseases Act, 1897.

The State Government is empowered, if it is satisfied that the State or any part thereof is visited or threatened with an outbreak of any dangerous epidemic disease if it is satisfied that ordinary provisions of law are insufiicient for the purpose, to take measures which it thinks fit and prescribe temporary regulations that would be required to be observed by the public or any class of persons necessary to prevent the outbreak and spread of such disease (Section 2, Epidemic Diseases Act). It further provides for the inspection of persons travelling by railway or otherwise and the segregation in hospital or temporary accommodation or otherwise of persons suspected by the Inspecting Officer of being infected with any such disease.

Under local municipal laws, every medical practitioner is required to notify the existence of any dangerous disease to the Executive Health Officer (Section 421, Bombay Municipal Corporation (BMC) Act). Persons infected with a dangerous disease can be removed to hospital or other places where other patients suffering from the same disease are received for medical treatment (Section 424, BMC Act). Persons suffering from dangerous diseases can be restricted from entering public conveyances without notice (Section 428 and 430, BMC Act).

There are no special brothel laws or laws relating to partner notification in respect of diseases or HIV.

5. Rights to Medical Information

Article 19(1)(a) of the Constitution provides the right to free speech to all citizens. It has been held that this right includes the right to isnpart and acquire information (See below).

As this right is available against the State and public authorities, the right to medical information is available against medical establishments and officers controlled by the State. There is, however, no specific statute conferring the right to medical information.

B. DISCRIMINATION

Introduction

The Constitution of India is anti-discriminatory and anti-arbitrary in its content. These provisions are contained in the fundamental rights chapter, including equal protection of laws (Article 14), Prohibition of Discrimination (Article 15) and Equal opportunity in matters of public employment (Article 16).

However, Articles 14, 15 and 16 are only applicable to the State and all the local or other authorities controlled by the State, which are considered to be 'State' within the meaning of Article 12 of the Constitution. They do not compel "purely private institutions performing private functions" to comply with the equality provisions.

1. Duty to Treat

Doctors in India have refused to treat HIV and AIDS patients in some institutions, including the All India Institute of Medical Sciences, the premier public medical institute in India.

There is no specific statute or rules or regulations obliging the doctors to treat HIV patients. However, all doctors and medical personnel have a common law duty to treat patients who are brought to them.

The Supreme Court has held that a doctor in a government hospital has an absolute duty to treat a patient to preserve his or her life (Parmanand Kataria v/s Union of India A 89 SC 20.59). But refusal on various grounds is commonplace.

In India, apart from that, in public hospitals, Article 14 will oblige a doctor not to refuse the patient on account of his specific illness and the doctor would be bound to treat the particular person, including an HIV positive person.

2. Accommodation ond Employment

The vast majority of the housing in India is in the private sector. There are no specific laws prohibiting discrimination against any particular individuals on any particular ground in the private sector. However, in the public sector i.e., where housing is built and/or allotted by the government or public sector, corporations or local authorities, the equality and anti-discriminatory provisions of Article 14 would apply.

In private sector employment there are hardly any statutory conditions of service which prohibit discrimination against individuals on the ground of ill health. However, arguments may be developed against the refusal of treating persons with particular ailments unfavourably if they are otherwise fit to carry out their duties. Vis-a-vis employment by the State, the public sector and other authorities controlled by the State, the equality and antidiscriminatory provisions of Articles 14, 15 and 16 would be applicable.

3. Migront Workers/Trovel

With the increased opportunities of employment in different parts of the country, there is large scale migration of population from various parts of the country to the others. So far as citizens are concerned, they have the right to move freely throughout the territory of India (Article 19(1)(d)) and to reside and settle in any part of the territory of India (Article 19(1)(e)). These are fundarnental rights. However, they are not absolute. So far as international travel is concerned, immigration into India of non-citizens is only subject to the non-arbitrary provisions of Article 14. However, despite this, long-term immigrants and students from overseas, unlike short-term tourists, are obliged to produce HIV-free certificates.

C. WOMEN'S ISSUES

1. Stotus within the Family and Society

Traditionally, in Indian families, irrespective of the community, women have had an inferior status to men. India is basically a patriarchial and patrilineal society, except for some parts of South India, particularly Kerala, where there has traditionally been a matrilineal society. Traditionally, in all Indian communities polygamy was common and continues to be so in the rural areas. In the case of Muslims, the law still sanctions polygamy and entitles a man to have four wives. The position regarding the right to inherit is discussed later.

After independence, the Constitution guaranteed equal rights to women in all spheres of public life . In fact, the Constitution sanctions law which may favour women. However, in practice, the situation is not much better for women. Inequality in public employment has been upheld (*Nergish Mirza v/s Air India. A 81 SC 1829*).

That apart, women in India have traditionally been subject to a number of derogatory practices such as dowry, *sati,* domestic violence and cruelty which in modern society have assumed new forms.

Cruelty by a husband or his relatives against the wife has been made a punishable offence (Section 498A, Indian Penal Code). Cruelty has been defined as: (a) any wilful conduct of a nature which is likely to drive a woman to commit suicide or to cause grave injury to life, limb or health (mental or physical) of a woman; or (b) harassment of the woman when such harassment is with a view to coercing her or any of her relatives to meet any unlawful demand or on account of failure to meet such a demand. The offence is cognisable, i.e., the police have the authority to arrest a person against whom a complaint is lodged, without a warrant of a magistrate.

Increasing incidents of rape, particularly in custodial situations, led to the law being amended substantially to provide for enhanced punishment in cases of custodial rape. Moreover, a rebuttable presumption is created to the effect that no consent was taken when sexual intercourse is proved and the woman says that there was no consent (Section 114, A: Indian Penal Code).

2. Economic Rights

Though nearly 50 per cent of the population consists of women, they have much lower access than men to the job market. According to the 1991 census, the work force constituted 37.68 per cent of the total population on an all-India basis. While 35.56 per cent of the male population is in the work force, only 22.73 per cent of the female population is in the workforce.

Economic rights of women in the family set up is discussed elsewhere. However, there is no right to the matrimonial property on the dissolution of marriage. The woman has the right to reside in the matrimonial home only during the subsistence of the marriage.

3. Role as Carers

Though women are the primary carers in the family set up, their rights as carers are not recognised in law to the fullest extent. An indicator in this behalf in the law is the rights of women as natural guardians. In all personal laws, women are not the natural guardians of the children throughout their minority. Amongst Hindus, the natural guardian of the male and the female child is the father. The same position obtains in laws applicable to Christians, Parsis and Jews. Under Muslim law, the mother is the natural guardian of a female child up to the age of puberty and male child only up to the age of seven years; the father is the guardian thereafter.

4. Strategy of Empowerment

The Government has recognised that the crucial factor in hindering development is the illiteracy of women. In this behalf, the total literacy programme has been taken up by the Central Government and State Governments with the help of NGOs to combat illiteracy. Marked success has been reported in some areas, whereas the programme has not taken off in other areas. However, in the realm of law, instead of progressing, the law seems to be taking a step backward, such as in the case of Muslims. Maintenance which was available to Muslim women under the ordinary law has been taken away under the Muslim Women's (Protection of Rights on Divorce) Act. It is, therefore, necessary that, apart from social mobilisation through programmes such as the total literacy programme, laws under which women are treated as second class citizens, particularly in the sphere of personal law, be changed as quickly as possible to give effect to the fundamental right of equality under the Constitution.

D. INFORMATION LAW

1. Right to Information

The Constitution of India guarantees the right to freedom of speech and expression to all citizens (Article 19(1)(a)). It is available only to citizens and against State action but not against private persons.

2. Obstacles to Information

There are as yet no specific statutes, rules or regulations governing HIV informaion. Obstacles to the general right to information would obviously he relevant in this behalf. In this context, it may be pointed out that the right guaranteed under Article 19(1)(a) is not an absolute right. Article 19(2) of the Constitution makes it clear that the right to free speech guaranteed under Article 19(1)(a) is subject to reasonable restrictions that may be imposed by a law in the interests of the sovereignty and integrity of India, the security of the State, friendly relations with foreign States, public order, decency or morality, or in relation to contempt of Court, defamation or incitement to an offence. For our purpose, i.e., regarding the law relating to HIV/AIDS information, a law against 'moral indecency' may be protected under this clause.

There are also specific statutes which restrict the freedom of information. Some examples follow:

a. Under the Official Secrets (OS) Act, 1923, wrongful communications in respect of information which is classified is an offence.
b. Under the Industrial Disputes Act, 1947, confidential information given during the course of adjudication proceedings is protected from being published to any other person, if a party supplying the information makes a request in this behalf.
c. Under the Indian Penal Code, a person is prohibited from publishing anything which would disclose the identity of a rape victim.
d. Sections 123 to 125 and 162 of the Indian Evidence Act protect the State from disclosure of documents and communications which are privileged, and publication of which would be prejudical to public interest.

3. Broadcosting/Censorship lows

In India, all radio broadcasting is under direct State control. Until recently All India Radio was the only radio broadcasting corporation and is bound by its own rules and regulations. These are not publicly available. However, criticism against the government and anything considered to be immoral or indecent is shunned.

The television media, until recently, was also entirely state controlled. Of late, satellite television has made a major entry, and operates largely outside state control.

India has the distinction of having the largest film industry in the world. All films before exhibition are subject to certification under the Cinematograph Act, 1952. A film shall not be certified if, in the opinion of the authority, the film or any part of it is against the interests of the sovereignty and integrity of India, the security of the State, friendly relations with foreign states, public order, decency or morality or involves defamation or contempt of court or is likely to incite the commission of an offence. Guidelines have been framed by the Central Government including a guideline stating that visuals or words depicting women in ignoble servility to man or glorifying such servility as a praiseworthy quality shall not be permitted. Moreover, the authority is to ensure that the film is examined in the light of contemporary standards of the country and the people to which the film relates.

4. Obscenity Laws

Section 292 of the Indian Penal Code makes the sale, hire, distribution, exhibition or circulation of obscene books, pamphlets, paper writings, drawings, paintings, representations, figures or any other objects and for that purpose possession of the same a punishable offence. Import or export for the aforesaid purposes, receiving profits from such ventures, advertising for such purposes or attempting to do such acts is also punishable. 'Obscene' is defined as that which is lascivious or appeals to the carnal interest or tends to deprave or corrupt those to whom it is addressed. However, exceptions are made if the publication is for scientific, literary, higher learning, or bonafide religious purposes or that which is sculpted, painted, depicted or represented on ancient monuments or temples.

Section 293 of the Indian Penal Code makes the sale of obscene objects to young people punishable, while Section 294 of the Indian Penal Code makes the commission of an obscene act and/or singing or reciting or uttering of an obscene song, ballad or words in or near a public place punishable.

5. Sex Education

There is no specific law pertaining to sex education. However, the *Strategic Plan For The Prevention And Control of AIDS* of the Government of India talks of the development of teaching material on sexuality and responsible behaviour for school children, youth in colleges and outside, as well as adult learners. The challenge, it points out, is to initiate a dialogue between teachers, parents and children on sex without moral overtones and without at the same time appearing to be supporting promiscuous or permissive behaviour.

E. FAMILY AND CARERS

Family laws and law relating to care and custody of children in India is governed by different personal laws. These are basically laws of various communities such as Hindus (Buddhists, Jains and Sikhs are also clubbed as Hindus), Christians, Muslims and Jews. All such communities have different laws relating to inheritance, marriage and divorce, maintenance, guardianship, custody, adoption, etc., i.e., family law or personal law.

1. Inheritance

(a) HIndu Law

In traditional Hindu law, a Hindu woman had a limited right to property. Although she could receive property either by gift or inheritance, she had no right to pass it on by will or any other means. This was changed under the Hindu Succession Act, which lays down that any property held by a female Hindu, whether acquired before or after the commencement of the Act, shall be held by her as a full owner and not as a limited owner (Section 14, Hindu Succession Act).

(b) Christians, Jews and Parsis

In India, Christian, Jews and Parsis are governed by the Indian Succession Act, 1925. There are separate rules for Parsis, Christians and Jews.

In the law regarding to Christians andJews, there is a distinction when a person dies intestate and has left a widow with lineal descendants or a widow and kindred or widow and no kindred. Specifically, when an intestate leaves a widow and lineal descendants, she gets one-third share and the two-third share goes to the lineal descendants. When there are no lineal descendants, the whole of the property goes to the widow. A widower has the same rights as a widow.

(c) Parsis

For all purposes there is a distinction in devolution of property intestate amongst the male and female heirs. In cases of male intestate leaving behind a widow and children or leaving behind no widow, but only children, the widow and the sons get double the share of the daughter, if the widow survives. On the other hand, in the case of a female Parsi dying intestate the widower and the sons and the daughters get equal shares. In other words, the property of the male Parsi preferrentially devolves on to the male lineal descendants.

(d) Testamentary Succession

Personal laws of all communities provide for the devolution of property by will. The whole of the property of the deceased can be willed away. However, the will has to be in writing and attested in accordance with the rules. In the case of Muslims, no Muslim can dispose of more than one third of the estate by a will.

2. Divorce and Separation

Again, different personal laws apply to different communities.

(a) Hindus

The law regarding marriage, divorce and separation is governed by the Hindu Marriage Act, 1955, (HMA). The conditions for a valid Hindu marriage inciude that the two parties must be Hindus, that neither is incapable of giving valid consent, and the man is at least 21 years and the woman 18 years of age.

Divorce and separation is available both to the husband and wife on various grounds, which includes adultery or cruelty or desertion for a period of not less than two years or conversion to another religion; or if the party is incurably of unsound rnind, or suffers from a mental disorder such that the other party cannot reasonably be expected to live with him or her; or if one party suffers from a virulent and incurable form of epilepsy or has been suffering from a venereal disease in a communicable form; or if one party has renounced the world by entering a religious order or has not been heard of being alive for a period of seven years (Section 13 HMA).

The wife has some other additional grounds, viz., if her husband has heen guilty of rape, sodomy, bestiality, or that an order of maintenance passed under various statutes has not been honoured, or the parties are living apart and cohabitation has not been resumed for a period of one year after the order.

Both parties can also obtain divorce on the ground of mutual consent (Section 13-B, HMA).

(b) Chrislians

The law for divorce and separation of Christians is based on the antiquated English law of the 19th Century. Whereas the husband can obtain divorce on the sole ground of adultery, the wife cannot obtain divorce only on that ground. The ground of adultery for a woman has to be coupled with one of the grounds which by itself is sufficient for a man to obtain divorce, viz. bigamy, incestual relationship, desertion, cruelty, change of religion, or rape, sodomy or bestiality (Section 10, Indian Divorce Act, 1869).

However, judicial separation can be obtained both by the husband or the wife on the ground of adultery or cruelty or desertion without reasonable excuse for two years or more (Section 22, Indian Divorce Act, 1869).

(c) Parsis

Parsi marriages and divorces are governed under the Parsi Marriages and Divorce Act, 1936.

Marriages can be annulled on the ground of impossibility of consumation of the marriage. Divorce is available on grounds very similar to those under the Hindu Marriage Act. Like in the Hindu Marriage Act, a party can sue for divorce if the spouse is suffering from an incurable venereal disease. Additionally, refusal to have marital intercourse for a period of two years after a Magistrate's award for maintenance is a ground for divorce.

(d) Muslims

Marriage and divorce under Muslim Law in India is in accordance with the Shariyat. Marriage in Muslim law is a contractual relationship for which a deed, a *nikahnama,* is drawn up setting out the conditions for the marriage. A Muslim man can divorce his wife unilateraly; the presence of the wife is not material. Divorce or *talaq* can be oral or in writing. Divorce by mutual consent is also recognised. Conversion to another religion *ipso facto* dissolves the marriage.

A woman can get a divorce under the Muslim Dissolution of Marriage Act, 1937. The grounds available include, among others, the whereabouts of the husband not being known for a period of four years, the husband neglecting or failing to provide maintenance, the husband being importent at the time of marriage and at the time of the petition, or the husband being insane or contracting a venereal disease.

(e) Special Marriage Act, 1956

Persons of different religions in India can marry under the Special Marriage Act. The grounds for divorce are practically identical to the grounds available under the Hindu Marriage Act. The main difference is the conditions of a valid marriage. Both parties need not be Hindus. The Act provides, like the Hindu Marriage Act, for the marriage to be declared void or voidable as well as for judicial separation. Divorce can also be obtained on the ground of mutual consent. Significantly, divorce is also available on the ground of the spouse suffering from a venereal disease in a communicable form.

3. Maintenance

Maintenance is available for both the spouses, i.e., husband and the wife, during the pendency of the marriage as well as on and after the dissolution of the marriage. It also depends on the religion that one belongs to. Apart from Muslim personal law, all the other personal laws mandate maintenance during the pendency of the marriage as well as on and after the dissolution of the marriage.

In addition to maintenance provided under various marriage and divorce and maintenance laws, under Section 125 of the Code of Criminal Procedure, 1973, old parents, women and children of a person having sufficient means who are unable to provide for themselves are entitled to maintenance from that person. The idea is to prevent vagrancy. By virtue of the passing of the Mulim Women (Protection on Divorce) Act, Mulims were taken out of the ambit of these provisions.

4. Age of Marriage

All laws relating to marriage provide for a minimum age for marriage; the woman is required to be 18 years of age and the man 21 years of age. There is no statutory law which requires a minimum age for a Muslim man or woman to get married. Under Muslim law the parties have to be able to have the capacity to enter into a contract of marriage i.e., attaining puberty.

5. Age of Consent end Non-consensual Sexual Intercourse

There is no legally defined age for consent to sexual intercourse under different personal laws. However, statutorily, under the Indian Penal Code, it is an offence of rape if a man has sexual intercourse with a woman under 16 years of age. However, if she happens to be his wife, it is not rape to have sexual intercouse with her after she attains the age of 15 years.

Punishment has now been increased for custodial rape. Moreover, under the Indian Evidence Act, a rebuttable presumption is created whereby in a prosecution for rape, when sexual intercourse by the accused is proved and the question is whether she has consented or not, if a woman states that she did not consent, the court is required to presume that the sexual intercourse took place without her consent (Section 114-A).

6. Termination of Pregnancy

Until 1971, the law relating to abortions was exclusively governed by the Indian Penal Code. Under that Act, anyone causing a miscarriage is, unless it is done in good faith to save the life of a pregnant woman, liable to imprisonment for three years.

Under the Medical Termination of Pregnancy (MTP) Act, 1971, the position changed radically, the effect being to legalise abortions carried out under the conditions specified under the MTP Act.

Pregnancy under the MTP Act is allowed to be terminated:

(a) if it is less than 12 weeks old on a certificate of one registered gynaecologist or obstetrician;

(b) between 12 and 20 weeks, on a certificate of two registered gynaecologists or obstetricians;

(c) the pregnancy would involve a risk to the life of the pregnant woman or cause grave injury to her physical or mental health; or

(d) there is a substantial risk that the child, if born, would suffer from physical or mental abnormalities so as to be seriously handicapped.

Anguish, either caused by pregnancy because of rape of a woman or caused by a failure of contraception by a married woman, is presumed to constitute grave injury to the mental health of a pregnant woman.

F. PRISONS AND INSTITUTIONS

1. Testing

There are no specific provisions for testing of HIV in prisons. However, as soon as possible after admission the prisoner is required to be examined medically. A record of the state of the prisoner's health is required to be kept in a register meant for the purpose.

It is not known how many prisons have the facilities to carry out testing of HIV. A question may arise, in view of the statutory provision (Section 24, Prisons Act), whether a non-consensual HIV test can be conducted in prisons. In this respect, great advances have been made in the law by decisions, particularly of the Supreme Court, which lay down that:

(i) prisoners retain all rights enjoyed by free citizens except those lost necessarily as an incident of confinement;

(ii) a prisoner wears the armour of basic freedom, even behind bars, and on, breach . . . the law will respond to his distress;

(iii) the right to life enshrined in Article 21 cannot be restricted to mere animal existence, and includes the right to live with human dignity and the bare necessities of life such as adequate nutrition, clothing and shelter over the head and facilities for reading, writing and expressing themselves in diverse forms, freely mixing and co-mingling with fellow human beings.

2. Segregation

Various prison manuals provide for segregation of prisoners who are suspected of having skin infections, or a contagious disease. Some prison manuals also require that certain categories of prisoners be kept together in a group to enable daily medical checks. These include:

a. permanently infirm prisoners;
b. prisoners discharged from hospitals and who are convalescing;
c. prisoners generally in poor health;
d. prisoners losing weight without any apparent reasons.

3. Counselling, Care and Support

All prisons have visitors. These include magistrates or district and sessions judges who have the right and duty to visit prisons and inspect them. They also hear prisoners' grievances. However, it is difficult to say whether the system works effectively. Prisoners also have access to the High Court and the Supreme Court through public interest petitions, mostly in the form of letters, ventilating their grievances. These worked quite well in the late seventies and early eighties when the Supreme Court had an activist judiciary. Most of the cases cited above developed in this manner.

Apart from counselling, care and support that may be bestowed by the medical officer and the medical team, few jails have institutionalised systems of counselling, care and support. Some jails have developed informal liaisons with social welfare and academic institutions whose visitors provide some counselling, care and support. However, this tends to be an exception rather than a rule.

G. EMPLOYMENT ISSUES

1. Introduction

Terms and conditions of employment in India are primarily contractual. However, they are largely superseded by terms and conditions of service imposed by statute. In areas where statutes are silent, common law applies. The precise terms and conditions depend on whether an employee is in Government, the public sector, the private sector, in an industry or in other sectors. For Government servants, the terms and conditions are entirely regulated by statutory and non-statutory rules framed under Articles 309 and 311 of the Constitution. Industrial establishments employing more than 100 workmen are covered by the Industrial Employment (Standing Orders) Act, 1946. Employees employed in an "industry" are covered under the Industrial Disputes Act, 1947.

Maharashtra has an additional Act, viz., the MRTU & PULP Act which allows both the employer and the employee to file a complaint in the Labour Court and Industrial Court alleging an unfair labour practice on the part of the other.

2. Work Place Testing

There is no statutory requirement for testing of HIV. However, an employee is required to be medically fit to carry on his or her employment. In fact, terminating the services of a workman on the ground of continued ill-health does not constitute retrenchment under the Industrial Disputes Act (Section 2(oo) (c) of the Industrial

Disputes Act). Under the general requirement of medical fitness, employers may test persons for HIV. However, there is no clear-cut policy being followed in this behalf. At the moment, only defence personnel are being 'regularly' tested for HIV.

3. Polides for HIV Infected Employees

There are no specific policies for HIV-infected employees. The Strategic Plan for 1992-96 of the Central Government makes it clear that the general policy is for the prevention of stigmatisation and discrimination of people with HIV through protection of confidentiality and partner notification. Under this general rubric it is presumed that the policy at the work place would be to not discriminate against HIV positive persons. However, unless there is a separate statute mandating this, it cannot be enforced.

4. Occupational Health

Both the Workmen's Compensation Act (Section 3) and the Employee's State Insurance Act (Section 52-A) provide that if employees in employments specified in the Schedules to the Acts contract a disease peculiar to the employment after being engaged in such employment for a specified period, the disease is deemed to be an 'employment injury' arising out of the course of employment for which compensation is payable. However, the rates of compensation are still low.

H. CRIMINAL LAW

Introduction

Under the Constitution of India, no person (citizen or non-citizen) shall be deprived of his life or liberty except according to procedure established by law (Article 21).

Further, no person can be detained in custody without being informed as soon as may be of the grounds of his arrest (Article 22 and Section 50, Code of Criminal Procedure). The person is entitled to be consulted and to be defended by a legal practitioner of his choice (Article 22). He or she is further entitled to be informed by the police of his or her right to bail in case of arrest in connection with a bailable offence (Section 50, Code of Criminal Procedure) .

Criminal law (substantive and procedural) in India, like in all common law countries, is based on the accusatory system as opposed to the inquisitorial system. The burden is entirely upon the prosecution to prove its case beyond reasonable doubt.

Unlike other common law countries, confessions to the police officer or made in police custody are not admissible in evidence and cannot be proved against the accused (Section 25 and 26, Evidence Act). Horvever, confessions which lead to a discovery of fact but only to the extent that they relate to the discovery of the fact are admissible (Section 27, Evidence Act). Confessions admissible are those made before a magistrate and made in the manner provided.

1. Transmission Offenses

There are no specific offences for transmitting HIV. However, a large number of offences ranging from murder and hurt to nuisance may be attracted depending on the facts and circumstances of the case. As transmission of HIV may cause death or hurt (grievous or simple), transmitting HIV with intention of causing death or hurt, or with the knowledge that it is likely to cause death or hurt, may attract the offence of murder (Section 302, Indian Penal Code), voluntarily causing hurt (Section 323, Indian Penal Code) or voluntarily causing grievous hurt (Section 325, Indian Penal Code). On the other hand, if the transmission is caused rashly and/or negligently, another set of offences may be attracted, via. Section 304 A, Indian Penal Code (causing death by a rash or negligent act), Section 336, Indian Penal Code (any act done rashly or negligently endangering human life or personal safety of others), Sections 337, and 338 IPC (causing hurt or grievous hurt to a person by any act so rashly or negligently performed as to endanger human life or the personal safety of others).

Moreover, under Section 133, Code of Criminal Procedure (for removal of nuisance), any person conducting any trade or occupation injurious to the health of the community can be prohibited from doing so by an order of a magistrate.

2. IVDU

There is considerable intravenous drug use in India, particularly in the North-Eastern States, bordering Myanmar. A large number of drug injectors have been found to have also contracted HIV.

The *Narcotics Drugs and Psychotropic Substances (NDPS) Act*, 1985 regulates as well as prohibits certain operations, viz., the cultivation, production, manufacture, possession, sale, purchase, transport, warehousing, use, consumption, inter-state movement;

import into and export out of India and the trans-shipment of drugs and narcotic substances. Unlike under ordinary criminal procedure, the NDPS Act provides that a statement made and signed by a person before a competent officer in the course of investigation is admissible in evidence if the court finds that it would be in the interest of justice, to do so. Also, a rebuttable presumption arises that the accused has committed an offence of possession if the accused is found in possession of a drug or a psychotropic substance.

3. Sex Workers

The Prevention of Immoral Traffic (PIT) Act, 1956 deals with sex workers. The Act was originally enacted in 1956 and dealt only with women and girl prostitution However, major changes were brought in by the 1986 amendment The Act now covers the sexual abuse and exploitation of both females and males, adult and children. Brothel keeping as well as abetment of brothel keeping are offences. Prostitution by itself is not an offence. However, living off the earnings of a prostitute, carrying on prostitution in a public place, abetting prostitution, soliciting or seducing for the purposes of prostitution are all punishable offences. Stringent punishments are liable to be meted out in the case of use of minors in prostitution. The presence of children in a brothel creates a rebuttable presumption that an offence of detention is committed. And if on examination the child is found to have been sexually abused, a rebuttable presumption is again created that the minor is detained for the purposes of prostitution.

4. Homosexuals

Traditionally, in India, homosexuality has been tolerated. The Kama Sutra contains an entire chapter entitled *Auparishtaka* (oral congress) on the subject. Vatsayana, its author, contends that the practice is permitted by the *Dharma Shastras* (religious scriptures). On the other hand, the Manu's Smritis (Manu's laws) prescribed severe punishment for male and female homosexuality. One of the forms that Shiva is worshipped is *Ardhanarishwara* (half-female god) containing both the male and female forms of energies.

The British with their Christian values obviously did not take kindly to the practice. Section 377 of the Indian Penal Code was enacted, dealing with 'unnatural offences' and provides 'that whoever voluntarily has carnal intercourse against the order of nature with any man, woman or animal' is punishable with imprisonment for life or ten years with or without a fine. The explanation to the Section provides that 'penetration' is sufficient to constitute carnal intercourse.

Though the vague definition of 'carnal intercourse against the order of nature' has been a subject matter of great debate, it has been held to include acts of oral as well as anal sex. Consent, of course, is irrelevant. Though the Section applies both to homosexual and heterosexual anal and oral sex, there are no reported cases of heterosexual anal or oral sex under this provision. A fair body of case law that exists shows that the vast majority of persons have been convicted for non-consensual acts of sodomy. Very few cases of consensual sodomy and none of oral sex between gay men have been brought to trial. However, the provision gives the police enormous powers to harass and blackmail the already stigmatised homosexual community.

I. THE LEGAL PROCESS

India is a common law country. The adversarial system prevails in civil litigation. The procedure followed in civil courts is laid down in the Code of Civil Procedure.

The accusatory, instead of the inquisitorial system, prevails in the criminal field. It is entirely up to the prosecution to prove its case beyond reasonable doubt. However, the burden shifts according to the evidence led or on the basis of rebuttable presumptions that are statutorily created under the Evidence Act. The accused has the right to remain silent and is always presumed to he innocent until proved guilty.

1. Legal Aid, Access to Low

The vast majority of the Indian population do not have access to the legal system. However, they are affected, more often than not adversely, by the legal system. Under the Advocate's Act, lawyers have a right to practice in all courts, tribunals and authorities to represent their client (Section 30, Advocate's Act, 1961). Though parties can appear in person, with complex substantives laws and even more complicated procedural laws and rules, it is advisable for litigants to be represented by lawyers. However, good lawyers are always available at a high price. Therefore, the poor are priced out of good lawyering.

The need for legal aid has been recognised by the Constitution (Article 39A). The right to legal aid has also been recognised as a fundamental right under Article 21 in various decisions of the

Supreme Court. However, except for criminal cases, there is no statutory right to legal aid.

Parliament has enacted the Legal Services Authority Act, 1987 to provide for legal aid and advice. However, that Act has still not been brought into force. A public interest petition filed in the Supreme Court has also not come up for hearing till today.

2. Acting for Someone with HIV

Very few HIV positive persons have gone to court. On the limited experience available, no guidelines can be worked out. However, given that a person with HIV is always conscious of the terminal nature of the illness, the positive person is very often demoralised, despondent and not very responsive or enthusiastic about his/her case. Thus, an HIV client has to be handled in a more sensitive and empathetic manner than an ordinary client would be handled. These are qualities that are essential in someone acting for someone with HIV. Moreover, the person acting for the person with HIV will also be required to take more initiative than an ordinary lawyer.

35

Law and Law Reform for HIV Prevention and Control in Indonesia

Dr. Herkutano
University of Indonesia
Indonesia

HIV Epidemic in Indonesia

Indonesia's first AIDS case was identified in 1987. By February 1995, 69 cases of AIDS out of 283 HIV positive people had been reported. However, WHO has estimated 50,000-60,000 cases -this suggests that the increase has been far more dramatic.

The development of the HIV epidemic in Indonesia has followed a pattern found in other Asian countries, i.e., appearing first in the homosexual community, and later in people in situations of risks, such as commercial sex workers, their clients and intravenous drug users. Ultimately, it has spread throughout the population, infecting both men and women. The largest percentage of infected people (96 per cent) is found in the productive age group (15-49 years). Sexual transmission is the primary mode of infection. Eighty per cent of the cases are assumed to be infected through this mode (55 per cent heterosexually and 25 per cent through homosexual and bisexual contact).

While the total number of reported HIV/AIDS cases is considered small, the reports have originated from 17 out of 27 province in Indonesia and cover all the socio-economic strata. Risk factors that contribute to the swift spread of HIV infection are present in Indonesia, i.e., a widespread commercial sex industry, high rates of sexually transmitted diseases (STDs), low awareness of STD and HIV infection prevention, high labour migration, and the prevalence of premarital and extramarital sexual activities.

AIDS Strategy in Indonesia

In 1986, even before the first case was found, the Indonesian government formed the National AIDS Commission. This was reorganized into the AIDS Prevention and Control Commission in 1994 through a Presidential Decree. The Commission is headed by the Co-ordinating Minister for People's Welfare, and consists of several ministers and other heads of government institutions.

A National AIDS Strategy was launched in June 1994. It provides the framework and guidelines for all preventive and control activities. It states that the government has the responsibility to lead and guide the efforts and to help create a supportive environment. Some important principles of the strategy, among others, are that all approaches should reflect the religious and cultural values found in Indonesia; all activities should mainly aim to strengthen the resilience and welfare of the family and the traditional social support systems rooted in the community; and that there should be no discrimination in providing services to people living with HIV infection, whose dignity and self-respect should be promoted and preserved.

An important step taken in February 1995 was the promotion of the concept of AIDS Conscious Prosperous Family. The government is of the view that the HIV epidemic awareness campaign should begin with the family because it is the first and foremost institution in forming people's attitudes and behaviours, including those pertaining to sexual matters; family is the basic institution for instilling religious and traditional national values. According to the Minister of Population, the number of AIDS conscious families to date is only 1,000-2,000, out of 40 million families (Kompas, 7 February 1995). Various programmes are being planned to increase this number.

Legal Developments Relating to the HIV Epidemic in Indonesia

Since the HIV epidemic is a relatively new problem in Indonesia, there are only a few laws and regulations that directly deal with it. Since the first reported AIDS case in 1987, several ministries, and the President himself, have enacted various law and regulations relating to the HIV epidemic.

In 1987, the Minister of Health (MOH) enacted Decree no. 484/ 1987 to establish a National AIDS Committee. This Committee was limited to representatives from various sectors in the Ministry of Health. In 1988 the MOH designated HIV/AIDS as a notifiable communicable disease and established guidelines for the reporting of AIDS and HIV positive cases. In 1989 the MOH enacted a new Decree - no. 301/1989 - to reorganize the National AIDS Committee.

The Director-General of Communicable Disease Control and Environmental Health of the MOH issued circular No. 5 of 3 January 1991 containing guidelines to be followed by port health authorities, indicating that HIV/AIDS infection should not interfere with international/tourist travel. In the same year, the Director-General - in his capacity as Chairman of the National AIDS Committee—also issued Decree no. 61/1991 which provided for the appointment, within the National AIDS Committee, of technical advisory groups dealing with health education, case management, surveillance, laboratories and blood banks, and research.

Between 1990 and 1992, some newly-enacted laws, e.g., Health Law and Immigration Law, had already covered the issue of HIV/ AIDS. In the same period the Minister of Health issued technical guidelines on the care of AIDS patient. In 1993-94, the President of the Republic of Indonesia issued a Presidential Decree on the National AIDS Prevention and Control Commission. The status of this Commission has been upgraded from ministerial level to the national level. In July 1994, the Co-ordinating Minister for People's Welfare, in his capacity as the Chairman of the Indonesian National AIDS Commission, released the Indonesian National AIDS Strategy. The strategy covers basic principles, programme areas, roles and responsibilities of the government and the community, international co-operation and financing.

The latest legal measure relating to the HIV epidemic is the Decree of the Co-ordinating Minister for People's Welfare/Chairman of the National AIDS Commission, No. 05, 22 February 1995, on the National HIV/AIDS Prevention and Control Programme for the Sixth Five year Development Plan. The programme for 1995-99 includes issues relating to information, education and communication, prevention measures, HIV testing and counselling, treatment, care and other health services, research and development, monitoring and evaluation, training, international cooperation, institutionalization, and laws and regulations. The section on each issue includes targets, strategies, activities, output indicators and coverage in units per year.

Besides the above law and regulations which directly related to the HIV epidemic, there are others which are indirectly related, e.g., the law on communicable disease control. Since it was enacted in 1984, HIV infection is not mentioned. The law, therefore, needs to be amended considering that the HIV epidemic is a new and developing social issue that can, among other things, pose a threat to human rights.

The legislative measures should cover all the issues emerging from the prevention and services efforts, as well as ensure protection for the community. The objectives of the Prevention Component of the National HIV/AIDS Prevention and Control Programme for the Sixth Five year Development Plan are: (a) to provide aid services and information for preventing the spread of HIV infection; (b) to provide and develop services for preventing and controlling STDs; (c) to perform screening procedures to prevent HIV infection through blood and blood products; and (d) to provide medical services that implement universal precautions.

Legislation should be enacted to deal with specific issues such as the provision of STD diagnostic and treatment facilities; standard procedures for applying HIV prevention measures including universal precautions; the procedures for blood and blood products screening; and the provision of health services to people living with HIV/AIDS without discrimination and stigmatization.

The objectives of the services component of the National HIV Programme are: (a) to provide facilities and continuing humane and non-discriminative treatment and care; (b) to ensure individual health and security for those who provide services to people with HIV/ AIDS in health facilities; (c) to develop skills and commitment at the family and community level, in providing services and care to people living with AIDS; (d) to create and develop laws and legislation relating to the standards of care and case management, which should be ethical, technically accurate, non-discriminatory and humane. Laws and regulations which may support these objectives include regulations on hospital standards of care for HIV/AIDS patients, non-discrimination in labour and education sectors, and a supportive insurance system for people living with AIDS.

These legal measures should also cover various issues arising from the implementation of the National HIV Epidemic Prevention and Control Programme, e.g., blood and blood products screening, blood testing, assistance to infants living with HIV, and counselling.

In conclusion, the upcoming reforms and new legislative texts should support the three approaches in the National AIDS Strategy:

(a) religious and cultural approach, (b) family function approach, and (c) public health approaches, which acknowledge public interest as well as individual rights. All laws and regulations should ensure protection for the entire community—the ones who are living with HIV/AIDS, the health providers, as well as the general community. However difficult it may be, attempts should be made to balance public interest and individual rights.

Finally, information on legal matters pertaining to HIV/AIDS should be made available among all levels of the government and its various sectors, and the general community throughout the country. The role of the press is crucial, as is of the law enforcement officers who should also be well-informed and skilled in dealing with legal cases relating to HIV/AIDS.

36

The Ethical and Legal HIV/AIDS—Related Issues in Indonesia

Djumhana Sumantri
Director
Department of Directly Transmitted Disease Control
Ministry of Health
Indonesia

Background Information

The Republic of Indonesia, lies between the Asian and Australian continents, and is an archipelago consisting of 13,000 islands. The unevenly distributed population lives in about 6,000 islands, particularly in five big islands: Sumatera, Java, Kalimantan, Sulawesi and Irian Jaya. The total population in 1993 is about 187 million, with more than 60 per cent living inJava island which is only 6 per cent of the total land area. As the fourth biggest nation in the world, Indonesia consists of about 300 ethnic groups with their own languages, but nationally the Indonesian language (which is basically similar to Malayan language) is used. Administratively, the republic consists of 27 Provinces, covering 302 Regency/Districts and about 6000 subdistricts (the lowest official governmental level of administration).

As a developing country, the Republic of Indonesia has to face a great deal of problems including health. Communicable diseases remain a major health problem, in particular. Malaria, Dengue, TB and sexually transmitted diseases are just some of the diseases whose propensity to affect the population is compounded by inadequate health awareness in certain segments of the population.

The first case of AIDS found in Indonesia was recorded as a foreign tourist who died in Bali, in 1987. Since then, cumulatively a total number of 31 AIDS cases including 22 deaths, and 109 HIV (+) have been found and recorded (from 1987 up to 31 March 1993).

To respond to the HIV epidemic properly, an appropriate legal and ethical environment is needed. But, bearing in mind that the introduction of HIV/AIDS to Indonesia is relatively new, it is a fact that up to this date no special AIDS law has been produced. Health-Legal approches in Indonesia are based on the available 1945 Basic Constitution, Epidemic Law, Quarantine Law, The Health Law, etc., implemented administratively and/or operationally through Government Regulations, Presidential Decree/Instruction, and implemented technically through a Health Minister's Regulation and/ or Decree, and through a Director General's Decree and/ or Instruction.

The following issues are intended as background information for establishing a legal and ethical network to address HIV/AIDS in Asia and the Pacific.

Public Health Versus Individual Rights

Surveillance and Notification of AIDS has been conducted in Indonesia as soon as the first case of AIDS was found in 1987. The legal aspect of those activities are based on the Health Minister's Decree.

Testing, Counselling for AIDS are implemented voluntarily. Consent is needed from each individual of the target group of a serological survey for HIV/AIDS.

Confidentiality of the HIV (+)/AIDS cases is guaranteed through the same Health Minister's Decree.

Compulsory treatment is not applied, except in relation to control measures during/related to certain epidemic diseases.

Prevention measures, e.g., quarantine is not allowed for HIV(+) and or AIDS cases. But it could be conducted if necessary for cases of other epidemic diseases stated in the Health Minister's Decree in relation with the implementation of the Epidemic Law mentioned above.

Brothel laws, upto this date, have never been produced, since prostitution is illegal in Indonesia.

Partner notification is conducted based on the CDC Director General decision related to NAC policy.

Rights to medical information The issue had been recently discussed in a workshop on "Medical Ethics and Rights of a Patient," held in Jakarta. Traditionally, doctors tend to keep the medical information confidential unless asked by the patients and/or their families.

There is no regulation on *Discontinuation of treatment* for non-communicable disease patients; it is considered as the right of the patient. But if it happened in cases of certain epidemic diseases (stipulated in the Health Minister's Decree) due to their reluctance to follow the treatment programme, the patient concerned could be charged as trying to endanger other people and could be punished according to the regulation.

Distrimination of People Living with HIV

To date, there exists no special law dealing with the right of people living with HIV in Indonesia. But according to The Epidemic Law, discrimination of people contracting certain epidemic diseases, if necessary, could be applied in efforts such as isolation and/or quarantine.

Legally, there can be no discrimination against people living with HIV/ AIDS. But factually, based on religious or cultural reasons, discrimination of people contracting certain diseases (not only HIV) postulated in those religions and/or specific cultures, to some extent, still exists in certain communities.

The Duty to treat (AIDS cases) has been applied to all government hospitals as a strategy of the national AIDS control programme. All general hospitals must accept/admit the hospitalisation of AIDS cases with no discrimination.

AIDS cases are subject to be treated as other infectious disease patients, for whom general precautions should be applied. People living with HIV/ AIDS have the same rights as other people in accommodation, employment, schools, and also have the same facilities as migrant workers and travellers.

International law is obeyed fully, and confidentiality is applied by the Indonesian Government.

Information Law

In Indonesia, there is no obstacle to HIV information, as long as it will not disturb the socio-cultural and or political stability and/or offend the ethnic religious norms.

Broadcasting/censorship laws, obscenity law, advertising regulations are to some extent subject to the guidelines stated in the existing criminal law. However, these are applied only to prevent the ill use of "freedom to speak and/or dissemination of information."

Sex education is essentially accepted by the community as long as it does not contradict ethics and/or religious norms.

Right to information is guaranteed by law and regulations, including the health aspect of information.

Family Law

Legal approaches to inheritance, divorce/separation, maintenance, custody/adoption, carer and survival support, age of marriage and sexual consent are enforced through the implementation of the civil law; legal approaches on non-consensual intercourse, termination of pregnancy (without medical reasons/ judgment) are enforced through the implementation of the criminal law. The termination of pregnancy due to medical reasons/judgment, and conducted by the right health professional, is made possible through the implementation of the health law (1993).

HIV/AIDS Policy in Prisons and Institutions

Principally, the HIV/AIDS policy in prisons and institutions in Indonesia is similar to the policy applied for the general population.

Testing, if required, should be conducted voluntarily. Segregation of prisoners living with HIV/AIDS is not allowed, except for reasons other than their HIV status (e.g., criminality). If hospitalisation is needed, the prisoner should be admitted to the nearest hospital. The provision of condoms and bleach is legal, but provision of needles is prohibited in relation to the antinarcotic regulation and/or safety reasons. Counselling, care and support is provided through collaborative efforts among the Ministries of Health, Social Affairs and Justice.

HIV/AIDS Legal Policy at the Workplace

Legal policy on HIV/AIDS at the workplace, up to this date, has not been produced, but is now in the process of being formulated.

Workplace testing may only be conducted in relation to a cross sectional survey on STDs, to be conducted anonymously and voluntarily by the authorised health team.

Policies on HIV infected employees, including sick leave,

disability support, and occupational health safety are similar to the policies which govern people living with other diseases.

HIV education at the workplace to some extent has been conducted and will be extended in the near future through intersectoral collaborations, involving non-governmental organisations.

Criminal Law and HIV/AIDS

In the existing Criminal Law, there are no legal statements concerning transmission offences. In certain cases (e.g., where the activities of sex workers and homosexuals are made public held to be against ethics norms), the performer could be charged legally.

37

HIV/AIDS Law and Law Reform in Kiribati

Dr. Takeieta Kienene
Acting Chief
Prevention and Public Health Services, Kiribati

Ms. Tiantaake Beero
Attorny General's
Chamber, Kiribati

Introduction

Kiribati consists of 33 low-lying islands scattered over 3.5 million square kilometres of the Pacific Ocean. The scattered nature of the islands causes considerable problems in administration, transport, communication and service delivery. It has a population of 72,355 (1990 census), of which 25,380 live on the capital island, South Tarawa, giving it a population density of roughly 1,000 per square kilometre. Fifty per cent of the population is below 6 years of age. The population growth rate is high at 2.24 per cent and the total fertility rate is 3.8 per cent. The adult literacy rate runs at 90 per cent.

There is a significant population drift from the outer islands to South Tarawa in search of employment. With this socio-economic shift, lifestyles are changing. The departure from small islands societal norms and separation from family units may contribute to a change in values and beliefs and an increase in risk taking behaviours.

More than 10 per cent of men aged 20-50 years are working overseas as merchant seamen away from their spouses and families, resulting in an increase in the number of marital rifts and divorces.

HIV/AIDS in Kiribati

The national response to the AIDS pandemic can be documented with regard to following phases:

1. *1987*: Formation of the National AIDS Committee (NAC) chaired by the Chief Medical Officer (CMO) and consisting of members nominated from all the government ministries, churches and non-government organizations (NGOs). The NAC meets on a regular basis. Lately, it has not been very active.
2. *1988:* Development of the Short-Term Plan (STP) with WHO support in grant and short-term consultant (STC), covering the period 1988-89.
3. *1989*: Development of the Medium-Term Plan (MTP1) to cover the period 1990-93.
4. *1993*: External review of STP (1988-89) and MTP1 (1990 - 93). This revealed that most of the activities were implemented as planned and the government was able to integrate most AIDS activities into the existing structures including primary health care (PHC). The review also formed the basis for the development of Medium-Term Plan 2 (MTP2), also called the National AIDS Plan (NAP) or the Strategic Plan, to cover the period 1994-98. MTP2 will be reviewed at the end of 1995 to coincide with the preparation of the next Kiribati National Health Plan.

Current HIV/AIDS Situation

To date, Kiribati has reported two HIV infections. The first was identified through blood donor screening and the second through a medical evaluation of an out-patient. It is highly likely that there are quite a few unidentified seropositive people in Kiribati, considering the limited testing activities and the universal nature of the under-reporting of HIV infections. No AIDS cases have ever been diagnosed. It is expected that Kiribati will have a few cases of AIDS during the next five to ten years.

Risk Factors

The geographical isolation and the current low prevalence of sexually transmitted diseases (STD) may have protected Kiribati from HIV infection. However, the high mobility of the population, a rapidly changing social culture, and the gradual development of tourism may increase the prevalence of HIV infection.

The close association between STD and HIV/AIDS is well-documented. The incidence of STD in Kiribati rises and falls in a curve, suggesting that perhaps this is not an endemic problem, but one that is frequently introduced from outside. As the number of people travelling to and from Kiribati rises, the chances of exposure to HIV/ AIDS will increase.

Males being treated for STD are often unwilling to name contacts for fear of reprisal and loss of status in the community. Women usually do not seek medical attention for STD because they are often asymptomatic or reluctant to be treated by male health workers. The lack of testing/screening facilities on all outer islands may also contribute to the problem.

More than 1,000 young men work on foreign shipping vessels, constantly travelling around the world, acquiring new ideas that may influence society, and undoubtedly engaging in risk taking behaviours. Occasionally drugs have been found in their possession but this has never been a problem.

Policies and Programmes

With the completion of MTP1, several important components of an effective HIV/AIDS programme are in place. This includes laboratory capacity, condom supply and distribution system, programme management, public education, and AIDS related policies.

MTP2 will maintain and strengthen these components while introducing new interventions. Recognizing fhat lifestyles are changing and that the threat of large numbers of I-Kiribati becoming infected is unlikely, MTP2 is focused on specific programmes/ projects.

Policies

The following AIDS-related guidelines for policy-making are being developed:

1. Transmission through blood:
   promote action to reduce the need for blood transfusion;
   promote safer blood supply;
   promote sterile conditions;
   promote safer drug-use behaviour.

2. Perinatal transmission.
3. Confidentiality.
4. Non-discrimination against HIV infected people.
5. The right of access to information, condoms, health care and public services.
6. STD clinical management and HIV/AIDS case management.

Existing Legal Framework and Reforms

There is no existing law or legal framework with respect to HIV/ AIDS in Kiribati. The guidelines currently in place are based on the existing laws dealing with human risthts and medical ethics.

38

Current Status of the Acquired Immunodeficiency Syndrome Prevention Act of the Republic of Korea

Dr. Kyung Chung
President
Korean Federation of AIDS Affairs, Inc., Republic of Korea

General Background

The Acquired Immunodeficiency Syndrome Prevention Act (HIV Law hereinafter) was first promulgated on 28 November 1987. It was supplemented by the Acquired Immunodeficiency Syndrome Prevention Decree (Presidential Decree) of 18 June 1988 and by the Acquired Immunodeficiency Syndrome Prevention Enforcement Regulations of 6 November 1990.

The HIV Law, as amended consists of 28 Articles in 6 Chapters that deal with general provisions, notification and reporting, medical examination, protection and control of the infected, supplementary provisions and penal provisions.

It must be pointed out that it is not always possible to respect everyone's human rights even though the Korean Constitution upholds the protection of the dignity and rights of everyone. The peculiarity of Korean HIV Law is that it places restrictions on the infected and mandatory duties on susceptible persons—these seem to be unavoidable and controversial as well. Ideally, a law must reflect the reality but insofar as the HIV Law is concerned, however, it seems never possible for us to have such a law. The reason for this negative view is that we do not have measures either to prevent or to treat persons with HIV/AIDS as yet. It is contradictory that some articles of the Korean HIV Law stipulate segregation, compulsory detention, and restriction of employment of the infected even though there are no specific measures for prevention and treatment.

The following aspects of the HIV Law need to be highlighted:

Underemphasis of the Importance of Educational Activities

A major weakness of the HIV Law is that it does not contain any article which stipulates mandatory duties for the state and the local governments with regard to educational activities.

For example, Article 3 of the Korean HIV Law merely states that:

1. The State and the local governments shall work out and execute counter measures to prevent AIDS and to protect and control those who are infected with HIV (hereinafter referred to as "infected"), and shall transmit information to those who are positive.
2. Citizens shall pay attention to prevention with adequate knowledge about AIDS, and co-operate actively in measures taken by the State or the local governments under this Act.

Given the vital importance of education activities, this type of article should stipulate specific items to be undertaken. For example, formal (school) education and non-formal(social) education can be stipulated. Furthermore, community organizations can be also mobilized by appropriate regulations.

Reinforcement of the Anti-AIDS Committee

Article 4 of the Korean HIV Law provides that in order to decide on important matters concerning the prevention of AIDS and protection, control, etc., an Anti-AIDS Committee shall be established in the Ministry of Health and Social Affairs. It is important to give more status to this Committee by placing it directly under the office of Prime Minister, for instance.

Necessity for Reforms in the Medical Examination and Control System

The importance of consent and anonymity of the person who receives medical examination for HIV test cannot be over emphasized. However, the Korean HIV Law appears to be rather vague in this respect, mentioning it only incidentally in various articles.

Testing of Foreigners

The Article concerning the regulation of testing of foreigners is very vague and impractical. Article 8 of the Korean HIV Law states that:

> "Foreigners entering the Republic of Korea from foreign countries, and who wish to stay for more than 91 days, must present to the Minister of Health and Social Affairs a written confirmation of the negative antibody test result issued within one month before entering the country. If it is impossible to present such document, the person must undergo medical examination at an institution designated by the Minister of Health and Social Affairs within seventy two hours after entering the country".

Although testing is prescribed by this Article, there is neither the procedure for informing foreigners nor a penal provision to meet instances of contravention. This Article is a typical example of the impracticability of some provisions of the Korean HIV Law.

Problem of Status of Women and the Young

International trends show that women are equally vulnerable to HIV/ AIDS and an increasingly juvenile population is exposed to this epidemic every year. Accordingly, the formulation of special articles in the HIV Law to deal with these issues should be seriously considered. Since the major reason for this problem is the low social status of women and children, we should reinforce articles which can help raise their social status.

Need for Legal Provision Concerning Support for NGOs

The AIDS programme of any country can never be carried out only by the government; the participation of the NGOs (non-governmental organizations) is essential. Unfortunately, however, there is no mention in the Korean HIV Law of support for NGOs.

There should be at least one article in the HIV Law which discusses the ways in which the state and local governments can extend financial and administrative support to the NGOs.

Conclusion

Since the AIDS programme itself is still young in Korea, it is understandable that many areas require to be reformed. Undoubtedly the Korean participants will be carrying back crucial lessons and information from this valuable workshop.

39

The HIV Epidemic in Malaysia: Legal and Ethical Issues

Mehrun Siraj
Advocate and Solicitor Kaula Lumpur
Malaysia

The Ministry of Health has prepared a Plan of Action that provides guidelines for the surveillance, prevention and control of HIV/AIDS in Malaysia. The policies enunciated in the Plan are more or less consistent with those of the WHO. What remains now is to examine how far existing law and practice reflect these policies and to consider whether it is necessary to enact, amend or repeal any law so as to satisfactorily address the legal and ethical issues arising from the epidemic. The term law as used in this paper includes administrative circulars and departmental directives.

A. PUBLIC HEALTH

The main statute in this area is the Prevention and Control of Infectious Diseases Act 1988, Act 342 (hereafter referred to as Act 342). The infectious diseases covered by the Act are specified in the 1st. Schedule of the Act. HIV is the only disease mentioned in Part 2 of the Schedule.

1. Surveillance

Act 342 defines surveillance as "the subjection of any person who is not isolated, to periodical examination or enquiry for the purpose of ascertaining his state of health and to conditions imposed by an authorised of ficer for such purpose" (section 2).

This definition refers to the surveillance authorised by section 15(1) of the Act which provides that authorised of ficers may order the contacts of any person with an infectious disease to undergo surveillance. Section 15(2) empowers the officer to use force to ensure compliance with his order relating to surveillance.

The Plan of Action defines surveillance as "the continuing scrutiny of the situation and the factors that determine the occurrence and distribution of HIV/AIDS in a given locality." It includes the collection, collation, analysis and distribution of relevant data for appropriate intervention. With regard to individuals, the Plan states that "all cases, carriers and contacts of HIV/AIDS are to be carefully and discretely investigated." The investigation involves collecting personal details and transmitting them to the Epidemiology Unit of the Ministry of Health. This raises the question of confidentiality.

2. Confidentiality

Section 3(3) of Act 342 provides that an authorised officer shall maintain confidentiality of all matters which come to his knowledge in the performance of his official duties under the Act and he shall not communicate any such matter to any person except for the purpose of carrying into effect the provisions of the Act. Under section 3(4) he may be punished with a fine or imprisonment for up to three years. This section, however, may not be enough to ensure that confidentiality is maintained, as it applies only to authorised officers. An authorised officer means any Medical Officer of Health, any Health Inspector, or any officer appointed by the Minister under section 3. Para-medics and other support staff who may have access to the same information are not subject to this provision. There are four alternatives that may he used to remedy this:

(i) Utilising the Official Secrets Act 1972, Act 88 which is an act for the protection of secrets. In addition to the documents specified in the schedule to the Act, "official secret" means any Official document, information and material as may he classified as "Top Secret", "Secret", "Confidential" or "Restricted" as the case may be, by a Minister, the Menteri Besar or Chief Minister of a State or such public officer appointed under section 2B. All information about HIV patients could be classified "confidential" under the Act. If the hreaches of confidentiality occur, the Act can be used and the procedure effected immediately by an administrative decision.

(ii) Issuing a departmental directive on confidentiality. Failure to abide by the order will constitute a disciplinary offence, as for example, under rule 4, Chapter D of the Government General Orders which deals with insubordination or the refusal to follow orders. Disciplinary action with the possibility of dismissal on the charge being proven may be an effective deterrent. The Disciplinary Rules of most agencies and organisations are worded so generally that it is possible to include this matter without further action.

(iii) Section 3 of Act 342 itself can be amended to apply to anyone having information that should be kept confidential. The information could be in relation to all infectious diseases or only those mentioned in Part 2 of the Schedule to the Act, i.e., only HIV infection. This alternative, however, requires legislative action and may take time to bring about.

(iv) Section 31 of Act 342 empowers the Minister to make regulations that provide for, *inter alia*, prescribing offences which may be compounded and the procedure for compounding. Section 3 can be left as it is and other persons not subject to section 3 may be brought under a new offence that will be created by the regulation, and therefore easier to effect than an amendment to section 3. If the fines that are imposed are high enough, it may be a deterrent.

The husband of a deceased AIDS patient drew attention to the burial procedures prescribed for people who have died from AIDS which raised questions among mourners at the funeral and led eventually to the revelation that his wife had died of AIDS.

Section 17 of Act 342 requires the burial or cremation of any person dying of an infectious disease to be in accordance with the directions of an authorised officer. The Plan of Action details the directions that are to be followed. At the funeral, an officer in uniform supervises the burial. Athough he is on duty, he would be less conspicuous if he were in *mufti*. Ultimately though, the aim of AIDS education should be to remove the stigma of death by AIDS so that there will no longer be a need for confidentiality whether at funerals or otherwise.

3. Notification

AIDS was first gazetted as a notifiable infectious disease in

May 1985. With the inclusion of HIV infection in all its forms in Act 342 in 1988, all the provisions of the Act relating to notification apply to HIV/AIDS cases.

Section 10(1) requires any person having knowledge of the existence of any infectious disease or the death of any person caused by the disease, to notify the officer in charge of the nearest District Health Office or government facility or police station or the nearest village head. Under section 10(2), a medical practitioner who treats or becomes aware of the existence of any infectious disease shall inform the Medical Officer of Health.

Persons in charge of boarding houses also have a duty to notify the nearest District Health Officer if he knows or has reason to know that a person in his boarding house has an infectious disease or has died of the disease (section 10(3)). The term "boarding house" includes a hotel, a hostel or any institution of refuge or rest for persons needing care.

Village heads and police officers who are notified must in turn notify the officer in charge of the nearest health office or government facililty (section 10(4)).

Failure to report is made an offence (section 10(5)). Section 10(6) creates a presumption of knowledge of the existence of the disease on the part of the person charged with the offence. The presumption is rebuttable by showing to the satisfaction of the court that he could not with reasonable diligence have obtained knowledge of the infectious disease or that he did not have reason to believe that an infectious disease existed.

4. Consent to Testing

It is the practice of all hospitals and clinics to obtain written consent from the patient or his/her guardian or next-of kin for all tests and treatment to he administered to the patient. In the case of patients with sexually transmitted diseases and tuberclosis, mental patients and patients with high risk behaviours like homosexuals bisexuals, prostitutes and intravenous drug users however, a signed consent form is not required for taking and testing blood. This is a directive in the Plan of Action.

It could he argued that the compulsory testing of blood without the patient's consent is authorised by section 14 of Act 342. The section provides for the removal to a quarantine station and the detention there for the purpose of treatment, any person believed to be infected. "Quarantine station" means any place where isolation or observaton is carried out and includes an infectious disease hospital. Section 2 defines "treatment" as including all such acts and procedures as may be necessary for the purpose of determining whether a person is infected with an infectious disease." Compulsory testing therefore may be carried out without obtaining consent it the patient is suspected of having an infectious disease. If this can be done for someone who has to be taken to a quarantine station, it can also apply to a person who is already in the hospital or clinic and who is suspected of having HIV/AIDS.

Prisoners, intravenous drug users detained in Drug Rehabilitation Centers, and women and girls in Places of Refuge are being tested for the purpose of identifying those who are infected with HIV so that they may be counselled against spreading it. The testing is done once before the person is released from custody. Signed consent is required for the taking and testing of blood. Such consent, however, is not too difficult to obtain in the case of persons in custody.

5. Compulsory Treatment

Sections 2 and 14 of Act 342, discussed above, imply that compulsory treatment may be carried out on persons suspected of being infected with HIV. Section 14 allows the authorities to detain a person "until he can be discharged without danger to the public."

In the case of HIV patients, the more relevant question relating to treatment is the right to receive treatment, including necessary medication. Government hospitals and clinics, limited in their financial resources, tend to prescribe drugs that are cheap. Patients who request the more expensive medication are expected to purchase it themselves from private pharmacies. Occasionally, an expensive drug is available but for certain classes of patients only. Such a practice creates discrimination in the treatment of patients. However, it is a practice that applies to all forms of illness and not just HIV.

6. Quarantine

Sections 14 and 15 of Act 342, discussed above, may be used to quarantine infected individuals and their contacts, respectively.

In addition, section 11(1) authorises the Minister to declare any area an infected area and by section 11(2) he may make regulations prescribing measures for the control and spread of infection within and from that area. Persons living in that area can then be subjected to treatment, isolation, observation, or surveillance for a period that may be specified according to circumstances (section 11(30)). To ensure compliance with directives given under section 11(3), authorised officers may use force with or without assistance and to employ such methods "as may be sufficient." The assistance that authorised officers can rely on is set out in section 5 which states that "police, customs and immigration officers and officers from other government departments and agencies shall render assistance if requested by authorised officers." There appears to be a great deal of subjective discretion that can be exercised by the authorised officers under this section. The medical officers, however, are in the service of either the government or local authorities and are therefore subject to their control. Abuse of power can be disciplined if brought to the attention of superior officers.

7. Control of Brothels/Massage Parlours as a Prevention Measure

The Women and Girls Protection Act 1973, Act 106, (hereafter referred to as WGPA) criminalises the sex sector with the aim of prohibiting prostitution. Section 20 of the WGPA is for the suppression of places of assignation and section 21 of brothels. Place of assignation is defined in section 2 as "any place where communication is established with any female person either directly or through an intermediary for purpose of prostitution." Section 20 itself mentions association, institution, club or place of public resort which may be used as a place of assignation. Place of public resort is any place to which the public has access and includes bars and massage parlours. The licensing regulations for such establishments, however, attempt to prevent them from being used either as a place of assignation or for actually dispensing sexual favours.

The Massage Establishments (Federal Territory) By-Laws 1980, (P.U (A) 87/1980 as amended by P.U. (A) 71/1991) were made under section 102 of the Local Government Act 1976, Act 171. A licence is required to operate a massage establishment (by-law 3) and the licence is revocable if the licencee contravenes any by-law or breaches any condition of the licence (by-law 12). A relevant prohibition is By-law 14(1)(b) which provides that "no licencee shall employ in his massage establishment any person whom he knows or has reason to believe to be a prostitute or a person of bad character." As a prevention measure, By-law 16 is more significant. It requires the licencee to ensure that all masseurs and masseuses undergo an annual medical examination. This will help to identify HIV positives and, it is anticipated, to control HIV and other health problems among the employees.

Section 21 of WGPA makes it an offence to keep or manage a brothel. Because brothels are totally prohibited, there is no provision for regular medical examination of sex workers despite the undisputed fact that brothels do exist and prostitution is a thriving trade. Sex workers who are picked up by the police in anti-vice raids are tested for HIV with their signed consent. Those who are below twenty-one years of age may be placed under the supervision of social workers (see discussion below).

8. Partner Notification

The Ministry of Health policy statement indicates that the attending physician should advise the patient to inform his/her sexual partner of one's HIV infection, but if this is not done within a reasonable period, say two weeks, the physician is to inform the Health Authority who will then notify the partner. Two questions arise from this. The first is: Should not the sexual partner be informed immediately? The second is: Who is liable if the infected person does not inform his/her partner and continues to have sex without the necessary precautions? This is one area where the partner's right to know must be weighed against the infected person's right to confidentiality.

That partner notification is in fact being done can be implied from two factors. The first is the investigation of all contacts of an infected person (discussed above) and the second is the counselling that is recommended to be given to sexual partners, family rnembers and carers of HIV patients. Specific mention is made of counselling for the prevention of pregnancy.

B. IMMIGRATION

The Immigration Act 1959/1963, Act 155, provides in section 8(1) that any person who falls within any of the classes of person mentioned in subsection 3 is a prohibited immigrant. Section 8(3)(b) refers to any person suffering from a contagious or infectious disease which makes his presence in Malaysia dangerous to the community. Under section 31, if a person arriving in Malaysia is found to be a prohibited immigrant, he/she can be detained in an Immigration centre and subsequently sent back to his/her place of origin. Under section 39A(1) a person can be required to submit to a medical examination. His/her refusal to do so will render him/her a prohibited immigrant (paragraph (c) of section 8(3)).

At present, tourists and other visitors are not being tested for HIV when coming into the country. People known to have HIV, however, may be refused entry if there is a possibility of the infection being spread.

Migrant workers are subject to strict immigration control. All foreign workers are required to undergo a medical examination including blood tests for HIV infection. Those that test positive are not given work permits and are sent home.

C. INFORMATION LAW

There is no right to information in Malaysia. There are instead many obstacles to information. The Official Secrets Act discussed above is one example of legislation that can prevent the acquisition of some kinds of information, although in the case of HIV it may be used in a positive way to maintain confidentiality. Other legislation may become obstacles in that they hinder the spread of HIV information.

1. Obscenity Laws

Section 292 of the Penal Code makes it an offence punishable with imprisonment for up to three years, to sell, let to hire, distribute, publicly exhibit or put into circulation in any manner, any obscene book, pamphlet, paper, drawing, painting, representation or figure or any other obscene object. An exception exists for bona fide religious purposes only. However, if materials carrying information on HIV/AIDS are genuinely educational in nature, it is not likely that any prosecution will be instituted under the Penal Code. Section 293 carries a punishment of five years imprisonment when the offence mentioned in section 292 is committed in relation to a person below the age of twenty-one years.

EMPLOYMENT ISSUES

1. Pre-employment Medital Examination

There is a long-standing practice of requiring prospective employees to undergo a medical examination before they are appointed. The justification for this is two-fold. One reason is that employers want to be sure that the employee will he able to carry out his duties and that productivity will not be reduced by frequent medical leave. The other reason is that establishments that provide medical care do not want to be burdened with the cost of treating an employee who is ill, particularly if it is a chronic illness that may require long-term treatment. Consequently, persons who are less than perfectly fit are sometimes not appointed despite the relevant qualifications and experience. This applies to all forms of illness and in all probability will apply to people with HIV as well.

At present there is no law that directly prohibits discrimination in employment. One such law has been proposed to eliminate discrimination against women. It could be made more general to include persons with HIV or other illnesses and persons with handicaps. To protect the interests of persons with HIV only, while others continue to suffer discrimination, may not be either justifiable or acceptable.

2. Contracting HIV in the Course of Employment

If an employee were found to be infected with HIV, can his employer terminate his services or is there sufficient legal protection for the employee?

Under section 12 of the Employment Act 1955, Act 265, an employer may terminate a contract of employment by giving an employee notice of four weeks if he has worked for less than two years, six weeks if he has worked for two to five years, and eight weeks if he has worked for more than five years. This provision may appear to give an employer an absolute right to terminate the services of an employee at any time and without any reason but it has to be read in conjunction with section 20 of the Industrial Relations Act 1967.

Although section 20 gives an employee who has been "dismissed without just cause" the right to make representation for reinstatement, the Eederal Court (now the Supreme Court) held in the case of *Goon Kwee Phoy v J. & P. Coats (M) Bhd. ((1981)2 MLJ 129)* that there is no material difference between termination of contract by due notice and the unilateral dismissal of a summary nature. The court stressed that "it is the duty of the court to determine whether the termination or dismissal is with or without just cause or excuse." An employee can conceivably challenge the termination of his contract if it were solely because he were found to be HIV positive. The Industrial Court personnel, however, need to be sufficiently informed about HIV/AIDS to ensure that they will decide that being HIV positive by itself is not a just cause for termination.

Section 14(3) of the Employment Act, however, raises an issue which could be problematical unless there is sufficient education about HIV in the workplace. The section allows an employee to terminate his contract of service where he or his dependents are immediately threatened by danger to him of violence or disease that he did not, by his contract of employment, undertake to run. Employees who are ignorant of the ways in which HIV is spread may be afraid to work with a colleague who has tested positive. They may threaten to resign, using this section, thereby forcing the employer to terminate the HIV positive employee. If the number of employees resigning will cause the employer difficulties, the Industrial Court may even hold that the circumstances provide a just cause for dismissing the HIV employee. Such a situation can be averted by disseminating relevant information about the disease at all workplaces.

CRIMINAL LAW

1. Transmission Olfences

The Penal Code has two sections dealing with the transmission of disease dangerous to life. Section 269 provides that whoever unlawfully or negligently does any act, and which he knows or has reason to believe to be likely to spread the infection of any disease dangerous to life, shall be punished with imprisonment for a term which may extend to six months or with fine or both. Section 270 increases the punishment to two years imprisonment where the act is done malignantly.

The Prevention and Control of Infectious Diseases Act 1988, Act 342 also provides penal sanctions for the transmission of disease. Section 12(1) which applies to all diseases covered by the Act, provides that "any person who knows or has reason to believe that he is suffering from an infectious disease, shall not expose other persons to the risk of infection by his presence or conduct." Section 12(2), which applies to HIV only, provides that he shall not do "any act which he knows or has reason to believe is likely to lead to the spread of such infectious disease."

Presumably, these provisions will be invoked only if people with HIV have been sufficiently counselled and, despite counselling, knowingly pass on the infection to others or put them at risk of contracting it.

2. Sex Workers

The law relating to the commercial sex sector is the Women and Girls Protection Act 1973, Act 106. Part IV, sections 16 to 22, of the Act deal with offences most of which are aimed at procurers and those who operate brothels. The sex worker herself does not commit any offence under the WGPA by earning income as a prostitute, unless she is caught soliciting. Soliciting appears to be punishable because it creates a nuisance. Hence, it is also punishable under the Minor Offences Act 1955 (Revised 1987) Act 336 under section 27 which falls within the part that is titled "Idle and disorderly persons."

If a sex worker is below the age of twenty-one years, she may be removed to a place of refuge (section 7 WGPA) where, by order of a Magistrate, made after an inquiry, she may be detained for up to three years for her protection (section 8(4)). The recommendation to detain or otherwise is made by the Protector in the Social Inquiry Report. Institutional rehabilitation is a last resort. The first step would be counselling and supervision by social workers while resident at home.

A sex worker who is detained in a place of refuge undergoes a rehabilitation programme to equip her for alternative employment. After her release, she may be subject to after-care supervision. Although this detention is regarded as a measure for the protection of young girls, it is nevertheless punitive, as the girls are deprived of their freedom and subjected to a programme of instruction that they may not enjoy.

If the sex worker is a Muslim, she will be open to prosecution under the Islamic Law legislation regardless of her age. Islamic Law is in the state list (9th Schedule of the Federal Constitution) and is therefore regulated by state enactments. The state of Kelantan is the most advanced in terms of enacting specific laws that deal with all aspects of the administration of Islamic Law. In relation to offences over which the Syariah Court has jurisdiction, Kelantan has enacted the Syariah Criminal Code, Enactment No. 2 of 1985.

Section 19 of the Code makes it an offence for women to be engaged in prostitution. Unlike the WGPA, the Code will punish a sex worker who takes on the role voluntarily. Poverty is not a valid excuse, as the state treasury or Bait-ul-Mal will provide financial assistance to destitute persons. The Religious Affairs Department will also assist in skills training and job placements for alternative employment.

3. Homosexuality

Homosexuality is not encouraged in Malaysia and homosexual relations constitute an offence under Malaysian Law. There are provisions in the Penal Code that address carnal intercourse against the order of nature. Section 377A declares "sexual connection by the introduction of the penis into the anus or mouth of the other person" an offence punishable with imprisonment for up to twenty years and whipping. The provision is intended for general application and could apply to a male-female relationship too.

The Syariah Criminal Code refers to the sexual act between two male partners as *Liwat Liwat* and is regarded as a serious offence carrying a fine of up to RM5,000 and imprisonment of up to three years as well as whipping with six strokes (section 14).

4. Drug Dependents

Under section 25A of the Dangerous Drugs Act 1952 (Revised 1980) Act 234, any social welfare officer or police officer not below the rank of Sergeant or officer in charge of a police station may take into custody any person reasonably suspected of being a drug dependent. The person must be produced before a Magistrate who may order him to be remanded and be medically examined or observed by a medical officer at a detention centre. If, after the examination or observation, the person is certified to be a drug dependent, the Magistrate may order the person to attend a Rehabilitation Centre for six months or supervised by a Welfare Officer for two years subject to the person executing a bond.

D. WOMEN AND FAMILIES

The role and status of women in the family can make them more vulnerable to HIV infection and to the adverse consequences that can result from it. It is necessary therefore to examine some relevant laws and practices to determine their effect on women faced with the HIV/AIDS epidemic.

1. Maintenance

For women who are not economically independent, the right to spousal support is of tremendous importance. Many women stay on in a marriage and put up with all kinds of mistreatment because they have no other source of income. For the same reason, women may not insist on safe sex even when they fear that their husbands may have contracted HIV or any other sexually transmitted disease. Knowing their rights to maintenance, and when they will lose them, may help protect women.

A Muslim woman who is either divorced or abandoned by her husband, whether or not she has HIV, is entitled to be supported by the male members of her family. And if she has no such relatives or if they themselves are destitute, the State Treasury or Bait-ul-Mal will provide an allowance. The same rights exist for any member of the family who may be incapacitated or suffering from ill health*.

2. Termination of Pregnancy

Before the 1989 amendments to the Penal Code, the termination of pregnancy was an offence unless it was done in good faith to save the life of the woman. The amendment to section 312 of the Penal Code deleted the general exception "in good faith for the purpose of saving the life of the woman" thus making the termination of pregnancy for whatever purpose an offence, and then added the following exception:

> This section does not extend to a medical practitioner registered under the Medical Act 1971 who terminates the pregnancy of a woman if such medical practitioner is of opinion, formed in good faith, that the continuance of the pregnancy would involve risk to the life of the pregnant woman, or injury to the mental or physical health of the pregnant woman, greater than if the pregnancy were terminated.

The final effect of the amendment, then, is to legalise the termination of pregnancies that are performed by registered medical practitioners. This ensures that all abortions will be carried out in a clinical manner and with minimum risk to the woman. From a legal point of view, therefore, people with HIV can be advised to terminate their pregnancies.

E. PRISONS, CUSTODIAL INSTITUTIONS AND WELFARE HOMES

Prisoners, intravenous drug users in Drug Treatment and

A Muslim woman who is either divorced or abandoned by her husband, whether or not she has HIv, is entitled to be supported by the male members of her family. And if she has no such relatives or if they themselves are destitute, the State Treasury or Balt-ul-Mal will provide an allowance.
The same rights exist for any member of the family who may be incapacitated or suffering from ill health.

Rehabilitation Centres, and sex workers in Places of Refuge are subjected to routine screening. Confidentiality is to be maintained and they are not to be discriminated against if found to be HIV positive. In prison and drug centres they are isolated either in a single cell where this is available or with others who may also be HIV positive. Given the overcrowding in the prisons and drug centres, this isolation is regarded as a privilege.

In one place of refuge where a sex worker with HIV has been placed, there is no isolation, in that the girl shares the same dormitory as the other girls but she was given her own bathroom, not to be shared by anyone. This inevitably raised questions among the inmates. Confidentiality in such a situation becomes illusory.

A major concern of officials responsible for persons in custody is that sexual activities continue, panicularly among male inmates. They question the right to confidentiality as they feel that the other inmates should be aware of the risks that exist. Alternatively, they feel that those with HIV should be segregated to prevent them from forcing themselves on the others .

The proposal that condoms be distributed and safe sex encouraged has been rejected by the government. Sexual intercourse not within a valid marriage is prohibited by Islam. To give effect to the proposal is tantamount to encouraging a person to go against the teachings of Islam and cannot be countenanced. The only accepatable way is by education and counselling with a view to bringing about a change in behaviour.

The same principles have been applied to injecting drug users. Assistance to them is not in the form of needle exchange and probably never will be. Counselling for them is aimed at changing their life styles. From an Islamic point of view, this is the only acceptable means of helping them.

Conclusion

There is an undeniable need for legislation to address specifically the issues arising from the HIV/AIDS epidemic. The interests of persons with HIV/AIDS, as well as the interests of persons either associated or working with them, need to be protected. To be protected, interests have to be expressed in the form of rights. While existing legislation can sometimes be

---

For a more thorough discussion of Maintenance, Divorce, Separation and Rape, see "Law, Traditional Family Customs and HIV" by the same author in Sector One of the present volume.

interpreted in a manner favourable to the rights of people with HIV/ AIDS it is better if these rights were declared clearly and unequivocably in the relevant legislation.

It must be remembered, however, that not all rights are universally acceptable. Some may conflict with religious norms and, where the religion has the force of law, as in the case of Islamic Law in Malaysia, such proposals can never hope to be enacted. In those areas, it is education of a kind that will succeed in changing attitudes and behaviour that will provide a more effective response to the epidemic.

Where rights are universally acceptable, then, having declared the rights, it becomes essential to provide remedies to protect those rights. Legislation should not be mere rhetoric. There must be clear procedures for enforcing the rights. Without a mechanism for enforcement, rights become illusory and interests fail to be protected.

Finally, to ensure that the prescribed remedies are available to all, there must also be provided the means of achieving them. Legal literacy programmes that disseminate information not only on rights but also on the means of enforcing the rights must be started. Access to legal aid and advice must be made easier. And to ensure that legal proceedings produce meaningful results, all persons involved in the administration of the law have to be sensitised and educated.

40

Law, Traditional Family Customs and HIV Infection—A Malaysian Perspective

Mehrun Siraj
Advocate and Solicitor
Kuala Lumpur, Malaysia

A. SOCIAL AND RELIGIOUS INFLUENCE SHAPING FAMILY LAW

The Family Law of Malaysia is a reflection of a plural society and its complex legal history. The law in force today comprises Islamic Law, Customary Law and legislation that is based on English Law. To understand how this has come about, it will be instructive to briefly trace the development of laws in the states that make up Malaysia. This exercise will also reveal the various influences that have helped shape Family Law.

Malaysia came into existence in 1963 with the union of Sabah, Sarawak, Singapore and the eleven states of Federation of Malaya—Johore, Kedah, Kelantan, Malacca, Negen Sembilan, Pahang, Penang, Porak, Porlis, Selangor and Tiongganu. Singapore separated from the Federation in August 1965 to become a Republic, leaving thirteen states in Malaysia. Kuala Lumpur and Labuan which are in the territories of Selangor and Sabah respectively are now Federal Territory.

Penang and Malacca were British colonies jointly known as the Straits Settlements. Penang was acquired by the British in 1786 and, as there was no known body of law in force then, the First Charter of Justice was granted in 1807, introducing the English Law and establishing a Court of Judicature that was to exercise Jurisdiction as an Ecclesiastical Court "so far as the several religions, manners and customs of the inhabitants will admit[1]." This established the principle that the religions and customs of the local inhabitants would be considered in all matters in which the application of English Law without modification would cause injustice or oppression to the local inhabitants.

The Undang-Undang Melaka or Hukum Kanun Melaka is the earliest known Code to contain provisions based on Islamic Law. The Code is believed to have been started by Sultan Muhamed Shah, sometime between 1424 and 1444. The first part of the Code is predominantly Adat or Customary Law but the influence of Islamic Law is seen in the many sections that refer to the law of God after stating the position according to the Adat. The Code was completed during the reign of Sultan Muzaffar Shah (1445-1448) and by then had two major parts that were exclusively Islamic Law, one of which was Family Law[2].

English Law ousted the Islamic Law as the basic law of the land, relegating it to the field of Family Law and to a few offences against the precepts of the religion. This occurred in the Malay states as well, when they came under the protection of the British through Treaties with the Sultans.

Although English Law was not introduced into the Malay states in the way that it was in the Straits Settlements, it was nevertheless brought in by means of new legislation that was either based on English statutes or on other models that had been based on English Law. Islamic Law was applied only to Family Law and to a few offences against the religion of Islam.

Sabah (which was formerly North Borneo) and Sarawak are the two states on the island of Borneo. They are sometimes referred to as East Malaysia; they were British Protectorates from 1888 but statutory reception of English Law came relatively late.[3] The 1928 Sarawak provision declared:

> "The law of England in so far as it is not modified by Order and other enactments issued by His Highness the Raja of Sarawak or with his authority, and in so far as it is applicable to Sarawak having regard to native customs and local conditions, shall be the law of Sarawak[4]."

The corresponding provisions in Sabah were sections 2 and 3 of the Civil Law Ordinance 1938, section 3 of which had this somewhat curious exception:

> "In the exercise of jurisdiction all courts shall have special regard to the laws and customs of the inhabitants of the state so far as they are not inhumane, unconscionable or contrary to public policy."

The extent to which customary law is applied in Sarawak was considered in the case of *Kho Lang Guan v Khoo Eng Guan*.[5] The Chief Justice acknowledged that certain laws and customs of races indigenous to Sarawak formed one of the three sources of law in Sarawak. This included Islamic Law, Dayak and other native law or customs concerning marriage and inheritance and certain customs by which criminal sanctions are imposed as, for example, for adultery and incestuous relations as understood by Malay and Dayak custom.

Chinese customary law is applied in Sarawak where the custom in question is expressly regulated by a Sarawak Ordinance, or by rules made under an ordinance; or where the custom is recognised, either expressly or by necessary implication, in a Sarawak Ordinance. Into the latter category fall two branches of Chinese customary law—matrimonial law and the law of inheritance.[6] The distribution of estates in the event of intestacy is according to the customary law of succession.[7]

In Sabah too, Islamic Law and the laws and customs of the indigenous people apply in relation to family matters.

This historical review establishes that in Malaysia, custom and religion have always played a major role in determining the law that governs family relations within a particular group. This can have both a positive and a negative effect in relation to the HIV epidemic. On the positive side, if the laws or customs provide a satisfactory solution to the issues arising from the ISIV epidemic, then the solution can be enforced with little objection and with much support from the community. In the negative situation, the laws and customs may have to be changed so as to provide a more suitable response to the HIV epidemic but if the required change goes to the very root of the custom or religion, it will not be well received and may be difficult to effect. Herein lies the difference between man-made statutes and laws based on custom and religion. The former can be amended at will, the latter only if the proposed change does not conflict with the basic values of the custom or the tenets of the religion.

This, however, does not mean that changes can never be introduced into Family Law merely because it is based on religion or custom. Some changes have heen effected quite successfully in the past and the experience can be repeated if deemed necessary. For example, the Law Reform (Marriage and Divorce) Act 1976, Act 164, abolished the long-standing practice of polygamy among non-Muslims, introduced a minimum age for marriage and made registration of all marriages compulsory. Although it allows marriages to be solemnised according to custom, such customary marriages must nevertheless comply with the above-mentioned requirements and can only be dissolved by a court. The provision for divorce had the effect of abolishing the Chinese husband's unilateral right to divorce his wife and gave the Chinese wife the right to seek a divorce so that she was no longer obliged to continue in a marriage until her husband chose to free her. This statute illustrates that, where necessary, Family Law regulated by custom can be modified.

Even in the case of Islamic Family Law where religion is involved, reform within the set parameters of Islam can be effected by employing the techniques that are permissible. Professor Tahir Mahmood has explained these techniques as follows:

1. Takhayyur which can take three different forms:
   (a) an eclectic choice between the corresponding legal principles of the various schools of Islamic Law;
   (b) enforcement of one of the conflicting solutions provided by various jurists in relation to controversial cases;
   (c) preference for an obsolete or lesser-known legal opinion over a generally accepted principle.
2. *Talfiq which* means the evolution of a new legal rule by combining two conflicting jurisdic views on the same problem or by blending certain parts of two or more such views.
3. *Siyasa shariya:* Under this principle the state can abandon a principle of the traditional law not by express supersession but by directing its courts that it shall not entertain any case based on such a principle. In the course of time such principles become obsolete.
4. *Ijtihad:* Under the doctrine of Ijtihad the settled legal principles may be interpreted by the jurists in accordance with the changed social conditions in any country at any point of time.[8]"

The Islamic Family Law therefore is not static and can be modified to meet new problems like those arising from the HIV/ AIDS epidemic. Such a change can be brought about by legislation. In Malaysia, legislative authority is divided between Federal and

State legislatures, with the Ninth Schedule to the Federal Constitution setting out the matters in each of the three Lists Federal, State and Concurrent List. Islamic Law, for example, is in the state list and therefore the Family Law that applies to Muslims is regulated by state enactments. Islamic Law is administered by the Shariah Courts which are state courts and have jurisdiction only over cases where all parties are Muslim .

Much existing legislation is a heritage of Malaysia's colonial past, so there remain laws in the statute books that apply to each of the three major components of Malaysia—Sabah, Sarawak and the Federation of Malaya.

In the Malaysian legal system therefore, and particularly in the area of Family Law, there are laws that can be classified into three categories:

(i) Federal Statutes that apply to the whole of Malaysia; for example the Law Reform (Marriage and Divorce) Act 1976, Act 164.

(ii) Statutes that apply to each of the three components of Malaysia:

(a) Guardianship of Infants Act 1961, Federation of Malaya Act 13 of 1961, which applies to all the eleven states of the former Federation of Malaya;

(b) Guardianship of Infants Ordinance, Sabah, Chapter 54, Laws of North Borneo, which applies only in the state of Sabah;

(c) Guardianship of Infants Ordinance, Sarawak, Chapter 93, Laws of Sarawak, which applies only in the state of Sarawak.

(iii) State Enactments of all the thirteen states, the application of which is restricted to the individual enacting state; for example, the Islamic Family Law Enactments which apply only to the Muslims who are resident in the enacting state.

In the case of the Islamic Law that is to be applied to Muslims resident in the Federal Territory, an Act of Parliament is passed but specifically limited in its application to Muslims in the Federal Territory.

It is against this backdrop that some HIV/AIDS related issues will be examined.

B. HIV/AIDS RELATED FAMILY LAW ISSUES

1. Support for Relatives During Illness

Malaysia is not a welfare state so, in the event of illness caused by HIV/AIDS, a major concern of individuals with no independent source of income is the right to financial support from family members.

In Islam, the responsibility to maintain a family rests entirely on the male members of the family. Hence a husband is to support his wife and a father, his children. The Islamic Family Law (Family Territory) Act 1984, Act 303 has codified these duties in sections 59(1) and 72 respectively. Islamic Law does not require a woman to support anyone other than an illegitimate child of hers (section 80). Many women however provide maintenance willingly and in many families they are the sole bread-winners.

A wife's right to maintenance is lost in certain circumstances. Section 59(2) provides:

> A wife shall not be entitled to maintenance when she *is nuzyuz* or unreasonably refuses to obey the lawful wishes or commands of her husband, that is to say, *inter alia.*
> (a) when she withholds her association with her husband;
> (b) when she leaves her husband's home against his will;
> (c) when she refuses to move with him to another home or place, without any valid reason according to Hukum Syara.

In relation to HIV/AIDS, this raises some significant questions. Would a woman who refuses to have sexual relations with her husband unless they practice safe sex be deemed *nuzyuz* if she has reason to believe from his activities that he may be at risk of contracting HIV? Likewise, if she chooses to leave the house for her safety, where for example her infected husband forces himself on her, should she be considered *nuzyuz?* If she is not *nuzyuz,* her husband must continue to support her; if she is, then she will lose her right to maintenance. In considering whether a woman is *nuzyuz* or not, it is important to consider whether she has any valid reason for acting the way she does. Ultimately, the question will be whether a wife has the right to protect herself from infection without losing her right to support. This issue is relevant only where the husband continues to receive an income despite his medical condition.

Where the infected husband has lost his source of income, it is the question of his support that arises. According to Islam, any person, male or female, who is unable to support himself/herself will be entitled to claim maintenance from any other person who is liable to support him/her. Such a person will be a male member of the family and the order in which these male members are responsible to support a relative is the same order in which they would have been entitled to inherit the estate of that relative had the issue been succession and not maintenance. Section 60 of Act 303 provides:

> "The court may order any person liable thereto according to Hukum Syara, to pay maintenance to another person where he is incapacitated, whally or practically from earning a livelihood by re physical injury or ill-health and the court is satisfied that having regard to the means of the first-mentioned person it is reasonable so to order."

A person with HIV/AIDS has a right to claim maintenance from his relatives and the only factor that should affect the court's decision is the means of the person from whom maintenance is sought. If there is no relative who is financially able to support, the State Treasury or Bait-ul-Mal will provide an allowance.

When it is the wife who contracts HIV, there is no excuse for the husband to refuse to provide maintenance. Some husbands may avoid their responsibility by alleging that the wives contracted the disease as a result of adulterous relationships. Such a situation would raise questions of evidence in establishing how the wife became infected when the husband is not. It is a relevant issue as adultery is viewed as a serious act of misconduct in Islam and the courts are bound to hold that a wife who commits adultery loses her right to maintenance.

A Muslim woman, however, is never without a right to maintenance. Whether her husband is no longer obliged to support her or has divorced or abandoned her, she is entitled to be supported by the male members of her family. And if she has no such relatives or if they themselves are destitute, the State Treasury or Bait-ul-Mal will provide assistance. This would apply whether or not she has HIV/AIDS.

In theory Islamic Family Law has sufficient provision to ensure that no HIV/AIDS patient is without a means of support. In practice, however, there may be many obstacles to obtaining this right, some of which are as follows:

1. The individual may not know that the rights exist or may not have the knowledge or means to enforce the right. In this regard, legal literacy campaigns addressing HIV issues should be conducted, utilising the media (especially the electronic media) peer group discussions and public talks and forums.
2. The wish to maintain confidentiality may prevent a person from claiming his/her rights. The desire for confidentiality

will be greater if he/she contracted the disease from a life-style that is condoned by Islam this will then manifest itself in a reluctance to appear in the Shariah Court.

3. There is no certainty that the courts will not consider an individual's lifestyle as a relevant factor in deciding the question of maintenance. The law itself emphasises need that arises out of an inability to support oneself because of illness. If a strict and literal interpretation is applied, an order for maintenance should be made without considering the way in which the disease was contracted. This section has not been tested yet, so there are no authorities that can be used as a guideline.

Despite the possible obstacles, there does exist under Islamic Family Law a provision for the support by family members of persons with HIV. The same is not true of the law applicable to non-Muslims where the obligation to support is limited to members of the nuclear family only.

The court can also award maintenance under the Law Reform (Marriage and Divorce) Act 1976, Act 164. The application under this law, however, can only be made if there are matrimonial proceedings pending.[9] If neither party wishes to obtain an order of judicial separation or dissolution of marriage, this section cannot be invoked. The section has made a significant inroad into the law of maintenance by giving the court the corresponding right to order a wife to pay maintenance to her husband where he is incapacitated, wholly or partially, from earning a livelihood by reason of mental or physical injury or ill-health.[10] This provision would give an HIV-infected husband the right to get maintenance, provided he applies for a divorce.

2. Divorce/Separation

(i) Islamic Low

A Muslim man can divorce his wife by the unilateral pronouncement of the *Talaq*. Under section 47 of Act 303, he must apply to the Sharjah Court for permission to do so. If the wife agrees to the divorce, he will be permitted to pronounce the *Talaq* in court. The divorce will be recorded together with the particulars relating to maintenance, the custody of children and the division of matrimonial property.

If the wife does not agree to the divorce, the parties will be sent for reconciliation. If the conciliatory body does not succeed in changing the husband's mind, they will recommend that the divorce be permitted. These procedures attempt to protect the wife's interest and ensure that in the event of a divorce she receives her entitlements. Sometimes a husband will refuse to wait and will pronounce the *Talaq*. Although his action is an offence, it is nevertheless effective in dissolving the marriage.

Should the divorce be for no just cause, the husband will have to pay a sum of money known as *muta'ah* which is translated as consolatory gift. The question that arises is whether HIV/AIDS will be regarded as a just cause for divorce. The manner in which the infection was contracted becomes relevant in deciding whether it is a just cause. This is because if the woman contracted the HIV infection through adultery, she can be divorced on the ground of her adultery. HIV is not the issue in such a situation; the adultery is. If HIV is raised as an issue, it may be regarded as an aggravating rather than a mitigating factor.

A Muslim woman can apply for a divorce under section 52(1)(f) of Act 303 which is the ground for various forms of illness including venereal disease in a communicable form. The section may be extended to include HIV/AIDS. This form of divorce is known as *fasakh*.

If a woman is unable to obtain a *fasakh,* she may apply for a *kholo'* divorce where she pays the husband a sum of money in return for her freedom. If she does not wish to do so, she may apply for a divorce under section 47 which regulates *talaq*.

Under section 47, the conciliatory committee will try to reconcile the parties, but if the wife is adamant, the committee will advise the husband to divorce her. If he refuses, the court may appoint another committee called *hakam* who will be given the authority to pronounce a divorce[11].

(ii) Law Applicable to Non-Muslims

For non-Muslims, the Law Reform (Marriage and Divorce) Act 1976, Act 164 allows divorce by mutual consent under section 52, when both parties are agreed that the marriage should be terminated. The difficulty in filing the joint petition lies in the fact that the parties must agree to the terms of all ancillary relief. If this can be settled amicably, this form of divorce is the best way of separating where one party has HIV/AIDS. The illness need never be revealed.

If the party who has HIV/AIDS refuses to consent to a joint petition, the other party may resort to section 53 where the ground for divorce is the irretrievable breakdown of marriage. To establish the breakdown, one of the four paragraphs in section 54(1) must be proved. Relevant to HIV/AIDS cases is paragraph(b) where the ground is that the respondent has behaved in such a way that the petitioner cannot reasonably be expected to live with the respondent. The manner in which HIV/AIDS was contracted becomes relevant in considering whether there was such behaviour as would justify the divorce. The illness by itself cannot be regarded as behaviour and would not be sufficient ground for the divorce[12].

If the parties do not wish to be divorced but do not want to continue cohabiting, either can apply for a decree of judicial separation under section 64 of Act 164. They may use the same grounds as mentioned in section 54.

The decree has two significant effects. The first is that when the wife dies intestate, her property will be divided as through her husband were dead.[13] This is important as under the Distribution Act 1958, the intestate estate of a woman devolves entirely upon her husband. The second significance is that although the woman is still married, she falls within the exception to the rule that there can be no rape between spouses. This is discussed more fully below.

3. Non-consensual Sexual Intercourse

Marital rape has become an important issue in the face of the HIV epidemic; the act not only constitutes violence against the woman, it also puts her at risk of contracting the infection if her husband has been infected. The law relating to rape has recently been amended to provide greater protection for women.

Sexual intercourse without the consent of a woman or against her will or in circumstances where her consent is obtained by duress or mistake amounts to rape under section 375 of the Penal Code. Where the girl is below sixteen years of age, then with or without her consent, it is rape. Thus the law fixes sixteen as the age of consent for sexual intercourse. For Muslims, marriage with a girl below the age of sixteen can only be solemnised with the permission of the authorities[14].

Section 375 provides that sexual intercourse by a man with his own wife by a marriage which is valid under any written law for the time being in force, or is recognised in the federation as valid, is not rape. There are three exceptions to this. One is where the woman has obtained a decree of judicial separation or a decree nisi for divorce. The second is where she has obtained an injunction restraining her husband from having sexual intercourse with her The third is where a Muslim woman is living separately from her husband during the period of *eddah* after the pronouncement of the divorce. In all these cases, the woman with not be deemed to be the man's wife and he can be charged with rape.

A decree of Judicial separation fees a woman from the obligation to cohabit with her husband. If she has no objection to staying with him but merely wishes to restrain him from molesting her in any way, she can obtain an injunction. The injuction, however, can provide protection only if the threat of prosecution for rape will have the effect of deterring the man from forcing himself on her. Ultimately, it is sense of responsibility on his part that will prevent him from inflicting himself on her. This sense of responsibility is more likely to be inculcated through counselling and education rather than through legal sanctions.

4. Custody of Children

When a couple with children separate or divorce, the custody of the children can become a bitter dispute. Where one parent has HIV, that fat may be used against him/her when deciding who should have custody.

Under the Islamic Law, a mother has first right to the custody of her infant children 15. This rule pre-supposes that she is fit to care for the children. If she is ill and in need of care herself, she may not be awarded custody. The difficulty that arises in deciding whether a person with HIV should be awarded custody is that, in the case of HIV infection, there are many degrees of illness. In some cases, despite being infection, there are many degrees of illness. In some cases, despite being infected, the person may function as usual and the performance of his/her duties will not be affected. In such cases, there is no justification for depriving the person of the custody of his/her children. In other cases, AIDS may develop and the person may then be in no condition to care for the children in such a situation the interests of the children may require a transfer of custody to a person who is better able to look after them.

It is possible, however, that a person with HIV/AIDS may not contest for custody if he/she is concerned about maintaining confidentiality, as is usually the case

For non-Muslims, Act 164 empowers the court to declare either parent unfit to have custody of any child.[16] This section can be invoked only when the court is making an order of either judicial separation or divorce If the ground for the divorce or separation is HIV/AIDS, then it is conceivable that the party getting the divorce or separation may insist on the declaration of unfitness for custody. Again, knowledge of attitudes to HIV will determine whether judges will use this provision in HIV cases.

Section 88(1) of Act 164 provides that "where there are exceptional circumstances making it undesirable that the child be entrusted to either parent the court may place the child with a relative of the child or with any association the objects of which include child welfare or with any suitable person." This section may be used by family members to prevent a person with HIV from obtaining custody.

5. Extra-marital Sexual Relations

Under Islamic Law, sexual relations not within a valid marriage are prohibited. This prohibition has been codified in legislation in Malaysia, though not in the Family Law Enactments.

The Administration of Islamic Law Enactment of all states have provisions that make extra-marital sexual relations of illicit intercourse, as it is usually termed, an offence. Some states have enacted a code that deals specifically with offences.[17]

These provisions are intended to be a deterrent. If they were successful in their objective, extra-marital sexual relations among Muslims would be controlled and consequently the spread of HIV/AIDS and other sexually transmitted diseases would also be controlled. In the face of the epidemic, it becomes even more necessary to retain such provisions in the law.

C. PROPOSALS FOR REFORM OF LAW AND PRACTICE

The legislative process is slow and cumbersome. Law reform is therefore not the quickest means of bringing about change. In some circumstances, administrative directives can be used to produce immediate results. In other instances, there is no alternative but to effect amendments to legislation.

Under the law applicable to non-Muslims, the provisions relating to maintenance could be amended by extending the duty to support to financially able wives of husbands who are unable to earn an income on account of any illness or incapacity. This general provision will probably be more acceptable than one that specifically mentions HIV/AIDS.

A provision could also be introduced to enable a non-Muslim to claim maintenance from a more distant relative, as in the case of Muslims. It may be necessary, however, to provide some incentive for the relative who is burdened with his additional responsibility. He/she could be granted tax relief, in the same way as tax payers are now entitled to claim relief for the medical expenses of their aged parents. Thus the provision in the Income Tax Act could be extended to the support of relatives who are incapacitated or ill. Such a change can be introduced fairly quickly as the next Budget, which will be announced in October, can include this as one of the tax incentives .

In relation to the other issues discussed, the actual effect of the relevant provisions will depend on the interpretations by the courts. It is only after the sections have been tested that it will be possible to determine the exact amendments that are needed.

Other measures that can be introduced administratively are:

1. Education Programmes

What is needed immediately is a programme for judges, and others involved in the administration of justice, that is designed to provide sufficient information about HIV/AIDS to assist them with the interpretations that they will have to make in cases where HIV is raised as an issue. Such sensitization programmes should be started soon before the issues are brought to the courts.

A special training programme should be introduced for parents to help them handle children with HIV. All other programmes on parenting skills should incorporate information about HIV.

2. Pre-marriage Courses

To target couples who are about to get married and start a family, the pre-marriage courses which are being conducted for Muslims in some states could include in their curriculum a talk about HIV, the means of transmission, the precautions to take and so on. These courses should be introduced in all states and possibly for non-Muslims too.

One topic that is already part of the course is "the rights of parties to a marriage.' This could be expanded to include the rights of spouses to protection from the risk of HIV as well as a discussion on the means of obtaining that protection. A practical instruction will be more beneficial for prospective marriage partners.

3. Counselling Units

At present only the Federal Territory of Kuala Lumpur has a Counselling Unit that is separate from the Shariah Court. This unit gives advice to anyone who seeks it, whether in person or by telephone. It also conducts counselling sessions, but this is restricted to residents of Kuala Lumpur only. The counsellors help couples with matrimonial problems. Given the demand for the services of this unit by the public, the following proposals should be considered:

(i) The counsellors presently attached to the unit should be given HIV-related training to assist in cases involving HIV-infected family members.

(ii) Similar units should be started in all states and all new staff recruited should be given training for counselling in HIV cases.

(iii) Counselling units specially geared for HIV counselling could be set up in places which are easily accessible to persons who may be in need of counselling, such as shopping complexes. People are reluctant to attend at government buildings or office blocks as their presence in such places may raise questions.

4 Family Life Courses in the School Curriculum

Information on HIV should be included in the courses on family life that are a part of the school curriculum.

In the final analysis, it is education that will have the greatest impact on efforts to control the epidemic.

References

1. Sir Roland Braddell. The Law of the Straits Settlements-A Commentary, Reprint of the 1915 Edition. Oxford University Press, 1982, p. 12.
2. Liau Yock Fang, Undang-Undang Melaka, The Laws of Melaka. The Hague. The Martinus Nijhoff, 1976, p. 38.
3. Ahmad Ibrahim, Towards a History of Law in Malaysia and Singapore, Dewan Bahasa dan Pustaka, Kuala Lumpur, 1992. p. 120.
4. Order L-4 Laws of Sarawk 1928, Section 2.
5. (1936) S. C. R. 60.
6. Chan Bee Neo v Ee Siok Chow (1947) S. C. R. I.
7. Section 17 of the Administration of Estates Ordinance specifically recognised law or custom and the courts have held that this includes Chinese custom.
8. Tahir Mahmood, Family Law Reform in the Muslim World, Tripathi Ltd. 1972, p. 12.
9. Section 77(I).
10. Section 77(2).
11. Section 48, Act 303.
12. See however Thurlow v. Thurlow (1975) 2 All E. R. 979 where it has been suggested that the risk to the health of the petitioner caused by the strain of the respondent's illness may be sufficient to hold that the petitioner cannot reasonably be expected to live with the respondent. (English cases are of persuasive authority in Malaysia).
13. Section 66(1).
14. Act 303, section 8.
15. Act 303, section 81.
16. Section 90(1).
17. See for example, the Shariah Criminal Code, Kelantan Enactment No. 2 of 1985.

41

Consultative Mechanisms for Law Review/Reform: A Malaysian Case Study

Dr. Abdul Rasid Kasri
Ministry of Health
Kuala Lumpur, Malaysia

Background

Government policies on issues related to HIV and AIDS can enhance or hinder AIDS prevention and care activities. For example, lack of educational and economic opportunities may mean an increase in the number of those who provide sexual services for money. Lack of confidentiality may create barriers for those who wish to take preventive measures or seek early diagnosis and treatment of AIDS and other STDs.

Consultative Process

HIV infection, a disease closely related to certain behaviours,.has a major socio-cultural impact on the affected community. The development of effective responses to the epidemic requires policies and measures which promote an environment that enables, encourages and sustains voluntary behaviour change and the care and support of those affected. This can be achieved by empowering individuals and communities to protect themselves against HIV and ensuring that people living with HIV remain integrated within society, are free from discrimination, and are involved and consulted during the process of policy formulation.

It is clear that the key objectives of preventing the spread of disease as well as limiting the impact of HIV infection on individuals, groups and societies cannot be achieved without the active support, co-operation and participation of many agencies and organizations both in the public and private sectors, which may have different but complementary roles to play. This includes people affected by the epidemic, the communities, and the legal, health and other professions. To facilitate the process of consultation, co-operation and collaboration, both formal and informal consultative structures need to be established.

Informal Consultative Forum

Informal consultative mechanisms such as seminars, workshops and conferences can facilitate the formulation of more comprehensive policies which take into consideration the view-points of all affected parties. Such policies stand a better chance of successful implementation and are less likely to meet with resistance. The recommendations of these informal consultative mechanisms are usually discussed in formal national level committees for further action.

Formal Consultative Forum

A high level formal consultative structure in the form of a multisectoral national committee can make a significant contribution to the efficacy of an AIDS control and prevention programme. It can overcome barriers among members by enhancing mutual knowledge and understanding. This can be achieved because deliberations and consultations take place. during discussions of certain issues or policies. Multisectoral national committees can also create synergy, which is sometimes available only through sharing or joint working, for example, in minimizing service gaps. Through outreach services, the NGOs complement governmental efforts in preventing HIV/AIDS because they have closer contacts with individuals and groups in the communities, especially those at high risk. These committees can act as co-ordinating bodies to avoid unnecessary duplication, maximizing the contribution of each agency and ensuring the efficient and effective use of skills and resources.

Government Administrative Structure on AIDS

The government is responsible for the development of national policies that form the framework within which intervention activities for HIV/AIDS take place. However, multisectoral involvement, co-operation and consultation is vital for the development of policies which reflect the needs and interests of various communities and individuals. Before contemplating the setting up of new and autonomous administrative structures, the government should consider strengthening existing structures.

In the case of Malaysia, it was decided that the prevention and control of AIDS should be integrated into the existing medical and health services and delivered through various outlets, i.e., through all government hospitals and health offices and centres. Recognizing that a high level multisectoral national committee is usually the most effective way to achieve multisectoral involvement, co-operation and consultation, a committee chaired by the Director of Health was constituted in the Ministry of Health in April 1985. The committee was subsequently renamed as 'The AIDS Task Force'.

The Task Force has the overall responsibility for formulating policies and co-ordinating the AIDS prevention and control programme. A total of 28 members representing various organizations-including Ministry of Education, Ministry of Information, Ministry of Youth and Sports, Prime Minister's Department, armed forces, Religious Department, universities, various medical bodies, the health sector, as well as non-government organizations-are on the committee. Assisting the Task Force are several standing and *ad hoc* committees. In every state, a state co-ordinating committee on AIDS has been established and made responsible for the implementation and co-ordination of AIDS prevention and control activities.

In 1992 a ministerial level committee on AIDS, chaired by the Minister of Health, was formed by the Cabinet. Its members include the Ministers of Information, Education, National Unity and Social Development, Justice and Law, Culture, Art and Tourism, Youth and Sports, Home Affairs as well as personnel from the Prime Minister's Department. The role of this committee is to advise the Cabinet on all matters pertaining to the prevention, control and management of HIV/AIDS in the country, as well as to facilitate interministerial co-ordination in this area.

In September 1993, the Health Division was reorganized and a Section on AIDS/STD was officially created within the Disease

Control Division. As a result the AIDS Task Force was reorganized into two main committees, i.e., the National Technical Committee and the National Coordinating Committee on AIDS. One of the functions of the AIDS Section is to serve as a secretariat to the ministerial level committee, National Technical Committee, National Co-ordinating Committee, and several national level subcommittees. The staff of the AIDS Section includes five public health doctors, two health education officers, and two supporting personnel.

The National Technical Committee, chaired by the Director-General of Health, is responsible for the formulation, monitoring and evaluation of policies and the review and approval of recommendations made by various subcommittees on technical matters relating to the prevention, control and management of HIV/AIDS. The members consist of chairmen of various subcommittees, representatives of various technical programmes, directors of the Ministry of Health, universities, and representative of various professional bodies.

The National Co-ordinating Committee chaired by the Secretary General of Health includes the secretaries-general of various ministries including those of Information, Education, National Unity and Social Development, Justice and Law, Culture, Art and Tourism, Youth and Sports, Home Affairs and the Prime Minister's Department, as well as the Deputy Secretary-General of Health, both finance and services, and the Legal Advisor to the Ministry of Health. This committee provides a platform for intersectoral consultations and discussions on social, cultural, religious, legal and other related issues. This committee also appoints working groups to review specific issues and evaluate and approve the recommendations of various subcommittees.

Collaboration with NGOs

The Ministry of Health in its effort to strengthen collaboration and consultation with NGOs working with HIV/AIDS issues responded to their call to assist in the formation of the Malaysian AIDS Council (MAC), which was registered with the Registrar of Societies in July 1992. The Malaysian AIDS Council is an umbrella organization which co-ordinates AIDS- related NGOs. The Council's educational, preventive and care activities complement, supplement and support the government's efforts. Among the co-ordinated projects and AIDS- related activities of its affiliates are submission of project proposals to the Ministry of Health for financial assistance and managing approved funds channelled through the council. The most important function is their participation in the national level committees and subcommittees representing the organizations, groups and individuals whose interests need to be taken into account.

Its affiliates are both AIDS specific NGOs and non-AIDS specific NGOs that have incorporated the AIDS agenda into their existing project structures. The Malaysian AIDS Council now has a membership of 22 NGOs induding various community based groups, health and legal professional associations, religious organizations, organizations addressing the needs of women and children, and social marketing affiliates, which are involved in various AIDS prevention and care efforts.

42

HIV/AIDS Law and Law Reform in Maldives

Mr. Husnu Al Suood
State Attorney
Attorney General's Office Male, Maldives

Maldives is a very small country with a population of about 250,000 people scattered over a number of small islands.

The Constitution and the laws of the country are based on the principles of Islamic law, which guarantees fundamental rights and freedoms of the individual and also places special emphasis on the rights of the public and society at large.

There are adequate laws to combat drug abuse, extra-marital sex etc. Such acts are illegal under Maldivian laws. Moreover, the Muslim population is very conscious of their religious duties and family values mainly because of the small size of the communities in which they live. Therefore, the spread of HIV is very limited in Maldives. This does not necessarily mean that there is no need to enact specific laws for the prevention of the spread of HIV and for the protection of HIV infected persons.

At present there is no HIV or AIDS related special legislation in the Maldives, nor is there even a single piece of legislation which mentions HIV or AIDS.

The first HIV case in Maldives was reported in 1991 and since then four more such cases have been reported.

The response of the Government to the HIV/AIDS problem has been very encouraging. It established a National AIDS Council which has a strong legal basis under Maldivian laws. Much has been done by this Council by way of developing and implementing action programmes for the prevention of the spread of HIV and for the protection of the HIV/AIDS infected persons.

Even though there is no specific HIV-related legislation in the country, there are administrative arrangements made to provide protection for the infected persons and to minimize possible discrimination.

Testing

There is no requirement for the compulsory testing or screening of any population sub-group. No particular group of the population is prohibited from donating blood. Initially when the first HIV case was reported in 1991 the media advocated mandatory testing for certain target groups, like seamen and those working in the tourist resorts.

Under Maldivian law there is no possibility for a person to face prosecution merely because he has contracted HIV. Therefore it is not likely for HIV infected persons to become reluctant to identify themselves or to undergo voluntary testing. A person might face prosecution only if there is evidence to show involvement in any illegal act or such person has been engaging in 'immoral conduct.'

Confidentiality

Confidentiality of information concerning persons infected with HIV has been preserved through administrative arrangements. But as the islands are very tiny, and the number of people living on each island is very small, it could be very difficult to preserve the identity of infected persons.

Equality in Employment

Administrative measures require that there be no discrimination of HIV infected persons with regard to employment. But this administrative order is only applicable to the civil service and government owned companies, and not to private sector employment.

Equality in Education

There is no rule or regulation with regard to enrolling in a school a child who is infected with HIV/AIDS. But the right to education of such children is well protected under the Fundamental Rights chapter of the Constitution.

Under the criminal laws it is an offence to knowingly or deliberately or recklessly spread HIV.

43

Legal Issues of AIDS in Mongolia

Dr. Gendensambuugiin Zuunai
Chairman
Standing Committee on Population, Health and Social Security Parliament of Mongolia, Mongolia

AIDS prevention and control is a priority for Mongolia. The National AIDS Programme was established in order to prevent the spread of HIV through skin piercing instruments, blood and blood products, and sexual means.

The Programme attempted to achieve those objectives in 1991-92 by:

— strengthening the National AIDS Reference Centre developing;
— development of HIV surveillance, including serosurveys of high-risk and sentinel population groups;
— training of health-care workers;
— conducting education activities, promoting condom use and safe sex, complemented by mass media campaigns and NGO involvement;
— mobilising additional resources; and,
— refining existing AIDS legislation.

The National AIDS Programme is being implemented at the same time as the health financing, management and organisational structure is changing as the country undergoes overall reform. At the same time, the view of Mongolia as being a low-risk country for AIDS most be revised. At present both external and internal factors are increasing the risk for the transmission and the wide-spread infection in the people of Mongolia. For example:

— Almost every country in the world, and particularly those countries close to Mongolia, have found their numbers of HIV positive and AIDS cases increasing;

— Mongolia's contacts with the outside world are also increasing. During 1990-1991 more than 200,000 Mongol citizens travelled to 40 countries, and 30,000 foreigners arrived in Mongolia. The number of international flights, trains, and local border communications, particularly with China and other Asian countries, has risen as well;

— Sexually transmitted diseases (STDs) in Mongolia during last few years show a tendency to increase. For instance, the incidence of gonorrhea doubled from 1985 to 1990.

Moderate increases in other STDs, such as syphilis, trichomoniasis, and chlamidia, have been observed. These trends may be explained by changes in Mongolian life styles, migration processes, the low cultural and educational level of the population, social unrest (i.e., unemployment, alcoholism, etc.) and obsolete facilities for the control and prevention of STDs.

So far, Mongolia is considered as one of the few countries in the world to remain AIDS-free. The first case of HIV infection in Mongolia was reported in Ulaanbaatar in August 1992. This case triggered strong and political commitment from the Government.

The Government in September 1992 discussed the situation of AIDS and proposed measures for preventing the spread of HIV. As a sign of its decision, the Government issued decree No.18 which renewed the National AIDS Committee headed by the Vice-Prime Minister. The deputy Chairman is the Minister of Health. Nine Deputy Ministers or Director Generals of other ministries and departments have been appointed as members of the Governmental Committee. The secretary of the Committee is the Deputy Minister of Health.

The new National AIDS Committee held its first meeting in September 1992 and approved the new version of the National AIDS programme, the plan of action for implementing the programme, and other important documents. The second meeting of the Committee is planned for December 1992.

As a follow up to the Government decree No. 18, the Health Minister issued decree No. 128. This decree created the Technical Advisory Board, which has 17 members under the chairmanship of the Deputy Health Minister. This board held its first meeting in

September 1992 and, thorough discussions, submitted the aforementioned documents to the National AIDS Committee .

The newly-approved plan of action for implementing the National AIDS Programme strengthens the capability of the National AIDS Reference Center, develops an AIDS laboratory network based on existing districts *(aimak)* and cities, establishes STD/blood bank serological laboratories, and creates AIDS patient wards in the Central Infectious Disease Hospital. The plan also calls for many educational measures. It calls for the inclusion of AIDS/STD in the school curricula, and incorporates AIDS into the teaching curricula of graduate and post-graduate training for medical students, doctors, and health personnel. The plan seeks to use education activities to promote condom use in sexual behaviour, as well as improving the commitment of the community and NGOs to anti-AIDS activities. The activities envisaged in the MTP were successfully implemented in 1991-1992 except for the KABP study which was not processed or analysed due to the lack of computers and trained personnel in the National AIDS Reference Center. WHO support is crucial to the success of the National AIDS Programme .

To date more than 90,000 serum samples, mainly from blood donors, pregnant women and other high-risk and sentinel population groups, have been tested for HIV. Only one test has been positive.

The draft law on AIDS was prepared jointly by the Ministry of Health and the Ministry of Justice and submitted to a working group of the Parliament. It is expected to be approved in 1993. While including regulations for preventing the spread of HIV/AIDS, the draft law emphasised the need to avoid discrimination against HIV/AIDS victims, their family members and relatives in accordance with World Health Organisation resolutions (41.24 and 45.35). The law is designed to replace decree No.103 of the People's Great Khural (the Parliament in the previous political system) which dealt with AIDS.

This draft law consists of many articles which regulate social relations as they affect state policies on the prevention, detection, and verification of AIDS and the treatment and counselling of HIV/AIDS patients. The law is also meant to provide people with sound information on HIV/AIDS.

The draft prescribes blood and medical interventions and increases the responsibility of medical personnel and establishments to halt spread of HIV. The draft also draws attention to the personal responsibility of HIV positive people to prevent the transmission of HIV. While it promotes voluntary screening tests, it also envisages coercive measures in case people with HIV or those suspected of having HIV fail to act responsibly. Finally, the draft recognises the importance of avoiding discrimination against HIV infected people while preserving their anonymity and right to confidentiality.

44

The AIDS Situation and Legal Issues Related to AIDS in Mongolia

Dr. G. Dashzaveg
Vice Minister of Health, Mongolia

Dr. D. Sagar
Vice-Minister of Justice, Mangolia

HIV/AIDS prevention and control is one of the priority health concerns of Mongolia. The first case of HIV infection in Mongolia was reported in Ulaanbaatar in August 1992. It triggered off strong and continuous political commitment from the government which in September 1992 discussed the AIDS situation in the country and proposed measures for its prevention and control. By issuing Decree No.18, the government decided to renew the composition of the National AIDS Committee headed by the Vice-Prime Minister. The Deputy to the Chairman is the Minister of Health and the secretary of the Governmental Committee is the Vice-Minister of Health. Nine Vice-Ministers or Deputy Chairmen of other ministries and governmental organizations have been appointed as members of the National AIDS Committee.

The National AIDS Committee has adopted the National AIDS Prevention Programme (NAPP). The main objectives of the NAPP are the prevention of the spread of HIV infection through skin piercing instruments, prevention of the spread of HIV and other blood borne infections through blood products, and the prevention of sexual transmission of HIV.

The National AIDS Prevention Programme is being implemented in the context of the overall continuing process of reforms in the country particula-rly in the field of health financing, management and its organizational structure, including those related to AIDS/HIV/ STD.

The present external and internal circumstances are conducive to the widespread transmission of HIV infection among the population of Mongolia.

In January 1994 the State Great Khural Parliament of Mongolia adopted the Law of Mongolia on Prevention of the Acquired Immunodeficiency Syndrome (AIDS), which was elaborated and modified along the lines of internationally recommended policies. This law consists of 15 articles.

In a subsequent governmental decree and Health Minister's resolution, the necessary recommendations for implementing the items of Law were adopted.

The purpose of the Law on the Prevention of AIDS is to determine the rights and duties of the state, health and other institutions, doctors, medical workers, citizens, and individuals infected and ill with HIV/AIDS; for the prevention and control of HIV; and to regulate relations connected with the realization thereof.

According to the Law the government and the governors shall have the following rights and duties with regard to the protection of the population from HIV/AIDS:

- To organize and supervise the implementation of the AIDS Prevention Law and regulations.
- To determine the state policy for the prevention and control of HIV/AIDS and take measures for its implementation.
- To determine the spheres of jobs and services where persons infected or ill with HIV/AIDS shall not work.
- To organize the medical examination of population groups at risk of infection and dissemination of HIV/AIDS.

The governmental central authority responsible for health and health institutions is to exercise the following rights and duties with regard to the prevention and control of HIV/AIDS:

- To elaborate measures for the prevention and control of HIV/ AIDS and organize the implementation of decisions taken on this matter.
- To bear responsibility for official information regarding HIV/ AIDS infection and morbidity.
- To determine population groups at risk of infection and dissemination of HIV/AIDS.
- To establish the terms of medical examination and investigation of persons at risk of infection and dissemination of HIV/AIDS and for clinical management in

cases of infection and disease; and to render medical aid and supervise implementation.

- To issue official instructions to persons infected with HIV and their guardians to prevent transmission of infection.
- To detect, confirm and treat HIV infection among the population.
- To ensure conditions so that HIV will not be transmitted through syringes and other medical instruments.
- To avoid using for the purpose of treatment blood products, tissues and organs not tested for HIV.
- To not refuse to render medical aid to persons infected or ill with HIV/AIDS on the grounds of incurability of the disease.

This Law attaches special attention to the personal responsibility and duties of persons infected with HIV. The duties of persons infected and ill with HIV/AIDS are as follows:

- To give health organizations accurate information about the conditions and causes of the infection and disease.
- To allow medical examinations to be conducted in conformity with the instructions of the concerned health organizations.
- To refrain from donating blood and other organs.
- To not transmit infection to others; to refrain from any acts and relations that may result in transmission of the virus.
- To strictly obey official instructions given by health organizations, doctors and medical workers.
- To inform upon entry into the country the frontier health inspection service about their infection and disease.

Citizens of Mongolia shall have the following duties with regard to the prevention and control of HIV/AIDS:

- To follow the official demands of the governor and health institutions on detection of and medical examination for AIDS.
- To actively participate in the measures on the prevention and control of HIV/AIDS organized by the responsible organizations and offices.
- To not violate the legitimate rights and interests of persons infected and ill with HIV/AIDS.
- To obtain accurate and comprehensive information about HIV/ AIDS and learn about prophylactic methods.

Confidentiality and anonymity, together with avoidance of discrimination and stigmatization of HIV infected persons, are other issues addressed by the Law on the Prevention of AIDS. Article 13 of the Law deals with the protection of human rights in connection with HIV infection. The following contexts are covered:

- Restriction of the inalienable human rights enshrined in the Constitution shall be prohibited on the ground of HIV infection or disease, unless otherwise provided for by the Law.
- Persons carrying out health examination and supervision in order to detect HIV infection can be asked for an official certificate that entitles them to do so.
- Citizens may voluntarily ask for clinical and laboratory examination to identify HIV infection.
- The institutions, officials and citizens who, by virtue of their official position or otherwise, have knowledge of any infected person(s) shall be prohibited from divulging their HIV status.
- In case of failure to fulfil the duties provided in this Law by a person infected and ill with HIV/AIDS due to inability to control himself/herself, the person shall be isolated and subjected to compulsory treatment.
- If a person whose infection or disease with HIV/AIDSis established becomes pregnant, the pregnancy shall be terminated on medical grounds.
- Blood, blood products, tissues and organs not guaranteed free of infection, shall be prohibited entry into the state and their sale shall be prohibited.
- If a foreign national or stateless person whose infection with HIV is established refuses to obey instructions of the concerned health organizations, that person shall be deported from the country as provided for in the legislation.

Activities envisaged in this law and in the MTP, which is based on Programme Management Policies of GPA are being implemented successfully. WHO support is crucial for the realization of the National AIDS Programme.

The recent social and economic changes in the country have in part contributed to an increase in prostitution, rape and high-risk sexual activities among the youth. The changes in sexual mores are also reflected in the increasing rates of STDs. It is necessary to redraft the law on the control of commercial sex and prostitution.

During recent years there have appeared on the market different sex and erotic publications which have an adverse influence on young people. There is a need to regulate the distribution of such publications.

Finally, it must be recognized that international and regional efforts aimed at worldwide exchange of experiences, globally developed policies, guidelines and advice on the prevention and treatment of HIV/AIDS, are useful for the implementation of national AIDS programmes in individual countries.

This Regional Workshop, through the exchange of various viewpomts, will provide valuable guidelines on the legal issues relating to AIDS in Asian countries, which in turn will greatly contribute to solving the legal and ethical problems with regard to AIDS.

45

The Current Status of AIDS Legislation in Myanmar

Mr. U. Saw Soe Phone Myint
Attorney General's office of Yangon, Myanmar

INTRODUCTION

The fight against AIDS has been given top priority by the Government of Myanmar and the importance of dealing with this problem in a multi sectoral approach has also been well recognized. Participation of non-government organizations in AIDS control activities is being encouraged and in the coming years it is hoped that they will play an important role in the fight against this dreaded disease.

Preventive measures relating to communicable diseases including AIDS, mainly undertaken by the Ministry of Health, are reflected in the newly-enacted law namely, the Prevention and Control of Communicable Diseases Law.

Although there is no legislation which deals specifically with HIV/ AIDS, certain provision concerning prevention of AIDS are contained in various laws.

LEGAL PROVISIONS CONCERNING HIV/AIDS

The Prevention and Control of Communicable Diseases Law

Until recently, the Epidemic Diseases Act was in force. It was enacted in 1897. The Prevention and Control of Communicable Diseases Law was enacted in March 1995.

The new law establishes an administrative mechanism in order to prevent the outbreak of communicable diseases; identifies functions and duties of the health officers as well as those of the public for environmental sanitation; identifies communicable diseases which require to be reported; prescribes measures to be taken in respect of an outbreak of a principal epidemic disease; identifies quarantine periods; specifies offences and penalties; and establishes the power to make rules (regulations) and procedures as well as to issue orders and directives.

Under this Law, AIDS is classified as a "principal epidemic disease".

Section 4 provides that when a Principal Epidemic Disease or a Notifiable Disease occurs:

(a) immunization and other necessary measures shall be undertaken by the Department of Health, in order to control the spread thereof;

(b) the public shall abide by the measures undertaken by the Department of Health under sub-section (a).

Section 5 prescribes the duties to be performed by the health officer when a principal epidemic disease or a notifiable disease occurs in an area to which he is assigned. Section 9 provides that the head of the household or any member of the household shall report immediately to the nearest health department or hospital principal epidemic disease cases. Section 10 provides that traditional medicine practitioners, health assistants and doctors shall report immediately to the nearest health department or hospital if a case of principal epidemic disease or a notifiable disease is found. Section 11 prescribes the measures to be undertaken by the health officer in order to prevent and control the spread of a principal epidemic disease. Section 13 provides that the health officer shall report immediately the source of the principal epidemic disease to the relevant Department of Health. Section 14 empowers an organization or an officer authorized by the Ministry of Health to issue a prohibitive order or a restrictive order in respect of matters mentioned in that section. Sections 15 to 18 provide penalties in respect of the failure to comply with or violations of the provisions of the Law. Section 20 provides that prevention, control of the spread, and necessary investigations in respect of AIDS shall be carried out in accordance with the orders and directives issued specifically by the Ministry of Health.

The Myanmar Excise Act

Under the above Act, no person may make, sell, possess or use any hypodermic syringe, or any other apparatus suitable for injecting any intoxicating drug, except under and in accordance with the conditions of a license granted under the Act. This prohibition, however, does not apply to medical practitioners, veterinary practitioners or persons who possess or use any syringe or apparatus on the prescription of a medical practitioner. Section 33 provides as follows:

Section 33. Whoever, in contravention of Section 13 makes, sells, possesses or uses:

(a) any hypodermic syringes, or

(b) any other apparatus suitable for injecting any intoxicating drug, shall be punished with imprisonment for a term which may extend to six months, or with fine which may extend to one thousand kyats, or with both.

It can be from the provisions of Section 13 that apart from the three kinds of persons provided in the proviso, no person has any right to make or sell or possess or use any hypodermic syringes or any other apparatus suitable for injecting any intoxicating drug.

Despite this legal prohibition disposable needles are now available in the market openly. In March 1992 the Ministry of Health issued a directive to the effect that proper sterilization of syringes, needles, surgical equipment, and other skin piercing equipment (boiled for at least twenty minutes) be undertaken in all health care centres in the country.

The Suppression of Brothels Act

This Act was enacted in 1949 and was amended in 1956.

Section 3 of the Act provides that any person who, in any public street or public place or place of public resort or within sight of, and in such manner as to be seen or heard from such public street or public place, whether from within any house, building, room, vessel, vehicle or not:

> by words, gestures, wilful and indecent exposure of her person or otherwise attracts or endeavours to attract attention for the purpose of prostitution; or solicits or molests any person for the purpose of prostitution shall be punished with rigorous imprisonment for a term which may extend to one year or with fine or with both.

Section 5 subsection (1) provides that any person who

knowingly lives, wholly or in part, on the earnings of prostitution shall be punished with imprisonment which may extend to three years. Subsection (2) provides that where a person is proved to be living with, or to be in the company of a prostitute, or is proved to have exercised control, direction or influence over the movements of a prostitute in such a manner as to show that he is aiding, abetting or compelling her prostitution with any other person, it shall be presumed, until the contrary is proved, that he is knowingly living on the earnings of prostitution.

Procurement as well as management of brothels are also offences under this Act.

The Penal Code

Section 377 of the Penal Code penalizes unnatural offences and is intended to punish the offence of sodomy, buggery and bestiality. The offence consists in having carnal knowledge against the order of nature by a man with a man, or in the same unnatural manner with a woman, or by a man or woman in any manner with an animal.

The Narcotic Drugs and Psychotropic Substances

With a view to strengthening the fight against the drug menace the Narcotic Drugs and Psychotropic Substances Law was enacted on 27 January 1993. The old law, namely the Narcotic and Dangerous Drugs Law, 1974 was repealed by the newly-enacted law. This law,contains 31 sections and was drafted to be in conformity with the United Nations Convention against Illicit Traffic in Narcotic Drugs and Psychotropic Substances.

Section 9 of the said Law provides for the registration of drug users at a medical centre recognized by the Government for the purpose of medical treatment.

Registered drug users undergoing medical treatment are requested to comply with the directives issued by the Ministry of Health.

Section 10 provides for the deregistration of drug users. Section 11 prescribed the measures to be carried out by the Ministry of Social Welfare, Relief and Resettlement in respect of the rehabilitation and after-care of drug users.

Under Section 15 of the law the failure to register at the place prescribed by the Ministry of Health or at a medical centre recognized by the Govemment for this purpose or to abide by the directives issued by the Ministry of Health for medical treatment is an offence liable to imprisonment for a term which may extend from a minimum of 3 years to a maximum of 5 years.

Thus, it will be noticed that whereas Section 9 prescribes a drug user to register and to abide by the directives issued by the Ministry of Health, Section 15 penalizes failure to comply with the provisions of Section 9.

Blood Screening

Although there is no specific law relating to blood transfusion, in fact, screening of blood donors is being carried out at the blood donation centres.

46

The HIV/AIDS Situation in New Zealand

Lady Jocelyn Smith
Chariperson,
New Zealand
Public Health Commission
Wellington, New Zealand

Prof. Peter Skegg
Department of Law
Ctago University Dinnedin
New Zealand

CURRENT HIV/AIDS SITUATION

HIV

Although HIV infection is not notifiable in New Zealand, laboratory reports of non-identifiable information are available. Statistics need to be interpreted with caution: not all people at risk will have been tested and testing may not be requested until many years after infection has occurred. Over the last 10 years, about 90-100 persons each year in New Zealand have been found to be infected. In 1994, 89 people were found to be infected, bringing the total to 997. Of these:

- 57 per cent were homosexual/bisexual males
- 3 per cent were intravenous drug users
- 2.8 per cent were recipients of blood products (1.2 per cent transfusion related)
- 0.2 per cent were infected perinatally.

In the fourth quarter of 1994, 26 people were newly-found to be infected with HIV. Of these 22 were male and 4 were female. No ethnicity data is available.

AIDS

AIDS is notifiable in New Zealand. The total number notified since monitoring began (on 31 December 1994) is 473. Of these 387 (81.8 per cent) are known to have died, 68 (14.4 per cent) were alive on that date; 390 (82.5 per cent) were European/pakeha, 52 (11 per cent) were Maori and 2.5 per cent were Pacific islanders.

RISK FACTORS

Of the twelve people notified with AIDS in the fourth quarter of 1994, all were male, and all reported having had sexual contact with other men.

Of the twenty-two men found to be infected with HIV in the fourth quarter of 1994, information is available on twenty of them. Thirteen were reported to have had sex with men. One was reported as an injecting drug user. Six were considered to have been heterosexually infected, five from parts of the world where heterosexual transmission is common.

Two of the four women were reported to have been heterosexually infected, one from a part of the world where this form of transmission is common. One women was reported to be an injecting drug user.

Use of Sentinel Populations

Sentinel populations are those in which HIV is or might be spreading, e.g., people attending STD clinics, injecting drug users. Prevalence surveys have been carried out using anonymous unlinked methods. Transmission through male-to-male sexual intercourse remains the largest group. This includes men who identify as gay or bisexual and others who do not identify as such but who have had sex with other men.

Although the number of those who have acquired HIV from hetrosexual intercourse remains low in New Zealand, the number of women infected continues to rise. In most cases, women are the sexual partners of men in other high-risk groups—bisexual men, injecting drug users, men from other countries where heterosexual transmission is common.

Injecting drug users are the third largest group, with transmission attributed to sharing injection equipment. No new cases of medically acquired HIV have been reported since blood donor screening was introduced in 1985.

There has been one case reported of mother to infant (vertical) transmission.

EXISTING LEGAL FRAMEWORK

Non-Discrimination Law

The Human Rights Act, 1993, specifies prohibited grounds of discrimination. These include discrimination on grounds of physical illness, the presence in the body of organisms capable of carrying disease and sexual orientation.

Privacy

The Privacy Act, 1993, and the Health Information Privacy Code, 1994, protect privacy interests, including those of people with HIV/ AIDS. Rule 11 of the Code deals with limits on the disclosure of health information. One circumstance in which it is sometimes permissible to disclose information without the consent of a person with HIV/AIDS is where there is reason to believe that the disclosure is necessary to prevent or lessen a serious and imminent threat to public health or safety, or to the life or health of another.

Needle Exchange

The Health (Needles and Syringes) Regulations, 1987, make provisions for a needle exchange scheme.

Criminal Offences

The Crimes Act, 1961, contains various provisions which have a bearing on the intentional, reckless or negligent communication of HIV/AIDS. It is an offence to wilfully and without lawful excuse cause or produce 'disease or sickness' in another person (Section 210), and, with reckless disregard for the safety of others, to cause 'actual bodily harm' to another person (Section 188(2)).

The Homosexual Law Reform Act, 1986, had the effect of decriminalizing anal intercourse between consenting persons over the age of 16 years.

PROPOSED LEGAL REFORMS

These include:

Health and Disability Services Amendment Bill

This legislation disestablishes the Public Health Commission and returns the responsibility to enhance, promote and protect public health (defined as the health of all the people in New Zealand or the health of a particular community) to the Ministry of Health. The Core Services Committee which has the responsibility for advising on national priorities for health will be expanded to ensure that public health and personal health needs are considered as a whole. The four regional health authorities will assume responsibility for purchasing services to address the prioritized health needs.

Review of the Health Act, 1956

This is currently underway and questions are being raised about the possibility of moving from the communicable disease model to a health promotion model. The new regulations will have to mesh with other legislation especially dealing with emergencies such as epidemic outbreaks. The progressive work on the harmonization of New Zealand's laws with those of Australia continues. Other legislation which has specifically been asked to be reviewed includes the Health (Needles and Syringes) Regulations, 1987 and the Misuse of Drugs Act, 1987.

Prostitution

The government has announced that it does not intend to proceed with legislation in this area.

Immigration

The Advisory Committee on STD/HIV/AIDS has advised that there should be no move to introduce mandatory testing of immigrants.

PROSPECTS

General

It would be fair to say that New Zealand is moving towards the maintenance mode regarding HIV/AIDS. Efforts to provide personal health services for people diagnosed with AIDS, in ways which suit them and those close to them will continue. This includes services for refugees who come to New Zealand. Voluntary testing associated with appropriate counselling and support is also being encouraged. At the same time (within the health public policy framework) attempts are being made to link the work on HIV/AIDS to the wider setting of sexual health. A paper advising the Minister of Health on STDs is in preparation. This paper will explicitly acknowledge the interface of HIV/AIDS with other sexually transmitted diseases. This in turn can be related to other work under way in the Ministry on unplanned pregnancy, cervical cancer and infertility. At the other end of the spectrum, work on bloodborne diseases, including hepatitis in relation to injecting drug users, transfused blood and blood products will be continuing.

It was recommended to the Minister in April 1994 that the Ministry of Health should undertake a review of the Health (Needles and Syringes) Regulations, 1987, and the Misuse of Drugs, 1978, in the context of the public health regulatory review. It was also recommended that the Departments of Justice and Police, and the Ministries of Health and Women's Affairs should prepare policy papers on legislation and law enforcement policies affecting prostitution, and public health policies related to the sex industry, for consideration by the government.

47

HIV/AIDS Law and Law Reform in Nauru

Ms. Elizabeth Amran
Chairperson
Nauru National AIDS Committee, Nauru

The AIDS Committee was established during 1992 under the umbrella of the Department of Health. Its main function is to create and sustain awareness concerning the HIV/AIDS problem.

In this respect the committee has endeavoured to give the AIDS issue high visibility through its activities of translating literature on the subject into local languages.

To mark World AIDS Day (1 December) the committee prepares a range of media presentations throughout the week leading up to the AIDS Day.

The AIDS Committee is made up of people representing the diverse ethnic groups of Nauru. In the production of radio and TV programmes, an attempt is made to include people from different age and interest groups and cultures. For instance, secondary level students, unemployed youth, Church deacons, women representatives, health educators and hospital staff, and people with differing ethnic backgrounds are encouraged to participate.

The Youth Affairs Work Skills Development Programme includes sessions which deal specifically with HIV/AIDS and STDs (sexually transmitted diseases). Over a hundred young unemployed people participate annually in this programme.

On the last World AIDS Day, a special prayer was dedicated during the Sunday service to HIV/AIDS victims the world over. The positive response of the Church is a great encouragement.

The first AIDS Committee had difficulty with the community response to the public discussion of HIV/AIDS. As recently as three years ago, people were reluctant to talk about AIDS. Today, people are becoming more receptive to discussions on the virus and its implications as more campaign material, including case-studies and documentary films developed around the theme of HIV/AIDS, are used.

The Department of Health has planned a series of workshops on STDs and HIV/AIDS in the near future.

48

HIV/AIDS Law in Pakistan

Mr. Shoukat Ali
Secretary-General
Pakistan AIDS Prevention Society Karachi, Pakistan

At present Pakistan has 800 HIV positive persons and 45 AIDS cases. Most of the AIDS patients are still surviving. The last known patient to die was a foreigner who died while being boarded onto a plane to return home.

All the factors that predispose a country to the growing spread of HIV/AIDS- like the influx of migrant workers, unregulated blood transfusion system, prevalence of prostitution, and homosexuality, travel to and from the country—are present in Pakistan.

HIV/AIDS Laws

Though the Constitution provides a certain degree of protection with regard to personal rights and liberties, there is no specific legislation which covers the area of HIV/AIDS.

There are laws like the Infectious Diseases Act, which indirectly provide for restrictive approaches in law.

Regulations

Among the administrative regulations in place are those covering quarantine and isolation (though not HIV specific); and travellers entering the country for a period exceeding six months.

New Laws

The provincial governments are engaged in formulating new

legislation covering blood transfusion and selected policies. The main features of these laws are the mandatory testing of all donated blood and the elimination of professional donors.

Notification

A notification law exists in terms of which HIV/AIDS has been specially declared as a notifiable disease by the government.

Laws of Other Countries Affecting Nationals

About 700 Pakistani HIV patients have been deported during the past two years from Middle East countries. Foreign embassies insist on a HIV-free certificate for processing visas.

General Laws

Some of the existing laws, though general in nature, cover certain HIV-related legal issues. Examples of such laws are:

1. Prohibition of Prostitution Law;
2. Child Abuse Law;
3. Hadood Ordinance;
4. Law relating to Medical Termination of-Pregnancy; and
5. Narcotics and Drugs Act.

Negative Laws

In the past, HIV/AIDS campaigns on the electronic media were not allowed. Following the recent changes in policy, the electronic media has begun to carry low profile AIDS prevention messages, with no direct mention of condoms and sex.

Law Reform

Among areas that require attention are the following:

1. The creation of legal/ethical committees at the national and provincial programme levels.
2. Integration of HIV counselling into legislation, more particularly workplace laws.

Pakistan is lagging behind in its understanding of the need for HIV-related laws because of less exposure to the issue in the past. Serious efforts need to be made to integrate HIV concerns into its legislative and quasi-legislative systems. Donor agencies, like the WHO, which are major financial partners in the National Programme, and are in the regular process of consultation with the National AIDS Committee, can play an important role in focusing the attention of the programme to the need for law review.

49

Existing Law on HIV/AIDS in Papua New Guinea

Christine Stewart
Legal Officer
PNG Legal Reform Committee
Papua, New Guinea

INTRODUCTION

Cultural Setting

Some 85 per cent of the population of nearly 4 million lives in traditional village settings in rural areas, which may be extremely remote and inaccessible. Access is often limited to poor bush roads, small plane airstrips or walking tracks only. In coastal and island regions, and on the major river systems, small boat and canoe transport is common. Despite this, there is a high casual flow rate between rural and urban areas. Cash cropping and access to money have intruded to varying degrees into the subsistence economy.

Village societies are small homogenous groups characterised by face to face relationships and group allegiance determined by one of the very wide variety of kinship systems, ranging from patrilineal/patrilocal through bilateral to various types of matrilineal society. Traditional values, rights and obligations pertain not to the individual but the group, from which the individual's status and position in society is derived.

Christianity is the professed religion of almost the entire population, with the Catholic, Anglican, Lutheran and United (Protestant) churches predominating, though a wide variety of fundamentalist churches are also present. Religious adherence tends to be determined by village or cultural group, rather than individual choice. Despite the advent of Christianity, traditional religious beliefs, including those of good and evil spirits, sorcery (white and black), telepathy, etc., persist at all levels of society, side by side or even syncretised with the introduced religious systems.

The country is governed by a Westminster-style National Parliament, elected by universal franchise, and Provincial Assemblies for each of the 19 provinces. Government authority is comparatively weak, which gives rise to constant demands from various sectors of the society for the imposition of draconian measures to combat social problems.

The depressed economy and the low level of national unity give rise to much violent crime, principally robbery, rape and murder. This is not confined to urban centres alone. Nation-wide cultural traditions of xenophobia and retaliation legitimise self-help measures for the redress of wrongs. This can take place on an individual or group level. Tribal clashes are frequent, even in "mixed" urban areas, and may continue for long periods of time.

Health services are provided mainly by the government. Private doctors practice in the larger urban centres, and missions operate their own services in remote rural areas. Large employers, such as mining companies, are required to provide medical facilities on site. Government health services, provided through the Department of Health and Provincial Governments, are relatively inexpensive, but problems are frequently faced with funding, staffing and drug distribution, etc.

Legal System

Papua New Guinea's legal system is adopted from the English common law adversarial system, with a typical appellate court hierarchy, principles of *stare decisis,* etc. Most overseas decisions have persuasive authority only. A substantial body of indigenous case law has developed since Independence in 1975.

The inferior courts consist of: District Courts, each declared for its own area which is in practical terms a province, and limited jurisdictionally in other ways as well; Local Courts with a more limited jurisdiction still; and Village Courts, which apply customary principles to village-level disputes and are subject only to the Constitution and to laws which are specifically applied to them. These courts operate with varying degrees of success and adherence to constitutional principles.

The formal courts are paying increasing attention to custom, which may be pleaded as a question of fact. Due to the diversity of cultures, however, a unified customary law is unlikely to develop, though general trends can be extracted.

The Constitution, adopted at Independence in 1975, is one of the world's lengthiest and most detailed. It is notable for its entrenchment of human rights, largely following upon the Universal Declaration of Human Rights. These are predicated on the concept of the rights (and obligations) of the individual, in contradistinction to traditional Papua New Guinea societies, whose mores are founded on the rights and obligations of the group.

Rights are classified into fundamental and qualified, with some of the latter applicable to citizens only. The independence of the judiciary and the comparative case of access by the literate and urban population to the courts has meant that rights are strenuously upheld, where adjudicated, and a considerable body of constitutional case law has already developed. The main inhibiting factors to this process have been widespread ignorance of constitutional rights and the legal process, and illiteracy and remoteness in the rural sector.

Fundamental Rights are:

- Right to Life (Section 35)
- Freedom from Inhuman Treatment (Section 36)
- Right to Protection of the Law (Section 37)

Other Rights are each defined in detail and at length, and may be qualified generally in the interests of defence, public safety, public order, public welfare, public health, the protection of children and persons under legal or practical disability, the development of underprivileged or less advanced groups or areas, or to protect the rights and freedoms of others, to the extent that the qualification is reasonably justifiable in a democratic society.

The HIV/AIDS epidemic has implications for nearly all human rights, but the primary operational right is the Fundamental Right to Life. AIDS threatens human life, and governments and the international community are obligated to take all measures to protect human life. Hence any action which prohibits or restricts an individual's ability to protect him or herself from contracting HIV contravenes this most fundamental of rights.

The most notable Qualified Right in the context of HIV/AIDS is Section 49, the Right to Privacy, in respect of personal and family life, communications and personal papers and effects.

Criminal law is codified, and is primarily governed by the Criminal Code (Chapter 262), which was adopted from the Code of Queensland. Much of it persists in its original form, with no modifications or adaptation to the country's circumstances.

Papua New Guinea's legal system, consisting of a body of imported law which is often paternalistic, outdated and inappropriate, a modern and detailed system of entrenched constitutional rights, and a growing recognition of general trends in customary law which are often in conflict with both of the foregoing, contains fundamental tensions and conflicts, many of which remain to be resolved.

Dimensions of the Epidemic in Papua New Guinea

By late 1992,127 HIV infections and 46 AIDS cases had been identified. The great majority of these were detected in the Capital. Slightly over half of infected persons are male, and the principal age category for both sexes is the 15-30 age group. A high rate of underreporting is suspected for Papua New Guinea.

A Medium Term Plan was developed in 1989 by WHO and the Department of Health. A review in 1992 found that excellent progress is being made, although much anticipated funding has not been forthcoming and the programme suffers lack of resources, staffing, etc.

Epidemic management is currently vested in the Department of Health, which has established a National AIDS Committee (originally the National AIDS Surveillance Committee, established in 1986) to advise the Departmental Secretary. Committee membership is drawn from the public and private sectors.

No public health legislation has yet heen enacted specifically in respect of HIV/AIDS. The existing Public Health Act (Chapter 226) contains separate Parts for: infectious diseases, with provision for proclamation of a disease; venereal diseases, which are exclusively defined in the body of the Act; and other special provisions for typhoid, Hansen's Disease and malaria. The Part most appropriate as it stands at present for HIV/AIDS would be Part-V—Venereal Diseases. Should it be considered appropriate to bring HIV/AIDS within the ambit of this Part of the Act, legislative intervention will be required. The decision to include or not will depend on the direction of policy formulation and the extent of its conformity with the existing provisions of the Act. For example,

Part-V includes provisions and procedures for treatment and cure which are inappropriate to HIV/AIDS, and some partner notification requirements which may run contrary to policies on confidentiality. Some amendment may be necessary to take account of such matters. Consequently, references to the Act in this paper are made for information purposes only, and should not be taken to refer to H HIV/AIDS .

A. PUBLIC HEALTH

1. Notification

There is no current legal requirement for notification of HIV infection. However, anonymous or coded test result reporting is collated at the STD/ AIDS Unit of the Department of Health. Reporting is relatively comprehensive, although substantial under-reporting is recognised. It is from these reports that the national database is compiled, and a quarterly report has been distributed since late 1990.

Part V of the Public Health Act provides for the appointment by the Minister of a Commissioner for the purposes of the Part (Section 49). There have been many departmental reorganisations and reclassifications since the Act was originally written, and the present-day equivalent of the position is Senior Medical Officer, STD/AIDS Unit.

Medical practitioners diagnosing a case of a venereal disease must notify the disease to the Commissioner (Section 52). The practitioner must also advise the sufferer of the dangers of infection and the “legal consequences” of infecting others, and warn him/her against contracting a marriage until cured (Section 53).

2. Testing

Under the Medical Code of Ethics, no-one may be required to submit him/ herself for medical examination unless the law requires it.

Test specimens are taken at STD clinics, provincial hospitals, health centres and subcentres, special survey sites, and private practitioner surgeries. Serodia and ELISA tests are performed in Papua New Guinea; Western Blot confirmation is carried out in Australia. Coding is used to identify specimens and other patient data are collected.

Mandatory nominal testing may infringe the Qualified Right to Privacy, unless it is carried out in an “optional” situation, e.g., for employment application. So far, such testing is performed in only three specific instances, on Defence Force servicemen, foreign work applicants and job applicants to one large mining company.

The Defence Force has instituted a policy of mandatory testing of all applicants for enlistment, and all servicemen as part of their Annual Medical Board. Voluntary testing of authorised civilians, and the families of servicemen, is encouraged. Alongside these testing policies, the Force has instituted strong awareness measures, including the promotion of its own brand of condom.

Where appiicants for entry visas are required to undergo medical testing before entry (e.g., applicants for work visas), an HIV test is now required as part of the medical.

Ok Tedi Mining requires a pre-employment medical examination for prospective employees. There is no obligation on existing employees to inform the company of their HIV status, nor are they required to undergo testing.

3. Compulsory Treatment

Under the Code of Ethics, no-one is compelled to submit him/herself for treatment unless the law requires it. It is the patient's consent which makes it lawful for the doctor to examine or treat.

Section 56 of the Public Health Act requires a person becoming aware that he is suffering a venereal disease to consult and place himself under the treatment of a medical practitioner, clinic or hospital within 3 days for the purposes of treatment, and must continue to present for treatment at prescribed intervals until certified cured.

4. Quarantine

Part IV of the Public Health Act provides various anti-infection measures including quarantine, for declared infectious diseases, although these have rarely been imposed in practice. In the light of the Constitutional Rights to Liberty of the Person in Section 42, and The Right of citizens to Freedom of Movement within the country in Section 52, the imposition of any legislative restrictions, such as quarantine, on people with HIV would prove difficult. Even if such measures were to be attempted on the grounds of public health, they may possibly be held unconstitutional.

B. CONFIDENTIALITY AND DISCRIMINATION

1. Confidentiality

Under the Code of Ethics, a doctor owes his patient absolute secrecy on all matters confided to him. There are some exceptions to the preservation of the bond of secrecy: where the patient gives consent; in the interest of all concerned; where required by law; where there is a question of danger to society. On the other hand, in serious illness where the likelihood of recovery is slight or absent, the doctor may, acting in the patient's best interests, inform a near and responsible relative of the true state of affairs and discuss how far to go in informing the patient. However, the Code does not have the force of law, and any statutory or judicial requirements of disclosure will override the Code's adjuration to preserve secrecy.

Under the Public Health Act, it is both an offence and professional misconduct for a medical practitioner to divulge personal particulars of a person suffering from a venereal disease other than in accordance with the Act. For other such medical matters, the imported legal system imposes the equitable duty of confidence on medical practitioners and so on, with the possibility of a tortious or contractual action for breach. The Constitutional Right to Privacy would extend to communications between a patient and a health care worker. The only proven exception so far to this is a situation where the patient chooses to take the matter to law, in which case medical information should be subpoenaed and come within the custody of the court in the first instance.

Ok Tedi Mining, which provides an industrial and a clinical medical facility in an isolated environment, specifically insists on a policy of confidentiality regarding medical records for all its employees.

2. Duty to Disclose/Rights to Medical Information

Under Section 19 of the Evidence Act, medical communications made by a patient to a medical practitioner or his delegate are privileged, except in criminal proceedings.

Section 51 of the Constitution, Right to Freedom of Information, guarantees to citizens the right of reasonable access to official documents, subject only to the need for secrecy in respect of, *inter alia*, the maintenance of personal privacy and security of the person. T9s is a Qualified Right and may be restricted by a law made in the interests of public health, public welfare, etc.

3. Partner Notification

No partner notification is currently required by law, although the presumption that a doctor has a responsibility to protect others from infection by tracing contacts probably operates. Positive test results are notified to the medical care provider or AIDS counsellor who ordered the test. Both are encouraged to involve the other in counselling, follow-up and partner notification.

A medical practitioner diagnosing a case of venereal disease as defined under the Public Health Act must warn the infected of the dangers of infecting others, and against contracting a marriage until cured. Where the practitioner has reason to believe that a person infected intends to contract a marriage, he may, after intimating his intention to his patient, warn the intended spouse or his/her parents or guardian, and the Commissioner.

4. Discrimination

The Constitution in Section 55, Equality of Citizens, guarantees to all citizens "the same rights, privileges, obligations and duties irrespective of race, tribe, place of origin, political opinion, colour, creed, religion or sex." Laws may however, take affirmative action for females, children, youth and the underprivileged or less advanced.

The Defence Force policy is to refuse admission to the Force of applicants who test positive. Servicemen testing positive who show no evidence of progressive clinical illness are not discharged, but are limited to base duties only within the country, as far as possible in non-combat roles. Those who demonstrate progressive clinical illness are downgraded accordingly and may be discharged for physical disability.

Ok Tedi Mining will employ HIV positive persons with no symptoms, and only discontinues employment when AIDS develops, on the grounds of unfitness to work, as is the case with other diseases such as kidney failure, terminal cancer, unstable diabetes, etc. Confidentiality is maintained and a policy of non-discrimination is pursued.

C. WOMEN'S ISSUES

1. Vulnerability to HIV

Despite Constitutional guarantees of equality, the status of women in Papua New Guinea, as in many other developing countries, is depressed in many of the ways which increase vulnerability (e.g., fewer educational opportunities, higher illiteracy, less access to the cash economy).

Specifically, most women cannot require fidelity from their male partners. Customary polygyny is legal and still widely practiced. Even where monogamy is the overt ideal, promiscuity is unsanctioned but widespread, and double standards between sexes are common. Women cannot usually compel condom use. Condoms are not always available, or affordable, in rural areas. Some churches oppose their use, or even promotion for safe sex. Finally, in the modern Papua New Guinea context, women's vulnerability is increased by the alarmingly high incidence of pack rape.

2. Status within Families and Societies

National Goal No. 1 (Integral Human Development) of the Constitution recognises the family as the basic social unit, and equality is guaranteed for all citizens by Section 55. Traditional societies are based on extended family or clan lines. Within the traditional social units, however defined in each culture group, women's status and roles are clearly defined, as different and separate from men's, but not necessarily inferior. Modern reality, however, differs markedly, with society tending towards the nuclear family and concomitant weakening of women's family status.

3. Economic Rights

Within traditional society, women played an important role in the subsistence economy as the principal food producers.

The Constitution in National Goal No. 2 calls for equal participation by women citizens in political, economic and developmental activities, but again, reality is different. Urbanisation, the tendency to formation of nuclear family units and economic development strategies which are largely targeted towards men, have depressed women's economic status.

D. INFORMATION LAW

1. Rights to Information

The Constitution in Section 46 guarantees Freedom of Expression. It is defined to include freedom to hold and communicate opinions and information and specifically guarantees freedom of the press and mass media. Papua New Guinea does in fact have a strong free press.

The Right to practice, manifest and propagate Conscience, Thought and Religion (including traditional religious beliefs and customs) may be exercised, provided it does not interfere with the freedom of others to do likewise, and there is no unsolicited intervention into another's religious affairs or religious harassment.

The dissemination of HIV/AIDS information is a priority of the NAC and the Health Department, and the area in which most action has been taken so far.

2. Obstacles to Information

The major legal obstacle to information comes currently from the Censorship Board, which has placed bans on information regarding condom use. Appeals to the Board have not yet been successful. This obstacle may be surmounted, however, by legal challenge on constitutional grounds or by HIV/AIDS-specific legislative action.

By Section 228 of the Criminal Code, it is an offence to publish an item which is obscene or might otherwise tend to corrupt morals, unless it can be proved as a question of fact that it was for the public benefit.

A major non-legal obstacle is presented by the churches, most of whom have so far refused to associate themselves with the dissemination of epidemic-related information other than by the preaching of chastity and fidelity. Some of the minor religious movements are actively spreading totally inaccurate and inflammatory messages, and there is currently no legal mechanism by which this tendency can be arrested.

E. FAMILIES AND CARERS

1. Marriage, Divorce and Separation

Family law in Papua New Guinea is in a very confused state, with imported and customary legal systems co-existing, and traditional constraints on the latter breaking down in the face of a changing social structure. Comprehensive reform has been impossible so far—even piecemeal improvement of the law has proved extremely difficult.

The National Goals of the Constitution recognise the family unit as the fundamental basis of society, and call for the promotion of the Melanesian family in every way.

Section 3 of the Marriage Act (Chapter 280) recognises both statutory (registered) and customary marriages. Polygyny is legal where customary. Most, but not all, customs require payment of a brideprice. Confusion and conflict between legal regimes leads to many situations of voluntary and involuntary de facto relationships.

Statutory marriages are dissolved in accordance with the Matrimonial Causes Act (Chapter 282). Either party may petition on the old Anglo-Australian fault basis. It is a very expensive process and few nationals embark upon it. Customary marriages are left to be dissolved by customary procedure. Many societies have no such procedure, or are vague about the process, as the concept of marriage dissolution was largely alien to pre-modern societies.

The law's inability to reconcile conflict between the imported legal regime and custom, and between different customary regimes in situations of "mixed marriage" is notable.

2. Non-consensual Sexual Intercourse

Forced sex, often with multiple perpetrators, is becoming increasingly common in Papua New Guinea. In the village setting, though, it is sometimes difficult to define the element of force when a young man is expected to "force" his attentions on a prospective marriage partner, and the girl is expected to submit to male demands on her sexual services.

In urban areas, though, where traditional social control mechanisms have been greatly weakened and economic and social depression are most prevalent, abduction and stranger-rape are common. It is a part of the ongoing street crime situation, which is steadily worsening.

Rape offences under the Criminal Code apply to females only, and there is no rape in marriage . An assault with intent to have anal intercourse carries a lesser penalty.

3. Termination of Pregnancy

By Sections 225 and 226 of the Criminal Code, all abortion is illegal. Although there is no Papua New Guinea case law directly on the matter, analogy may be drawn from Queensland decisions on the interaction between the equivalent of these sections and that of Section 280, surgical operations, which make lawful operations for the patient's benefit, or on an unborn child for the preservation of the mother's life. The Queensland cases have held that this section must be negatived by the prosecution in order to prove an unlawful abortion. In practice, this principle is applied in Papua New Guinea.

F. PRISONS, CUSTODIAL INSTITUTIONS AND WELFARE HOMES

No specific laws have been enacted in relation to HIV and prisoners, though group testing is under discussion and counselling planned.

Although detailed provisions are laid down by law regarding the operation of corrective institutions, prison discipline and management in Papua New Guinea is in reality by no means perfect. This should be borne in mind when examining the details of statutory requirements laid out below.

1. Testing

The corrective Institutions Act (Chapter 63) requires that a medical officer "examine" all prisoners upon admission to, and discharge or removal from, prison on a regular basis, and where a prisoner "appears to require medical attention." He may also examine warders where he thinks it necessary and both warders and detainees must submit to any medical treatment ordered. Nominal medical records are kept on prisoners and warders.

Compulsory testing of prisoners may contravene the constitutional Right to Privacy.

2. Segregation and Preventive Measures

There is a high incidence of homosexual activity, both consensual and forced, amongst male prisoners and possibly warders as well. Secret self-circumcision and other genital mutilation practices have sprung up among male prisoners as a sub-culture ritual. They use whatever cutting implements are available, usually shared rusty razor blades, and general infection often results.

A prison should have an infirmary for sick prisoners. Ill prisoners may be removed to hospital, but must be returned to prison if their sentences are not expired.

According to the Act, where a medical officer suspects a prisoner of having an infectious or quarantinable disease (not defined), he must inform the Commissioner and the Department of Health, and institute "all necessary measures" to ensure that other prisoners are not infected. Additionally, the common law duty of care owed by those in authority to their charges means that all prison authorities are bound to ensure that prisoners are protected from danger of infection.

Segregation of prisoners may contravene the fundamental

Right to Liberty. It may, however, be the only viable preventive measure available in a situation where behavioural change proves too slow, although in reality it may not be economically feasible (recent calls for the establishment of a maximum security prison are defeated on financial grounds).

The illegality of all homosexual activity means that it is hard to distinguish between consensual and non-consensual sex, and victims of forced sex may be reluctant to cornplain, particularly in prison situations. It is also an impediment to condom distribution in prisons. Prison authorities could be held liable for condoning illegal acts.

3. Early Release

Prisoners undergoing life sentence are to be reviewed after 12 years by the VisitingJustice who reports to a Reviewing Committee, and after 15 years by the Reviewing Committee itself. Where a life prisoner reaches 55 years of age, he is to be reviewed annually. Health reasons constitute a ground for the Reviewing Committee to recommend to Cabinet that the life sentence be commuted. In practice, though, the operations of the Reviewing Committee, like those of Visiting Justices, have largely lapsed.

A visiting medical officer must report to prison authorities any case of a prisoner whom he considers may not survive his detention, who is unfit for detention, or whose life may be endangered by imprisonment.

G. EMPLOYMENT ISSUES

1. Workplace Testing

The Defence Force has instituted compulsory testing for servicemen as part of the Annual Medical Board. In the private sector, Ok Tedi Mining requires testing for employment applicants only, as does the Department of Foreign Affairs for non-citizen work visa applications.

2. Policies on Infected Employees

The Constitution in Section 48 guarantees to every person the Qualified Right to Freedom of choice of Employment, subject only to laws relating to the employment of non-citizens. This Right refers to choice, not practice, of employment.

All employment *is* deemed to be by contract unless othervvise regulated by statute, and basic employment is governed by the Employment Act (Chapter 373) which lays down minimum standards for the contract of employment. The Act may be displaced by other legislation pertaining to employment (e.g., Employment of Non-Citizens Act, the Public Services (Management) Act, etc.). The Act is supervised by the Department of Labour and Employment, via Labour Offices and Inspectors. Employees in urban centres are quick to seek recourse to the protection thus offered.

Unless displaced by the terms of a contract or legislation, the Act provides that employment may be terminated according to the common law principle of the right to hire and fire in the employer, with a period of notice dependent on the method of salary payment.

No employment legislation has been enacted specifically for the protection of HIV infected employees.

In reality, paid employment is available to only a small section of the population, and unemployment is a major contributing factor to the depressed economy, offset only by reliance on subsistence economy survival in rural areas. Even if laws were to be put in place preventing dismissal on grounds of infection alone, it is likely that they will be circumvented, by the use of real or spurious threats to force resignation. In most situations, though, the ease of termination offered by the Employment Act and the principles of common law will suffice.

Ok Tedi Mining pursues a policy of confidentiality, no discrimination and no limitation on fitness to work unless HIV-related illness is present. An exclusion clause may be placed in the company-provided medical insurance plan, on the same basis as other medical conditions which do not impair fitness but show a high risk of a re-occurrence of a medical or surgical condition .

3. Disability Support

There is no social security system in Papua New Guinea, nor is there likely to be one. Concern here centres on persuading rural dwellers to integrate people with HIV into the village community. There are reports that this has happened in some instances, but for other areas, discrimination and stigmatisation have surfaced.

Both the Defence Force and Ok Tedi Mining will repatriate people with AIDS upon their becoming unfit for work.

Most employment contracts (including Public Service) do not appear to provide for the employee's right to terminate on disability grounds.

4. HIV Education in the Workplace

The Defence Force has instituted a rigorous system of HIV education and awareness amongst servicemen. Private enterprise is being encouraged to follow suit on a voluntary basis.

The Ok Tedi Mining policy stresses the need for information and education promotion in order to ensure protection from discrimination and prejudice.

H. CRIMINAL LAW

1. Transmission Offences

The Public Health Act provides for offences of marrying while suffering a venereal disease in an infectious stage (Section 64); knowingly infecting another person; or knowingly doing or permitting the doing of any act which is likely to lead to any other person's infection (Section 66). It is also an offence for the owner or occupier of premises to knowingly permit a female suffering a venereal disease to use the premises for prostitution (in addition to any other legal liability for keeping a brothel etc.: Section 67).

The Criminal Code Part V, Division 1 codifies the common law range of offences against the person, ranging from murder to common assault. Some of these may be applicable to HIV transmission, depending on the resolution of matters of causation, *mens rea* in the accused and implied consent in the victim. The year and a day rule applies to unlawful killing by Section 297, so that the greatest offence chargeable for a deliberate act intended to transmit infection would be attempted murder. The act of unlawfully, and with intent to injure or annoy, administering poison or other noxious thing to a person, which may possibly be extended to cover situations of malicious acts intended to transmit infection, is found under the offence of wounding in Section 322.

In the light of a recent report of a pack rape in a rural area allegedly carried out with the expressed intention of transmitting HIV infection, the matter of transmission offences has assumed high importance in Papua New Guinea.

2. Sex Workers

Although prostitution *per se* is not an offence, it is against the law to live off the earnings of prostitution, or to keep a brothel, or to procure. The National court has construed the Summary Offences Act so as to apply the offence of living on the earnings of prostitution to the prostitute nerself. However, this interpretation was not applied in a subsequent case of receiving money for an isolated prostitution association, which was held not to constitute living, even partly, off earnings.

Both male and female prostitution are now common in towns, and female prostitution in rural areas also. However, it is often difficult to define prostitution clearly, along a continuum from casual sex given for favours to clear-cut commercial sale of sexual favours. Urban sex workers are not visually organised into brothel situations, but rather, free-lance around bars and discos. Organisation is more prevalent in rural areas, for example in the village drinking clubs established along the major highway artery to and through the highland region, and along the shores of the coasts and major rivers. Some villages in various regions of the country are renowned for the fact that the entire adult female population is available for sex work.

3. Homosexuality

Ritualised homosexuality occurs in a few societies in Papua New Guinea. More widespread, though, is homosexual activity as a transitional phase in the development of the individual. Thus it can be said that bisexuality, rather than exclusive homosexuality, is the norm.

The Criminal Code in Part IV, Division 2 retains its original terms of outlawing all homosexual activity try making crimes of all "carnal knowledge against the order of nature" (anal intercourse), and "acts of gross indecency" between males. Although actual prosecutions are not common, the illegality situation gives rise to practices of blackmail and discrimination, e.g., threats of exposure and prosecution are used to force resignations in the workplace.

The Code provisions may well conflict with the constitutional Right to privacy in Section 49, the Right to Equality of citizens in Section 55 (which includes equality regardless of sex, although not specifically sexual preference). For those whose traditional cultures include ritualised homosexual practices (and there are several in the country) they may constitute an infringement of Freedom of Religion in Section 45.

4. Illegal Treatment and Advertising

Only a medical practitioner, or a person acting under his direct instructions, may prescribe for and treat a venereal disease.

The Public Health Act in Section 140 contains a general offence of the publishing statements promoting the sale of any medicine, instrument or appliance for the alleviation or cure of venereal diseases, complaints or infirmities arising from or relating to sexual intercourse, diseases affecting generative functions, etc., (this does not apply to publications in relation to medical research, and publications sent to medical practitioners or pharmacist for the purposes of their businesses, or advertisements, etc., approved by the Commissioner for Venereal Diseases). This provision is not confined to defined venereal diseases alone, and could therefore apply to the advertising of false cures for HIV/AIDS.

I. THE LEGAL PROCESS

1. Legal Aid and Access to the Law

Section 37 of the Constitution guarantees to all persons the fundamental Right to Protection of the Law. No person may be charged with an offence that is not defined by a written law. Determination of civil rights and obligations must be made by a court or similar impartial authority within a reasonable time.

In many situations persons may obtain free legal representation from the Public Solicitor. However the office is under-resourced and its first priority is criminal defence. Even this is only available at National and Supreme court level. The Public Solicitor and the Law Society administer a means-tested legal aid scheme for situations where the Public Solicitor is unable to act.

Where violations of Constitution. Rights are concerned the National Court will act of its own initiative to protect them. The court has instituted simple procedures whereby rights violations may be brought speedily before the court.

2. Evident

The Evidence Act Section 19 prohibits a medical practitioner (which has been held to include all persons) from divulging in any civil proceedings any communication made to him by a patient unless the patient consents. The privilege has also been held to attach to any information given to persons specifically or impliedly delegated by the practitioner to obtain information from the patient for the purpose of medical treatment. On its wording this protection may not extend to medical information the practitioner has about the patient.

Spouses are not compellable to disclose communications during the marriage in any legal proceedings except divorce and matrimonial causes proceedings .

3. Courtroom Procedure

Under the Constitution all court proceedings shall be held in public unless the parties agree otherwise. A court may be closed where it is empowered to do so by law in the interests of *inter alia* the protection of the private lives of persons concerned in the proceedings. Under the District Courts Act (Chapter 40) which was enacted prior to the Constitution a court may be closed in " the interests of public morfaity."

The Judicial Proceedings (Regulation of Reports) Act (Chapter 51) prohibits the publishing of any "indecent medical, surgical or physiological details the publication of which would be calculated to injure pubic morals." However, this does not apply to the communication of the content of pleadings, transcripts of evidence or similar documents to "a person concerned in the proceedings."

4. Sentencing

Judges take many factors into account in sentencing, including age, medical infirmity and likelihood of surviving a prison sentence. As no case involving a person known to be HIV-positive has yet come before the courts, no specific sentencing policy has evolved in respect of any crime. However, guidance may be drawn from the 1989 case of *The State V. Thomas Pipon,* in which the judge noted in sentencing that knowingly attempting to infect a victim of sexual assault with HIV would constitute an aggravating factor of more extreme seriousness than infection with gonorrhoea, a curable disease.

50

Law, Custom and the HIV/AIDS Epidemic in Papua New Guinea

Christine Stewart and Pascoe Kase
Legal Officer
PNG Legal Reform Committee
Papua, New Guinea

Pascoe Kase
Legal Officer
PNG department of Health
Papua, New Guinea

INTRODUCTION—THE SCENARIO

The Papua New Guinea tourism promotion slogan, appearing on glossy posters around the world, reads "Papua New Guinea - Land of the Unexpected." The slogan has caught on within the country, too. We use it to explain many things.

For example, here are three stories which illustrate how Papua New Guinea can indeed be the Land of the Unexpected.

The Goroka Contact-trading Incident

The Defence Force is virtually the only body in Papua New Guinea which has so far established any sort of thorough policy on AIDS. Part of this policy requires that all servicemen undergo an HIV test as part of their Annual Medical Board. A soldier was thereby found to be HIV-positive. Questioning on his sexual contacts led to a former girlfriend, now married and living in Goroka, in the Highlands. The lady was tested, and also her new husband, and both were found to be positive. Without any concern for trying to determine who originally infected whom, the husband immediately demanded cash compensation from the soldier.

The Awareness Video

As part of the public awareness campaign already instituted in the country, a man living with HIV from the Highlands area volunteered his services in various outreach programmes. He did an excellent job, travelling around villages all over the remote and rugged Highlands area, explaining, demonstrating, counselling. A video was made in which he starred in his role as an outreach worker. Shortly afterwards, he died. The video has had to he suppressed. The subject is dead, and a dead person has passed into the spirit world and it is vital that his privacy be respected. If the video were to be released for public showing, his angry relatives would object and ask for compensation for the infringement of sacred taboos.

Protector Condoms

A cheap line of condoms is being packaged and sold in Papua New Guinea under the brand-name "Protector." The packaging includes instructions for use in the Papua New Guinea lingua franca, Tok Pisin, and cartoon-style line drawings, essential in a largely illiterate society. The National Censorship Board, which is influenced by a fundamentalist Christian outlook, objected to the instructions, not because they depicted condoms, but because a few lines in some of the drawings suggested the possibility of sexual intercourse. This was unacceptably erotic, and a circular was sent to every pharmacy in the country directing removal of the instructions from every packet of Protector condoms before sale.

These Stories at first glance may be comparable to similar stories from other countries, other cultural systems. But each also demonstrates some problems of the interaction between certain customary traditions and laws, and a new social problem which has an unsettling impact on them.

The Multiplicity of Legal Systems'

In Papua New Guinea, there are conflicts and tensions between the pre-Independence received common law, which is often paternalistic, outdated and inappropriate, and in application, frequently irrelevant; the nation's Constitution, which entrenches many of the internationally-recognised Rights and Freedoms of the individual; and customary law, which is declared by the Constitution as one of the bases of the underlying law which legislators and the courts are bound to take into account in the development of the country's system of jurisprudence.

What, then, is Papua New Guinea's customary law? Customary law in Papua New Guinea is really a multitude of different, sometimes wildly different, sets of customs, traditions and community beliefs. Papua New Guinea is a land of rugged mountain ranges, great swamps, scattered islands. It is not a terrain which is easily traversed. 85 per cent of the nation's population lives in scattered and geographically isolated small village communities, surviving on the produce of subsistence horticulture. There are nearly 800 language groups in the country. This means 800 different societies, each with its own social constructs, its own culture, its own set of customs. Papua New Guinea is an anthropologist's paradise, displaying every conceivable type of social and kinship structure, from extreme patriarchal societies to a wide variety of matrilineal systems, which govern clan allegiance, land and property distribution and inheritance, who one may or may not marry, where one may or may not live, how one owes and is owed work obligations—all the things by which a given community regulates its behavioural interactions. So you will never hear a Papua New Guinean speak of "my country's custom." Instead, he will say "in my custom" or "in my area," and what he then describes may well sound as strange to his fellow countryman as to a visitor from the other side of the world.

It is therefore impossible to make any kind of authoritative statement about a single phenomenon labelled "Papua New Guinea custom." Any such pronouncement will invariably be wrong for one, if not more, of Papua New Guinea's diverse social systems. Any commentator can only hope to extract some general trends and principles, and hope in the process not to make too many mistakes.

Along with diversity, Papua New Guinea is undergoing dramatic social change, all in no more than a generation or so. With European contact, which effectively commenced last century, gradually penetrating to the Highland areas a mere 50 years ago, Christianity in its many and varied forms has become the professed religion of the country. The early missions made inroads on many cultural practices to which they took exception, such as initiation ceremonies and ritualised homosexuality, and customs thus affected were wiped out or survived in altered and attenuated form. The twentieth century has made further general inroads on traditional structures and belief systems.

Consequently, the customary regimes which have operated very well for several millennia in regulating and harmonising societies are themselves being changed and distorted to suit new social forms and even individual ends. The consequence of so many such systems impacting upon each other has been a cultural syncretism of the old and the new, the accommodating of sometimes diametrically opposed traditional systems, a ready acceptance of new concepts, imported and adapted (sometimes almost beyond recognition) to suit present needs. The newly emerging patterns of custom are considered equally as valid as the old. This acknowledgement of the dynamic nature of Papua New Guinea's customary systems is even found in the Constitution, which declares specifically that custom need not have pertained since time immemorial[2].

HIV LEGAL POLICY AND CUSTOMARY LAW

It is most important that customary law be examined in relation to the development of HIV legal strategies. The HIV epidemic involves two matters which affect people deeply and personally, namely sex and death. To be at all effective, HIV legal policy must take good account of customary beliefs and practices. Certain general trends may be discerned in the diverse range of customary legal systems in Papua New Guinea. An apparent factor in these customary systems is their sharp divergence from the basic precepts of the introduced law, both the "traditional" common law and the constitutional framework of entrenched individual Rights and Freedoms.

(a) Egalitarianism

Most traditional societies in Papua New Guinea are politically unstratified —all members have at least the potential to assume a leadership role within the community. Such a role is achieved by prowess in such matters as participation in community activities, skills in sorcery, mediation of internal conflicts and, most importantly, by the accumulation and redistribution of wealth in the form of food items, though ceremonial objects may also be significant. This redistribution process does not occur at random, hut according to strictly determined patterns based on kinship ties. The apparent consequence of this is that a network of mutual economic support is established within each customary group. Trade in scarce, location specific resources was also traditionally widespread, and wide networks of economic interdependence were thus established.

Even in the handful of societies which have hereditary

chieftainships, there is very little to distinguish the chief from his followers, and his authority is far less than the absolute which is often presumed from the use of the term "chief." Societies with chiefs continue to display most of the features of those societies where status and power must be achieved, not inherited.

The principal consequence of this is that, whereas the political structures of hierarchical societies evolved simultaneous checks and balances on the exercise of power (concepts such as noblesse oblige, for example), egalitarian societies are at a loss to handle the sudden devolution of exceptional power onto a chosen minority. Politicians and senior public servants have no general basis on which to discriminate between use and abuse of these powers. The perceived ability to alter society's behaviour and direction through legislation, or at least high executive decision, means that many unnecessary legislative and policy interventions, often of dubious constitutionality, are proposed and even implemented. Successive governments recently, have tended to formulate increasingly draconian measures to deal with perceived social ills. No culturally accepted effective mechanisms have yet evolved in the modern nation to provide a system of checks and balances to the exercise of political power. Papua New Guinea's leaders are currently going through a denial phase in relation to the epidemic. No amount of reasoned argument, even couched in objective economic terms, seems to be getting through. Political reaction, if there is any at all, tends to follow the repressive, contagious disease confinement model. And consequently also we are faced with a reaction such as that of the Censorship Board to the Protector condoms.

There exist some good sides to the basic egalitarian principle underlying society. Firstly, the fundamental social mechanism of redistribution of wealth gives a continual process of social levelling. Secondly, with the continued importance and relevance of non-cash wealth in customary societies, the disparities in wealth, status and power between the top and bottom strata of society, those most vulnerable levels, are by no means as great as they may first appear to be, if measured purely in monetary terms and other formal indices.

Egalitarianism in each given community means that the people believe that they have the right to take responsibility for their own destinies, and the ability to claim their rights, however those rights may be defined in each instance. And what is more, they do not hesitate to establish a claim, by direct and sometimes even violent means, when they perceive the need to do so[3]. The new leaders may attempt to move in harsh and repressive ways, but the legitimacy of their authority rests on tenuous grounds. No matter how much the nation's leaders may attempt to impose their sometimes excessively authoritarian wills on the people, the people do not wait too long to make their displeasure felt. Attempts at punitive measures will be ignored, and on the other hand apathy and inertia at the national level can be circumvented by effective and positive action at the village level of society. This is already happening. What we have to do is ensure that when people take the law into their own hands, as they are only too ready to do, that this law is good law.

(b) The Commission of Wrongs

Liability and Rights

The imported Western legal system relies on the rights and responsibilities of the individual. When a wrong is committed, the common law is concerned with the adjustment of rights as between the individual perpetrator and the actual victim. Only the individual to whom the links of the injury can be traced is held responsible, with the exception of clearly delimited areas of vicarious liability. Hence, if the link is traced to an individual whom the law does not deem a responsible person (a minor, or a mentally deficient person) or who is incapable of making redress (a poor or bankrupt person) then the injured party receives only an empty victory in the court process.

Melanesian society, on the other hand, believes in group membership, group allegiance, group support, group responsibility. Rights pertain not to individuals but to groups. All negotiations and decisions regarding redress for wrongs are conducted between groups. Any individual may call on his or her group for support in financial obligations, in seeking redress for injuries. Retaliation for an individual's wrongdoing may fall upon any member of the individual's group.

There are both advantages and disadvantages in this system of group rights and responsibilities. Where blame is laid at a person's door, retribution may be exacted against anyone who is perceived to be a member of that person's group. On the other hand, the intra-group responsibility ethic means that the prospects are good for the acceptance and caring of those with AIDS, at least at the village level. There are already a couple of reports that this is happening.

This phenomenon of the cohesiveness of the group raises another interesting question—how great is the need for confidentiality in the Papua New Guinea context? Papua New Guinea already exhibits an unusually high level of acceptance of the impaired. The ethic of loyalty to the group is highly persuasive in virtually all situations. The fear reaction will be, and already is, we will find that the need to maintain strict silence regarding a person's HIV status is not so high as in the individualised societies of the west. Differentiation does not necessarily lead to automatic stigmatiation—rather the reverse. Village societies tend to adapt readily and in ingenious ways to people with differences[4].

Causation

The introduced common law system contains certain clear limits to determining liability for a wrong. A causational chain must be shown, and this chain has a clear cutout point. Usually, there must be in the causer an element of *mens rea,* be it downright malicious intent or at least neglect of a duty of care. But Melanesian tradition believes, firstly, that there is no such thing as an accident[5]. Every injury has a cause in some person or action— even sometimes in the very person who is injured. There is always a causal link. To determine the link, the evidentiary net must he cast much wider than the common law could countenance. A baby's deformity may be caused by the father's adultery during the pregnancy. The electrocution of a worker on the job may be caused by sorcery worked by an envious enemy clan, etc.

The tendency to belief in a virtually unlimited chain of no-fault responsibility will create enormous problems in Papua New Guinea in the context of HIV. The common law system has already been obliged to reconcile itself with this in various ways. The Motor Vehicles (Third Party Insurance) (Basic Protection Compensation) Act, for example, provides an immediate and swift payment for injury by a motor vehicle on an absolute liability, no-fault basis. A belief system which cannot accommodate the concept of accident, of innocent causation, means that much time and energy is devoted to attributing blame, and the logic systems which underly the imported law often consider that such blame is attributed unfairly. HIV-related deaths, particularly if they occur by wasting disease, which is already the predominant mode, provide a fertile ground for sorcery accusations. As can be seen from the Goroka contact-tracing incident, logical considerations did not necessarily play a part in the husband's decision to demand compensation. And compensation, in the end, can do little to remedy the situation. Intensive, on-going awareness education and counselling must play a vital role in suppressing the worst of the trauma.

Retribution

Once the cause has been established, social harmony is restored by some form of retributive and conciliatory measure. For small injuries, small redress, whether in goods, or even just a confession, a public shaming, a promise to behave better in future, may suffice. For larger injuries, a larger redress is required—either massive amounts of wealth, or equivalent retaliatory injury. And there is no escaping the obligation to make redress, no pronouncement by a higher authority that some technicality has voided or reduced the causer's obligation. If the redress is not offered, and fast, it will usually be claimed, and, if necessary, taken by some form of retaliation. If this process happens to exceed the mark, then retaliatory action will be taken in return, and an often lengthy process of adjustment and readjustment, sometimes involving violence, ensues.

This is the mechanism which drives the famous payback system and the tribal fighting which is constantly going on in some parts of the country. These tribal wars have already escalated from traditional affairs of spears, bows and arrows to situations of high-level damage with the use of guns, both factory-made and home-manufactured. Once blame has been attributed, retribution may be swift to follow, as can be seen from the and the Goroka contact-tracing incident. Coupled with the causation factor described above, and the willingness of people to demand their rights from all segments of society, we have the ingredients in Papua New Guinean society for some potentially explosive situations to emerge from the epidemic.

(c) Family law

It is in the field of family law that one of the greatest breakdowns in the reconciliation of customary law with introduced law becomes apparent. The imported law itself has been imported piecemeal, adapted in an *ad hoc* way, and is hopelessly out of date, cumbersome and expensive to apply. Its basic precepts are in many ways completely at odds with the many and diverse customary regimes, which are themselves often in conflict as between different societies[6].

It is here also that the effects of social change are taking one of their highest tolls. The fact of diversity between traditional systems is being used in a rapidly changing society to justify some very dubious ends. For example, polygamous marriage is customary in many Papua New Guinean societies. Traditionally, this practice had a sound economic basis and, moreover, required the consent of the previous wife, or wives, before embarking on it. Any objections to the new marriage were taken seriously and usually carried the day[7]. But the imported law, as adapted to the circumstances of Papua New Guinea, recognises a customary marriage as valid[8]. A customary polygamous marriage is not illegal, provided it does not follow a statutory marriage (although the Criminal Code still retains the offence of bigamy, but prosecutions are rare and usually involve expatriates). The recognition by law of polygamous marriage means that many men, even though not necessarily from an area where polygamy is a valid customary marriage form, may, and often do, claim to have more than one "wife"—and in many instances, believe truly that this claim is quite legitimate.

The wide-scale revision and updating of family law in Papua New Guinea has been tackled sporadically over the years, but has proved to be a mammoth, almost impossible task. Continued piecemeal reform seems to be the best that we can hope for. Meanwhile, customary societies themselves continue to regulate, as best they can, family law matters amongst their members, and as between group members and outsiders associating with them. The tensions that arise from interaction between people from different customary groups, and from the dynamics of modernisation, have already given us the dispossessed, the homeless, the destitute. The epidemic, falling as it does mainly on the economically active, will exacerbate this greatly. Papua New Guinea will increasingly be confronted with situations which no current legal system can handle. However, the ability of customary systems to change and adapt rapidly to new circumstances could well throw up some ingenious and positive new coping mechanisms which the formal legal system would do well to heed.

(d) Sexual Learning, Belief and Behaviour[9]

Young people in village societies learn about sex from their same-sex parents and other older same-sex relatives. The content of these lessons varies in detail, from the vague warnings given to many girls to avoid young men for fear of pregnancy, to the detailed descriptions given to boys about the "correct" methods of bodily contact during sex with their future wives. By and large, the accuracy of information is low and mainly derived from traditional beliefs. Young people therefore obtain much further informal education from their peers, and it is via this channel that the bulk of the nation's youth can be reached for HIV education. Not surprisingly also, older members of society bemoan the waning influence of custom on young people and blame many negative aspects of modern culture on their lack of respect for tradition. By themselves, however, villagers are unable to reverse this trend.

A feature of many societies is the male initiation ceremony, usually performed on teenage boys. Such ceremonies are by no means universal, and in many places, were to a greater or lesser extent stamped out by mission and colonial government influence. However, they have persisted in several notable instances, and have even revived in modern forms among newly developing urban subcultures, for example amongst prisoners[14]. The first notable feature of such ceremonies for our purposes is that they often involve penile and other bodily cutting. Tattoos and cicatrices are important identity markers and fashionable bodily features amongst people from many different traditional groups, and often performed by teenagers upon each other even when there is no association with a formal initiation. These skin penetrations were originally carried out with bamboo or thorn blades or needles, which blunted easily and were usually changed for each subject. However, modern steel implements are now used, and as they do not blunt as easily, they are often frequently re-used. In the current absence of injecting drug-use in Papua New Guinea, these practices constitute the greatest danger of HIV transmission through blood contact, and educational programmes must pay special attention to warnings of the dangers of using shared instruments.

Paralleling the male initiation ceremonies are many variations of menarcheal ceremonies for girls. A feature of both the male and the female ceremonies, where they occur, is that they are usually an important venue by which the initiates are educated about sexual practices and behaviour. They could therefore provide a good means of transmission of information about safe sexual behaviour. Education of parents and elders, who are responsible for the teachings performed at these ceremonies, is as important as the education of young people. It is also important that the forces of the church, the formal education system and the state via its national legal system discontinue any efforts to attenuate or obliterate these practices.

Forced sex, often involving more than one perpetrator, is unfortunately an all too common occurrence in the country. Psychologically, it has its roots in cementing male bonding and to emphasis domination and control of female sexuality. In some areas, the traditional and acceptable acts of aggression in tribal fights are to burn the enemy's houses, destroy his food gardens, steal or slaughter his pigs, and rape his women. Unfortunately also, in some traditional societies gang rape was a mechanism sanctioned by customary law as punishment for women's transgression of certain taboos, usually related to sex and marriage. These practices continue in modern guises. Many such incidents are the outcome of the desire for male bonding by initiating younger cousins etc. into sexual activity. The prevalence of rape is a major problem in relation to the AIDS epidemic, and particularly gang rape, as it endangers not only the woman involved, but also places each of the male perpetrators at risk of infection from any of the others, due to semen contact.

For some societies, group sex activities formed part of traditional religious practices, usually as fertility and renewal rites. It has been reported, though not very commonly, that women may actually take pride in their ability to take on a multiplicity of sexual partners. Non-forced group sex is as high a risk activity as forced group sex, and requires a similar degree of attention for the formulation of deterrent measures. Unfortunately, this will not be easy. The law already condemns rape, particularly where multiple offenders are involved, and recent years have seen a significant increase in the severity of prison sentences being handed out for this crime. But prison sentences alone are never a fully effective instrument for behavioural change.

Multiple sexual partners, both before and during marriage, are usually disapproved both by tradition and in the modern Papua New Guinean society, although a certain amount of latitude was accorded to men before marriage—though not to women. However, the reality is that the average of multiple partners is sufficiently high throughout the nation as to provide the principal means of HIV transmission. Adultery was strictly forbidden in most customary systems[11], and in some areas the punishment exacted was particularly brutal. Adultery in the indigenous population was a crime under the formal legal system well before Independence, and it is only in recent years that it has been decriminalised, by the Adultery and Enticement Act 1988, and made the subject of a civil suit for compensation. One widespread traditional belief which is claimed to contribute to adultery rates is the conviction that sex during pregnancy and lactation should be avoided, as it will harm the baby. Many men justify adultery or the buying of sex on these grounds, although in actuality most of these men have extramarital affairs at other times also. In the face of such deep-rooted beliefs and common practices, the mere preaching of chastity within marriage will not resolve the dangers of infection caused by multiple sex partners.

(e) Women and Custom

The traditional status of women in Papua New Guinean society was in many respects better than it is today under the onslaught of twentieth century living. In village society, women were "separate but equal," and although their political influence and status may not be immediately apparent, in fact may appear virtually non-existent in the public sphere, women as the principal producers of food have a very great influence in society's processes and decisions[12]. This is breaking down now as families enter the cash economy, usually by the male's exclusive assumption of breadwinner role, either as wage-earner, business entrepreneur or cash-cropper, and the status of women is consequently eroding. Urbanisation and modernisation are steadily disempowering women, and the trend is proving virtually impossible to stop, let alone reverse.

However, the positive side to these sensitive gender issues is that women in general are willing to speak up for their own protection and strengthening. Women's groups are active at all levels of society and all over the country, and their success may well be based on the traditional belief that they have the right to organise their own intra-gender affairs. Traditional values such as the protection of fenility and the stability of family and marriage are as accepted by men as by women and provide a base upon which women can assume significant roles as protectors and upholders.

SUMMARY

As with all legal regimes, Papua New Guinea's many customary systems contain both negative and positive features for the formulation of successful jurisprudential strategies for the management of the AIDS epidemic.

Negative Aspects

The poor understanding by those who wield power in a modern nation state of their roles and functions means that it may prove particularly difficult to determine and implement effective epidemic policy. On the material side, the rising levels of corruption amongst leaders means that the ability to provide already scarce social services is further eroded.

Processes by which disputes were traditionally resolved and social harmony restored, factors such as the continual apportionment of blame, and the exacting of retribution by and against groups rather than individuals, can work very much against the needs and concerns of an individual. The HIV virus infects individuals on the basis of their private behaviour, in contrast to other diseases which strike generally in given environmental circumstances. Communities already driven by fear of the supernatural may be all too ready to incorporate the fears, born of ignorance, that typically surround the HIV epidemic, and hence react accordingly, to the detriment of many. Widespread ignorance about the facts of sex, reproduction and disease, coupled with complex systems of traditional beliefs and practices in these matters, do not make the task of educators any easier. Misconceptions readily arise, with received messages becoming instantly distorted when combined with and translated through the medium of community. Official (in the form of state and church) opposition to customs such as initiation ceremonies serves, as most opposition does, only to drive these things underground and make contact, admission and change harder. The various cutting and tattooing customs still widely practiced constitute particular dangers for infection if shared implements are used. Opposition to, and denial of, such behaviour patterns as adultery and promiscuity also pose obstacles to a clear-headed approach.

Continued failure to acknowledge the importance of empowering women to fight the epidemic will have disastrous effects. A society which finds it easy to undervalue women must nevertheless be made to realise that the consequence of infecting women is the infection of other men, and of children, and the subsequent disintegration of society as a whole.

Positive Aspects

The egalitarian nature of Papua New Guinean societies in general means that the worst efforts of political leaders can be countered by a grounds well of opinion which opposes those measures, and effectively chooses to ignore them. The mutual support systems which still flourish, even if in forms somewhat altered from the traditional, in village society, and the general tendency for acceptance of the different and the disabled, mean that the chances are good for family and clan support for infected members.

The general failure of the imported law to reconcile itself with customary family law could possibly prove to be an advantage, as societies evolve their own methods of coping with the new problems posed by the epidemic. Some traditions, such as the puberty ceremonies which provide sexual education to the young, may be adapted and built upon as a venue for teaching young people. Fertility, family and children have traditionally been held in high regard, and a message which emphasises the saving of children and family life will be well-accepted.

Conclusion

Attempting to devise legal interventions which take full account of the multiplicity and diversity of Papua New Guinean cultures will not only be largely unsuccessful and a waste of precious time, they may also be largely unnecessary. Beliefs, traditions and laws of whatever kind are not by themselves enough to make or change behaviour. Ultimately, the decision to maintain or modify a set of actions must lie in each individual. But Papua New Guineans rarely yet, if ever, are obliged to operate in situations of social anomie such as are found in the highly urbanised societies of the First World. Successful interventions will hopefully achieve their own snowball effect.

Papua New Guinea is not yet in a position to formulate clear recommendations for successful epidemic management. Work has begun, but there is far to go. It is clear, though, that the impact of customary law on the people's thinking is a factor which must never be sidestepped in the process of formulating legal interventions.

REFERENCES

1. For further details, see Stewart (1993) Country Background Paper, published as "Law, Ethics and HIV/AIDS" Department of Health, Port Moresby.
2. Schedule 1.2.
3. It is submitted that this is the essence underlying PNG's current conflict situations. Bougainville is essentially an expression by a highly articulate people, pushed to extremes of dissatisfaction by a situation pushed on them by outsiders (originally the colonial power) that they will no longer tolerate the erosion of their traditional right to control their own destinies, their own resources. And the same dissatisfaction is being expressed, in different forms, by other peoples across the country-roadblocks on the Highlands Highway,

exorbitant load compensation claims for the use of traditional land for public purposes, even if that land is no more than a small unusable area of a remote mountaintop where a telegraphic repeater station has been built.

4. Personal observation from Dr. Carol Jenkins, Institute of Medical Research, Goroka.
5. Personal observations of the authors.
6. For further detail see Stewart (1993) Country Background Paper, published as "Law, Ethics and HIV/AIDS" Department of Health.
7. See for example some of the stories in : Kyakas and Wiessner (1992)" From Inside the Women's House" Robert Brown and Associates (Qld) Pty. Ltd.
8. Marriage Act Section 3.
9. This paper is indebted for much of the information in this section and elsewhere to Dr. Carol Jenkins, of the Institute of Medical Research, Goroka, conveyed through personal communication and to be found in her "Study of Sexual and Reproductive Knowledge and Behaviour in Papua New Guinea", Child Survival Support Project Special Report Number 2, (in press).
10. Personal communication from Anne Borrey, criminologist, National Research Institute, and others.
11. See also Strathern, M. (1975) "Report on Questionnaire relating to Sexual Offences as defined in the Criminal Code", prepared for the Department of Law.
12. See for example Kyakas and Wiessner *op cit.* and the summary and various citations contained in Borrey, A. (1992) "Ol Kalabus Meri- A Study of Female Prisoners in Papua New Guinea", Law Reform Commission Occasional Paper No. 21.

51

The HIV/AIDS Situation in the Philippines

Dr. Evelyn Grace B. Gacad
Programme Manager
National AIDS/STD Prevention and Control Programme
Department of Health, Philippines

Historical Backgrounds

The first case of AIDS was diagnosed in December 1984. Serosurveys commenced in 1985 but have been limited primarily to female commercial sex workers who are required by law to submit regularly for testing for sexually transmitted diseases (STDs).

Epidemiological Situation

As of February 1995 there had been a cumulative total of 616 HIV seropositive cases in the Philippines as reported to the National AIDS Registry of the Department of Health. Out of this number, 194 (31 per cent) are AIDS cases. More than 90 have died.

The spread of HIV infection in the Philippines has the following characteristics:

1. There is a steady increase of HIV infection.
2. Heterosexual transmission accounts for most HIV infections.
3. The male to female ratio is almost 1:1.
4. Among the female population tested, the majority of those

infected are between the ages of 20 and 29 years, while among males the vulnerable age group is between 30-39 years.

According to data the most common reported mode of HIV transmission is sexual intercourse between men and women. About 70 per cent of reported HIV infections were contracted through sexual transmission; 52 per cent were between men and women. Perinatal transmission and transmission through blood transfusion or injecting drug use is limited.

Despite the relatively low incidence of HIV infection and number of AIDS notifications, the threat of widespread HIV transmission is real. The increasing number of reported cases from 1984 up to the present indicates that considerable HIV transmission is taking place. The general expectation is that these rates will increase markedly in the next few years.

A high prevalence of risky behaviours has been documented through an established surveillance system. The National HIV Sentinel Surveillance has recently completed its third round of activities in six sites in the country involving six selected groups: registered female sex workers, freelance female sex workers, male sex workers, male STD patients, men who have sex with men, and injecting drug users. The surveillance studies have established that injecting drug use is a potential mode of transmission.

The high prevalence of syphilis among the selected groups in these areas is indicative of the great danger of potential widespread transmission if HIV is introduced into these groups. Low condom use, sharing of injecting drug equipment, and of course multiple sex partners, were common among all groups tested, further compounding the already high risks of HIV transmission.

It is estimated that there are 15,000—50,000 Filipinos who are HIV infected. Without preventive efforts, the Philippines will have 90,000 HIV infected Filipinos, with about 15,000—20,000 AIDS cases, by the year 2000.

The National Programme

The National AIDS Prevention and Control Programme, which was formally launched in 1988 by the Department of Health, has had Medium-Term Plans or MTPs. The first MTP was for the period 1988-93, with a mid-term review in 1990. The second Medium-Term Plan was drafted in 1994 and provides the framework for activities from 1994 to 1999. Compared to the first MTP, which was more vertical, there is more multisectoral involvement in the second—with the participation of various government and non-government agencies.

There are four main strategies identified in MTP II: prevention of sexual transmission; prevention of transmission through blood; prevention of perinatal transmission; and reduction of impact on individual, family, community and society. The fourth strategy, is further categorized into: (a) impact on the individuals and their families, and (b) impact on the health care structure and services. To reduce the impact on individuals and their families, several interventions have been identified, such as protecting the rights of individuals; making social and health care services accessible to individuals and their families; and providing community-based social support, and counselling.

Interventions to meet the impact on the health care structure and services include: mobilizing communities providing care for the infected and social support to individuals and their families; safeguarding rights of the individual; accessing social services; promoting human resources development not only for government health personnel but also for community based health providers; and upgrading of facilities for diagnosis and care.

At present, all these planned interventions are yet to be translated into a clear-cut schedule of activities to meet the objectives of the National Programme, which is consistent with the global thrusts in the prevention and control of HIV infection.

52

Philippine Laws and Jurisprudence Relevant to HIV/AIDS

Glenda T. Litong
Director Human Rights Desk
Integrated Bai of the Philippines
Philippines

Julita Espartero
Attorney
Integrated Bar of the Philippines
Namila , Philippines

A. PUBLIC HEALTH

In 1986, the Department of Health decreed AIDS as a notifiable dtsease and directed the reporting of its incidence. Ministry Circular No. 2 of the Department of Health, dated 2 January 1986, adopted the definition of the Conference of State and Territorial Epidemiologists at its annual meeting in Madison, Wisconsin, onJune 2-5, 1985 and added refinements in the case definition of AIDS for purposes of national reporting which are: (1) anyone found positive in serologic or virologic test for Human Immunodeficiency Virus (HIV); and/or (2) anyone exhibiting manifestations of opportunistic infections like chronic diarrhea or kaposi's sarcoma. Thereafter, the Department of Health issued several circulars and orders providing the mechanism for surveillance, notification and monitoring of the disease[1].

The National AIDS Programme, as formulated by the Department of Health, has five components, namely: (a) Communication and Health Education; (b) Surveillance; (c) Laboratory Services; (d) Care of HIV infected individuals and people with AIDS; and (e) Programme Management. The Programme aims to reduce HIV transmission and the impact of HIV and AIDS on the individual, family, community and society.

Modest strides have been made in the implementation of the programme despite the fact that no law directly addressing the problem of HIV/AIDS has been enacted except the fore stated administrative circulars and policy statements.

Executive Order No. 39, creating the Philippine National AIDS Council (PNAC), was signed into law by President Fidel V. Ramos on 3 December, 1992. The PNAC shall serve as the national policy and advisory body to the President in the prevention and control of HIV infection and AIDS in the Philippines.

B. HUMAN RIGHTS AND DISCRIMINATION

Article II, section 2 of the Philippine Constitution provides that generally accepted principles of international law form part of the law of the land. Some of the rights embodied in the Universal Declaration of Human Rights that are pertinent and relevant to the issue of HIV/AIDS are as follows:

Right of all to Faire and Equal Treatment (Art. 2)

The rights and freedoms listed in the Declaration are guaranteed to every human being, regardless of race, creed, sex or beliefs, including people infected with HIV and with AIDS. It should be emphasised that the campaign to stem the spread of the disease is a fight waged against the virus and not against the individual.

Right to life (Art. 3)

Right to life includes the right to live in dignity, freedom and safety.

Right to be Regarded as a Person (Art. 6)

Men are human beings and inherent in men is the right to be treated by law was a person and not just a thing. One does not cease being a human when infected with HIV.

Right to Equality before the Law (Art. 7)

Men are equal before the eyes of the law and the law must be applied equally in the same manner for everyone. The law must not discriminate merely by reason of race or sex or way of life.

Right to Legal protection (Art. 8)

An individual has the right to redress and secure effective remedy through the courts and other appropriate agencies for acts violating his fundamental rights granted by the Constitution or law.

Right to Freedom (Art. 9)

No one has the right to restrict a person's liberty without a valid and just cause. Such rights include the right to exist and the right to be free from arbitrary personal restraint or servitude; it is deemed to embrace the right of man to enjoy the faculties with which he has been endowed by his Creator, subject only to such restraints as are necessary for the common welfare (*Rubi v. Provincial Board of Mindoro. .49 Phil 704*).

Right to Privacy {Art. IV)

This right safeguards the dignity of one's person, including his honour and reputation, and the privacy of his home and effects from unjust intrusion, attack and interference. Confidentiality of information relating to an individual with AIDS or infected with HIV is protected under this right. Autonomy of decision-making by an individual also falls under this fundamental right.

Right to Freedom of Movement (Art. 13)

This is the right to locomotion, the right to choose one's domicile and the right to travel and to return to one's country. Nobody has the right to quarantine or isolate an individual in the absence of compelling reasons therefore.

Rights to Marry and have a Family (Art. 16)

The decision whether to get married and found a family is a decision that only the individual can make for himself. Requiring an HIV clearance certificate, for example, curtails the right of individuals who are otherwise capable of contractipg a valid marriage but, for one reason or another, would refuse to undergo a test.

Right to Social Security (Art. 22)

The individual has the right, as a member of the society, to serial security sufficient for a decent living, including shelter and medical assistance.

Right to Work {Art. 23)

Everyone has the right to gainful employment and to receive the just fruits of his labour without discrimination, save for reasonable standards that the nature of work entails.

All of the foregoing fundamental rights are guaranteed to every human being, regardless of race, sex, beliefs or ways of life. These rights cannot be abridged without compelling reasons. The same rights cannot be denied even to persons infected with HIV or those who have AIDS. However, neither can the rights of other individuals, who are at the same time exposed to the possibility of infection, be neglected and/or sacrificed in the process of trying to find a solution to the epidemic. These rights, guaranteed by the State, clearly indicate the pre-eminent role of the individual which every government is mandated to protect. Intrusions by the government in the exercise of these rights by the individual are very limited and defined.

In furtherance of its international commitment, Articles II, III and IV of the Philippine Constitution embody and safeguard the aforementioned rights[2]. These Articles relate to issues pertaining to maintenance of peace and order, the sanctity of family life, privacy of communication, the States approach to health, etc.

C. POLICE POWER

The aforestated constitutional guarantees, however, are neither absolute nor inflexible. They may give way to the requirement of public interest allowing government to intervene in certain instances but in a very restricted manner through police power.

Police power is an inherent power of the State and embraces the power to prescribe regulations to promote health, morals, education, good order, safety, or the general welfare of the people (*Ermita-Malate Hotel Association v. City Mayor of Manila*). An inquiry into the reasonableness of legislation enacted in pursuit of police power must consider the individual's right to due process. The legislation must involve public interest and a public purpose, for this alone will ensure the reasonableness of the legislative purpose. It is essential that the Act not be unreasonable, arbitrary or oppressive; it must have sufficient foundation or reason in connection with the matter involved. Nor should there be a capricious use of the legislative power; the aim conceived must be achieved by the means used and not merely an unjustified interference with private interest. (*Ichong v. Hernandez. 101 Phil 115.*)

Primordial in any inquiry is the avoidance of injustice by eliminating arbitrariness. Laws are merely man-made and man is not infallible; man has his own individual prejudices and biases. In the task of controlling and stemming the epidemic, judgment may be clouded and objectivity sacrificed by reason of the ignorance in the nature and epidemiology of the HIV. Therefore, any legislation that directly addresses the problem posed by the epidemic has to stand the test of reasonableness.

In a landmark case, *Villavicencio v. Lukban. 43 Phils 778 (1919)*, the Supreme Court rebuked the action of the city mayor in rounding up the prostitutes of Manila and shipping them to Davao to rid the city of vices. It was held that the city mayor had no authority to do the same, since no law, order, or regulation allows him to do the same. The Court ruled that "these women despite their being, in a sense, lepers of society are nevertheless, not chattels but Philippine citizens protected by the same constitutional guarantees as are other citizens". No individual can have such arbitrary power as to deny another individual his liberty of abode. The same principle may be invoked to protect the rights of an individual infected with HIV.

D. IMMIGRATION RULES ON AIDS

Several pieces of legislation require an AIDS Clearance Certificate for the entry into and continued stay of certain classes of aliens in the Philippines[3]. Just recently, however, these regulations were suspended by the Bureau of Immigration through Office Memorandum No. 030-93 issued on 5 March 1993 pending the submission of a report by the Committee tasked with reviewing said requirements.

E. LAWS ON DOCTOR-PATIENT RELATIONSHIP

The Code of Ethics of the Medical Profession of the Philippines provides that, "while recognising that it is the prior right of the patient to choose his physician, a physician is under no obligation to accept a patient unless the situation is an emergency or he is the only physician in the community (Art. II: 2). " It can be argued, however, that the right to medical treatment is implicit in the right to life and the same cannot be denied to an individual afflicted with a disease whatever the gravity of the illness may be. More particularly, one who has HIV may not be denied his right to medical treatment.

The Physician is obliged to respect the confidentiality of all information acquired in the discharge of his professional duties. As a matter of evidence, information divulged to a physician during a relationship cannot be admitted in evidence without the consent of the patient (Rule 130, sec. 24, Rules of Court). Doctors, however, are required to report any AIDS cases they attend. In order to protect the fundamental right of privacy of an individual with AIDS or infected with HIV, the reporting must be limited to the number of AIDS cases and other statistics without divulging the identity of the person unless the patient agrees in writing to the disclosure.

F. WOMEN AND AIDS

Philippine society and culture lay the burden and responsibility of providing for the family upon the male spouse. In a society where the majority of its populace live below the poverty line, economic dependency and cultural and social role-playing render Filipino women more vulnerable to HIV infection.

Filipino wives are expected to remain in the home and take care of the children and their husband. Many wives do not have economic autonomy and become economically dependent on their husbands.

While the wife is expected to remain loyal to her husband, the same is not expected of the husband. In the matter of engaging in sexual activity, the wife has very little latitude in determining the sexual relationship with her husband. The moral ascendancy of the husband over the wife as influenced and molded by culture makes the wife prone to accepting the desires and wishes of her husband. Worse, some husbands batter and abuse their wives if they do not accede to their wishes. The wife cannot even cry rape for forcible sexual intercourse under Philippine laws. At the most, the husband can only be held liable for coercion. Neither can a Filipino wife exercise much freedom in adopting measures that will protect herself from infection of a sexually transmitted disease.

The situation is no different for women outside marriage, especially those engaged in the sex industry. Here, too, the man dictates the sexual relationship and can insist on the non-use of condoms.

Women are also expected to be carers for the sick and the dying. They will bear the burden of having to deal with the virus at great emotional, physiological as well as psychological cost.

The situation remains true up to this day despite provisions in the Family Code of gender-equality rules (e.g., joint responsibility between wife and husband for the support of the family, joint management and administration of the household affairs and property regimes, among others) and declarations in the Philippine Constitution on the role of women.

G. THE RIGHT TO MARRY

The right to marry and found a family are basic human rights guaranteed to all adults, including people infected with HIV. Article XV of the Philippine Constitution recognises the value of the family and marriage as basic social institutions.

A law that will make an AIDS Clearance Certificate condition precedent to the issuance of a marriage license would effectively negate the right of an individual to a valid marriage. The intent of the law, which is to prevent transmission of the virus to the prospective spouse and children, is valid and proper. The means proposed, however, cannot pass the test of reasonableness for the following reasons:

1. HIV tests are not reliable because of the so called "window period;"
2. The denial of a marriage license based on the individual's refusal to undergo an HIV test does not guarantee the absence of sexual intercourse between applicants that would abate the transmission of the virus. On the contrary, it might even encourage promiscuity which runs counter to the purpose of the legislation.

On the other hand, a married person whose spouse is infected during the effectivity of their marriage is entitled to an annulment of the marriage under Art. 45 (6) of the Family Code. Since the reference is to a sexually transmissible disease found to be serious and which appears to be incurable, at present it would refer only to HIV infection or AIDS.

The law does assure certain rights and privileges to an individual with AIDS and persons infected with the virus such as support and maintenance[4], inheritance[5], adoption[6] and parential authority[7].

H. CRIMINAL LAW AND AIDS

Philippine law criminalises certain activities associated with the spread of HIV, as prostitution, vagrancy and the possession, manufacture, sale and use of prohibited drugs. Such criminalisation has discouraged participation in preventive measures.

The criminalisation of prostitution has contributed to the difficulty of combating the disease as it discourages individuals engaged in this highrisk activity from openly participating in the formulation of approaches to control the epidemic.

Nightclubs, bars and sauna parlours are widely known as fronts for prostitution. Recent clean-up initiatives of the Manila city government have only forced the relocation of the activity to other areas within Metro Manila and further pushed prostitution underground. This has presented a problem to several non-governmental organisations which have initiated modest information campaigns on safe sex practices and the use of condoms directed towards sex workers.

There are provisions of the law which may have a bearing on the issue of discrimination, breach of confidentiality, and other violations of the rights of affected groups. Aside from civil damages under the Civil Code, an aggrieved individual can resort to filing of criminal cases for libel, slander, oral defamation, intriguing against honour, malicious mischief, and unjust vexation.

In the matter of terminating a pregnancy by reason of HIV infection, there is no law that allows abortion at any stage, even if sought by the mother herself, for any reason. Terminating a fetal life is a criminal act and is liable to penalisation.

In case of transmission by negligence, the Penal Code sanctions injury caused through reckless imprudence. Thus, blood transfusions done without required HIV blood screening despite the knowledge of said requirement and the possibility of transmission is an act punishable as reckless imprudence. Having sexual contact despite knowledge of infection and the risk of transmission may constitute reckless imprudence.

By and large, the penal laws of the Philippines have not anticipated a situation characterised by a deliberate transmission of a disease similar to HIV/AIDS. Certain quarters in the legal profession insist that a wilful transmission of HIV/AIDS should be included as one of the aggravating circumstances which, if present in the commission of any of the listed crimes, will increase the penalty to its maximum period.

I. THE LEGAL PROCESS AVAILABLE

The Philippine Constitution guarantees that access to the courts as well as to adequate legal assistance shall not be denied to anyone for reasons of poverty.

Violations of human rights as well as other rights granted by law give rise to civil as well as criminal liabilities. The Civil Code of the Philippines (Republic Act No. 386) on Human Relations provides the basis for redress of human rights violations in its Articles 19, 20, 21, 26 & 32. An individual whose rights are violated is entitled to indemnification in the form of damages. A criminal act gives rise to civil liability.

The refusal of health carers to provide necessary medical assistance to a patient is a matter that can be brought to the attention of the Profession Regulatory Commission. Malpractice suits against doctors, however, are very rare in the Philippines due to the reluctance of other members of the medical profession to testify against their fellow doctors.

As to the right of an individual infected with the virus or one who has AIDS to confidentiality of his condition, the rules on evidence provide a safeguard that renders evidence inadmissible if it falls under what is termed as privileged communication. Rule 130, section 24 of the Revised Rules on Evidence guarantees the confidentiality of the information by reason of the relationship of confidentiality existing between the individuals at the time the information was given as between husband and wife, a lawyer and his client, a physician and his patient, a priest and a confessant.

Conclusion

Current legislative responses have been slow and inadequate. Neither are proposed laws to address the problem integrated, or comprehensive. They tend to neglect the psycho-social aspects of the epidemic in terms of the possible repercussions and impact of the measures on the rights of the individual, family, community and the society in general. These propositions tend to promote stigmatisation resulting in the individual's displacement and discrimination. It is imperative that any measure aimed at addressing the HIV/AIDS epidemic should take into account all aspects and factors that contribute to the dynamism of the problem at hand—a solution that should focus on policies that encourage voluntary control and behavioural change.

REFERENCES

1. The circulars and orders refer to specific fiats issued with reference to reporting of HIV infections, research, surveillance and health and social assistance, and revocation of licenses of sex workers.
2. See Article II, Sections 5, 11, 12, 15 & 18, Article III, Sections 1, 2, 3, & 6; Article; XIII, Section 3 & 11; and Article XIV, Section 1 thereof.
3. Immigration Regulation Instructions No. 14 of the Commission on Immigration and Deportation issued on 17 February 1989 supplemented by Immigration Regulation Instruction No. 21 issued on 13 April 1988.
4. Art. 194-195 of the Family code.
5. Art. 887 of Civil Code amended by the Family Code.
6. Art. 183 & 184 of the Family Code.
7. Art. 211 & 288 of the Family Code.

53

Information Law, Privacy and HIV/AIDS in the Philippines: A Case Study

Cecilia Jimenez
Attorney,
Philippines Alliance of Human Rights Advocates Manila
Philippines

INTRODUCTION

The issue of HIV/AIDS is controversial because of its impact, or potential impact, on the socio-cultural, economic and political fabric of any given society and of the world in general. In this context, the law may be seen as a tool that ought to be used in the prevention of the spread of HIV and in minimising the impact of HIV/AIDS on the people. Corollary to this is the care that must be given to those infected with the HIV virus and to persons with AIDS (PWA).

Given the low threshold of awareness and understanding of the real nature of HIV/AIDS, the law in itself can be used, and is being used, as a tool to oppress and violate the rights of the individuals and of society whom the law is supposed to protect. This concrete reality is facilitated by the fact that it is usually a powerful elite that controls the law of a given society, a situation which does not help in the over-all protection of the rights of a marginalised majority in a developing or underdeveloped country.

The Philippines is no exception to this general rule. The role of the law in the context of the HIV/AIDS issue may therefore be either positive or negative.

The field of information law and privacy in relation to the issue of HIV/ AIDS has been little examined. The positive role that information law and law protecting privacy rights can play in the attainment of the objectives of reducing transmission of HIV infection, and of minimising its impact on society should be encouraged and developed.

This paper attempts to survey the status and potential of information law and privacy law, as it relates to the issue of HIV/ AIDS in the Philippines. It will therefore include not only a description and analysis of the existing law and attempted legislation but general recommendations as well.

Information law is generally treated in this paper as dealing directly with public access to information, including the publication, circulation and broadcast of such information. It also includes restrictions to such access and circulation, as far as they relate to the rights of the individuals and of society in general.

The law on privacy, on the other hand, deals with the right of the individual to be left alone. This right includes protection of data relating to that individual and the use of those data as they relate to public welfare.

At this point it must be stressed that, in the Philippines, information law, specifically the law on mass media and obscenity, is fully developed within the context of the freedoms of expression, speech and the press. Philippine privacy law, on the other hand, leaves much to be desired. This is not only because of the low threshold of awareness and education of the general public and policy-makers on the issue of HIV/AIDS as it affects privacy rights; it is also because, at this point of time, the development of the law on privacy in this country is still at an incipient stage.

A. INFORMATION LAW

The Philippine National AIDS Prevention and Control Programme being undertaken by the Philippine government, as implemented by the Department of Health, has as its primary objective the following: "to reduce transmission of HIV infection, reduce mortality and morbidity and reduce impact. "

A major element of the programme is the national HIV/AIDS awareness campaign that includes Information, Education and Communication (IEC)[1].

Access to information on HIV/AIDS by the public is therefore a *sina* qua non for the success of the programme. Such information and education must be directed to both the society as well as to individuals who are at the highest risk of infection. Such information must be aimed at effecting behavioural changes that will attain the basic objectives of reducing transmission of HIV infection and minimising impact on society.

The role of information law, therefore, must be construed as empowering the society and concerned individuals with sufficient information necessary to equip themselves for their own welfare and benefit.

1. Freedoms of Speech, Expression and the Press; Access to Information; Freedom of Circulation and Publication

In the Philippines, the right of the individual and of society to information is explicity provided for as "the right of the people to information on matters of public concern." Such rights, however, have been integrated into the 1987 Philippine Constitution within the context of political developments ensuing from the Philippine national experience of more than decade of one-man dictatorship. In the ensuing jurisprudence, therefore, this right has been interpreted to cover government records and documents that should be accessible to the general public.

However, despite this initial, restrictive constitutional interpretation, Philippine information law should be seen as including the mass media law, the jurisprudence of which has developed to such an extent that the freedoms of speech, expression and the press have been adequately described and guaranteed[2]. The recognition over time of this role of the mass media as a manifestation of the freedoms of speech, expression and the press has resulted in what is generally known as legal media privileges, the most important of which is the privilege of publishing and broadcasting news and newsworthy accounts. Such privilege applies to articles of informational and educational value, which include truthful accounts of events in good faith and occurrences of legitimate interest to the public. Such major interests include public health, public education and other aspects of public welfare.

Information on HIV/AIDS is definitely part of this largely defined "public concern." Indeed, the role of the mass media as an effective conduit for HIV/AIDS awareness and education cannot be underestimated. Such a role of the mass media can be appreciated as a vehicle in influencing and effecting behavioural change and in initiating appropriate action on the part of Philippine policy-makers.

The ancillary rights of the freedoms of speech, expression and the press include free discussion as well as every accessory right essential to the purpose. Since the aim is to allow the widest possible broadcast or circulation of the best tracts available on problems of public concern, freedom of access to information and freedom of circulation or publication have received parallel protection under Philippine law and jurisprudence. The reason is that such freedoms of access to information and circulation are vital to the education of the public.

As concerns access to information, Philippine law and jurisprudence attempt to balance the right of the individual to one's privacy and reputation, with the media's right to report on a matter of public concern. In this case, the International Covenant on Civil and Political Rights, the 1987 Philippine constitution and the Philippine Civil Code all secure the privacy of communication and correspondence except upon a lawful order of the court. The Philippine Civil Code further provides for the respect of the dignity, personality, privacy and peace of mind of one's neighbour and other persons in general. The right of the individual to one's reputation and privacy is further enhanced by penal restrictions on defamation (provisions on libel, slander and the like) as provided for by the Revised Penal code of the Philippines.

The media's privilege of reporting and publication is therefore also restricted by the same laws on privacy and defamation. Law and jurisprudence are quite explicit that since persons are entitled to be left alone, the publication of private facts unsuited for publicity, though not necessarily libelous (i.e., malicious), is actionable where it causes embarrassment and may injure one's interaction with fellow persons. Definitely, given the present stigmatisation of the issue of HIV/AIDS within Philippine society, such media privileges are restricted as such.

In the field of evidence, any privileged matter is presumed to have been published with good motives and for justifiable ends without the necessity of proof. However, such privilege is defeasible and may be overcome by a showing of actual malice. In such event, the privilege immediately disappears and the defamatory matter becomes actionable not only civilly but also criminally.

Another restrictive component in Philippine law and jurisprudence is the law on obscenity. Among the time-honoured limitations to the freedoms of speech, expression and the press is the law penalising any publication that is "offensive" to public morals, i.e., to the values of the society at large. The Revised Penal Code of the Philippines prohibits the expression and circulation of immoral doctrines, obscene publications and exhibitions. Given the nature of the issue of HIV/AIDS, the question is: is the Philippine obscenity law applicable in this regard?

Taking after US law interpreting freedoms of speech as it relates to obscenity law, which Philippine jurisprudence usually follows, the answer seems to be no. Philippine jurisprudence provides that obscenity is not within the constitutionally protected speech because obscenity is utterly without redeeming social importance. Therefore, if a publication or broadcast can be proved to be of public value, i.e., with redeeming social importance or value, such may not be deemed as obscene or immoral. Periodicals and primers, which may be illustrated, for example, may claim such privilege as being within the protection of constitutional guarantees for the benefit and welfare of the public.

The development and state of mass media in the Philippines should therefore be seen positively as having a great potential in spreading awareness and information on HIV/AIDS. In the ongoing debate on the issue, the role of the media and the laws and jurisprudence guaranteeing its privileges prove indispensable in effecting change.

The breakthrough in Philippine mass media came last year with the publication of the story of a person with AIDS (PWA), Dolzura Cortes, later followed by the publication of the story of another PWA, Rachel Reyes. These media publications ensured the effective use by the media of its privileges while, at the same time, respecting privacy rights of the individuals concerned. These media features put faces on the issue of HIV/AIDS which consequently caught the attention of the nation, involving as they do young women with families, jobs, etc. The interest shown by the media and the public was bolstered by the media coverage of the Department of Health Secretary whose controversial statements and actions caught the ire of the more conservative sectors of Philippine society. The media fortunately proved to be essential in the public monitoring of the debate among these various sectors.

One must cite, however, that the media is presently covering these issues because of the controversies they entail and, therefore, their consequent "newsworthiness."

A prime example of such media coverage is the condom tug-of-war between the condom "endorsers," headed by the Health Secretary, and the conservative sectors, headed by the Catholic

Church[3]. These groups espouse opposing policies: the former considers the use of condoms as necessary, though not limited to the overall national HIV/AIDS prevention campaign; the latter considers it as promoting behaviour contrary to moral values that the Catholic Church tries to develop. Considering that Philippine society is predominantly Catholic, this clash of policy statements between two power blocks in Philippine society is a matter not only of public interest or concern but also of being good, saleable news.

Pending Philippine legislation recognises the role that the mass media has to play in the information and awareness campaign on the issue of HIV/ AIDS. House Bill No. 8077, for example, proposes for the conduct of an information dissemination campaign on AIDS in media at least once a week during primetime in television and radio, and once a week in all commercial newspapers and magazines.

2. Formal Education

An essential component of any national programme on HIV/ AIDS is education. The right to education is provided for by both international obligations of the Philippine government as well as by the 1987 Philippine Constitution. Thus, one of the most important policy statements in the Philippine National AIDS Prevention and Control Programme is the integration of HIV/AIDS education into the existing formal school curricula (elementary, high school and college levels), the implementation of which shall be the responsibility of the Department of Education, Culture and Sports (DECS). In pursuance of this policy statement, the DECS has been conducting experimental modules in certain regions of the Philippines. Based on evaluation, these modules shall be implemented starting in the coming schoolyear 1993-1994.

Legislative response to the need to integrate HIV/AIDS education formally into the existing curricula manifests itself in several pending bills in both the House of Representatives and the Philippine Senate. On the other hand, legislative counter reactions can also be seen in Senate Resolution No. 314 which, while recognising the necessity of teaching HIV prevention and control and integrating it into the high school curriculum, opposes the DECS programme of integrating into the First and Second Year High School's "Physical Education, Health and Music" Programme the promotion of the use of condoms, on the ground that such plans promote promiscuity among teenagers who should be taught moral values and standards instead.

Indeed, the issue of HIV/AIDS education and the approach of its integration into the formal school curricula is a current subject of debate, fueled again by the clashing values between and among sectors of society over moral standards.

3. Role of Non-Government Organisations

At this point, after an examination of information law, the role of non-government organisations must also be seen as contributing to such a campaign and as enhancing the implementation of the law on access to information and circulation. A primary example of such private endeavours is the project called "Remedios AIDS Information Center" which, through its AIDS Hotline and Counselling Center, provides free anonymous as well as face-to-face counselling, with guarantees of confidentiality to any interested member of the general public. Other NGOs enhance this capacity with publications, training courses and the like.

Conclusions

One should take the opportunities provided by the strength of information law in the Philippines in so far as it concerns the mass media. Moreover, the institutionalisation of such opportunities should seriously be adopted, such as the regular use of the various media outlets for information dissemination campaigns. This is important in order that information on HIV/AIDS will not be limited to, or based on, the commercial value of newsworthy accounts or coverage. In so doing, the general public shall be more systematically provided with the necessary information on the issue of HIV/AIDS and developments thereof.

Also, the integration of HIV/AIDS education into the formal curricula is a matter of utmost importance and even urgency. The ongoing debate on the adequacy or approach to HIV/AIDS education, especially for the young people, should be settled by a firm policy statement and action by the Department of Education, Culture and Sports, without prejudice to the constitutional right of the parents to choose the education they wish for their children.

Lastly, more institutional support and legislative recognition should be given to the role of non-government organisations that provide much needed information and training components in the campaign to increase the awareness on the issue of HIV/AIDS and thus to effect positive behavioural change.

B. LAW ON PRIVACY

1. The Law on Privacy in the Philippines, Confidentiality and Data Protection

As already mentioned, the law on privacy rights in the Philippines can be found in various statutes. In general, these laws provide for the guarantees of the dignity of one's person and his family, including one's honour, peace of mind and reputation, and the privacy of one's home, communication and correspondence, and effects from unjust intrusion, attack and interference. In short, the right to privacy entails the right to be left alone and the protection of data relating to the person concerned.

It must also be pointed out that international standards and the Philippine Constitution provide the right not to be a witness against oneself (i.e., the right against self-incrimination). This includes the right not to be subjected to the seizure of substances of one's body without the person's express and informed consent. The violation of such a right is also considered by Philippine jurisprudence as an intrusion of privacy and a violation of security of one's person.

Another important component of the right to privacy is confidentiality. Such confidentiality refers both to testimonies and to relevant data. In the Philippines, the Revised Rules of Evidence provide a safeguard that renders as inadmissible any evidence of confidential information falling under the "privileged communication" rule. The privileged communication rule guarantees the confidentiality of information, at the time the information was provided, within the following relationships: between husband and wife; between a lawyer and the client; between a person authorised to practice medicine, surgery or obstetrics and the patient; and between a minister/priest and the confessor. Philippine law is more explicit on the confidentiality of medical information, as already provided by the law on evidence and further by the code of Ethics of the Medical Profession of the Philippines[4] as promulgated by the Philippine Medical Association.

On the other hand, such privilege of confidentiality of medical information does not extend to other medical workers such as nurses. Nor does it exist where the patient brings an action for damages against the physician or where there is express waiver by the patient in the form of consent for disclosure. The privilege also does not apply in criminal cases for the maintenance of public order and where the life and liberty of the citizens are deemed more important than the purpose for which the privilege was created. Lastly, the Labour Code provides for the disclosure by the physician to the Social Security System or Government Service Insurance System of any information relevant to a medical claim by the patient for compensation or medical benefits.

It should likewise be pointed out that Philippine law is deficient in data protection which should guarantee that data obtained for a specific purpose cannot be used for another purpose. Neither does the insurance law of the Philippines provide for any confidentiality of medical information provided by the insured to the insurance company, nor for any prohibition against the demand of such insurance company for medical information.

As can be seen, the law on the right to privacy in the Philippines is still at an incipient stage where privacy rights, while provided for in general but limited terms, have not been explicitly nor adequately developed. Furthermore, data protection is a legal issue that must be addressed further in order to adequately protect the privacy rights of any given individual from mis-use and abuse that will entail further encroachments of other individual human rights, especially the right against discrimination.

2. The Police Power of the State

Philippine law and jurisprudence on the police power of the state has been adequately provided for and developed. In the Philippines, police power as an inherent power of the state has been upheld where public interest allows government intervention. At the same time, jurisprudence has also emphasised that such powers should be exercised with the end view of securing the individual's freedom to exercise one's rights and should be aimed at emphasising the inviolability of human rights rather than at their restriction. Moreover, the act of police power must be for a public interest and purpose and must be reasonably necessary for the accomplishment of the purpose for which it was conceived. The test of reasonableness can also be measured by the rule on non-arbitrariness. In the case of the HIV/AIDS issue, these are principles that must always be kept in mind in measuring the constitutionality of any infringement of privacy rights.

In the government campaign to prevent the transmission of HIV/AIDS, the Department of Health (DOH) has issued several circulars that effectively decreed AIDS as a notifiable disease and set up monitoring structures for the surveillance of the state of HIV/AIDS in the Philippines. At the same time, the DOH also specifies that for purposes of surveillance, statistics on the incidence of infection shall be maintained by the Department.

3. The issue of Testing and Disclosure of Results and their Implication on Privacy Rights and other Rights and Freedoms

The objective of surveillance has been defined by the Department of Health as the assessment and monitoring of the status of HIV infection and AIDS so that information derived shall guide decision-makers in the institution of appropriate interventions for specific target groups and individuals. As a component of the HIV/AIDS programme of surveillance, the issue of testing, especially mandatory testing, has assumed monumental proportions of controversy precisely because testing and the consequent disclosure of the results directly affect the right to privacy of the individual concerned. In this case, the absence of consent, or of informed consent for that matter, is by itself a violation of the right to privacy.

On such matters of testing and disclosure of testing results, DOH Circular No. 57-A therefore explicitly provides that:

(a) no mandatory testing shall be required except for those persons already being treated under existing law;

(b) persons who engage in high-risk behaviour shall be encouraged to undergo voluntary testing;

(c) information on the testing and counselling shall remain confidential;

(d) tourists shall not be required to undergo testing for HIV unless there are medical indications for testing;

(e) visa applicants who have undergone previous testing will be required to disclose the results of such tests upon visa applications.

For a time, the Philippine commission on Immigration and Deportation, based on the Philippine Immigration Act[5], required the production of AIDS Clearance Certificates(ACC) from certain classes of aliens. Among those required to undergo mandatory HIV testing were: an alien whose visa or application for visa allows him to stay in the Philippines beyond six months; alien seamen regardless of length of stay; an alien entering the country on a permanent basis or applying for permanent residency; alien refugees and illegal aliens.

The requirement by the Commission on Immigration and Deportation of such mandatory testing was opposed by the Department of Health for the following grounds:

(a) there is no firm scientific reasons for such requirement;

(b) there is no satisfactory enforcement; and

(c) the violation of the ethical issue of confidentiality as the prerogative of patients to keep information about their illness a secret and as the imperative placed on doctors in the exercise of their profession. In March 1993, after official protests were lodged by the foreign business chambers in the Philippines, the Phiiippine commissioner on Immigration and Deportation ordered the suspension of the requirement of HIV testing.

Unfortunately, the issue of mandatory testing in the Philippines as it affects privacy rights has not yet been settled. Legislation pending in both the House of Representatives and the Philippine Senate reveals a general trend of requiring compulsory HIV testing for surveillance and control purposes, as follows:

(a) as condition precedent in entry or continued stay of aliens in the Philippines or the deportation of aliens found positive for HIV/AIDS[6].

(b) as a requirement for the issuance of working permits to hospitality girls, dancing partners for hire, massage parlour attendants, waitresses and the like[7].

(c) as a requirement for graduating students in the secondary and tertiary levels and for students in the tertiary levels for promotion to the next level[8],

(d) as a requirement for marrying couples[9] among others.

Moreover, pending legislation also requires the creating of a Central AIDS Registry[10] where a listing of all persons infected with the HIV virus shall be "discreetly but effectively" kept. Other proposals infringing on privacy rights are the forced segregation of prison inmates infected with HIV and the establishment of special communities for people with HIV[11].

It must be stressed that, should these requirements be enacted into law, the violation of privacy rights shall also lead to the violations of other rights and freedoms, i.e., the right not to be discriminated against, right to marry and found a family, freedom of movement, right of education, freedom of movement, etc.

Recommendations

There is an apparent case of the lack of legislation and

institutionalised protection of privacy rights in the Philippines,not cnly within the context of the issue of HIV/AIDS hut also in general terms as well. Moreover, the propensity of pending legislation to propose draconian measures that will weaken the national campaign to prevent transmission of HIV, and that will effectively violate privacy rights and other rights and freedoms as well, only serve to underline the following needs:

(a) instill the necessary understanding of the nature, epidemiology and implication of HIV/AIDS on persons tasked with policy-making, including those in the legislature, and on those tasked with the interpretation of the law, i.e., the iudiciary;

(b) empower the general public of their awareness and knowledge of human rights and freedoms, including privacy rights;

(c) ensure that the exercise of the police power of the state, in so far as it relates to the prevention of the transmission of HIV,is in accord with the requirements of necessity, reasonableness and non-violation of fundamental rights and freedoms.

(d) enact general principles for the protection of privacy rights that will cover both confidentiality and data protection. A general law on privacy and data protection, and a privacy law specific to the handling of medical information related to HIV/AIDS, should include strict provisions on the collection, storage/security and use of information (including alteration and disclosure) that will guarantee the respect of the privacy rights of the individual concerned.

Over-All Conclusions

The above treatise attempted to make a general survey and analysis of information law, privacy and HIV/AIDS in the Philippines. In conclusion, the urgency of the campaign for the control and prevention of the spread of HIV in the Philippines, as in any other given society, should be constantly assessed with the continuing need to respect the rights and freedoms of the individuals and the society for whose benefit the campaign is being conducted. As human rights advocates, we must discourage the tendency of the law as an imposition from above which consequently results in the marginalisation of the intended beneficiaries of the law and in fact violates human rights. Instead, we must aim at the participation of the society in the discussion on the issue of HIV/AIDS so that we can substantially attempt a meaningful interaction between the policy-makers and the constituency.

Nowhere in the field of law can this necessity be seen as well as information law and privacy. One must maximise and strengthen the use of information law in the national HIV/AIDS campaign in order to guarantee the respect of privacy rights, just as it is necessary to be aware of privacy rights and requirements so that we can have a meaningful participation in creating an enabling environment that will prevent HIV transmission and minimise its impact on ourselves and our societies.

REFERENCES

1. Department of Health Administrative Order No. 574 dated 4 January 1987.
2. See Philippine Bill of Rights. Philippine State International Obligations are also provided for in the International Covenant on Civil and Political Rights.
3. Early 1993, the Philippine Catholic Church issued a Pastoral Letter read in Catholic Churches all over the Philippines and published in the media, assailing the government campaign on the use of condoms as promoting promiscuity among the youth of the country.
4. Article II (5) provides that: "The physician is obliged to respect the confidentially of all information he acquired on the basis of his professional capacity, and not to divulge this information unless there is a signed consent from the patient or when the common good so requires it (as defined by specific instances)."
5. Section 29, paragraph 2, subparagraph 1 provides: "The following classes shall be excluded from entry into the Philippines... (2) persons afflicted with a loathsome or dangerous or contagious disease."
6. House Bill No. 2844 entitled "An Act Requiring All Aliens and Balikbayans to Submit Themselves to an AIDS Test as a Condition Precedent for Entry or for Continued Stay in the Country" introduced by Representatives Bakunawa and Dragon and pending with the Committee on Health; House Bill No. 8077 entitled "An Act to Control the Spread of AIDS and other Sexually–Transmitted Diseases in the Philippines" introduced by Senators Tatad and Herrera and pending with the Committee on Health, Constitutional Amendments and Revision of Codes and Laws.
7. House Bill No. 8077.
8. House Bill No. 8077.
9. House Bill No. 8077 and Senate Bill No. 8077.
10. Such as that proposed in House Bill No. 8077.
11. Senate Bill No. 8077.

54

The Law and HIV/AIDS at the Workplace: A Case Study on the Philippines

Johannes L. Ignacio and Manuel M. Goyena
Attorneys
Alternative Law Centre Manila
Philippines

RATIONALE

There is no doubt that HIV/AIDS is not just a health problem, but a development problem as well. The fact that the disease affects the most productive segment of society (ages 20 to 35), and is incurable and debilitating, makes it a threat to a country's economic growth. Its negative impact is felt more seriously by the poor and the marginalised. In the context therefore of underdeveloped countries where the majority are poor, the disease can shake the very foundations of civil society.

The foregoing underscores the need for a rational, well-studied response to the problem of HIV/AIDS in the workplace. There is, in particular, a need to know how HIV/AIDS affects the working force. To what extent does the law address the emerging problems of HIV/AIDS at the workplace? Are the existing legal mechanisms adequate? What recommendations can be drawn up to make the law more responsive to these issues?

Hopefully, a case study on the Philippines will generate more interest on the subject, and can be the basis of similar policy papers on other countries and, eventually, for the entire Asia-Pacific Region.

The legal and ethical implications of HIV/AIDS as a whole has not been the subject of serious study in the Philippines. There is a need to extrapolate, anticipate, and project, what will be the key issues of HIV/AIDS in the workplace, as it relates to the Philippine legal system. This kind of extrapolation is necessary in order to make a more meaningful assessment of the readiness of the Philippine legal system to deal responsively and responsibly to the inevitable conflict between public health concerns and the protection of the rights and welfare of groups affected by the HIV/AIDS epidemic.

SOCIO-ECONOMIC-CULTURAL CONTEXT OF HIV/AIDS IN THE PHILIPPINES

The Philippines is a country of 60 million people. The economy is agriculture based, export oriented, and free enterprise. Despite the replacement of a corrupt and authoritarian regime in 1986, the economy has remained stagnant, and the majority of the people remain poor. The legislated minimum wage for urban industrial workers is P118.00 ($4.72) per day. Average monthly income for production workers average from P2,000.00/month to P4,000.00/month ($80.00 to $160.00 per month). Current minimum wage rates are not sufficient to sustain a family of six persons.

Social ethics and morality in the Philippines is of the western "conservative" type. This is due to more than four hundred years of Spanish rule, and another fifty years of American tutelage. The culture considers sex, and matters surrounding it, taboo.

The conservatism is strengthened by the pervasive influence of the Catholic Church on the populace (82 per cent of Filipinos are Catholics). The Church considers the following practices to be "sinful", perverse, or as socially reprehensible:

Extra-marital relationships.

Pre-marital sex.

Homosexuality.

Drug abuse.

Contraception, other than by natural means.

It has stated that a condom use and "safe sex" policy condones promiscuity and sexual permissiveness.

To a large extent, sexually liberated behaviour, as well as certain behaviour associated with HIV/AIDS, is prohibited by law. Proposals such as the legalisation of prostitution, abortion, and the encouragement of condom use have met with strong opposition in the legislature.

UPDATE ON HIV/AIDS IN THE PHILIPPINES

As of February 1993, a total of 287 cases of HIV infection have been reported to the Department of Health. Of this number,91 have been reported as AIDS cases. Official estimates by the Department of Health places the total number of HIV infections at anywhere between 30,000 to 35,000.

These statistics are of course in no way indicative of the extent of the problem. Several factors contribute to masking the extent of the epidemic, as well as the potential threats thereof. These include:

1. Lack of education and information on the disease of the public in general, including doctors and other health workers.
2. Negative attitudes towards people with HIV, as well as behaviour associated with HIV/AIDS (e.g., prostitution.)
3. Negative attitudes towards safe sex practices, coupled with a culturally influenced reluctance to discuss sexual behaviour openly.

The official response of the government to the HIV/AIDS problem, at least at the policy level, has been relatively progressive. However, official pronouncements notwithstanding, much has to be done by way of developing and implementing viable action programmes for prevention and alleviation of the negative socio-economic impact of HIV/AIDS.

REVIEW OF EXISTING LAW AND JURISPRUDENCE BEARING ON HIV IN THE WORKPLACE

General Considerations

1. *Individual Rights versus the Police Power of the state: The Perpetuat Tug-of-War*

The Philippines has a long constitution and is history, which includes a Bill of Rights (Art. III of the 1987 Constitution) and is among the most liberal in the world. In addition, there is a full fledged article on social justice, and economic, social and cultural rights (Art. XIII). The Philippines is a signatory to the significant international documents on human rights, as well as to ILO conventions on the protection of workers rights.

At the same time, however, Philippine law and jurisprudence displays a strong tendency towards upholding the police power of the state vis-a-vis human rights. Particularly with respect to public health issues, the balance is tilted in favour of police power.

Under The Revised Administrative Code, the Director of Health is empowered to cause the segregation of persons suffering from leprosy. There exists at present a leper colony in Cullion, in the island of Palawan, which is run by the government.

Such authority was challenged in the case of *Lorenzo vs. Director of Health 50 Phils: 595*, on the ground that it violated the constitutional rights to liberty and equal protection of those stricken by leprosy. The Supreme Court, acting on the denial by a lower court of a petition for a writ of Habeas Corpus, against the Director of Health, upheld the validity of compulsory segregation, as well as the authority of the Director of Health to effect quarantine, detention and segregation of those affected by leprosy'.

2. *Management Prerogatives, the Rights of Workers and the Power of State Regulation*

Under the general principles of law, the government can enact labour and welfare legislation regulating the conduct of businesses in relation to terms and incidents of employment. This is balanced by the inherent right of management to set the terms and conditions of employment, adopt internal rules and policies, and to exercise its prerogative to hire and fire, subject to reasonable limitations provided by law.

For instance, management has the prerogative to terminate the services of a person suffering from disease. However, the legislature can set guidelines for its exercise. Art. 284 of the Labour Code provides that for dismissal to be valid, it must be shown that continued employment of the employee is prohibited by law or is prejudicial to his health and the health of his co-employees. Such employee must be paid separation pay equivalent to at least one month salary to one-half month salary for every year of service, whichever is greater, a fraction of at least six months being considered as one whole year.

In addition, Sec. 8, Rule 1, Book VI of the Rule and Regulations implementing the Labour Code provides that the disease must be of such nature or of such stage that it cannot be cured within a period of six months even with medical treatment, as certified by a competent public authority. In actual cases, the Department of Labour, and ultimately the courts, may pass upon the validity of management action.

Labour Legislation HIV/AIDS Related Issues

I. Discrimination in the Workplace

The Labour Code of the Philippines cites specific instances of discriminatory acts of the employer and/or a labour organisation denominated as "unfair labour practices". These are:

(a) For management to discriminate in regard to wages, hours of work, and other terms and conditions of employment in order to encourage or discourage membership in any labour organisation, or to dismiss, discharge, or otherwise prejudice or discriminate against the employee for having given or being about to give testimony under this Code.

(b) For the labour organisation to cause or attempt to cause an employer to discriminate against an employee (Art. 248-249, Labour Code of the Philippines).

It is immediately apparent that the acts contemplated are those which are union related. These provisions are designed to protect and promote the workers right to self-organisation, and do not provide protection against all types of discrimination. Discrimination related to gender, ethnic affiliation, political belief, or status is not dealt with by the Labour Code.

Another observable characteristic of these acts defined as "discriminatory" is that they speak of a post-employment setting, or discrimination in the exercise of the prerogative to terminate. There has been no substantial erosion of, nor serious opposition to, this aspect of management prerogative, despite the 1987 Constitution and the passage of the "Hererra Law", RA 6750 which strengthens protection to labour and the constitutional rights of workers. This perhaps can be traced to the fact that the present Constitution recognises the freedom of contract as a constitutional right. The state will generally not intervene in the contractual relations between labour and management unless in the exercise of the police power. In this particular instance, there must be a determination by the legislature that the intervention is justified.

The large labour surplus gives management greater leverage to dictate terms and conditions of work, and further enhances its legally recognised prerogatives. At the pre-employment stage, compliance with any management requirement, including undergoing mandatory medical examinations, is left to the decision of the applicant. If he/she does not agree or refuses to comply with any of the requirements of management, then he/she has to face the risk of losing the job opportunity.

Given the above observations, it is seriously doubted that existing labour laws can provide the necessary protection against HIV/AIDS-related acts of discrimination.

The Labour Code's provisions protecting the workers from discriminatory acts of the employer have not developed beyond relating it to the worker's right to self-organisation. Thus, for such other discriminatory acts which do not fall within the concept of "unfair labour practices" as define by the code, workers have to seek protection under Article III of the 1981 constitution, protecting individual liberties. In terms of labour legislation recourse will have to be made on the general provisions of the Code enunciating the basic policies of the state to: (a) ... ensure equal work opportunities regardless of sex, race or creed and (b) to just and humane conditions of work.

2. Mandatory Medical/Physical Examinations

There is no statutory basis for the conduct of mandatory medical examinations either as a pre-employment requirement, or as a condition for continued employment.

The Philippine Labour Code deals largely with standards specifying the type of medical personnel required to be present in the workplace depending upon the size of the employers' workforce. Benefits and services for workers are couched in very general terms. The only reference to mandatory examinations found in the law is regarding compulsory medical examinations, in the Employees Compensation Act (Presidential Decree No. 626, as amended).

This medical examination is designed to monitor the health status of employees, particularly in workplaces which constitute a high-risk environment of injury and/or illness. Employers may use these examinations to check on their workers' capacity to perform their jobs. It should be noted, however, that these provisions cannot be used to justify compulsory testing for HIV/AIDS.

The law can be used to determine if exposure to HIV is work related, thus entitling someone with HIV to the benefits of the law. It does not authorise the employer to include HIV testing as part of a routine medical examination. The law is meant to benefit workers, not prejudice them.

In the Philippines, there is a long standing recognition of the employer's "right" to conduct mandatory medical examinations either as a pre- or post employment requirement. Challenges to this "right" have been limited to the use of medical examinations and results thereof by management as devices to screen-out and/or terminate an employee due to his union activities or exercise to the workers' constitutional right to self-organisation. (See discussion on discriminatory acts).

In the case of a job applicant, management, as general rule, may deny his application by reason of failure to submit himself to medical examination. In the course of employment, while non-submission of medical requirements is not *per se* a ground for termination, a deliberate failure or refusal to submit medical requirements, and undergo medical examination as part of an internal management policy, may be construed as insubordination, which is a cause for termination. Here, there will be some debate as to whether HIV testing can lawfully be done, as part of general management prerogative. The employer seeking to impose mandatory HIV testing will probably invoke its inherent right to determine internal policy, to choose its own employees, and to protect its' corporate image from the "stigma" and the perceived "dangers" of having HIV positives in its workforce.

Other special sectors of the Philippine workforce (i.e., overseas contract workers) are compelled to undergo mandatory clinical examinations for Sexually Transmitted Diseases (STD) and/or HIV. The results of this examination have a direct bearing on their job applications and/or their present employment status.

In the case of workers in the entertainment sector, municipal ordinances exist which require them to undergo regular monthly venereal and sexually transmitted disease tests. Particularly affected are workers labelled as hospitality men and women, receptionists, beer house entertainers, sauna bath masseurs, or similarly situated workers who are exposed to the sex trade. If found negative of VD or STD, they are issued a "pink" card, or a municipal permit/license allowing them to pursue their trade. If found positive, their permit/license will not be processed and/or revoked, and will be prohibited from working.

It is anticipated that the demand for mandatory HIV antibody testing will grow, in direct proportion to reported increases in the incidence of such cases. This incipient clamour can be attributed to a conservative public health tradition that has relied upon the government's exercise of police power to address perceived public health threats.

This pre-occupation with mandatory HIV antibody testing as a method of screening-out individuals is not only inefficient and ineffective, but also violates basic individual rights, particularly to privacy and freedom from degradation of his dignity as a person. In the workplace setting, such an approach shall only encourage discriminatory action against individuals and facilitate their stigmatisation in society.

Extensive research has repeatedly shown that, in general, the workplace setting does not contribute to the increase in the risk of contracting or transmitting HIV. There are only three prevalent ways of contracting the virus: (1) sexual intercourse, (2) blood transfusion and use of needles containing infected blood, and (3) perinatal transmission.

Casual contact, as that generally experienced in the course of performing ordinary responsibilities arising from work, does not result in transmission of the virus. While indeed there are certain workplace settings wherein the employee may be exposed to infected blood, syringes and other medical paraphernalia which may increase the risk of transmission, these are exceptional instances that must be addressed particularly.

A negative result in an HIV test does not guarantee that a person is not infected because the test may have been performed during the "window period" when the infection cannot be detected in blood testing. Moreover instead of discouraging or preventing high-risk sexual behaviour, negative test results may lead to the reverse. In addition, the conduct of periodic mandatory testing will not achieve the management's desire to cut expenses on medical benefits of infected employees.

3. Confidentiality of Medical Information

Article II (5) of the Code of Ethics of the Medical Profession of the Philippines States:

> The physician is obliged to respect the confidentiality of all information he acquires on the basis of his professional capacity, and not to divulge this information unless there is a signed consent from the patient or when the common good so requires it.

Further legal bases for the principle are given in the Law on Civil Damages, the Revised Penal Code and the Rules of Court governing pleading and practice.

The responsibility to preserve the absolute secrecy on all information about the patient extends even after the patient has died. In support of this position, one can cite certain provisions of the International Code of Medical Ethics adopted by the World Medical Association in 1949 and the 1948 Declaration of Geneva.

The Philippine Law on Evidence classifies as privileged information any communication or information arising from a doctor-client relation. The purpose of the rule is to inspire confidence in the patient and encourage him to make full disclosure to the physician of his symptoms and condition. By preventing the physicians from making known to the public the ailment of their patients, particularly when affected by diseases which might bring reproach, criticism, unfriendly comment or disgrace upon the patient, disclosure is encouraged.

There are exceptions to this rule, such as:

(a) The privilege does not apply in criminal cases for the maintenance of public order;
(b) The ban in secrecy is extended only to information given to those authorised to practice medicine, surgery or obstetrics. In general, the privilege does not include the testimony of a nurse or other attendants assisting the physician;
(c) The rule is inapplicable when the patient brings an action for damages against the physician; and
(d) Being a personal privilege, this could be waived by the patient.

Ironically, the other instances when the confidentiality rule is deemed inapplicable are in the Labour Code itself. Article 187 seeks to validate the claim of a worker for compensation arising from a work-related illness or injury, in which case all medical information can be made available.

At present, the custody and control of medical records and information is freely granted to the employer. Most often, the test results of medical examinations of employees form part of the file record (201 File) of the employee to which the personnel manager or his staff has access, especially true when the person conducting the medical examination is a company retained doctor. The extent to which these medical records may be considered as property of the company, or the limits on the proper and valid use and dissemination thereof, has not been laid down by law.

In the Philippines, the right to privacy has not developed beyond providing the individual with protection from interventions or incursions of public authority in arrest, search and seizure situations, and presently does not directly cover unwarranted intrusions by employers in the exercise of management prerogatives.

The absence of standards for care and custody of medical records make very real the threat of unauthorised disclosure of such information, whether through deliberate action or negligence, which will expose the individual to serious social consequences, particularly when there exists a host of misconceptions about the cause and mode of transmission of the disease as in the case of HIV/AIDS.

4. *Disease as a Ground for forced Leaves and/or termination from Employment*

Under Article 284 of the Labour Code, the following standards are thus laid down by law for the lawful termination of an employee afflicted with a disease:

1. Continued employment is prohibited by law;
2. Continued employment is prejudicial to the health of the employee or the health of his co-workers; or
3. Certification by competent public health authority that the disease cannot be cured within a period of six months even with proper medical attention.

It must be emphasised, however, that a causal relation between continued employment and the resulting prejudice to the health of such employee or that of his co-workers has to be established. Even in the case of employees suffering from HIV/AIDS, management's prerogative is clearly circumscribed by the above standards.

Seropositivity does not necessarily affect the capacity of the employee to continuete performing his work. In fact, seropositive individual are known to carry-on with their usual life activities for a period in excess of six to ten years before succumbing to some debilitation as a result of HIV -related the illness or AIDS. HIV-related illness should be treated as any other illness and the infected individual allowed to continue in his employment as long as he is medically fit for appropriate work.

5. *Works' sickness Benefits*

There are three social welfare laws that govern the social security benefits of the Filipino working class. These are the Social Security Law (Republic Act. No. 1161, as amended), the Revised Government Service Insurance Act of 1977 or GSIS Law (Presidential Decree No. 1146 amending Commonwealth Act No. 186) and the Employees Compensation Act (PD 626, as amended).

The main policy considerations of the first two law i members a comprehensive social security and insurance benefit package for sickness, disability,, death, retirement and similar situations.

Membership to the System is compulsory in character for employees less than sixty years of age.

In case of actual occurrence of any of the listed contingencies, the employee's entitlement to medical benefits, such as confinement and hospitalisation, surgery and doctors' fees, is not qualified by the nature of the illness or disease afflicting him/her. The entitlements to the above social security packages are not directly affected by the issue of HIV/AIDS, as there are no other pre-requisites other than the contributions of the employee.

Benefits provided under the Employees Compensation Act (PD *626)*, can be availed of only if the injury or illness is work related. The law is applicable to employees belonging either to the private or government sector. It should be noted that HIV/AIDS is not listed as a work-related or occupational disease that is compensable under the Employees Compensation Act. PD 626 nevertheless provides for situations when an employee can claim for compensation, benefits and services even if the disease is unlisted, so long as the employee can prove that such working conditions to which he has been exposed contribute to the increase in the risk of acquiring a specific illness or injury. (In the case of HIV, this may be true of health workers).

The law will also continue to benefit workers suffering from certain opportunistic illnesses, such as pneumonia or tuberculosis, which commonly affect HIV/AIDS patients, and which may be aggravated by certain working conditions.

6. Labour Relations

One of the main pillars of the Philippine economic development plan is the promotion of "export-oriented, labour-intensive" industries. The core of this approach is to attract foreign corporations and interests to invest and/ or set up industries in the country particularly in economic enclaves by offering tax holidays/incentives; available local capital; and cheap labour.

To reduce the tensions in this kind of situation, the Labour Code has institutionalised the concept of "tripartism" or partnership among the major actors in the workplace setting: labour, management and government. The purpose of adopting this kind of approach in labour relations is to promote the spirit of partnership and to provide a mechanism for balancing the oftentimes contentious relations between labour and management.

A similar approach can be considered in dealing with HIV/AIDS in the workplace. Efforts can initially be focused at educating the leaders of labour and management on the nature, causes, methods of transmission, and other data pertinent to the HIV/AIDS problem.

On a national scale, the greater responsibility will fall upon the shoulders of the government in making use of existing institutions, in particular adjuncts of the Department of Labour to propagate this national consensus.

The Government may also solicit the support of the employer, through existing employers' associations or labour federations for activities such as lectures/seminars at the company or industry level, on a co-operative basis.

CONCLUSIONS AND RECOMMENDATIONS

The current situation of Philippine Law and HIV/AIDS in the workplace can be described as one of apprehension and hope.

On one hand there exists a strong legal framework for the protection of individual rights against discrimination, and intrusions on privacy. This posture of respecting the right to privacy and against discrimination has been adopted by the government, particularly the Department of Health, as an integral part of the national HIV/AIDS prevention policy.

On the other hand, there exists a strong tendency in the law to uphold police power vis-a-vis human rights in dealing with public health issues. In particular, there is a need to review, if not overhaul, existing legal mechanisms that deal with epidemics and infectious diseases. The law on the subject is half a century old, and has not been updated since then. In relation to HIV/AIDS, existing laws are not only outmoded; they represent obstacles to a rational and compassionate approach to HIV/AIDS-related issues.

There is cause for concern for the sweeping prerogatives open to management in dealing with HIV/AIDS-related issues. There is clearly a need in this regard to spell out specific policies, standards and/or guidelines for the exercise of management prerogatives with a view to protecting the rights of affected sectors, as well as leading employers towards a more appropriate and enlightened means for dealing with the epidemic in the workplace.

The legal framework in dealing with HIV/AIDS in the workplace should have two basic features:

A. Adherence to the following fundamental principles:

1. People living with HIV should in all respects be treated as a "normal" worker. Workers with HIV-related illnesses, including AIDS, should be treated just like

any worker suffering from a disease.

2. The protection of human rights and dignity of HIV-infected persons, including persons with AIDS, should be integral to prevention and control programmes at all levels. HIV-infected persons should not be subjected to any from of discrimination. Their basic rights to liberty, privacy, equal protection and due process must always be respected.

B. A set of recommendations for the modification of existing laws in order to ensure a more responsible and compassionate approach to HIV/AIDS related issues in the workplace.

1. Discrimination:

   Expand the definition of discriminatory acts to include those acts, direct and indirect, which have a tendency to cause discrimination against a worker, including his/her termination from employment, because of a condition or disease which does not affect his/her capacity to continue performing work, nor poses a threat to co-workers in the ordinary performance of work assignments. The protection should also include the preservation of rights and benefits to education, travel, continuing health care and medical services.

   Access to the benefits provided by existing social security and insurance legislation in the area of medical services and health care, including rehabilitory services, should be ensured and should not be denied because a person has HIV or AIDS.

2. Mandatory Testing

   Compulsory testing for HIV, either as a requirement for employment or for the continued enjoyment of tenure, should be prohibited by law.

   All medical (clinical or diagnostic) testing should be voluntary in nature, and must be carried-out only after acquiring the informed consent of the individual.

   Any voluntary testing must be preceded by pre-test counselling and post-test counselling.

3. Confidentiality of Medical information

   Incorporate into the Labour Code the confidential character of, medical information, especially in situations where the doctor is a company-retained doctor, including medical corporations engaged by management to conduct the medical/physical examinations of its employees.

Provide for standards and procedures for maintenance of medical records to prevent unnecessary disclosures of medical information, including the expansion of the persons covered by the privileged communication rule. Emphasis of such a law on confidentiality should focus on inculcating in the patient his responsibility, compatible and concurrent with that of his right to privacy, to inform his familv, spouse or sex-partner of his HIV-positive status.

4. Occupational Health and Safety Standards

Medical institutions of whatever size, including clinics, should be obliged to provide personnel with protective gear, disposable and properly sterilised equipment, including information material and/or lectures and seminars on the care and handling of patients, particularly those infected with HIV.

First-aiders, nurses, and other medical personnel designated, hired or retained by management to act as such in the workplace must be provided with the proper information on open wounds and body injuries, including making provisions for protective medical equipment, in the handling of accidents or injuries suffered by the employees in the workplace.

In addition to the above recommendations for law reform, complementary non-legal approaches may also be considered:

C. Initiate the conduct of national level consultations or conferences, preferably initiated by the Department of Health, with the leaders of national employer's organisations or associations and national labour federations to discuss the issue of HIV/AIDS in the workplace. Invite noted experts from international agencies or organisations and local medical experts as speakers. The purpose is to encourage and promote a tripartite dialogue, consistent with a multi-sectoral, preventive approach to the problem of HIV/AIDS at the workplace.

The creation of tripartite bodies can result from these dialogues that can pursue multi-sectoral initiatives, such as a national information campaign to be implemented at various levels.

Management and labour should be encouraged to initiate deliberations on a company or industry level on HIV/AIDS-related issues at the workplace.

D. Government may consider involving the broadcast industry to develop an educational campaign on HIV/AIDS and laying the foundations for support, compassion and assistance to HIV/AIDS patients. Tax credits or other incentives may be considered.

55

The National AIDS Control Programme in Singapore

Prof. Chao Tzee Cheng
Director
Institute of Science and Foamic Medicine, Singapore

HIV/AIDS Situation in Singapore

As of 31 December 1994, 308 Singaporeans have been reported to be HIV infected. Among them, 44 are AIDS cases, 180 are asymptomatic carriers, and 84 have died. The number of reported cases of HIV infection has increased since the first HIV infected Singaporean was detected -from 2 cases in 1985 to 17 cases in 1990, and 86 cases in 1994.

Modes of Transmission of HIV Infection Among Singaporeans

Of the 308 HIV infected Singaporeans, 295 (95.8 per cent) contracted the infection through sexual transmission, 7 (2.3 per cent) by intravenous drug use, 4 (1.3 per cent) through renal transplant overseas, 1 (0.3 per cent) through blood transfusion overseas, and 1 (0.3 per cent) through the perinatal route. Since 1991, heterosexual contact has become the most common mode of HIV transmission among Singaporeans. In 1994, it accounted for more than 72 per cent cases of HIV transmission. Most people have contracted the infection through casual sex with commercial sex workers in Singapore and overseas.

Characteristics of HIV Infected Singaporeans

Among the 308 Singaporeans who have been detected to be HIV positive, 281 (91.2 per cent) are males and 27 (8.8 per cent) are females. At the time of diagnosis, 78 per cent were between the ages of 20 and 39 years. They are mostly single (71 per cent). Only 21 per cent were married, while the rest were either widowed or divorced.

National AIDS Control Programme in Singapore

The control and prevention of AIDS comes under the purview of the Ministry of Health with the active involvement of other government agencies and community groups fighting against AIDS in Singapore. The National AIDS Control Programme was formulated in 1985.

The programme addresses issues dealing with:

- Public education
- Legislation
- Protection of the national blood supply through routine screening of blood and blood products
- Managing the infected
- Counselling those with high risk of infection
- Monitoring the disease
- Training personnel
- Conducting research and studies

Two Committees were formed to assist the programme: the National Advisory Committee on AIDS, which provides community feedback on the AIDS education prograrnme, and the AIDS Task Force, which advises the Ministry of Health on medical and scientific matters relating to AIDS.

Legislation

While efforts are constantly being made to educate the public on HIV infection/AIDS, certain legal measures have also been taken to combat the disease in the interest of both the infected as well as the general public. HIV infection and AIDS were made notifiable diseases under the Infectious Diseases Act in 1985. To further tighten the control of AIDS in Singapore, the Infectious Diseases Act was amended in 1992 to include the following provisions:

1. The Director of Medical Services is empowered to require any person who has been diagnosed as having AIDS or being infected with HIV to undergo counselling or to comply with specified safety measures.

2. It is an offence for any person who knows that he is infected with the HIV or has AIDS to commit any act which is likely to transmit the disease to another person, e.g., sexual intercourse with another person or donating blood at any blood bank in Singapore.

In addition, the Infectious Diseases (Amendment) Act also protects the identity of a HIV infected person, so as to prevent discrimination against such person as well as encourage those who are at risk of infection to come forward for counselling and HIV testing.

Protection of the National Blood Supply

Stringent measures are being undertaken to safeguard the national blood supply from HIV infection and other bloodborne diseases. These measures include:

- Testing of blood and blood products for HIV, syphilis and Hepatitis B and C.
- Stringent donor selection at the pre-donation stage is carried out using a specially designed questionnaire. All potential donors are interviewed and have to complete a detailed questionnaire on past and present risk activities associated with HIV infection. Persons at risk of such diseases are to exclude themselves from donating blood. The potential donor is then counselled by a doctor, after which he signs a declaration saying that he has not made a false statement. Offenders with false declarations may face prosecution. This is to deter anyone indulging in high-risk behaviour from donating blood that may be infected.

Singapore also has facilities for autologous blood donation to allow persons to store their own blood for elective operation. This measure has eliminated the risk of a patient contracting bloodborne diseases, such as AIDS, from other people's blood.

Managing the Infected

Individuals who perceive themselves to be at risk of infection are encouraged to undergo HIV screening. Cases are managed at the Communicable Disease Centre by doctors and other staff who are specially trained to manage such cases. Patients are counselled to ensure compliance with treatment, care and follow-up measures. All patients with AIDS/HIV infection are counselled regularly. Infected persons and their sex partners are counselled and screening is carried out for those who have been exposed to the infection. Person to-person counselling is provided for those with high-risk behaviour.

An AIDS Telephone Helpline was started in 1987 to provide anonymous personal counselling to the public. Recorded information on AIDS in the four main languages is also provided.

Monitoring the Situation

Surveillance of the AIDS situation in Singapore is based on the collated results of:

1. Voluntary confidential blood testing.
2. Screening of prostitutes.
3. Unlinked sentinel surveillance of selected groups in the population at a higher risk of the infection, such as patients with sexually transmitted diseases, Hepatitis B and tuberculosis, and pregnant women.

Training Personnel

The Ministry of Health works closely with other relevant ministries, community groups and international bodies in the training of personnel for the effective control of AIDS. All medical and paramedical personnel have been issued with 'Guidelines for Preventing Transmission of Bloodborne Infection in a Health Care Setting'. They are constantly reminded of the importance of proper infection control procedures based on universal precautions.

Workshops have been held for prison and drug rehabilitation officers to educate them on AIDS, how to handle infected inmates, and how to counsel those engaging in high-risk activities. Teachers have been trained to conduct educational programmes on AIDS/ HIV infection for students in their schools and institutions.

Community Involvement

A voluntary organization, Action for AIDS, Singapore, was formed in 1988. Its activities complement the government's efforts in controlling AIDS. Its objectives are to promote educational activities relating to AIDS and HIV infection; support welfare activities to prevent discrimination against patients and families; and promote research in areas related to HIV infection and AIDS.

56

Solomon Islands National AIDS (HIV Infection) Prevention and Control Programme

Prime Afeau
Solicitor General
Attorney General's Chambers Solomon Islands

INTRODUCTION

The Solomon Islands has a population of approximately 360,000, with 47 per cent being below the age of 15 years.

Homosexual behaviour does not have cultural and religious sanction in most communities, but no objective study had been undertaken to determine its extent. Tattooing is a traditional practice in some communities, often using traditional instruments of questionable sterility. No incidence of intravenous drug abuse has been reported and this practice is deemed very rare.

STDs are on the increase, especially in the urban areas—no special programmes deal with STDs; they are covered by the general health services.

In the past decade, the number of visitors to Solomon Islands, has increased—particularly those from Asia, Australia and New Zealand, either as tourists or as business persons, labourers or fish earner. Also, the number of Solomon Islanders going abroad has increased.

Epidemiological Situation of HIV Infection/AIDS

The epidemiological situation regarding HIV infection/AIDS has not been fully established due to the absence of regular and continuous surveillance and representative serosurveys.

The current limited surveillance activities have yielded no AIDS cases (as of 30 April 1995). However, one HIV positive case has been detected from tests carried out on 10,575 individuals.

Problems Encountered in HIV Epidemiological Surveillance

1. Justification to carry out surveillance on grounds of AIDS is inadequate as it has been given a low priority.
2. Inadequate HIV testing facilities and trained manpower, especially in the provinces.
3. Lack of support services such as counselling, expertise in management of HIV infection, and outreach services.
4. Difficulty in identifying persons engaging in risk behaviour and obtaining their cooperation.

The AIDS/HIV Infection Prevention and Control Programme

The National AIDS Policy was adopted in April 1988 with the formation of the National AIDS Committee (NAC) and a Short-Term Plan (STP). The National AIDS Committee is an intersectoral committee consisting of sixteen members and a core action group comprising health personnel and non-government organizations (NGOs).

The Short-Term Plan (STP)

The Short-Term Plan was implemented with effect from March 1988. The main objectives of the STP were:

1. to establish a National AIDS Prevention and Control Programme and a NAC;
2. to inform, educate and create awareness about AIDS and HIV infection with regard to modes of transmission and means of preventing infection;
3. to educate health personnel with regard to HIV infection, especially its epidemiology, clinical diagnosis, management and counselling; and
4. to prevent transmission of HIV infection.

To achieve these objectives, some 29 activities and strategies were planned to be undertaken from March 1988 to March 1989. The STP activities were funded by WHO and the EEC.

Assessment of the STP

The assessment of the STP in 1989 showed that 40 per cent of the planned activities has been accomplished, 28 per cent were partially completed, and 32 per cent were yet to be implemented. The STP budget utilization was 65 per cent. As of December 1989, only 12 per cent of the planned activeness had not been completed, while the budget allocated for the STP had been fully utilized.

Constraints In the Implementation of the STP

The main constraints encountered in the implementation of the *STP* were as follows:

1. Relative lack of support to the programme such as inadequate manpower, and HIV testing equipment.
2. Difficulties in identifying individuals with risk behaviour.
3. No favourable opportunities to undertake KAPB studies and sero prevalence studies.

Medium-Term Plan 1990- 94

A Medium-Term Plan (MTP) was formulated in July 1989 for the period 1990-94. Its objectives were:

1. to prevent the kansmission of HIV infection;
2. to reduce the morbidity and mortality due to HIV infection; and
3. to reduce the social and economic impact of HIV/AIDS on individuals, families and society.

Risk Factors

Solomon Islands recorded its first HIV positive case in January 1995. This confirms that the HIV epidemic has reached these islands. The possible important risk factors that may fuel the epidemic further include:

- The increasing incidence of STDs, especially in urban centres.
- Increase in the number of visitors to the country from other parts of the world where HIV / AIDS is a problem.
- Increase in the number of Solomon Islanders that travel overseas.
- The absence of the testing of all blood for HIV before transfusion, especially in rural health centres which lack such facilities.

- The poor socio-economic situation of the country.
- The increase in teenage pregnancies and alcoholism, with the erosion of socio-cultural values.

Despite these risk factors, there are certain positive features that will help control the spread of AIDS/HIV in Solomon Islands:

- The absence of intravenous drug abuse.
- The very low incidence, if any, of homosexuality.
- The presence of cultural, traditional values and norms.
- The strong extended family system and support structure.

AIDS Policies

The National AIDS Policy was formulated and adopted in 1988 with inputs from international experts and the World Health Organization; government officials; legal, church, youth and women representatives; the NGOs and community leaders.

The National AIDS Policy, apart from setting out a programme approach and management structure, clearly adopts the following principles:

1. The principle of adopting the normal public health approach to disease control utilizing known facts and experiences. In this regard, there is no mandatory screening for HIV of visitors, foreigners seeking employment, etc. Blood products are screened prior to transfusion.
2. The principle of non discrimination vis-a-vis persons with HIV/AIDS.
3. The principle of respect for human and individual rights; above all upholding medical/professional ethics and codes of practice.
4. The principle of upholding confidentiality with respect of patent information and health condition.
5. The principle of compassion, tolerance, respect and care for those in need and the sick (based on socio cultural and religious values).

The policy addresses most of the controversial issues issue surrounding HIV/AIDS. While it may appear that the policy favours persons with HIV/AID this is not so, as there are provisions to protect the public as well (for e.g., infected expatriates who knowingly infect others can be repatriated).

Existing Legal Framework

The individual rights and freedom of the citizens of Solomon

Islands are guaranteed by the Constitution. The Public Health Act, 1970 specifically authorizes doctors and health workers to do what is appropriate, in terms of patients' needs and requirements and also in the public interest.

The Medical Code of Practice also respects patients' rights and upholds the principle of confidentiality.

The Health Services Amendment Act. 1988, empowers the Minister of Health to formulate policies regarding patient care, management and treatment. It is under this Act that regulations on various aspects of health care, including prevention of spread of infections, promotion of safe practices, and confidentiality of patient information, can be formulated.

Legal Reforms and Problems

The need to reform the legal system and policies to deal with the problem of HIV/AIDS has not been felt so far because there has been only a single HIV positive case in the Solomon islands. In other words, the current polig on AIDS ant the legal system have not been challenged as yet.

However, when the news of the first HIV positive result was mate public, there were mixed public relations. Despite demands for the name of the person to be disclosed confidentiality was maintained. To allay any fears and entreaty the Health Ministry strengthened its awareness campaigns and urged the public to be constructive and not to get emotional. The Government is continuing with this intensified public awareness carnpaign.

57

The Legal Framework for HIV/AIDS in Sri Lanka

Indunil Abeysekera
Professor of Law University of Colombo, Sri Lanka

AIDS—a castastrophe of major proportions, with an estimate of 10 million infections in the world—has posed a serious threat to humanity. With the magnitude sharply rising, the disease requires the development of legislation within the legitimate rights of the patient. To meet this challenge, there are many legal and ethical issues to be resolved.

As there are no specific laws in Sri Lanka relating to AIDS, we have to take into consideration the rubric of the prevailing laws, of which the relevant are:

1. *Contagious Diseases Ordinance No. 8 of 1866*—which states that every case of smallpox, cholera or other disease which may from time to time be named by the Minister should be notified to a police officer or *grama seva niladhari.* Although no regulation has been made under this ordinance to cover AIDS specifically, the executive has still to make use of the broad statement ("other disease") in the section of the law to the benefit of solving AIDS-related issues.
2. *Venereal Diseases Ordinance No. 27 of 1938*—permits only registered medical practitioners and specially authorised ayurvedic practitioners to treat persons for venereal diseases. Under this Ordinance, "venereal disease" means

syphilis, gonorrhoea of soft chancre and includes any complication of any such disease. By virtue of interpretation, HIV infection would not be one of them.

3. *Quarantine and Prevention of Diseases Ordinance No. 3 of 1897*—is the most pertinent in this context. The Quarantine and Prevention of Diseases Ordinance in Sri Lanka governs the rights and obligations of the health authority in respect of identification and control of contazious diseases. Through this Ordinance, the Minister of Health has been empowered to issue regulations specifying a disease as contagious. The Ordinance establisnes the prevention and spread of disease in and outside Sri Lanka.

The Ordinance requires a medical practitioner who is reporting a case of HIV infection to identify the individual who is the subject of the report, by name, race, sex, age and place of residence and the nature of the disease. It shall be made in writing to the relevant authority before the expiration of 12 hours from the time the patient was first treated. Provision is also made in the regulations for the medical practitioner to take action based on a doubtful diagnosis rather than a positive diagnosis, giving him time to confirm his doubts to the authorities. Here the legislation is definitely helping the medical practitioner to go about his duty towards the public with confidence.

It also empowers the authority to remove the infected person or person suspected of being infected to some public hospital or other place for such period as the proper authority shall direct.

In view of the sensitivity attached to HIV-related personnel, information and the potential for discrimination should unauthorised disclosure occur, it is vital that the confidentiality of such information be assured. There is no section in the Quarantine and Prevention of Diseases Ordinance to safeguard the confidentiality of personally identifying information pertaining to cases of certain specified diseases.

VOLUNTARY HLV-RELATED TESTING

Consent to Treatment

The law of consent to medical treatment is in the process of continuous evolvement. The application of this area of the law raises many unresolved questions of particular concern and the question whether a physician must obtain a patient's specific informed consent before an HIV-related test can be legally administered or whether a physician could rely upon a patient's implied or tacit consent to perform an HIV-related test, so long as the patient provides the general consent necessary to obtain a blood sample for diagnostic purposes, is still questionable.

Discussions with some physicians in Sri Lanka revealed that HIV antibody tests are being done without obtaining specific informed consent, relying instead on the implied consent or treatment and blood tests that hospital patients typically provide.

Testing of Individuals at High Risk

It is sometimes suggested that many of the problems associated with universal mandatory HIV testing could be avoided if mandatory testing were confined solely to individuals at high behavioural risk with a comparatively high incidence of infection, such as men who are gay, bisexual, injecting drug users, haemophiliacs and their sexual partners.

Some of the laws which have a bearing on high risk behaviours are those which were enacted in the last century such as the Vagrants Ordinance No. 4 of 1841 where indècent behaviour of persons in public is deemed guilty of an offence liable for prosecution, and the Brothel's Ordinance No. 5 of 1880 deeming brothels as illegal and any person who manages or assists in the management of one shall be guilty of an offence.

The Penal Code No. 2 of 1883 is of vital importance wherein whoever maliciously, unlawfully or negligently does any act which has reason to believe to be likely to spread the infection of any disease dangerous to life shall be punished. These are cognisable offenses, in which a police officer could arrest without a warrant and conduct an investigation according to the Criminal Procedure Code No. 15 of 1979.

The Children and Young Persons Ordinance No. 48 of 1939 resolves to safeguard young persons from being exploited for immoral or indecent purposes. Furthermore, necessary legislation is to be implemented to tighten and strictly forbid prostitution, homosexuality, paedophilia, child abuse and sexual exploitation of children. Since there is great potential for the spread of HIV through the above-mentioned offences, invoking the Act and implementing the laws therein would certainly facilitate the reduction in the spread of infection.

Testing of Immigrants and Emigrants

Under the Immigrants and Emigrants Act No. 20 of 1948, *prima facie* the authorities could deny entry of persons to the country for medical reasons. This could involve a person with HIV being refused entry into the country. However, in an attempt to invoke this section of the Act, one could find the law inadequate to cover this aspect.

Applicants for Health or Life Insurance

There are two types of private insurance: employee group insurance and individual insurance. In most group cases, all members of an employee group are eligible for group coverage without any medical inquiry. HIV related tests could be performed on applicants for individual policies, but it is not a requirement.

However, even if an HIV test were not done and if the application is aware that he is HIV-positive, it is his duty to disclose every, fact within his knowledge that is material to the insurance, failing which will render the contract voidable by the insurer.

Testing in the Workplace

Since HIV transmission is sexual or blood borne and not casual, there is no effective risk of transmission in the majority of workplaces. As knowledge regarding limited transmissibility of HIV infection has increased, anxiety as to risk of transmission in the workplace has correspondingly decreased. However, Middle-East recruits from Sri Lanka have to undergo a compulsory HIV anti-body test.

Donors of Blood Products or Bodily Tissues

The mandatory HIV anti-body testing of donors of blood, organs, tissue, ova, semen or other human body parts and Quids, has been universally endorsed by public health officials as an essential and effective means of preventing the spread of HIV infection. With the development of the HIV anti-body test, the normal practice in Sri Lanka is to screen all blood donors.

The current regulation and practice in the area of human tissue donation is less clear. The transplantation of Human Tissues Act No. 48 of 1987 deals with the donation of human tissue for transplantation purpose. Tissue includes "any human flesh, organ, bone, or body fluid or part thereof." In the wake of the AIDS epidemic, several countries have amended their legislation relating to transplants and transfusions to make HIV screening mandatory prior to any transplant or transfusion. It may be desirable to amend the transplantation of Human Tissues Act by introducing a similar requirement.

Fundamental Rights Issues in Relation to AIDS

The Constitution of 1987 of Sri Lanka has devoted an entire chapter which deals with "Fundamental Rights." It enumerates many rights, the violation of which is justifiable in a court of law. For instance, according to Article 14 (g), (h) and (i) of the Constitution, every citizen is entitled to the freedom to engage by himself or in association with others in any lawful occupation, profession, trade, business or enterprise, the freedom of movement and of choosing his residence within Sri Lanka and the freedom to return to one's own country, which means even an HIV-positive citizen has all the above rights.

But, according to Article 15(7), these rights shall be subject to such restrictions as may be prescribed by law in the interest of national security, public order and the protection of public health or morality, or for the purpose of securing due recognition and respect for the rights and freedom of others or of meeting the just requirements of the general welfare of a democratic society.

Therefore, even though an HIV-positive citizen has all the above rights of any other, they could be restricted mainly for the protection of public health, and thus other rules, regulations and laws that facilitate identification of AIDS patients and thereby control the spread of the disease should not in any way be seen as a violation of anyone's fundamental rights.

However, this restrictive clause under Article 15 does not cover Article 11, namely that "no person shall be subjected to torture or to cruel, inhuman or degrading treatment or punishment." Therefore, by virtue of interpretation, Article 11 confers upon any individual (even an AIDS patient) a fundamental right that is non-derogable.

58

HIV-Related Laws of Sri Lanka

Ms. C. Narasinghe
Faculty of Law
University of Colombo
Sri Lanka

A. Public Health Laws/Provisions of other Laws Relating to the Prevention and Control of Infectious Diseases

Quarantine and Prevention of Diseases Ordinance No. 3 of 1897

The Act empowers the Minister of Health to make regulations to provide amongst other things:

- For isolating all cases of disease and diseased persons.
- For prescribing the mode of burial or cremation of any person dying of disease.
- For regulating the removal of diseased persons to hospitals or other places for medical treatment, and for their detention until they can be discharged with safety to the public.
- For prescribing the reporting to such officer or officers as may be named in the regulations, by medical practitioners and persons professing to treat diseases, of cases of disease treated by them.

Regulations require every medical practitioner who attends on any person suffering from AIDS to notify to the proper authority the' name, race, sex, age, and place of residence. This notification has to be made within 12 hours.

Contagious Diseases Ordinance No. 8 of 1866

An Ordinance to provide against introduction and spread of contagious or infectious diseases.

- Householders and medical personnel are required to report cases of smallpox and cholera to the officials mentioned in the Ordinance.

Venereal Diseases Ordinance No. 27 of 1938

- An Ordinance to prevent the treatment of venereal diseases other than by registered medical practitioners or specially authorized practitioners of ayurvedic medicine.
- The Ordinance places restrictions on advertisements to treat any person for venereal diseases.
- Venereal diseases mean syphilis, gonorrhoea or soft chancre and includes any complication of such diseases.

Immigrants and Emigrants Act No. 20 of 1948

- No endorsement or visa shall be granted or issued to any person who is certified by a prescribed medical practitioner to be a person whom for medical reasons it is undesirable to admit into Sri Lanka.
- The Minister may make a deportation order requiring a foreigner to leave Sri Lanka, where that person is shown, by evidence that, for medical reasons, it is undesirable to allow him to remain in Sri Lanka.

B. Law Relating to Transplantation and Grafting

Transplantation of Human Tissues Act No. 48 of 1987

- This Act provides for the donation of human bodies and tissues upon death for therapeutic, scientific, educational, and research purposes; for the removal of such tissues and their use on living persons; and, for the preservation of such tissues.
- Tissue' means any human flesh, organ, bone or body fluid or part thereof.

Corneal Grafting Act No. 38 of 1955

This makes provisions with respect to the use of eyes of diseased persons for therapeutic purposes.

Law Regulating Public and Private Health Institutions
Health Services Law No. 3 of 1977
Nursing Homes (Regulation) Act No. 29 of 1953
Private Medical Institutions (Regulations) Bill (1994)

- A Bill to provide for the regulation, management, supervision and inspection of private medical institutions.
- Private Medical Institution means 'an institution or establishment used or intended to be used for the reception of and the providing of medical and nursing care and treatment for persons suffering from any sicknesses, injury or infirmity, a hospital, nursing home, maternity home, medical laboratory, dispensary and surgery, consultation room.'

The Bill seeks to achieve the following objectives:

1. To develop, manage and monitor standards of private medical institutions.
2. To improve, manage and evaluate the performance of private medical institutions.
3. To regulate, recruit and train personnel employed in private medical institutions.
4. To promote, improve and regulate working conditions and general welfare of the personnel.
5. To ensure the quality of services rendered or provided by private medical institutions.

C. Laws Restricting High-Risk Behaviour

Vagrants Ordinance No. 4 of 1841

- Every common prostitute wandering in a public street or highway in any place of public resort and behaving in a riotous or indecent manner is liable upon conviction to be imprisoned with or without hard labour for any term not exceeding fourteen months or to a fine not exceeding ten rupees.
- Any person in or about any public places soliciting any person for the purpose of the commission of any act of illicit sexual intercourse or indecency, whether with a person soliciting or with any other person is liable on summary conviction for imprisonment for a period not exceeding six months and/or to a fine not exceeding Rs. 100 or both.

Every person causing, encouraging seduction or prostitution or unlawful carnal knowledge of a girl shall be liable to a summary conviction for imprisonment to a fine for a period not exceeding six months or not exceeding Rs. 100 or both.

Brothels Ordinance No. 5 of 1889

- Any person who
  1. keeps or manages or acts or assists in the management of a brothel, or
  2. being the tenant, lessee, occupier or owner of any premises used as a brothel or for the purpose of habitual prostitution,
  3. being the lessor or landlord of any premises used as a brothel

is liable to a penalty of five hundred rupees or imprisonment for a term not exceeding six months or both.

- On a second or subsequent conviction the punishment is a penalty not exceeding one thousand rupees or imprisonment not exceeding one year.

Children and Young Persons Ordinance No. 48 of 1939

- If any person having the custody, charge or care of a girl under sixteen causes or encourages seduction or prostitution in respect of her, such person is guilty of an offence and is liable to imprisonment for a term not exceeding two years.
- If any person having the custody, charge or care of a girl who has attained the age of four years or a girl under sixteen allows that child to reside in or to frequent a brothel such person is guilty of an offence and is liable to a fine not exceeding two hundred and fifty rupees or imprisonment for a term of not exceeding six months or both.

Penal Code

- Any male person who in public or private commits or is a party to the commission of, or procures or attempts to procure the commission by any male person of, any act of gross indecency with another male person is guilty of an offence and is liable to be punished with imprisonment for a term of two years or with a fine or both.

- Whoever unlawfully or negligently does any act which is, and which he knows or has reason to believe to be, likely to spread infection of any diseases dangerous to life is liable to be punished with imprisonment for a term of six months or with a fine or both.
- Whoever maliciously does any act which is, and which he knows or has reason to believe to be, likely to spread infection of any diseases dangerous to life is liable to be punished with imprisonment for a term of two years or with a fine or both.
- Whoever knowingly disobeys any quarantine rule is liable to be punished with imprisonment for a term which may extend to six months or a fine or both.

Protective Laws

Constitution of Sri Lanka

- Under the Constitution, all persons are equal before the law and are entitled to the equal protection of the law.

The Constitution guarantees:

- Freedom of thought, conscience and religion;
- Freedom from torture;
- Freedom from arbitrary arrest and detention and punishment; and
- Freedom of speech, assembly, association, occupation and movement.

Labour Laws

- Industrial Disputes Act No. 27 of 1966.
- Termination of Employment of Workmen (Special Provisions) Act No. 45 of 1971.
- Workman's Compensation Ordinance No. 19 of 1934.

Protection of Housing Rights

- The Protection of Tenants (Special Provision) Act No. 28 of 1970.

Social Security

Poor Law Ordinance No. 30 of 1939

- An Ordinance for the relief of the poor
- 'Poor Persons' mean persons of either sex unable to

maintain themselves owing to physical or mental infirmity or incapacity and in need of relief.

Medical Ordinance No. 26 of 1927

Sri Lanka Nurses Council Act No. 19 of 1988

Criminal Procedure Code Act No. 15 of 1979

Where a swept does not consent to taking of finger impressions, [8]pecimens of saliva, urine, hair or finger nails the Magistrate may make an order authorizing a police officer to take such impressions or specimen.

Poisons, Opium and Dangerous Drugs Ortinanec No. 17 of 1929

Excise Ordinance No. 8 of 1912

Custom Ordinance No. 6 of 1890

59

Law Review/Law Reform: Models of the Consultative Process in Sri Lanka

Mr. Nalin Abeysekera P.C.
Legal Draftsman
Sri Lanka

Legislation as an instrument of social policy depends to a large extent on the acceptance of the policy underlying the legislation by the people who will be affected by it. This paper describes some of the available mechanisms for consultation which serve to secure this acceptance.

Consultations

The source of most legislation is the administration. Administrators in the course of administering or in furthering government policy or what has been described as the momentum of administration find gaps in the legislative framework or entire areas that are not regulated by legislation. They then take steps to plug what they perceive to be gaps in the law or to bring in new legislation to regulate the unregulated areas. In doing so, they consult the people who will or who are likely to be affected by the legislation. These consultations generally are at an informal level. It is inconceivable, for example, that any legislation in the field of industrial relations can be prepared without some sort of consultation with organizations representative of the employers and the workmen. Where the affected parties are organized in a centralized manner, like in the case of the federation of trade unions or the federation of employers, the task of consultation is much easier. A question that might strike the policy-maker at this stage is whether the net should be cast wider. Should, for example, in the case of industrial relations, the public be consulted?

When interest groups are well-organized they themselves may provide the impetus for legislative change. Good examples are environmental groups. They have been highly effective in many countries in promoting policies and legislation which protect the environment and in discouraging those with detrimental effects. In these cases, it is always prudent for the policy-maker to consult other groups before deciding on the policy or legislation.

These consultations between policy-makers and interest groups take place at an informal level and, generally, on an *ad hoc* basis if and when the need for consultation arises. Some statutes, however, provide for permanent advisory committees that can serve as very useful conduits for consultation. One such body is the Fisheries Advisory Board set up under the Fisheries Ordinance, whose duties include advising the Director of Fisheries on all matters relating to fisheries and the fishing industry in Sri Lanka and on matters relating to the administration of the Fisheries Ordinance.

Green Papers and White Papers

Another mechanism for consultation is the use of green papers and white papers. Green papers are not commonly used in Sri Lanka but white papers are. A white paper gives a broad outline of the proposed government policy and sometimes has attached to it a draft bill giving effect to this policy. This device is useful when the government is not committed to a policy in dealing with a particular social problem or in cases where it is not certain how it should address itself to the problem. The purpose of green and white papers is to elicit a response from the public as to what shape government policy should take in addressing itself to the problem. It is a very effective mechanism for consultation for more than one reason. Firstly, it enables the broadest possible consultation. Consultation is not restricted to the stronger and better organized interest groups as any member of the public can make representations for or against the policy outlined.

Secondly, it serves to clarify the issues which underline the proposed policy. As often is the case, things may not be as simple or clear-cut as they appear to be at first glance. A social problem has to be viewed at several levels. To take an example, a policy that addresses the problems of drugs or HIV purely as a law and order problem will be less effective than a policy that takes account of the several social factors which give rise to such problems. A current example of a white paper is the government policy paper on the goods and services tax. After the paper has been circulated, responses from the public are elicited through means of seminars and other informal meetings. The discussions these will generate will enable the government to get an overall view of the possible impact its policy may have and could lead to modifications in its policy on the tax, or even to its abandonment. The use of green papers and white papers should be encouraged, whilst keeping in mind that in situations which require quick policy or legislative responses this mechanism may not always be feasible.

Commission of Inquiry

Another mechanism for enabling the participation of the public in the formulation of policy is the commission of inquiry. In Sri Lanka, there are three types of commissions—a departmental commission, a commission of inquiry under the Commissions of Inquiry Act, and a Special Presidential Commission of inquiry under the Special Presidential Commissions of Inquiry Act. Departmental commissions are very much the vogue in the United Kingdom as investigative bodies preceding the formulation of policy or legislation. They have superseded royal commissions in this respect. Royal commissions were a notable feature of nineteenth century England and have been described as the chief instruments of government investigation and preparation for numerous innovations in social and industrial policy. Many of the legislative reforms in public health, education, housing and local government in that period can be traced to the investigations and recommendations of these commissions. Departmental committees are not known in Sri Lanka. There are a few in the Ministry of Health, including one on mental health consisting of officers of the ministry, academics and representatives of NGOs. The departmental committees have three advantages over the formal commissions of inquiry: their proceedings are more informal and participation in them is less inhibited; they are easier to set up, for example, by an administrative fiat; and unlike commissions of inquiry, the membership can be expanded from time to time to accommodate interests which have inadequately or not been represented

Among the commissions of inquiry, the presidential commissions of inquiry have to be presided over by sitting judges. They may not be an appropriate vehicle for the consultative process. Apart from the difficulty in getting them to serve on these commissions, judges may not be the best equipped to perform this function. They may have the expertise to ascertain the facts, but recommending policies based on an evaluation of facts may require a multi disciplinary approach.

Commissions of inquiry appointed under the Commissions of Inquiry Act do not have these drawbacks. Compared to a departmental committee, a commission of inquiry has greater visibility, by reason of the fact that the members are appointed by the President, and a vast panoply of powers—to summon witnesses, to call on persons to give evidence on oath, to produce documents, etc. Thus it is invested with all the powers needed to investigate a problem with great thoroughness. These powers also enable a commission of inquiry to have a wider reach. While commissions of inquiry call for representations from the public, by means of advertisements in newspapers and the like, they have been described as providing a unique channel through which private individuals and interest groups can participate directly in the making of public policy. On the other hand, the formal procedures of a commission of inquiry may deter affected parties from making representations before it.

The recent Commission of Inquiry on NGOs has, it appears, made some useful recommendations on the regulation of NGOs by legislation. It may be cited as an example of a commission of inquiry being used in the consultative process.

Law Commissions

Finally, mention must be made of the Law Commissions. The statue which instituted it enjoins the Law Commission to bring the law under review, both procedural and substantive, with a view to its systematic development and reform. While the selection of subjects for law reform is left to the commissioners, the commission is empowered to receive and consider any proposals which may be made or referred to them. Certainly, in those areas of law review or law reform which appear to be neglected, the focus of this workshop, interest groups have a particularly important duty to prod the Law Commission into action. In formulating proposals for reform, the commission endeavours to consult as broad a range of interests as possible and, certainly, the ministries concerned. The proposals for reform made by the Law Commission are, of course, subject to ratification by the Minister of Justice.

Reforms in the Area of HIV Law

When governments embark on law reform in sensitive areas like HIV, they should so after the broadest possible consultation. A few years ago in Sri Lanka when several cases of HIV were reported, there were proposals to rush legislation. In situations like this, governments resort to legislation to demonstrate that they are doing something about the problem, without seriously addressing the issues involved. The public also tends to take the view that once the law is in place, the problem is mitigated to some extent or that it is under control. In fact, the opposite may be true. Hastily enacted legislation may be conceptually flawed and its mechanics of implementation may not be well thought-out. This could lead to problems in interpreting, administering and implementing the law. More importantly, if the people at whom the legislation is targeted, like the medical profession or persons suffering from HIV, have not been consulted, there is bound to be resistance to its implementation. Instead of addressing some of the problems posed by the HIV epidemic, this may aggravate them further.

60

HIV/AIDS, Ethics and the Law: The Case of Thailand

Vitit Muntarbhorn
Associate Professor of Law
Chulalongkom University Bangkok
Thailand

INTRODUCTION

The advent of the Human Immunodeficiency Virus (HIV) and Acquired Immunodeficiency Syndrome (AIDS) has posed increasing dilemmas to Thai society. As estimates of those with HIV/AIDS approach the half a million mark out of a population of approximately sixty million, controversies abound concerning not only the epidemiological nature of the disease and related issues of vaccine trails, but also the socio-economic, political and legal consequences.

Issues of poverty, discrimination, budgetary tug-of-war, and the presence of draconian practice indicate clearly that HIV/AIDS is not simply a medical disease. It is also a socio-economic and political disease. From the angle of law, HIV/AIDS is exposing loopholes and pitfalls as never before. In a word, HIV/AIDS is equally a "legal" disease.

The function of law and its interrelationship with ethics pose several challenges to the dimension of HIV/AIDS. In this society, as in many other developing societies, the formal national law in the shape of parliamentary statutes and executive decrees, coupled with the judicial system of courts and lawyers, tends to be distant from the majority of the population. As there is already a pervasive problem concerning access by the people to the legal system, particularly in their quest for redress, a similar problem faces those who wish to use the law to address issues of HIV/AIDS. Will they have real access to the law and the formal legal system?

On another front, existing laws tend to be remedial by nature. More often than not, they address grievances after the event, rather than provide for preventive action. As will be seen below, sanctions against various acts abound in the legislation available, but they fail to tackle the root causes of the problem. While many laws seek to proscribe and punish, there is a paucity of laws and related measures that seek to assist, protect, and prevent.

A related issue is that in many developing settings, law enforcement is poor. Even where there could be remedies against malpractices, the low quality of law enforcement personnel, at times compounded by corruption, detracts from the potential efficacy of the law. There is thus a huge divide between the law and law enforcement, no less in the area of HIV/AIDS.

By contrast, it should be noted that in many instances where the law fails to provide the answers, it is to policies, often in the guise of national development plans, that one must look for guidelines concerning ethical conduct, even if they are not binding as such. In this light, it should be observed that currently Thailand has a National Plan for the Prevention and Control of AIDS (1992-96). It is this plan which establishes the more enlightened and humane framework for action on HIV/AIDS. It is much more progressive that the existing legal framework, and as a policy document, it paves the way for revamping the latter.

Yet, there lingers a pervasive doubt at the end of the day. Even with the existence of forward-looking policy guidelines, will the gap between principles and practices ever be bridged? Can a balance between certain traditional public health rationales and universal human rights standards ever be established?

Scrutiny of specific areas of concern provides various clues to the responses.

Public Health

The main law in this sector is the Infectious Diseases Act 1980. Particularly for "the disease requiring notification" to the authorities, the Act provides for broad discretion on the part of the medical authorities to take measures, even those verging on the draconian. By section 8, the authorities are empowered to order infected persons to appear for examination, to detain them, and to order measures of protection. They may also order them to desist from action which may lead to the spread of the disease (including presumably sexual intercourse). Non-compliance may lead to fines. Moreover, by section 10, the Minister of Public Health or provincial governors may cause infected persons to leave their employment. Violations of these orders may lead to fines and/or imprisonment.

Subsequent legislation under the umbrella of the 1970 Act dealt with the question of reporting and notification. By ministerial announcements of 1985 and 1986, AIDS was classified as one of the "the diseases requiring notification," indicating that householders, doctors in charge of hospitals or the equivalent had to report information on infected persons to the health authorities within twenty four hours of discovering the illness or suspicion of illness. Fines could be imposed on those who did not report such cases. This obligation overrode the general confidentiality principle concerning doctors and patients discussed below.

It is clear from this Act and subordinate legislation that at the time when AIDS was classified as one of "the diseases requiring notification," the public health authorities had broad powers to subject those with AIDS to their discretion, including coercion and draconian measures. These were in conflict with international human rights standards espoused by the World Health Organisation, which advocate voluntariness and humane measures with safeguard against discrimination.

Matters were compounded by a certain lobby that sought enact an even more reactionary law in the 1990-91 period. An AID bill which would have adopted stricter measures and punishmen against those with HIV/ AIDS was introduced. It purported to do th following, *inter alia*:

— establish a national committee to supervise and prevent AIDS.
— compel reporting of those with AIDS to the medical authorities.
— order those with AIDS to appear for medical check-up and supervision.
— oblige those with AIDS to report their movements to the medical authorities.
— compel those with AIDS to be detained in certain areas or prohibit them from entering certain areas.

— prohibit those with AIDS from spreading the disease.

— punish those who violate the law, including those with AIDS, by means of imprisonment and fines.

The bill was heavily attacked by many quarters and was never passed. Criticisms of the draconian approach of the Infectious Diseases Act also led to the deletion of AIDS from the list of "the diseases requiring notification" in 1991. Currently, there is thus no compulsory notification of those with HIV/AIDS to the authorities.

As regards surveillance, the issue falls under policy rather than law. It is part and parcel of the research priorities recognised by the National Plan for the Prevention of AIDS noted earlier. The two major sources of information are linked with the Public Health Ministry, namely:

— the AIDS/ARC (AIDS related complex) voluntary reporting system.

— the Biennual Sentinel Seroprevalence Surveillance system.

As reporting is done on a voluntary basis and through sentinel surveillance, it is difficult to establish the exact national statistics in regard to those with HIV/AIDS.

The National Plan for the Prevention of AIDS lays down guidelines on the type of testing permitted. While screening of donated blood is ensured, testing of persons for HIV/AIDS must only be carried out voluntarily with informed consent on the part of the person tested. A few exceptions are provided for in regard to various professions such as the military and the police. Pre-and post-test counselling are also advocated by the Plan.

The realities are still a far cry from that which is advocated by the National Plan. Reports of compulsory or hidden testing without informed consent continue to appear. Examples of those compelled to undergo testing without consent include pregnant women, employees and prostitutes. Insurance companies also impose the condition of HIV/AIDS testing without which they will refuse to insure candidates. On another front, access to counselling is not always guaranteed, and the quality of counsellors leaves much to be desired. This is aggravated by insufficient facilities for training counsellors to become attuned to personal, local, and cultural situations.

On the relationship between doctors and patients, by reason of national medical ethics, doctors are obliged to care for their patients. However, in practice, there are instances where doctors and hospitals shun those with HIV/AIDS. A related problem is that there is [illegible]al social welfare legislation or provision to provide free medical care to the needy. The lengthy nature of HIV/AIDS could ultimately lead to the situation where many of those affected would not have the means to pay for medical expenses on a long-term basis. Even if at the outset they may have some access to doctors and hospitals, ultimately they will be unable to cover their own expenses. Enpassant, it may be added that even if they had some access to medical facilities, the poor tend to suffer from a lower quality of medical treatment.

The issue of vaccine trials has led to heated debate in Thai society. In 1992 a National Plan for HIV/AIDS Vaccine Development and Evaluation was adopted with national guidelines for reviewing HIV/AIDS vaccine studies in Thailand. It recognised the role of various national institutions in considering whether to approve the trials of specific vaccines in the country.

Public debate continues. Some argue that certain groups are liable to be tested as "guinea pigs," while others favour a proactive approach so as to enable Thailand to be in the forefront of vaccine trials with potential longterm benefits.

The dispute is dependent upon resolution through various governmental committees concerning the green light for the vaccines to be tested. The National AIDS Committee is, in theory, the primary entity for guiding the process but it has not met since 1991. The fact that there is an overlap between the lower rungs of sub-committees on technical and ethical issues militates against efficacious decision-making. This bureaucratisation has led to a long waiting period for decision-making on whether to test vaccines in Thailand. On another front, it is unclear to what extent those tested with vaccines will be assisted with support facilities from firms that produce the vaccines and the national authorities after the trials are undertaken.

Discrimination

A key weakness is that there is no general law providing redress against discrimination in Thai society. The nearest one comes to a law on the subject is the Thai Constitution. Yet, this national instrument is illusory for a variety of reasons.

Since 1932, Thailand has witnessed 22 coups and failed coups, and fifteen Constitutions—mostly drafted (and overturned) by those allied to coup-makers. The latest Constitution was drafted in 1991 after the coup in the same year. Like its predecessors, it has a chapter on citizens rights, including equality of treatment, which could, in principle, be used to counter discrimination.

However, this Constitution suffers from the constraints of most of the previous Constitutions. It does not confer direct rights—no "justiciable rights"—upon individuals to enable them to challenge the validity of laws and administrative action in the courts. For that purpose, individuals have to resort to others laws, such as the law on employment, to concretise their rights under the Constitution.

Moreover, all the rights stipulated under the Constitution are constrained by the notion of national security (including public health), and the rights recognised do not include those of non-Thais. In effect, the Constitution does not help those claiming discrimination at the hands of the authorities and employers unless there are other laws which confer protection specifically.

Therefore, if there is discrimination concerning treatment, accommodation, education and access to services and facilities, there are generally no legal provisions to help the affected parties. The main exception is the presence of the labour legislation, such as Revolutionary Decree No. 103 of 1972, which has provisions against discrimination in employment, and a special labour court to provide redress. However, no case concerning discrimination by reasons of HIV/AIDS has yet come to court, even though it is common knowledge that several employers have been dismissing those with HIV/AIDS from employment. One can surmise that an essential reason for this is the fear of exposure of one's identity if one takes action in court.

In the realm of immigration, one has also witnessed discriminatory action in recent years. The most infamous concerns action taken to exclude foreigners with HIV/AIDS from entering the country. In this context, the Immigration Act 1979 confers broad powers upon the Minister of Interior to control entry into and exit from the country. By Announcement No. 11 of 1986, foreigners with HIV/AIDS were prohibited from entering the country or becoming residents. Due to much public criticisrn lodged against these measures, the Announcement was revoked in 1991.

More specifically on matters of confidentiality, the criminal and civil law in the guise of the Criminal Code and the Civil Code provide a degree of protection for personal privacy, even though there is no substantive law on privacy. Confidentiality on the part of medical personnel and other authorities in caring for those with HIV/AIDS is proffered by section 323 of the Criminal Code which states as follows:

> whoever discloses any private secret which became known or communicated to him by reason of his functions as a

> competent official or his profession as a medical practitioner shall be punished with imprisonment not exceeding six months or fine not exceeding one thousand bath, or both.
>
> Civil action may also be taken under section 420 of the Civil Code which establishes tortious liability as follows:
>
> A person who, wilfully or negligently, unlawfully injures the life, body, health, liberty, property or any right of another person, is said to commit a wrongful act and is bound to make compensation therefore.

In practice, these provisions have not been used against doctors and others who have violated the rights of those with HIV/AIDS. The reasons include general reticence to sue doctors, inaccessibility of the judicial system, and fear of exposure of one's identity.

An innovative input at the national level is provided by the National Plan for the Prevention of AIDS already mentioned. It has a specific section on human rights and social assistance which calls for measures against discrimination and to protect confidentiality. However, these aspirations are not reflected in the current law and practice in terms of effective redress.

More specifically on the role of international law concerning these issues, it should be noted that the Thai legal approach is based upon a dualistic system; international law is not automatically part and parcel of Thai law. In order for international law to be invoked in Thailand, it is necessary to transform such law into local law through parliamentary legislation or the equivalent.

However, it may said that in terms of national policies, exemplified by the National Plan for the Prevention of AIDS, international principles which have emerged from treaties and customs, as well as through various decisions and recommendations of the World Health Organisation, are accepted in Thai policy-making. The main constraints are the practices which are often amiss and the lack of effective remedies at the local level.

Women's Issues

Women's vulnerability to HIV/AIDS has emerged to the fore more prominently in recent years. This is due to a variety of reasons. First, there is increasingly a cross-over link of the disease into the family system. More women are now affected, principally due to the male spouse who brings the disease to the family. Second, there are large numbers of female sex workers in Thailand, and the spread of HIV among this group is most disconcerting. Third, due to ingrained socio-cultural impediments, women's role in sexual negotiation, including their choice in taking universal precautions against HIV (e.g., whether to wear a condom, and whether it should be a male or female condom), is constrained. The male is often seen as entitled to take an active role in such negotiation while the female is relegated to a more passive stereotype.

Although there have been many legislative improvements concerning the status of women in Thailand in the past decade, witnessed most recently in 1992-93 by the Cabinet's approval of 90 day maternity leave for those in the private sector and women's access to the post of sub-district officials, there remains much discrimination in practice. Women are also victims of the pressures of a triple burden—domestic work, child care, and agricultural, industrial or service-related work, all part and parcel of socio-economic needs. One is witnessing continued migration from rural to urban areas, and disintegration of the extended family system.

At a time when there is a decline of the family, HIV/AIDS is posing an additional question for Thai society. Who is to care for women who have HIV/AIDS, especially when the traditional social welfare system through the family network is no longer available? What support system is there to help promote care within the family?

Although the National Plan for the Prevention of AIDS calls for the provision of assistance and care for all those with HIV/AIDS and their families, in reality the answers are not yet forthcoming. The state has not intervened to offer family subsidies, on the one hand, and there is no general social welfare assistance for needy persons, on the other hand. The only widespread form of social security is in regard to those employed in the formal sector. There is no such equivalent for those doing domestic chores and working in the non-formal sector, or for the unemployed.

The issue is related to both prevention and cure, particularly to assist women to protect themselves and the family from harm. This entails measures to counter gender discrimination within society and within the home. The role of the husband is at stake, especially as it is he who all too often brings the disease home to the family, on the one hand, and who fails to share in the household obligations, on the other hand. The state action required is necessarily linked with the call for national provision for the needy, such as through social security and a fund to help those with HIV and AIDS. Empowerment of women also requires mobilisation of women's groups to help the women affected, and the elevation of their educational capacity as well as improved sexual negotiating skills so as be on par with their male counterparts.

Information Law

There is no specific law guaranteeing access to official information in Thailand, even though the past two years have witnessed the rise of a proposal to enact a Freedom of Information Act. At the personal level, although the expectation is that doctors will provide patients with all the necessary information, there is little that the patient can do if the doctor refuses to divulge all the relevant information. As with everyone else, doctors are under the umbrella of the criminal and civil law in the case of wrongful acts and negligence. However, in regard to non-release of medical information, there is practically no effective legal remedy. A more accessible means of redress would be to resort to social sanctions such as by complaining to the medical council and/or the medical boards of hospitals. Yet instances of complaints by patients against doctors are rare in this country, as there is much reverence towards them.

More specifically on broadcasting, censorship, pornography and advertising, there is a myriad of laws on these subjects. Both the Criminal and Civil Codes pertain to them, while provisions on defamation in these Codes may be invoked in the cases where reputations are jeopardised. The Criminal Code has specific provisions against pornography. On a related front, television and radio stations are to a large extent controlled by the state under the Radio and Television Broadcasting Act 1955 which requires all broadcasters to obtain a license from the Government. By contrast, the press in Thailand is in the hands of the private sector; it is the freest of the mass media (and some of the freest in Asia). However, still on the books is the Press Act 1941 which confers power upon the executive to control and suppress publications deemed to be contrary to the public interest.

There has been a variety of educational programmes on television, radio and the press on the prevention and control of AIDS. These have included advertisements, films, plays and publicity spots to raise public awareness of HIV/AIDS and promote precautions, such as the use of condoms. However although people are generally aware of HIV/AIDS, behavioural change in terms of changed habits in favour of safer conduct is difficult to measure. Many programmes do not have proper impact assessment. Also missing is the nurturing of a humane attitude, such as learning to live with AIDS and the prevention of discrimination, among large sectors of the community. There remains a rampant negative syndrome towards those with HIV/AIDS.

More generally on the educational process, it must be noted that culturally there has been a reticence towards sex education, particularly at school. However, AIDS-related information is now inserted at various levels of formal education, for example through "family life education" programmes. Students at the lower levels of education are encouraged to undertake consciousness-raising activities, such as by writing essays on AIDS and taking them home to discuss related issues with their parents and/or to leave copies in libraries for dissemination.

At the tertiary level of formal education, it is interesting that administrators tend to assume that university students already have access to information on AIDS. Some universities also fail to act as suitable role models for non-discrimination; they compel foreign teaching staff to be tested for HIV.

In terms of non-formal education, a range of campaigns is carried out by non-governmental organisations, bolstered by various mass media programmes. Here, the challenge of education concerns not only how to nurture a change of sexual habits among certain target groups but also how to sustain the dissemination efforts. This would then help to create a multiplier effect within the community, and to provide concomitant facilities and help for those in need.

Families and Carers

As already noted, the family is breaking up and breaking down for a number of reasons. AIDS is a contributing factor. As the numbers of infected persons increase, one can foresee enormous pressures placed upon families and carers. Currently one is witnessing reports of mothers abandoning their infected babies in hospitals. The gloomy picture strikes particularly at the fate of children—they are becoming abandoned, orphaned and/or discriminated against in the progression of the pandemic.

There is no law to provide subsidies for the family, and there is no general social security provision to help the poor. However, such facilities are now advocated by the National Plan for the Prevention of AIDS, and decisive commitment is awaited among national leaders.

More specifically on family law, the provisions pertaining to the family arise under the Civil Code. Death for those who are intestate leads to the division of property among the next of kin. Half the property belongs automatically to the surviving spouse, and the other half is divided in equal shares between the children, the parents of the deceased and the surviving spouse. Adoption matters are regulated by a special statute, namely the Adoption Act 1979. Custody matters are now supervised by a newly established family court.

The family law remains distorted in favour of men. Several provisions are discriminatory. For example, while it suffices for a man to prove adultery on the part of his wife so as to obtain a divorce, the same does not apply to a woman in a parallel situation. The woman has to prove not only her husband's adultery but also the fact that he has treated another women as though she were his wife (e.g., by appearing in public with her). More specifically on AIDS, there is a provision of the Civil Code which provides a ground for divorce in regard to diseases as follows: by section 1500 (8), "if one spouse is suffering from a communicable disease which is incurable and may cause injury to the other spouse, the latter may enter a claim for divorce."

In practice, the provision has not been used; this is again probably due to the fear of exposing one's identity in relation to HIV/AIDS. En passant, it should be noted that the law does not recognise the crime of rape when it is committed by a husband against his wife. However, where one spouse is infected with HIV, there remains a moot point concerning whether the infected spouse must inform the other spouse and what responsibility would be incurred if the one infects the other. The preferred solution would be to look at how the system treats situations involving other serious diseases, and treat AIDS accordingly. Criminal and civil liability may thus ensue from the general context of infectious diseases, including AIDS.

On the related issue of maintenance, while the courts have the power to order maintenance payments, in practice these are difficult to enforce. In terms of the age of marriage, the minimum age is seventeen years. However, in the Muslim community in Southern Thailand, the age criterion is more flexible due to prevalence of religious law.

On another front, in criminal law, the age of consent is set at fifteen; consent of the child is no defence to sexual assault if the child is under fifteen years of age. This is particularly relevant to the issue of children in prostitution; customers are criminally responsible for sexual acts committed against those under fifteen.

There is the additional issue of abortion. At present, by the Criminal Code, abortion is illegal except for two reasons, namely where the health of the mother so demands, and where the conception was due to crimes such as rape. In practice, however, several doctors are known to encourage those with HIV/AIDS to have abortions. Strictly speaking, these are illegal because they do not fall neatly into the two exceptions noted. The ethics of such practice are also open to query. The abortion in such context should depend upon the woman's choice rather than coercion. Moreover, the fact that the pregnant woman has HIV/AIDS does not necessarily mean that the child will be born with HIV/AIDS.

Prisons and Related Institutions

The main law on the subject is the Corrections Act 1936 which gives great divscretion to the Corrections Department to deal with prisoners. By section 11, it is empowered to divide the prisoners into groups and separate them. The Director General of the Department also has discretion to send prisoners to other places for treatment.

Until recently prisoners were tested for HIV/AIDS without their consent and were segregated if they tested HIV-positive. However, the more liberal policy of the Public Health Ministry and the National Plan for the Prevention of AIDS has now influenced the prison system to take a more humanitarian approach. In theory, there is now no compulsory testing and segregation. In practice, however, reports suggest the contrary, particularly in the smaller prisons. One source indicates that those segregated before the advent of the new policy remain segregated, but new arrivals are not segregated even if they are HIV-positive. This ambivalence is part of the invisibility factor surrounding prisons. This calls for greater openness of monitoring, precisely because the prison system is also an environment where needles are shared between those who inject drugs and unprotected sex is a corollary of the environment—all of which lend themselves to the risk of contracting HIV.

Condoms are not generally available in prisons, but prisoners are given three condoms upon discharge from these institutions. Needles and other implements affiliated with drug injection are prohibited. For those infected with HIV, early release is sometimes sought, particularly as annual national celebrations provide for the pardoning of prisoners. Although some education on AIDS is available in prison, it tends to be *ad hoc*. Counselling is also constrained by the limited facilities provided to those in prison.

The current situation remains nebulous. Ideally, it would be best if prison authorities could follow the National Plan for the Prevention of AIDS strictly for the purpose of implementation.

Employment

There is differentiation between the pre-employment and post-employment stages. The current labour protection law covers the latter and not the former. Therefore, where there are cases of discrimination and abuses in the pre-employment stage, there are few remedies. The affected party could try to invoke various provisions of the Criminal and Civil Codes based upon intention, negligence and harm. However, access to courts is difficult and slow.

A key concern is that, despite the National Plan for the Prevention of AIDS which rejects compulsory testing of potential and actual employees, transgressions abound. Rejections of potential employees on the basis of HIV/AIDS and dismissals of actual employees due to HIV/AIDS are commonplace. The latter practice is also in violation of the National Plan which prohibits dismissal of employees with HIV/AIDS. Hence the recurrent gap between policy and practice.

Is the labour law of any use in this area? There are a number of laws on employment with implications for HIV/AIDS. These range from the provisions on the Civil Code on employment contracts to specific laws on labour protection and labour relations. The most pertinent is probably Revolutionary Decree No. 103 of 1972 which stipulates the rights of employees in regard to unfair dismissal, remuneration and safe working conditions. However, even though employees dismissed by reason of HIV/AIDS could sue the employer under such labour protection law, this has not taken place for the reason already noted, namely fear of exposure of identity.

In regard to sick leave, by the same law, employees are entitled to take a thirty day leave with pay. With respect to disability support, prior to the Social Security Act 1990, there was a provident fund for employees, and disability support was given only for harm incurred in the course of employment. In 1990 a new law was enacted to provide extensive social security to workers and their families through the establishment of a social security fund to cover injuries and diseases suffered by workers even if they are not related to the work. The law applies to establishments with ten or more employees.

It provides for different rates of support and periods of payment, depending upon whether they pertain to unemployment benefits, disability payment or other support.

Although there is some HIV/AIDS education in the workplace, the expectations of the National Plan for the Prevention of AIDS which call for extensive education have yet to be realised. However, on a more positive front, various employers are now linking up to form a kind of coalition to promote education and voluntary testing in an exemplary manner.

Criminal Law

The criminal law affects the HIV/AIDS issue in a variety of ways. In general, according to the Criminal Code, criminal liability arises from intentional acts. However, negligence may also give rise to criminal liability in some situations. These are relevant to those who transmit HIV to other persons.

A key concern of criminal law in the country is the suppression of narcotics. The Dangerous Drugs Act 1979 allows the authorities to send a drug addict to rehabilitation centres if the person has been indicted for drug addiction on three or more occasions. The provision could also be used to detain those with HIV/AIDS where they are related to drug addiction. The powers of the authorities were broadened in 1991 with a new law on the rehabilitation of drug addicts. A new committee has been established to oversee the process of rehabilitation for drug addicts. Those accused of drug addiction can be sent to rehabilitation centres without waiting for a court decision. However, when the case comes to trial, the court will bear in mind the period already spent in the rehabilitation centres for the purpose of sentencing.

On the issue of sex workers, there is a variety of pertinent laws. The Criminal Code has already been mentioned in the context of the provision which prohibits sexual intercourse with those under fifteen years, even if they consent. Two other laws are relevant: the Prostitution Suppression Act 1960 and the Entertainment Places Act 1966.

In regard to the 1960 Act,- although the law does not refer directly to infectious diseases, it has great impact upon a trade which lends itself to the possibility of diseases. According to this law, prostitution is illegal in Thailand. The Act catches both prostitutes and procurers, but customers are exempted from its scope. Courts are also empowered to send prostitutes to rehabilitation programmes, impliedly covering those with HIV/AIDS.

Despite this legislation, prostitution is rampant in Thailand, indicating poor implementation of the law. When the Act is enforced, it tends to be the prostitutes themselves rather then the procurers who are punished. The law also fails to take into account the root causes of the prostitution, thereby being confined to a remedial approach. If there are no real incentives for prostitutes to change their profession, particularly through alternative livelihoods, medical risks may be only a step away, and the legal framework may aggravate the situation. Current proposals to reform this law include suggestions to incriminate the actions of those who exploit children under eighteen years of age for sexual purposes.

The 1966 Act covers entertainment places such as massage parlours and bars which could be haunts for prostitution. It compels those wishing to set up these institutions to request permission from the authorities, and by section (6.4) of the Act, those seeking permission must not be infected with infectious diseases, impliedly including HIV/AIDS. The Act fails to deal with the issue of the health of the prostitutes themselves.

The prostitution trade in the country affects both men and women, although the figures are larger among women. A worrying trend also is the sale and trafficking of children into prostitution. Recent instances point to an underground trade of children and women trafficked for prostitution between China, Laos, Burma, Cambodia, Vietnam and Thailand. Many are then infected with HIV.

En passant, it should be noted that homosexuality is not illegal in Thailand. Although this group was initially the most affected group at the start of the epidemic in Thailand, this is no longer the case. By contrast recent trends highlight the problem of prostitution as the factor most closely linked with the exponential spread of HIV.

Legal Process

Although the Thai legal process adheres to the maxim "ignorance of the law is no excuse," it is peculiar that an obligation upon the state to disseminate the law to the people is lacking. Thus many people simply do not know the law. This is aggravated by the physical and mental distance between the formal system embodied in courts and lawyers and the people at large. It should not pass unnoticed that 70 per cent of the population are rural based with few means of access to the legal structure which is situated in towns. The people are not litigious in the sense of the developed world—disputes tend to be settled at the local level rather by means of formal courts of law. Limited legal aid and assistance provided by both governmental and non-governmental sectors are available under the formal system.

It does not suffice to presume that the formal courts system will provide the relevant remedies. The capacity to settle disputes at the local level is equally pertinent. On the one hand this implies the potential and actual use of local mediation-and the intervention of respected persons for example village headmen and para-legal personnel in providing redress. On the other hand it implies that the urban judicial system and lawyers needs to be decentralised to rural areas. They should aim to be more efficacious cost effective and speedy in their deliberations.

However there is a need to ensure that the informal system also abides by the national law and procedure. Too much discretion on the part of the informal system may lead to a conflict between the informal system and the formal structure based upon legislation and the judiciary. For this reason training of local mediators is important to ensure that they are conscious of the parameters of national law.

Conclusion

In retrospect it may be observed that as in many other countries Thailand has a myriad of laws relevant to HIV/AIDS. In several instances they are remedial rather than preventive. At times they are reactive indeed reactionary rather than proactive and humane. Legislative aspirations are plagued by poor law enforcement.

The current guiding light for better performance towards those with HIV/AIDS is the National Plan for the Prevention of AIDS with its multipronged strategies of public relations and education rehabilitation and medical help protection of human rights and social assistance and research and evaluation. However the Plan suffers from the fact that it purports to be persuasive rather than binding. It is also threatened by lack of continuity when there is a change of government. A key challenge will be how to ensure that the Plan itself is able to transcend such change and avoid the internecine skirmishes between some bureaucrats who view AIDS-related budgets and programmes as another source of power.

The law alone will never suffice. It can only respond effectively to the needs of the people, including those with HIV/AIDS, if it encompasses and bolsters an inter-disciplinary and cross-sectoral perspective. It has to be posited in the framework of both preventive and remedial strategies. It should move away from the reactive to become proactive. It should shun inhumane action but espouse humane principles and practices. Some of the needed measures for improving the law thus include the following:

- the establishment of a proper fund to help those with medical problems, including HIV/AIDS;
- the provision of assistance to families in need of care and protection, including the possibility of family subsidies;
- the setting up of hospices, half-way houses and other facilities to help those with medical and other problems, including those with HIV/AIDS and their families;
- the adoption of legal and other measures to counter discrimination, with effective redress based upon access to both formal and non-formal systems of dispute resolution;
- the maximisation of programmes to empower women, and to protect women and children from AIDS, with the aim of re-orienting fathers to take precautions against HIV/AIDS as well as to share in shouldering the responsibilities in the home;
- the promotion of international human rights and humane standards set by the United Nations, in particular the World Health Organisation, at the local level, and the conclusion of bilateral, regional and multilateral co-operation to curb the sale and trafficking of women and children;
- the encouragement of community action and information dissemination to enhance universal precautions and empathy for those with HIV/AIDS and their families;
- the formation of more alliances between community groups, nongovernmental organisations, the business sector and governmental authorities to prevent draconian measures and to nurture humane responses;
- the adoption of a code of ethics not only among doctors but also lawyers, the business sector and others who have impact on those with HIV/AIDS so as to promote greater self-scrutiny, incentives for good behaviour, and social sanctions among professional and other peer groups;
- the enhancement of participation among those with HIV/AIDS in planning, implementing, and evaluating all programmes relating to them, thereby ensuring their inputs in decision-making and benefit sharing; and
- the acceleration and coordination of decision-making between policymakers so as to ensure that essential issues such as vaccine trials and provision of help to those with HIV/AIDS are accorded priority attention in terms of programming and budgetary allocations.

With these in mind, one can move away from a purely legalistic and jurisdical approach to law to adopt a more comprehensive and people centered vision of desired laws, policies and practices in the tapestry of alliance-building. The law may then learn to be less judicial and more judicious.

61

HIV/AIDS Law and Law Reform in Tonga

Ms. Linda Folaumoefee'
Crown Law Office, Tonga

Dr. Taoruru Tebana
SPAFH Nukualofa, Tonga

Current HIV/AIDS Situations

Tonga has so far had six cases of HIV/AIDS (5 males and 1 female). Of these five had full-blown AIDS and all have died, while one person has HIV.

Two of the six patients had acquired the infection locally, one from a homosexual relationship and the other from a heterosexual one. The rest had contracted the infection overseas.

Risk Factors that May Fuel the Epidemic

1. High divorce rate
2. Increase in teenage pregnancy
3. Increase in alcohol consumption
4. Breakdown of family structure

Policies and Programmes in Place

The HIV prevention programme was developed in 1988. A review in *1990* found that excellent progress had been made by health officers involved in the educational campaign, which targets church groups, Police and non-government organizations.

A survey revealed that approximately 8-90 per cent *of the* population had comprehensive knowledge about AIDS. But knowing about AIDS does not necessarily mean that knowledge is translated into practice.

Blood Transfusion

Screening of all blood donors is compulsory. However, antenatal screening is not available.

Public Health Act

No public health legislation has yet been enacted specially in respect of HIV/AIDS. The existing Public Health Act, 1992 [Cap 74] includes HIV/AIDS in Part X as one of the notifiable diseases listed in Schedule 4.

Section 138 (1) lists HIV/AIDS as a notifiable disease.

Section 139 provides that there is a duty to notify cases of notifiable diseases.

- Section 139 (1) provides that where any person is suffering from an illness which creates a reasonable suspicion that he/she is suffering from a notifiable disease, it shall be the duty of that person forthwith notify a medical practitioner or a nurse or an authorized officer or a health officer of a district where that person is residing.
- Section 139 (2) provides that other persons which includes friends/relatives who are aware that a person described in subsection (1) may be suffering from a notifiable disease shall enquire of that person whether notification has been made. Otherwise, they should immediately notify a medical practitioner.
- Section 139 (3) provides that a medical practitioner, nurse, authorized officer or health officer shall immediately record the information prescribed under Schedule 5 and deliver the information to the Director of Health within 12 hours.
- Section 139 (4) states that 'any person who contravenes the provisions of this section is guilty of an offence'.
- Section 140 provides that the medical officer in charge may order that person to; be isolated or removed to hospital. Section 141 provides for a medical practitioner or an authorized officer to notify the Director of Health on the prescribed form under Schedule 6.
- Section 143 provides that on receipt of the notification of a

case or suspected case of notifiable disease, the Director of Health shall require an authorized officer to take all steps in conjunction with the medical officer to prevent the spread of the disease. These measures include provision to:

(a) examine the patient and determine the best practicable means of dealing with the case.

(f) order the patient or contacts or carriers to be detained in hospital or isolated in a suitable place until the medical officer with the approval of the Director of Health is satisfied that there is no risk of the patient or any contact or carrier spreading the disease.

(s) prohibit the patient or his contacts or anyone else whom he considers might spreat the disease from engaging or being employed in the sale, preparation, storage, packing, conveying or delivery of food or of an ingredient or package for such food.

Section 144 states any person who knowing or believing that he is suffering from a notifiable disease exposes other persons to the risk of infection by his presence or conduct in any street, public place, public transport, vehicle, place or enuinnmt, assembly, dub, hotel restaurant or shop shall be guilty of an offence.

Section 145 provide that where the patient is suffering from one of the diseases subject to the current International Health Regulations, the Director of Health shall immediately bring into operation all or any of those measures necessary to prevent the spread of disease as are recommended therein.

Section 16 states that a person convicted of an offence under this Act for which a special penalty is provided shall be liable:

(a) in the case of a first offence, to a find not exceeding $100 or to imprisonment for a term not exceeding 3 months or to both.

(b) in the case of a subsequent offence, to a fine not exceeding $200 or imprisonment for; a term not exceeding 6 months or to both.

Problems

1. Section 139(1) of the Public Health Act creates fear of be trayal by the family ant discourages an infected person from seeking much needed emotional support from his family and loved ones.
2. Certain sections of the Public Health Act require persons

suffering from a notifiable disease to be isolated, but within the Ministry of Health there are conflicting views on this issue. First, there is the view that patients should be given the freedom to move without restrictions of any kind. The other view is that people who are suffering from notifiable diseases should be confined in or isolated at the hospital. At present, although, the Act favours isolation, in reality HIV/AIDS patients are not isolated and individual rights override public health protection.

3. Another problem in the context of the debate over the issue of confidentiality is whether everybody should undergo testing for HIV.

62

HIV/AIDS Prevention and Control in the Republic of Vanuatu

Staff of STD/HIV/AIDS Section
Disease Control Unit
Department of Health
Republic of Vanuatu

BACKGROUND

In response to the global concern for and danger of the rapid spread of AIDS, the Government of the Republic of Vanuatu formed the National AIDS Committee (NAC) in September 1987 and formulated a Short-Term Plan (STP) for the prevention and control of AIDS beginning March 1988.

In the same year the STD/HIV/AIDS Section in the Department of Health was established. The Section is currently linked to the Disease Control Unit within the Prevention Services of the Department of Health.

The STP was successfully completed and provided the basic background for the first Medium-Term Plan (MTP), which was finalized in November 1990 for the period 1991-93. This MTP for the HIV/ AIDS programme was in fact implemented as the STD, HIV and AIDS Prevention and Control Programme.

The MTP 2 covers the period 1994-96.

The current programme staff comprise a National STD/HIV/ AIDS Programme Manager, an Assistant Co-ordinator and a clerical assistant. Presently only the Programme Manager is a full-time government employee. The remaining staff is paid on a daily basis, with limited job security. The programme has in real terms expanded to the point that all positions are needed to sustain activities and their effectiveness.

Risk Factors that may Fuel the Epidemic

The National AIDS Programme (NAP) identified three major determinants and their underlying behaviours for the spread of HIV/AIDS and STD in Vanuatu. The population most likely at risk are:

1. *Youth (13-25 years)* who make up about 20 per cent of the population.
2. *Ni-Vanuatu who travel overseas* for study, business, government work, conferences and other reasons may engage in high-risk behaviour and return home with STD or HIV infections.
3. *The clients seen in STD clinics,* (the majority of whom fall in the youth group\.
4. *People who exchange sex for money or status.*

HIV/AIDS POLICY

In 1993 the Vanuatu National HIV/AIDS Policy was formulated by the Department of Health and presented to the Council of Ministers for approval.

The policy statement highlighted four main areas:

Health and Safety

It is the government policy:

(a) to screen blood for HIV;

(b) to take standard precautionary measures in respect of persons receiving first aid, emergency, medical or surgical treatment and nursing care;

(c) to train health personal in universal precautionary measures.

Confidentiality

It is the government policy:

(a) to require the notification of cases of HIV/AIDS without disclosing names of the infected persons;

(b) to provide voluntary testing for HIV/AIDS;

(c) to provide for partner notification only by the person with HIV; and
(d) to use a coding system to ensure confidentiality.

Access to Information, Education and Training

It is the government policy:
(a) to provide education and training at all levels to ensure that entire population is fully aware and participates in the control and prevention of HIV/AIDS; and
(b) to guarantee access to goods and services to persons with HIV/AIDS.

Discrimination

It is government policy:
(a) to ensure that policies or laws implemented address behaviours that spread the risk and not to target individuals or groups;
(b) to ensure appropriate care, tolerance, compassion and support from the family and the community at large for persons with HIV/AIDS; and
(c) to provide legal protection against discrimination.

Present HIV/AIDS Situation

Upto May 1995 Vanuatu has not reported a single HIV/AIDS case. With increasing global mobility, however, the spread of the disease into Vanuatu is only a matter of time. Because HIV testing among high-risk groups has been limited, it is possible that HIV infection may already exist in the population.

Vanuatu is experiencing a socio-economic transition. A growing tourist industry, increasing number of Ni-Vanuatu travelling abroad, and the urban drift are elements of this change. The increasing number of teenage pregnancies, STD infections and the low usage of condoms by Ni-Vanuatu males suggest a high potential for HIV transmission.

Sexually Transmitted Diseases (STD) cause a significant amount of morbidity and their presence will facilitate the spread of HIV/ AIDS once the virus is introduced.

Vanuatu's close proximity to countries with higher prevalence of HIV, such as Australia, New Zealand, Papua New Guinea and New Caledonia will increase the risk of HIV infection. It is expected that this will occur within the next three to four years. Without an intensive programme for condom use, the incidence of STDs will continue to rise.

Existing Legal Framework

The Public Health Act, No.22 of 1994 deals with notifiable diseases. Since HIV/AIDS is regarded as a notifiable disease, a legal framework for this disease is provided by this legislation.

The relevant sections are Sections 18-21 under Part 3 of the Act.

Considering the modes of transmission of HIV/AIDS it is felt that the present legislation is inappropriate.

Proposed Legal Reforms

The National AIDS Policy document in its conclusion seeks the approval of the Council of Ministers for the formulation of appropriate legislation to support the implementation of the policy and to provide protection and security for infected people.

The present Public Health Act No. 22 of 1994 will need to be amended to delete HIV/AIDS from the First Schedule of the Act in the event that more specific legislation is introduced providing for the special circumstances presented by HIV/AIDS.

Problems

Shortage of Staff

With limited staff for coordinating and implementing the AIDS control programme for the whole nation, it is extremely difficult to implement activities within the planned time-frame.

Lack of Governmental Financial Support

The only contributions given by the Government are the salary of the Programme Manager and the office building. Otherwise the programme is funded by the World Health Organization's Global Programme on AIDS. Since GPA has already reduced the level of funding, many of the budgeted activities have not been implemented.

Lack of Full-time STD Clinics

At present there is only one full-time STD clinic; this cannot adequately provide all the services required.

High Prevalence of STD Infections

The National AIDS Programme has done an excellent job in raising the public's awareness about HIV/AIDS and STDs. At the same time, however, there has been an increase in the number of STD cases and teenage pregnancies. The most affected population is the youth in the age group 16-20 years.

Poor Monitoring of STD Cases

The health information system is not very efficient in providing accurate data when it comes to reporting STD cases.

Inadequate Screening of Blood

Although blood is screened before it is transfused there are urgent cases—this usually happens in remote areas—where the usual practice is for the dose relatives of the patient to donate blood which is transfused without screening. However, district hospitals have been requested to order screened blood to Vila/ Luganville hospitals for long-term patients.

While a National Blood Committee exists, it is not yet functioning.

Prevailing Cultural Taboos and Religious Constraints on Sex Education

Although the national programme has carried out a major awareness campaign on AIDS/STD prevention, traditional and religious barriers against sex education still persist.

CONCLUSIONS

Vanuatu urgently needs an appropriate HIV/AIDS legislative framework, firstly to support the implementation of its HIV/AIDS policy, and secondly to provide protection and security in the likely event of an HIV/AIDS epidemic.

63

Law on Prevention and Control of HIV/AIDS in Vietnam

Dang Thanh Son
Legal Expert
Ministry of Justice, Vietnam

Dang Van Khoat
Chief of Information Education
Communication Unit
National AIDS Commitee Honoi,
Vietnam

Introduction

Since the first case of HIV/AIDS in Vietnam was reported in December 1990, the number of those affected has dramatically increased—as of 30 March 1995, there were over 2,000 HIV positive cases, 131 AIDS cases and 54 deaths. Thus, although the epidemic reached this South-East Asian country relatively late, it is spreading very rapidly. If Vietnam does not adopt timely and effective measures to arrest its spread, it will have to shoulder a heavy social-economic burden. It is estimated that the number of people infected with HIV/AIDS in Vietnam in the year 1998 will be about 570,000.

The pattern of HIV/AIDS infection in Vietnam is characterized by a high rate of transmission through intravenous drug use (approximately 72.2 per cent). Transmission through unprotected sexual intercourse accounts for only 4.4 per cent of the cases. Males have been disproportionately infected (86.1 per cent).

The first significant step taken by the Vietnamese government was to create a Vietnamese National AIDS Committee (NAC) for the prevention and control of HIV/AIDS. The Minister for Health is it's president. The NAC is responsible for co-ordinating state bodies, social organizations and the public in preventive activities.

A strategic policy on prevention and control of HIV/AIDS has been formulated by the Vietnamese government, incorporating short term and long-term plans which have been derived from the general policies of the international community on prevention and control of HIV/AIDS. An important point stressed by the National Programme on prevention and control of HIV/AIDS is that HIV/ AIDS is not merely a medical issue. To control the danger of the spread of HIV/AIDS, it is necessary to ensure the participation of social organizations, state bodies and community groups.

Legal Texts Directly Related to the Prevention and Control of HIV/ AIDS

On 2 December 1989, the Chairman of the Council of Ministers, in anticipation of the danger of HIV infection, issued instruction No. 339/CT, for the prevention and control of HIV/AIDS. In this document, he entrusted ministries, branches and provinces the responsibility of informing the public about the measures necessary to prevent the disease.

The document also provides for the close surveillance of groups at high risk, such as prostitutes and intravenous drug users.

Decree No-16/CP, issued by the Vietnamese government on 18 December 1992, confirms the principle of non-discrimination towards HIV/AIDS patients. It also encourages Vietnamese and expatriates to undergo HIV testing.

The Decree recognizes the principle of right to confidentiality with regard to name, age and address and of the result of tests, if requested. Furthermore, health institutions are responsible for testing for HIV blood and semen donors and donors of tissues or other organs.

Another important issue is the rights and obligations of persons infected with HIV/AIDS. The Decree provides that it is strictly forbidden for anyone who has HIV/AIDS infection to deliberately transmit the infection to others. They are responsible for protecting the community.

The Decree sets out the responsibilities of doctors and health staff. It also provides for state incentives for them.

Legal Texts Indirectly Dealing with the Prevention and Control of HIV/ AIDS

- Law on the protection of people's health provides for the compulsory treatment of diseases which are transmitted through unprotected sexual intercourse and intravenous drug use.
- Ordinance on immigration, residence and travel by expatriates in Vietnam provides the conditions for issuing visas, consistent with the prevention and control of diseases and the safety of the community.
- Ordinance on marriages between Vietnamese citizens and expatriates, issued by the Standing Committee of the National Assembly, provides the conditions, subject to which marriages can take place.
- Penal Code makes the violation of the rules of confidentiality in HIV testing an offence.

The Constitution contains a provision in Article 61 dealing with social evils such as prostitution and intravenous drug use. Their regulation can play an important role in the prevention and control of HIV/AIDS. Resolution No- 05/CP deals with the control of prostitution and resolution 06/CP with the prevention, control and supervision of drug use.

The Vietnamese government has taken steps to curb prostitution in any form, especially in cities and tourist and industrial centres. It has also launched public awareness campaigns on the harmful consequences of prostitution, particularly the transmission of HIV.

The government has entrusted the ministries and its branches responsible for the prevention and control of drug abuse and prostitution the special task of limiting the spread of HIV.

Decree No- 53,CP issued by the government provides for the actions to be taken against state employees especially directors of hotels and owners of restaurants, involved in prostitution and drug related crimes—e.g. they can be dismissed.

Legal Texts Relating to Professional Rules in Medical Settings

The Ministry of Health has issued regulations on blood transfusion and on treatment of HIV/AIDS infection. Health professionals are responsible for consulting with persons infected with HIV/AIDS so that these patients understand their disease; for encouraging them to seek treatment and actively participate in communication strategies on the prevention and control of HIV/AIDS; and instructing the patients' families to look after them and avoid discrimination.

Conclusion

The Vietnamese government has taken several steps, including legal measures, for the prevention and control of HIV/AIDS.

While the legal texts issued by the government and its branches so far have, by and large, specially addressed the prevention and control of HIV/AIDS, these texts are not very effective or systematic. Vietnam urgently needs laws promulgated by a legislative body, which address basic matters in the prevention and control of HIV/AIDS.

A new draft Ordinance on Prevention and Control of HIV/AIDS Infection is aimed at meeting these requirements. Its formulation has highlighted several difficulties, especially in balancing the rights of the individual against public interest in matters concerning the prevention and control of HIV/AIDS. For example, concrete provisions need to be provided so that they not only satisfy the requirements of non-discrimination of the infected, but also ensure the safety of the community.

64

HIV Law: The United States

Prof. Lawrence O. Gostin
Director
Johns Hopkins/Georgetown Programme on Law and
Public Health, Washington, D.C., U.S.A.

The Acquired IMMUNO Deficiency Syndrome (AIDS) epidemic poses a serious threat to public health, but its impact goes far beyond health. The burden of the disease in the United States falls predominantly on disfavoured populations intravenous drug users and gay men. Moreover, racial minorities—African-Americans and Hispanics are disproportionately burdened by the disease. Although HIV infection is spreading more rapidly among heterosexuals, they account for a relatively small section of the infected population.

Many argue that governmental and public health officials have failed to implement strong measures in deference to the civil liberties of persons at risk for HIV. Others argue that society has overreacted to the epidemic and imposed penalties and discriminatory treatment that would never have occurred if the primary targets of intervention were more popular. Not surprisingly, these two contradictory viewpoints are espoused by groups at opposite ends of the political spectrum. A deeper dimension of the AIDS epidemic, then, is political and is manifested in legislation.

Legislation related to AIDS has been enacted in every state and the District of Columbia. This AIDS-specific legislation is superimposed on a large body of existing, often obsolete, legislation governing communicable and sexually transmitted diseases.

Problems exist relating to the lack of clear criteria, fair procedures, and consistent structures.[1]

Legislation can make a rich contribution to health efforts by promoting professional standards through reasoned guidelines; by mandating and/or funding appropriate health care services and public education, particularly in sensitive areas such as sex education in schools, condom advertising, and outreach programmes for drug-dependant people; by funding research and policy development; and by safeguarding confidentiality and protecting against discrimination. Legislation, however, can also seriously inhibit health efforts by dictating the content of educational messages based on moral disapproval of sexual practices and drug use; by enacting a patchwork of exceptions to the principle of confidentiality; and by succumbing to political pressures to "get tough" on persons at increased risk of HIV through compulsory screening, isolation, and criminalizahon of HIV transmission.[2]

No other infectious disease in recent history compares with HIV in the ways it has affected our relationships with each other and with our social institutions. Sharp differences in perceptions of public health, ethics, and civil liberties have created the largest body of legal cases attributable to a single disease in the history of American jurisprudence.

Litigation related to AIDS has powerfully impacted major social institutions in the United States—schools, health care, the blood supply, the judiciary, prisons, and the military. The litigation has left an equally strong impress on cherished constitutional principles of privacy, freedom of speech and association, and liberty. The HIV epidemic has even reached into intimate personal relationships, sparking litigation against sexual partners and family members.

This chapter discusses AIDS legislation and litigation in the United States. While an essay of this length cannot provide a systematic examination of the law relating to HIV, it does touch on some of the central areas of AIDS law and policy in the United States.

AIDS Education

From the earliest moments of the HIV epidemic, educational messages were influenced not only by public health need, but also by morality and politics.[3,4] Consequently, federal funds could not be used to provide AIDS prevention materials that "promote or encourage" homosexual activities or used to support educational content that could be "judged by a reasonable person to be offensive to most educated adults."[5] Similar legislation has been enacted in the states.

The conflict between public health and morals is nowhere more evident than in educational programmes in schools. A devout religious group challenged New York's mandatory AIDS education programme as a violation of its freedom of religion. New York's highest court ordered a full hearing on the group's challenge because "we cannot summarily brush aside the passionate assertions of a unique religious group that exposure to [AIDS education] could destroy the foundations of their faith."[6] In another case, a New York court invalidated a free in-school condom distribution programme. The court found that condom distribution violated the parents' right to raise their children as they saw fit. In addition to being educational, the programme was considered a public health service and, therefore, required parental consent.[7]

Liability of Blood Collection Centres and Hospitals

Reported cases of *Pneumocystis carinii* pneumonia in persons with haemophilia[8] and blood transfusion recipients[9] in late 1982 first brought into question the safety of the national blood supply. By March 1983, the US Centers for Disease Control (CDC) had recommended self-deferral of donors who had engaged in high-risk behaviour. A test to detect antibody to HIV was not commercially available until early 1985.[10] Much of the blood supply litigation in the United States has concerned the failure of blood collection centres and hospitals to recommend self-deferral and/or screening for HIV during the early years of the epidemic. The Institute of Medicine issued a critical report about the role of the federal Food and Drug Administration (FDA) in safeguarding the blood supply after it became known that HIV was blood-borne.[11]

The major public policy issue is whether blood suppliers should be held to a standard of negligence or strict liability. Most states have blood-shield statutes that treat blood as a service rather than a product, thus avoiding strict liability. The clear trend is to use a standard of negligence, which means that no liability will ensue if the supplier complied with industry standard at the time.[12] By adopting a standard of negligence rather than strict liability, courts support the important state goal of assuring the integrity of the voluntary blood supply.[13] Some juries, however, have awarded substantial damages.[14]

Even where a blood supplier has exercised due care, there remains a small chance of receiving HIV-contaminated blood. Infected patients have brought claims for relief including failure to warn about the risk of transfusion-associated HIV-infection before obtaining consent, and failure to inform the patient about alternatives to transfusion from the general blood supply, such as directed or autologous donations.15

Epidemiological Surveillance and Disease Control

The evidence demonstrating the efficacy of zidovudine, aerosolized pentamidine isethionate, and other emerging pharmaceuticals such as dideoxyinosine has resulted in increased interest in epidemiological surveillance and disease control.[16] The ability of public health departments to identify persons exposed to HIV expeditiously through testing, reporting, and partner notification is thought to be important to effective therapeutic intervention. The evidence is mixed, however, as to whether therapeutic intervention early in the course of HIV infection is highly beneficial.[17,18,19]

The finding that perinatal transmission of HIV can be significantly reduced through the administration of zidovudine has also fuelled calls for surveillance among pregnant women and newborns, including renewed interest in routine or involuntary screening.

Reporting

While all states require reporting of CDC-defined AIDS, slightly more than half the states require reporting of HIV-positive test results. Several of the larger states, such as New York and California, still do not require reporting of HIV infection, reasoning that named HIV reporting could discourage persons at higher risk of HIV to avoid testing. New York's highest court upheld the decision of the health commissioner not to require HIV reporting.[20] Many states have adopted a parallel system in which a person can be tested anonymously for HIV infection with no reporting requirement.

Testing and Screening

HIV testing or screening of persons or populations has been challenged in a wide variety of settings, including the judiciary, corrections systems, health care, public health, insurance, and employment. Testing or screening programmes have been challenged under several legal theories, including common law informed consent, discrimination under the Americans with Disabilities Act, and search and seizure under the Fourth Amendment of the US Constitution.

The judiciary has been deferential in reviewing federal screening programmes. Federal courts have upheld screening in the Departments of State21 and Defense,[22] and in the Job Corps.[23] Courts have also upheld testing requirements of emergency service personnel such as fire fighters and paramedics.[24]

The courts have been permissive in allowing health care providers to test physicians and nurses for HIV infection, particularly where they are involved in invasive, exposure-prone procedures.[25] However, where health care providers are not engaged in invasive procedures, some courts have invalidated testing or screening programmes.[26]

Some courts have found that testing of persons for HIV infection is unlawful, where there is no clear public health rationale. For example, an Alabama court ruled that a state statute that permitted compulsory HIV testing of persons at "high risk" of infection denied them equal protection of the laws.[27] In addition, many states have enacted statutes requiring written informed consent for HIV testing.

The Criminal Law

Numerous prosecutions for risking transmission of HIV have been undertaken in the United States. Many of these cases have been brought under the general criminal law for attempted murder, assault with a dangerous of deadly weapon, or simple or aggravated assault. From a public health perspective, a threshold question in assessing the value of prosecuting persons infected with HIV is whether their behaviour poses a significant risk of viral transmission. Several cases involve sexual assaults, needle-sharing, or prostitution where there is a risk of transmission. The majority of cases, however, involve behaviours that are unlikely to transmit HIV infection. These include biting, spitting or splattering of blood.

While several prosecutions have been successful even in cases of biting or spitting,[28] many have been difficult to prosecute. It is hard to prove that a person intended to transmit HIV. People enter sexual relationships with many different intentions, desires, and fears. Causing harm through sexuality is seldom consciously planned, although both partners may be aware of the risks. Sometimes cases involve hopelessness rather than premeditation, such as a man who splattered his blood on emergency workers. He had just made a serious suicide attempt, and his first words to the emergency workers were, "Let me die, I have AIDS." He was convicted of attempted murder, and the sentence was ultimately upheld.[29] In other cases, prosecutors were unable to prove that HIV-infected blood donors attempted to kill any particular person or poison the community.[30]

Federal courts of appeal have held that the mouth and teeth of an HIV-infected person could be regarded as a "dangerous'(or "deadly" weapon.[31, 32] This is so despite the fact that the risk of transmission of HIV infection through spitting or biting is *de minimis.*[33]

Because it is not always possible to prove that an HIV-infected person intended to kill, many state legislatures have enacted AIDS specific criminal offences. These statutes make it a crime for persons to engage in specified behaviour such as sex or needle sharing knowing that they are infected with HIV; the statutes usually require persons with HIV infection to inform their partners of their serological status. Courts have upheld these HIV-specific criminal statutes.[34]

HIV Testing of Persons Charged or Convicted of Sexual Ottences

Federal law requires states to test sex offenders postconviction as a condition for receiving 10 per cent of the funds allocated to each state under the Federal Bureau of Justice Assistance Grant Programmes.[35] As of 1994, thirty two states explicitly .authorized compulsory HIV testing of sex offenders. Fifteen states allowed postconviction testing only; five permitted preconviction testing only; and seven authorized both pre- and postconviction testing. These statutory provisions vary widely on a number of key variables, including whether the survivor, through a request, may trigger the testing; and the persons who may view the results.[36]

Legislators and courts face a dilemma in deciding when, or even whether, to impose HIV testing following sexual assault. The dilemma arises because the usefulness of the information to the survivor, and the strength of the accused's privacy interests, shift over time. The survivor's strongest claim of benefit is in testing the accused as early as possible after the assault. At this point in time, the survivor will not yet have seroconverted, and may use the knowledge of the accused's serological status to decide about sexual relationships, childbearing, and treatment. However, the accused's strongest claim to protection is also early in the criminal process. Testing an accused person prior to coniction amounts to a significant invasion of autonomy and privaby without the corresponding benefit of trial to establish guilt. Yet testing the accused after conviction provides little benefit to survivors, who could then undergo their own serological testing. Consequently, any solution either diminishes the value of the information to the survivor or infringes on the legitimate interests of the accused.

Private Tort Actions

The United States has become a highly litigious society. Contracting a disease used to be perceived to be a matter of chance or inadvertent misfortune. Today, it is not unusual for an ill person to search for fault and with it, liability. Claims of lack of due care, even bad faith or betrayal, by those who have been exposed to HIV have found their way to the courts. The depth of mistrust spans many relationships: patients against their hospitals or physicians, health care professionals against the facility that employs them, one health care professional against another, and sexual partners against their heterosexual or homosexual partners.

Perhaps the most interesting line of cases involves the duty to inform sexual and needle sharing partners of the risk of HIV infection. Most courts that have heard such cases have held that persons who know they have a sexually transmitted infection have a duty to protect their sexual partners.[37,38] This duty is ordinarily taken to mean abstaining from sexual relations or, minimally, disclosing the infection prior to intercourse. For example, in the widely publicized case of Christian v. Sheft, a jury rendered a verdict against the estate of Rock Hudson for $ 14.5 million.[39] The jury concluded that at the time Mr. Christian and Mr. Hudson were engaging in "high risk" sex, Mr. Hudson knew he had AIDS, concealed that information, and intentionally misrepresented his physical condition to induce Mr. Christian to continue sexual relations.

Mr. Hudson's insurer later filed a declaration in a federal court, contesting its indemnity for the underlying state action. Accepting the lower court's findings, the Ninth Circuit Court of Appeals held that the insured's intentional misrepresentation to induce participation in "high-risk" sex constituted inherently harmful conduct under California law. The court further ruled that the insured was precluded from indemnification of the $ 14.5 million jury verdict under a statute prohibiting coverage for the wilful acts of an insured.[40]

The duty to protect a sexual partner from a known sexually transmitted disease (STD) apparently is accepted in most United.States jurisdictions. However, in another celebrated case (involving Erwin "Magic" Johnson), the court held that a similar duty does not extend to persons who *should have known* they were infected.[41] Thus, if a person has engaged in sex with multiple partners, he may not be liable for failing to inform his partner, provided he has not been tested and does not know his HIV-status.

Special Populations: Prisons

The HIV epidemic in the corrections systems, particularly in high prevalence areas, is disturbing. A closed environment in which there may be homosexual contact,.needle sharing, and sexual assaults may be conducive to the spread of HIV. Surveys in the United States have demonstrated high levels of HIV infection in the federal and state corrections systems.[42] The critical policy question is whether the usual public health strategy of testing and treatment on a fully consensual basis can work in closed institutions. Most of the litigation in the prison system concerns decisions whether to screen for HIV and isolate those infected; other litigation has involved claims that persons infected with HIV were not provided with adequate medical treatment.

Courts have tended to uphold the decisions of prison officials to screen the inmate population as well as decisions not to screen. Inmates concerned about the risk of contracting HIV in prison have sued corrections systems to require them to institute screening and segregation of HIV-positive inmates. These claims are based on the Eighth Amendment of the Constitution which prohibits cruel and unusual punishment. The Eighth Amendment has been construed to require corrections officials to protect inmates form contracting communicable diseases.[43] HIV-negative prisoners argued that compulsory screening and segregation are necessary to prevent the spread of HIV infection in prison. Most courts have rejected these claims on the grounds that the evidence was insufficient both to demonstrate a real risk of transmission and to show that screening or segregation would reduce the risk.[44]

Many courts have also rejected claims by HIV-positive inmates that their civil rights were violated when corrections officials required screening and segregation.[45] These courts reason that control of disease within prisons and jails is largely within the discretion of correction officials. Still, courts have struck down segregation in an "AIDS unit" because it violated the privacy rights of inmates infected with HIV.[46, 47]

Inmates have complained that they have not received adequate medical treatment for HIV disease. The complaints in these cases included failure to diagnose HIV disease, misdiagnosis, and refusal to treat *Pneumocystis* pneumonia and to provide zidovudine. Prisoners with HIV claimed they were deprived of social, recreational, and rehabilitative opportunities, family visits, and education.[48, 49] The Supreme Court has set a highly permissive standard under the Eighth Amendment for prison officials, and courts have rarely upheld claims of mistreatment or inadequate treatment by HIV-infected inmates.[50]

Policies designed to control the spread of HIV in prisons should consider the terms of progressive consent decrees which provide that no housing area can be specifically designated for HIV-infected inmates. Infected inmates must be given primary and specialized health care, counselling, prophylaxis for HIV-related conditions, recreation, association, and privileges.[51]

Privacy and Confidentiality

Strong ethical reasons exist for protecting the privacy of persons with HIV infection.[52, 53] An important justification for privacy resides in the principle of respect for autonomy. To respect the privacy of persons with HIV/AIDS is to respect their wishes not to be observed or to have intimate information about themselves made available to others. Privacy also enhances the development of trust in the physician. One of the defining characteristics of the doctor-patient relationship is that it involves the sharing—freely given—of private information. Failure to respect the confidentiality of patient drives patients away from HIV testing, counselling and treatment, and discourages patients from confiding in their physicians.

Unwanted disclosure of intimate health information can cause patients a great deal of emotional, social, and economic harm. Stigmatization may be a consequence of such disclosure, particularly when HIV infection reveals the person's sexual orientation or use of illegal drugs. Disclosure can cause embarrassment, social isolation, and loss of employment or employability, insurance or insurability, or housing.

The majority of states have statutes protecting the confidentiality of HIV-related information. The early states were very explicit in prohibiting disclosure of an HIV test result without written consent. State legislatures at that time had given little thought to the public health responsibility to identified third parties from unknowing exposure to HIV. More recent statutes have been much more permissive in authorizing disclosure to third parties. They often allow disclosure to sexual or needle sharing partners. Many statutes, however, have so many exceptions that they swallow up the rule of confidentiality. They may permit disclosure to emergency workers or "first responders" (e.g., ambulance workers or emergency room personnel), police, prisons officials, funeral workers, health care workers, laboratory workers, and school officials.

The Media

Although most states have statutes protecting the confidentiality of information concerning an individual's HIV infection, the courts have allowed the media considerable leeway in presenting information to the public. In a criminal case in Florida, an individual was accused of biting a store owner during an attempted robbery. The court decided to make the hearing public since the issue was already discussed in some public documents.[54]

When a defendant's identity has already become public, he may not even be covered by a specific confidentiality act. Accordingly, a television station was permitted to broadcast the name of a person charged with the criminal transmission of HIV.[55] In another case, a newspaper was allowed to publish the names of three nurses injured by an HIV-positive patient. The court felt that the matters were not private and that, in fact, they were of legitimate public concern.[56]

The "Right to Know"

The HIV epidemic has posed two powerful, and conflicting, legal and ethical obligations. The first obligation, just discussed, is to respect the privacy of persons with HIV infection. The threat of stigma and discrimination has had a profound impact on the extent to which persons with HIV/AIDS have demanded iron-clad legal protections of confidentiality. The second obligation is the duty to inform persons who may be exposed to HIV. The public claims the right to know if their sexual or needle sharing partners are infected with HIV. Persons have a legitimate ethical claim that they ought not be exposed to significant danger without their knowledge and consent. Courts, moreover, have found physicians liable for failure to inform persons of the risk of HIV infection. Thus, physicians face dual ethical loyalties and legal obligations: to maintain the confidences of patients and to reveal confidential information to persons at significant risk of contracting HIV infection. In countries with a litigious culture, like the United States, physicians are caught in an inescapable dilemma.

Consider the case of Jennifer Lawson, recently decided by an appellate court in California. The day after 12-year-old Jennifer received a transfusion, her doctor discovered that the blood was contaminated with HIV. Jennifer, however, was never informed. Three years later Jennifer began dating Daniel Reesner, and she still was unaware of her infection. Later she was diagnosed with AIDS and died one month after the diagnosis. After learning of his girlfriend's death, Daniel tested positive for HIV. Did the physician have an obligation to inform Jennifer? If he failed to inform Jennifer, could he be held liable to her boyfriend many years later? The California court answered both questions in the affirmative. There exists little doubt that in most United States jurisdictions, physicians have a legal duty to disclose a positive-HIV test result to his or her patient. All patients have the right to be informed of relevant information about their own body and health. It is likely also that many courts would find it a duty to warn known sexual and needle sharing partners. Nearly two decades ago the California Supreme Court, in the landmark case of *Tarasoff v. the Regents of University of California,*[57] found that physicians have a legal duty to inform known third parties of significant risks posed by their patients.

Is there any principled way to reconcile the dual obligations of the right to privacy and the right to know? If one takes the ethical and legal right to privacy seriously, then it ought to yield only where it is absolutely necessary to avert a serious harm. Accordingly, the right to confidentiality ought to be near absolute in cases where the risk of contracting HIV is remote. Thus, claims by health care professionals, emergency workers, prison guards, and others for this sensitive information ought to be denied if the patient refuses to consent to the disclosure.

The strongest claim to a right to know exists where there is an ongoing sexual or needle sharing relationship. In such cases, the law should give health care professionals a power, not a duty, to disclose if in their judgment it is necessary to avert a significant risk of transmission. Health care professionals should first counsel the patient to make the disclosure himself or herself. Framing the law in this way permits health care professionals to exercise their judgment; they can decide whether maintenance of the confidence and trust of patients overrides the rights of their partners. If the health care professional exercises a diligent good faith judgment, he or she ought not to risk legal liability in a case where society itself is unable to resolve this powerful ethical and legal dilemma.

Discrimination

Every major government,[58] medical,[59] and public health[60] organization to issue a report on the HIV epidemic has condemned discrimination because it violates basic tenets of individual justice and is detrimental to public health. Discrimination based on an infectious condition is just as inequitable as discrimination based on race, gender, or disability. In each case, people are treated inequitably not because they lack inherent ability, but solely because of a status over which they have no control. Complex and often pernicious mythologies develop about the nature, cause, and transmission of disease. Society's accumulated myths and fears about disability and disease are just as handicapping as are the physical limitations that flow from actual impairment. Few aspects of handicap give rise to the same level of public fear and misapprehension as contagiousness,[61] as the US Supreme Court has recognized.

Persons with HIV infection have to endure not only archaic attitudes that they present a health menace, but also moral disapprovai of their behaviour. The public association of the disease with traditionally disfavoured groups—gay men, intravenous drug uses, and commercial sex workers—only compounds the bigotry.

In the United States, at least two different classes of statute proscribe discrimination. The first, HIV-specific antidiscrimination statutes, have been enacted in most states. These statutes make it unlawful to discriminate against persons with HIV infection in jobs, public accommodations, housing, and other areas. The second group of statutes prohibi discrimination against persons with disabilities. Disability dis crimination statutes have been widely enacted at state and local levels. More importantly, several disability discrimination statutes have been enacted at the federal level, including the Rehabilitation Act, the Fair Housing Act, and the Americans with Disabilities Act.

By far the most important statute prohibiting discrimination against persons with HIV/AIDS is the Americans with Disabilities Act of 1990 (ADA). A finding of discrimination under the ADA requires adverse treatment of the person in employment (Title I), public services (Title II), or public accommodations (Title III). The person must: (i) have a *"disability"*; and (ii) be *"qualified"* (or be qualified if *"reasonable accommodations"* were offered).

Disability is defined broadly in the ADA to mean: (i) a physical or mental impairment that substantially limits one or more of the major life activities (i.e. a current disability); (ii) a record of such impairment (i.e., a survivor of a past disability); or (iii) being regarded as having such an impairment (i.e., a perception of a disability, even if the person is in fact not disabled).[62]

"Physical or mental impairment" includes: (i) any physiological disorder or condition, disfigurement or anatomical loss affecting any of the major bodily systems; or (ii) any mental or physiological disorder, such as mental retardation or mental illness. The legislative history as well as the prior caselaw, make clear that "disability" includes diseases and infections which are communicable (e.g., tuberculosis and hepatitis) as well as those which are not (e.g., cancer, heart disease, arthritis, diabetes and epilepsy). In particular, it is clear that persons with HIV infection, even if asymptomatic,[63] are covered by the ADSA.[64]

A person is "qualified" if he or she is capable of meeting rhe essential performance or eligibility criteria for the particular job, service, or benefit. Thus, a person with a disability is not protected unless he or she is qualified to hold the job or to receive or benefit.

Qualification standards can include a requirement that the person with a disability does not pose a direct threat to the health or safety of others. The "direct threat" standard means that persons can be excluded from jobs, public accommodations, or public services, if necessary, to prevent a "significant risk" to others.

The ADA or other disability legislation has been used, for example, to require health care providers to reasonably treat persons with HIV infection; to require employers to treat them fairly at work; and to require landlords or owners of public accommodations not to unfairly exclude them.

Non-discrimination for persons infected with HIV is consistent with a prevailing sense of justice. With continued AIDS education, rigorous enforcement of disability laws, and increased tolerance and respect for all persons associated with HIV—gay men, women, drug users, and others — discrimination can be reduced and, with it, public health advanced.

Conclusion

This review of AIDS legislation and litigation in the United States reveals a mixed record. Many jurisdictions in the United States have come to accept the health service research showing the sometimes remarkable efficacy of well-targeted education and counselling and the promise of therapy. So too there has been wide acceptance of the critical public health importance of confidentiality and guarantees of anti-discrimination. Even here, however, state legislatures are reducing the confidentiality protections offered, and the federal government is considering amendments to the ADA. Ensuring the privacy and equal treatment of persons with HIV/AIDS is essential to the success of public health programmes. Public health officials will not gain the confidence and co-operation of affected individuals if these individuals are not legally protected from stigma and irrational prejudice.

While legislators and the judiciary have responded reasonably well in the areas of confidentiality and anti-discrimination, they have often succumbed to political pressures. Government has sometimes posed obstacles to effective education, making morality more important than health; and it has used coercive powers and criminalisation in cases where the risk of HIV transmission was negligible.

Legal reform in the HIV epidemic ought to be guided by one overriding maxim: *Good law ought to follow sound scientific* and *ethical principles.*

REFERENCES

1. Gostin L.O. The future of public health law. *American Journal of Law and Medicine,* 1987; 12(3-4): 461-90.
2. Gostin L..O. A decade of a maturing epidemic: as Assessment and directions for future public policy. *American Journal of Law and Medicine,* 1990; 16(1,2): 1-32.
3. Bayer R. *Private Acts, Social Consequences: AIDS and the Politics of Public Health.* New Brunswick, New Jersy: Rutgers University Press, 1989.
4. Barnes, M. Towards ghastly death: the censorship of AIDS education. *Columbia Law Review* 1989; 89: 698-724.
5. Pub. L. No. 100-706.
6. *Ware v. Valley Street High School District,* 1989 WL 156177 (NY 1989).
7. *Alfonso v. Fernandez,* 606 N.Y.S. 2d 259 (N.Y. App.Div. 1993).
8. Centres for Disease Control. Pneumocystis carinii pneumonia among persons with hemophilia A. *Morbidity and Mortality Weekly Report* 1982: 31: 365-7.
9. Centres for Disease Control. Possible transfusion-associated acquired immunodeficiency syndrome-California. *Morbidity and Mortality Weekly Report* 1982; 31: 652-4.
10. Centres for Disease Control. Provisional public health service interagency recommendations for screening donated blood and plasma for antibody to the virus causing acquired immunodeficiency syndrome. *Morbidity and Mortality Weekly Report* 1985; 34:1-5.
11. Government is blamed in AIDS deaths, New York Times 1995, July 14: A15 (col 5).
12. *Coffee v. Cutter Biological,* 809 F.2d 191 (2d Cir. 1987).
13. *Spence v Miles Laboratories,* 27 F.3d 1185 (6th Cir. 1994).

14. *Carroll v. Blood Centre of SE Wiseconsin, Wis.* Cir. Ct.: *AIDS Litigation Reporter,* March 24, 1989.
15. *Valdiviez v. United States,* 884 F.2d 196 (5th Cir. 1989).
16. Volberding P.A., Lagakos S.W., Grimes J.M. *et al.* The duration of zidovudine benefit in persons with asymptomatic HIV infection: prolonged evaluation of protocol 019 of the AIDS Clinical Trials Group. *Journal of the American Medical Association* 1994; 272: 437-42.
17. Ho DD. Time to hit HIV, early and hard. *New England Journal of Medicine* 1995; 333: 450-1.
18. Kinloch-de Loes S., Hirschel B.J., Hoen B. A controlled trial of zidovudine in primary human immunodeficiency virus infection. *New England Journal of Medicine* 1995; 333: 408-13.
19. Volberding P.A., Lagakos S.W., Grimes J.M. *et al.* A comparison of immediate with deferred zidovudine therapy for asymptomatic HIV-infected adults with CD4 cell counts of 500 or more per cubic millimeter. *New England Journal of Medicine* 1995; 333: 401-7.
20. *New York State Society of Surgeons v. Axelrod,* 77 N.Y. 2d 677 (1991).
21. Local 1812, *American Federation of Government Employees v. United States Department of State,* 662 F, Supp. 50 (D.D.C. 1987).
22. *Batten v. Lehman,* No. CA 85-4108 (U.S.D.C. Jan. 8, 1986).
23. *Dorsey v. U.S. Department of Labour,* No. 88-1898 (D.D.C.).
24. *Anonymous Fireman v. City of Willoughby,* 779 F. Supp. 402 (N.D. Ohio 1991).
25. *Leckelt v. Board of Commissioners of Hospital District No.1, 909* F.2d 820 (5th Cir. 1990).
26. *Glover v. Eastern Nebraska Community Office of Retardation,* 686 F.Supp. 243, affirmed, 867 F.2d 461 (8th Cir. 1989).
27. *Hill v. Evans, U.S.* District Court for the Middle District of Alabama, No.91-A-626-N (1993).
28. *State v. Smith,* 262 N.J. Super. 487, 621 A.2d 493, cert. denied, 134 N.J. 476, (1993).
29. *State v. Haines,* 545 N.E.2d 834 (Ind. Ct. App. 1989).
30. *People v. Markowitz,* Super Ct, LA Cal; *AIDS Litigation Reports* March 11, 1988.
31. *United States v. Sturgis,* 1995 U.S. App. LEXIS 3925.
32. *United States v. Moore,* 846 F.2d 1163 (8th Cir. 1988).
33. Gostin LO. The politics of AIDS: compulsory state powers, public health and civil liberties. *Ohio State Law Journal* 1989; 59(4):1017-58.
34. *State v. Gamberella,* 633 So. 2d 595, cert. denied, 640 So. 2d 1341 (La 1994).
35. 42 U.S.C. @ 3756(f) (1993).
36. Gostin L.O. *et al.*, HIV testing, counselling, and prophylaxis after sexual assault. *Journal of the American Medical Association* 1994; 271: 1436, 1439.
37. *Meany v. Meany,* 639 So. 2d 229 (La. 1994).
38. *Zysk v. Zysk,* 239 Va. 32, 404 S.E. 2d 721 (S. Ct. Va. 1990).
39. No. C 574153 (Cal. Super. Ct. Feb. 17, 1989).
40. *Aetna Casualty & Sur. Co. v. Sheft,* 989 F.2d 1105 (9th Cir. 1993).
41. *Doe v. Johnson,* 817 F. Supp. 1382 (WD Mich. 1993).
42. Hammett T. *et al.* 1992 *Update: HIV/AIDS in U.S. Prisons and Jails,* Washington D.C.: U.S. Department of Justice, 1994.
43. Gostin L.O. The resurgent tuberculosis epidemic in the era of AIDS: reflections on public health, law, and society. *Maryland Law Review* 1995; 54:1-131.
44. *Holt v. Norris,* 871 F.2d 1087 (6th Cir. 1989).
45. *Harris v. Thigpen,* 941 F.2d 1495 (11th Cir. 1991).

46. *Doe v. Coughlin,* 697 F. Supp. 1234 (NDNY 1988).
47. *Nolley v. Country of Erie,* 776 F.Supp 715 (WDNY 1991).
48. *Feighley v. Fulcomer,* 1989 U.S. Dist. LEXIS 9913 (MD Pa.).
49. *Doe v. Coughlin,* 521 N.E. 2d 446 (1988).
50. *Turner v. Safley,* 482 U.S. 78 (1987).
51. Burris S. Prisons, Law, and public health: the case for a co-ordinated response to epidemic diseases behind bars. *University of Miami Law Review;* 1992; 47:291.
52. Gostin L.O., Turek-Brezina J., Powers M. Privacy and security of personal information in a new health care system. *Journal of the American Medical Association* 1993; 270:2487-93.
53. Gostin L.O. Health information privacy. *Cornell Law Review* 1995; 80:101-84.
54. *State v. Jenki* , 1993 WL 556594 (F1.Cir. Ct., Sept. 17, 1993).
55. *In re Application of Multimedia KSDK,* 581 N.E.2d 911 (111.App. Ct. 1991).
56. *Dinkel v. Lincoln Publishing,* 638 N.E.2d (Ohio Ct. App. 1994).
57. 551 P.2d 334 (S.Ct. Cal. 1976).
58. *Report of the Presidential Commission on the Human Immunodeficiency Virus Epidemic.* Washington D.C.: U.S. Government Printing Office, 1988.
59. Institute of Medicine. *Confronting AIDS: Directions for Public Health Care and Research.* Washington D.C.: National Academy Press, 1986.
60. Centers for Disease Control. *Recommended Additional Guidelines for Antibody Counselling and Testing in the Prevention of HIV Infection and AIDS.* Washington D.C.: US Public Health Service, 1987.
61. *School Board of Nassau County v. Arline,* 107 S. Ct. 1123 (1987).
62. 42 U.S.C. 12111 (1992).
63. *Doe v. Centinela Hospital,* 57 U.S.L.W. 2034 (C.D. Cal. 1988).
64. *Chalk v. United District Court,* 840 F.2d 701 (9th Cir. 1988).

65

HIV/AIDS Law and Law Reform in Western Samoa

Dr. Kamuta Seuseu
Director
Preventive Health Services
Apia Western Samoa

Fagaloa Tufuga
State Solicitor
Attorney General's Office
Western Samoa

National Programme

The AIDS programme was formulated jointly by Government officials and WHO consultants in 1987. The Short-Term Plan was approved and implemented from 1988 to 1990. A Medium-Term Plan was formulated to cover the period 1991 to 1993.

Legal Framework

Due to the colonial historical background some of the existing laws reflect measures that were perhaps seen relevant by the legislators at the time but questionable today. The existing Health Ordinance from 1959 is one example of that colonial legacy. AIDS is not listed as one of the infectious diseases in the schedule of the Health Ordinance, 1959. However, the Western Samoa Government in 1987/88 specified, by notification in the Government Gazette HIV/AIDS as an infectious disease. Infectious disease is defined in the Ordinance as:

"any disease for the time being specified in the First

Schedule to this Ordinance, and includes any other disease which may be declared by the Minister by notice in the Western Samoa Gazette to be an infectious disease."

Part IV of the Ordinance deals specifically with infectious diseases.

The following sections are relevant in the context of HIV/AIDS:

Section 29 - The Director has special powers subject to Minister's approval for the purpose of preventing the outbreak or spread of any infectious disease.

Section 29 (c) - The Director may require persons to report themselves or submit themselves for medical examination at specified times and places.

Section 29 (h) - The Director may forbid persons to leave the place in which they are isolated or quarantined until they have been medically examined and found to be free from infectious disease, and until they have undergone such treatment as prescribed.

Section 36 - The Director has the power to isolate persons likely to spread infectious diseases. That is, the Director may do such things if expedient to do so in the interest of public health.

A new Bill entitled "The Health of the People Bill 1995/96" has already been drafted and is now ready to be tabled in Parliament. This Bill is an attempt to amend and consolidate the laws relating to the health of Samoan people. It is also an attempt to bring together all laws relating to the health of Samoan people instead of isolating different aspects relating to health of the people. In short, the Bill, amongst other things, covers dental practitioners, medical practitioners, nurses, etc. AIDS is not listed in the schedule as an infectious disease.

Immigration Act 1966

This legislation is also relevant in relation to HIV/AIDS issues.

There was a recent incident in Western Samoa when two visitors (tourists) were ordered by the Minister of Immigration to leave Western Samoa pursuant to S.13(1)(a) of the Act. One of the tourists was HIV positive according to information relayed by New Zealand authorities to the immigration authorities in Samoa. Both health and immigration authorities interviewed the two tourists and they also subsequently found some drugs in their possession. They claimed and voluntarily admitted that such drugs were used to re lieve pain. The relevant authorities, therefore, advised the Minister to exercise his powers under Section 13(1)(a) of the Act.

In terms of this section the:

> "Minister may, by order signed by him and served on any immigrant, stating one or more of the grounds set out in this subsection, order the immigrant to leave Western Samoa within a period from the date of service to be stated in the order, if he is of the opinion, based on the information or advice received from a source considered by him to be reliable:
>
> (a) that the immigrant is disaffected or likely to be in danger to the peace, order, or good Government of Western Samoa, or to be otherwise an undesirable immigrant".

The action taken has been the subject of debate. Under the Act the decision of the Minister is final and conclusive and cannot be questioned in proceedings before a court of law.

Law Reform

Western Samoa does not have a mechanism such as a Law Commission. Although the Attorney-General's Office plays a major role in screening, revising and drafting legislation, Government Departments would usually instruct the Attorney-General's office to draft amendments before draft laws are presented in Parliament and the Attorney-General does not have the manpower to do such tasks. There is only one Parliamentary Counsel who deals specifically with drafting legislation. It would be ideal to engage a group of lawyers to focus entirely on making recommendations on what amendments are needed for any legislation. Solicitors working in the Attorney-General's Office do not have the time for revising legislation as they have other duties, especially litigation on behalf of the State.

Problems

1. Funding—rely on outside financial aid.
2. Expertise/consultants limited—there is a need to engage outside expertise.
3. No guarantee that draft legislation or amendments will be approved by Parliament.

Prospects

It is possible that, in responding to AIDS, the country will be forced to face up to realities, and to adopt urgently more realistic, honest and sensible laws and policies.

Any specific legislation that deals with HIV/AIDS must follow policies already established by the National AIDS Co-ordinating Council (NACC).

It is impossible to lay down universal rules for HIV prevention because of the diversity of the region. Law responds to local needs and reflects local culture. It grows out of local institutions. But such laws must incorporate the right principles in accordance with the regional standards and also the global standards. The laws should have the "right mix" of both the local and external factors.

While it is easy to pass legislation it is necessary to look at the consequences and the resources necessary for implementation.

Conclusions

It is not known as to what extent political leaders will be willing to face the very hard choices that will need to be made if there is to be a real effort at AIDS prevention, as distinct from enacting oppressive or ineffective laws.

The existing legislation, namely the Health Ordinance 1959 and the Immigration Act 1966, are inadequate.

People are free to travel to Samoa, but they do not declare their HIV status, etc. Therefore, there is a risk that carriers of the virus would transmit the virus to the locals.

There is a debate over the issue of confidentiality and right of the public to know. The nature of traditional Samoan society makes it hard for any individual to maintain his/her privacy or confidentiality (i.e., the conflict between individual rights and the public rights).

66

Facts for Moot Case (Trial)

FACTS

Mr. A regularly donates blood as a meritorious deed. He last donated blood two months ago. A few days later the public health officer of his village had come to the factory where he was the manager and had directed him to report to the general hospital. He had been taken away in a police jeep and had not returned home that night. His friend Mr. B had informed Mrs. A, his pregnant wife, that Mr. A had been taken away in a police jeep. It was only after unsuccessfully trying to track him down for two days that Mrs. A had come to know that her husband was being detained at the Infectious Diseases Hospital.

When Mrs. A had presented herself at the Hospital to see her husband she had been asked as to when the baby was due. When she had replied that she was seven months pregnant she too had been detained in another ward in the same hospital. On hearing what had happened to Mr. A, his father, had consulted the District Medical Officer who had refused to intervene on the ground that under the new AIDS Prevention Law he cannot disclose any information concerning patients at the Infectious Diseases Hospital. This law provides for detention upto six months of persons engaging in "high-risk" activities.

On returning home Mr. A's father had informed his wife that there was nothing more that he could have possibly done to help his son and daughter-in-law, but his wife had insisted that he should seek your help to file action.

Action is filed by Mr. A's father against:

(a) the Attorney-General as representing the Government; and

(b) the District Medical Officer.

On the day of hearing, a newspaper reporter is present in the court premises and threatens to publish the names and photographs of Mr. A and his wife, Mrs. A.

HIV-Ralated Specific Laws

The only statute in the country specific to EB is HIV is the new AIDS Prevention Law. This law has only two provisions. Section 1 empowers the health authorities to detain upto six months any person engaging in "high risk" activities. Section 2 states that no information can be provided to any member of the public concerning persons detained at the Infectious Diseases Hospital.

General Law

Under the general law an action can be institute; against the Attorney-General for any legal complaint against the Government The Constitution provides for the validity of laws to be challenged even after the law has come into operation. In addition to the remedy for damages, the law provides for the following: actions:

(1) writ of habeas corpus (for the release of persons held illegally or without authority);

(2) declaration of 'right' or 'status';

(3) writ of mandamus to compel a public authority to perform a duty; and

(4) an injunction to restrain from performing any act.

Admissions

The Counsel for the Plaintiff must first set out the facts, the reliefs claimed and the law applicable. All parties admit the facts stated on page 1, but the Counsel for the 1st and 2nd Defendants do not agree that there has been any violation of the law or any irregular or unauthorized act.

67

Hypothetical Legislative Measures

You are the Minister of Health. A committee headed by the Minister of Justice has prepared a draft HIV/AIDS Prevention and Control Bill. The other members of the committee were the Attorney-General, the Director General of Health, the Director General of Social Services, the Chief of Police, a senior Judge of the Supreme Court and representatives of associations of lawyers, doctors, social workers and non-governmental organizations. At a Cabinet Meeting, you are requested by the Prime Minister to express your views on the desirability of including the following provisions proposed unanimously by the committee:

1. A requirement to subject to compulsory testing for HIV "any person" whom a police officer or a public health inspector suspects to be a drug addict, a homosexual or a sex worker.
2. A requirement for foreign visitors intending to reside for more than two weeks to be tested for HIV within 10 days of their arrival, and thereafter at intervals of six months.
3. A requirement to quarantine all nationals who are HIV seropositive and to deport all seropositive foreign nationals.
4. A requirement to prohibit nationals from marrying foreigners.
5. A requirement to provide free needles, syringes and condoms to all drug addicts who are registered with the

police.

6. A requirement to permit commercial sex establishments to employ as sex workers only those in possession of a HIV free certificate issued by a government doctor during the past six months.
7. A requirement to compulsorily pre-screen for HIV all job applicants and new university undergraduates.
8. A requirement for the compulsory teaching of sex education from the primary school level upwards.
9. A requirement to make the presence of infection with HIV or STD a ground for divorce.
10. A requirement for the compulsory use of condoms in all commercial sex encounters.
11. A requirement that medical practitioners who are HIV seropositive must inform all patients with whom they come into physical contact their HIV status at the earliest possible opportunity.
12. A requirement to prohibit newspapers from reporting the names of persons with HIV or AIDS.

68

Paris AIDS Summit (1 December 1994) Declaration

The following is the text of the Declaration adopted by the Heads of Government or Representatives of the 42 States which participated in the Summit (which was organized by the French Government and WHO):

"We, the Heads of Government or Representatives of the 42 States assembled in Paris on 1 December 1994:

I. Mindful

* that the AIDS pandemic, by virtue of its magnitude, constitutes a threat to humanity,
* that its spread is affecting all societies,
* that it is hindering social and economic development, in particular of the worst affected countries, and increasing the disparities within and between countries,
* that poverty and discrimination are contributing factors in the spread of the pandemic,
* that HIV/AIDS inflicts irreparable damage on families and communities,
* that the pandemic concerns all people without distinction but that women, children and youth are becoming infected at an increasing rate,
* that it not only causes physical and emotional suffering but

it is often used as justification for grave violations of human rights,

* that obstacles of all kinds—cultural, legal, economic and political—are hampering information, prevention, care and support efforts,
* that HIV/AIDS prevention and care and support strategies are inseparable, and hence must be an integral component of an effective and comprehensive approach to combating the pandemic,
* that new local, national and international forms of solidarity are emerging, involving in particular people living with HIV/AIDS and community-based organizations,

II. Solemnly Declare

* our obligation as political leaders to make the fight against HIV/AIDS a priority,
* our obligation to act with compassion for and in solidarity with those with HIV or at risk of becoming infected, both within our societies and internationally,
* our determination to ensure that all persons living with HIV/AIDS are able to realize the full and equal enjoyment of their fundamental rights and freedoms without distinction and under all circumstances,
* our determination to fight against poverty, stigmatization and discrimination,
* our determination to mobilize all of society—the public and private sectors, community-based organizations and people living with HIV/AIDS— in a spirit of true partnership,
* our appreciation and support for the activities and work carried out by multilateral, intergovernmental, nongovernmental and community-based organizations, and our recognition of their important role in combating the pandemic,
* our conviction that only more vigorous and better co-ordinated action worldwide, sustained over the long-term—such as that to be undertaken by the joint and co-sponsored United Nations programme on HIV/AIDS—can halt the pandemic,

III. Undertake in Our National Policies to

* protect and promote the rights of individuals, in particular

those living with or most vulnerable to HIV/ AIDS, through the legal and social environment,

* fully involve the non-governmental and community based organizations as well as people living with HIV/AIDS in the formulation and implementation of public policies,
* ensure equal protection under the law for persons living with HIV/AIDS with regard to access to health care, employment, education travel, housing and social welfare,
* intensify the following range of essential approaches for the prevention of HIV/AIDS:
    - promotion of and access to various culturally acceptable prevention strategies and products, including condoms and treatment of sexually transmitted diseases,
    - promotion of appropriate prevention education, including sex and gender education, for youth in school and out of school,
    - improvement of women's status, education and living conditions,
    - specific risk-reduction activities for and in collaboration with the most vulnerable populations, such as groups at high risk of sexual transmission and migrant populations the safety of blood and blood products,
* strengthen primary health care systems as a basis for prevention and care, and integrate HIV/AIDS activities into these systems, so as to ensure equitable access to comprehensive care,
* make available necessary resources to better combat the pandemic, including adequate support for people infected with HIV/AIDS, nongovernmental organizations and community-based organizations working with vulnerable populations,

IV. Are resolved to step up intonational co-operation through the following measures and initiatives. We shall do so by providing our commitment and support to the development of the joint and co-sponsored United Nations programme on HIV/AIDS, as the appropriate framework to reinforce partnerships between all involved and give guidance and worldwide leadership in the fight against HIV/AIDS. The scope of each initiative should be further defined and developed in the context of the joint and co-sponsored programme and other appropriate fora:

1. Support greater involvement of people living with HIV/

AIDS through an initiative to strengthen the capacity and coordination of networks of people living with HIV/AIDS and community-based organizations. By ensuring their full involvement in our common response to the pandemic at all—national, regional and global-levels, this initiative will, in particular, stimulate the creation of supportive political, legal and social environments.

2. Promote global collaboration for HIV/AIDS research by supporting national and international partnerships between the public and private sectors, in order to accelerate the development of prevention and treatment technologies, including vaccines and microbicides, and to provide for the measures needed to help ensure their accessibility in developing countries. This collaborative effort should include related social and behavioural research.
3. Strengthen international collaboration for blood safety with a view to co-ordinating technical information, proposing standards for good manufacturing practices for all blood products, and fostering the establishment and implementation of co-operative partnerships to ensure blood safety in all countries.
4. Encourage a global care initiative so as to reinforce the national capability of countries, especially those in greatest need, to ensure access to comprehensive care and social support services, essential drugs and existing preventive methods.
5. Mobilize local, national and international organizations assisting as part of their regular activities children and youth, including orphans, at risk of infection or affected by HIV/AIDS, in order to encourage a global partnership to reduce the impact of the HIV/AIDS pandemic upon the world's children and youth.
6. Support initiatives to reduce the vulnerability of women to HIV/AIDS by encouraging national and international efforts, aimed at the empowerment of women: by raising their status and eliminating adverse social, economic and cultural factors; by ensuring their participation in all decision-making and implementation processes which concern them; and by establishing linkages and strengthening the networks that promote women's rights.

7. Strengthen national and international mechanisms that are concerned with HIV/AIDS related human rights and ethics, including the use of an advisory council and national and regional networks to provide leadership, advocacy and guidance in order to ensure that non-discrimination, human rights and ethical principles form an integral part of the response to the pandemic.

We urge all countries and the international community to provide the resources necessary for the measures and initiatives mentioned above.

We call upon all countries, the future joint and co-sponsored United Nations programme on HIV/AIDS and its six member organizations and programmes to take all steps possible to implement this Declaration in co-ordination with multilateral and bilateral aid programmes and intergovernmental and non-governmental organizations..."

Paris, 1 December 1994

Argentina
Australia
Bahamas
Belgium
Brazil
Burundi
Cambodia
Cameroon
Canada
China
Cote D'Ivoire
Denmark
Djibouti
Finland
France
Germany
India
Indonesia
Italy
Japan
Mexico
Morocco
Mozambique
Netherlands
Norway
Philippines
Portugal
Republic of Russia
Romania
Senegal
Spain
Sweden
Switzerland
Tanzania
Thailand
Tunisia
Uganda
United Kingdom
United States of America
Vietnam
Zambia
Zimbabwe

69

United Nations Commission on Human Rights Resolution on HIV/AIDS

(Resolution 1994/49 Adopted on 4 March 1994)

Resolution 1994/49 on the protection of human rights in the context of human immunodeficiency virus (HIV) and acquired immunodeficiency syndrome (AIDS) (adopted on 4 March 1994):

"The Commission on Human Rights,

Convinced that HIV-AIDS related discrimination is a contravention of the fundamental principle of non-discrimination as reaffirmed in the Vienna Declaration and Programme of Action, adopted by the World Conference on Human Rights,

Recalling General Assembly resolutions 46/203 of 20 December 1991 and 45/187 of 21 December 1990, Economic and Social Council resolution 1990/86 of 27 July 1990, World Health Assembly resolutions WHA 41.24 of 13 May 1988, WHA 43.10 of 16 May 1990, WHA 45.35 of 14 May 1992 and WHA 46.37 of 14 May 1993, general recommendation 15 of the Committee on the Elimination of Discrimination Against Women and other relevant resolutions and decisions adopted by organizations of the United Nations system, as well as by other competent forums,

Recalling its resolution 1990/65 of 7 March 1990, in which it endorsed the appointment by the Sub-Commission on Prevention of Discrimination and Protection of Minorities of Mr. Luis Varela Quiros to undertake a study on problems and causes of discrimination against people infected with HIV or people with AIDS, and its resolutions 1992/56 of 3 March 1992 and 1993/53 of 9 March 1993 concerning discrimination against people with HIV infection or AIDS,

Acknowledging the significant role of the World Health Organization, within the framework of the global strategy for the prevention and control of AIDS, in combating discrimination against HIV-infected persons, including people with AIDS,

Recognizing the major contribution made by national and international non-governmental organizations in particular organizations of people with HIV/AIDS, and the International Federation of Red Cross and the Red Crescent Societies in fighting discrimination against and advocating the rights of people living with HIV/AIDS,

Noting with appreciation the Rights and Humanity Declaration and Charter on HIV/AIDS, transmitted to the Commission at its forty-eighth session by the Permanent Mission of the Gambia to the United Nations (E/CN.4/1992/82),

Recognizing that the challenges presented by HIV/AIDS require renewed efforts to ensure universal respect for and observance of human rights and fundamental freedoms for all,

Concerned that lack of full enjoyment of their fundamental rights by persons suffering from economic, social or legal disadvantages heightens their vulnerability to the risk of HIV infection,

Noting that, according to a report submitted to the Commission on the Status of Women at its thirty-third session (E/CN.6/1986/6/Add.1), women are especially vulnerable to the risk of HIV infection and to the economic and social impact of AIDS ass a result of their disadvantageous legal, social and economic status,

Alarmed at discriminatory laws and policies and the emergence of new forms of discriminatory practices which deny people with HIV infection or AIDS, their families and associates enjoyment of their fundamental rights and freedoms,

Concerned that the fear and ignorance surrounding AIDS are leading to increased stigmatization and prejudice against people with HIV/AIDS or presumed to be at risk of infection, sometimes resulting in intimidation, harassment or violence against such individuals, as well as to arbitrary detention and deportation,

Bearing in mind that, as recognized by the World Health

Assembly in its resolution WHA 45.35, there is no public health rationale for any measures that limit the rights of the individual, notably measures establishing mandatory screening,

Recognizing that anti-discrimination measures form a component part of an effective public health strategy,

Stressing that discrimination and stigmatization are counter productive to measures to prevent and control HIV/AIDS,

Emphasizing the responsibility of Governments, in a spirit of human solidarity and tolerance, to counter social stigmatization of and discrimination against those affected by HIV/ AIDS, their families and those with whom they live, and people considered to be at risk of infection,

1. *Calls upon* all States to ensure that their laws, policies, and practices, including those introduced in the context of HIV/ AIDS, respect human rights standards and do not have the effect of inhibiting programmes for the prevention of HIV/ AIDS and for the care of persons infected with HIV/AIDS;
2. *Also calls* upon all States to take all the necessary steps, including appropriate and speedy redress procedures, to ensure the full enjoyment of civil, political, economic, social and cultural rights by people with HIV/AIDS, their families and those in any way associated with them, and people presumed to be at risk of infection, with particular attention to women, children and vulnerable groups, in order to prevent discriminatory action against them or their social stigmatization, and to ensure their access to the necessary care and support;
3. *Urges* all States to include in their AIDS programmes measures to combat social stigmatization, discrimination and violence directed against persons with HIV/AIDS, and to take the necessary steps to develop the supportive social environment necessary for the effective prevention and care of AIDS;
4. *Also urges* all States to review their legislation and practice to ensure the right to privacy and integrity of persons with HIV/AIDS and those presumed to be at risk of infection;
5. Invites the Human Rights Committee, the Committee on Economic, Social and Cultural Rights and other similar bodies to give full attention to monitoring States parties' compliance with their commitments under the relevant human rights instruments regarding the rights of people infected with HIV/ AIDS, their families and people with whom

they live, or people presumed to be at risk of infection;

6. Urges relevant working groups and special rapporteurs to consider in their reports the impact of HIV/AIDS on the enjoyment of human rights;
7. *Welcomes* the preliminary, progress and final reports of Mr. Luis Varela Quiros, Special Rapporteur of the Sub-Commission on the Prevention of Discrimination and Protection of Minorities, on discrimination against HIV-infected people or people with AIDS (E/CN.4/Sub.2/1990/9, E/CN.4/Sub.2/ 1991/10, E/CN.4/Sub.2/1992/10 and E/CN.4/Sub.2/1993/9), and requests the Secretary-General to bring these reports to the attention of the relevant bodies of the United Nations system, specialized agencies, working groups and special rapporteurs, as well as to the human rights treaty bodies, the World Bank and other relevant financial institutions, and those concerned with the status of women;
8. *Also welcomes* resolution EB93.R5 of 21 January 1994 adopted by the Executive Board of the World Health Organization, in which the Executive Board recommended the development and eventual establishment of a joint and co-sponsored United Nations programme on HIV/AIDS and urged that human rights concerns be incorporated into the strategies implementing the new programme;
9. *Expresses its grave concern* about the risk which the continuing exploitation of children and child prostitution pose for the transmission of HIV, and calls upon the Special Rapporteur on the sale of children, child prostitution and child pornography, the Committee on the Rights of the Child and the Working Group on Contemporary Forms of Slavery to pay sustained attention to this question;
10. *Calls upon* relevant professional bodies to re-examine their codes of professional practice with the view of strengthening respect for human rights and dignity in the context of HIV/AIDS, and calls upon the relevant authorities to develop training in this regard;
11. *Requests* the Secretary-General to prepare for the consideration of the Commission at its fifty-first session a report on international and domestic measures taken to protect human rights and to prevent discrimination in the context of HIV/AIDS and to make appropriate recommendations thereon."

70

United Nations Commission on Human Rights Resolution on HIV/AIDS

In the course of its fifty-first session, held in Geneva on 30 January—10 March 1995, the Commission on Human Rights adopted the following resolution on the protection of human rights in the context of human immunodeficiency virus (HIV) and acquired immune deficiency syndrome (AIDS) (resolution 1995/44, adopted on 3 March 1995).

"The Commission on Human Rights,

Recognizing that the increasing challenges presented by HIV/AIDS require renewed efforts to ensure universal respect for and observance of human rights and fundamental freedoms for all, as well as the avoidance of HIV/AIDS-related discrimination and stigma.

Mindful that respect for the principle of non-discrimination is the key to the protection and realization of human rights and fundamental freedoms as recognized in international instruments.

Recalling General Assembly resolutions 45/187 of 21 December 1990 and 46/203 of 20 December 1991, Economic and Social Council resolution 1990/86 of 27 July 1990, World Health Assembly resolutions WHA 41.24 of 13 May 1988, WHA 43.10 of 16 May 1990, WHA 45.35 of 14 May 1992 and WHA 46.37 of 14 May 1993, General Recommendation 15 of the Committee on the

Elimination of Discrimination against Women and other relevant resolutions and decisions adopted by organizations of the United Nations system, as well as by other competent forums,

Welcomes the Final Declaration of the Paris AIDS Summit, of 1 December 1994, in which the participants pledged to promote and protect the rights of people infected and affected by HIV/AIDS,

Also welcomes the progress made in the establishment of a joint and co-sponsored United Nations programme on HIV/ AIDS,

Recalling its resolutions 1992/56 of 3 March 1992, 1993/53 of 9 March 1993 and 1994/49 of 4 March 1994 concerning discrimination against people with HIV infection or AIDS,

Acknowledging the significant role of the World Health Organization, and other bodies of the United Nations system, and the major contribution made by national and international non governmental organizations, in particular organizations of people living with HIV/AIDS, and the International Federation of Red Cross and Red Crescent Societies, in fighting discrimination against and advocating the rights of people living with HIV/AIDS,

Noting with appreciation the Rights and Humanity Declaration and Charter on HIV and AIDS transmitted to the Commission at its forty-eighth session by the Permanent Mission of the Gambia to the United Nations (E/CN.4/1992/82),

Concerned that lack of full enjoyment of their fundamental rights by persons suffering from economic, social or legal disadvantage heightens their vulnerability to the risk of HIV infection,

Noting that, according to a report submitted to the Commission on the Status of Women at its thirty-third session (E/CN.6/1989/6/ Add.1),women are especially vulnerable to the risk of HIV infection and to the economic and social impact of AIDS as a result of their disadvantageous legal, social and economic status, and concerned at the increasing rate of HIV infection among women and girls,

Expresses its- grave concern that the continuing exploitation of children, including child prostitution, poses the risk of transmission of HIV,

Concerned at evidence indicating that groups in society suffering discrimination in the enjoyment of their fundamental rights, and disadvantage with respect to their access to education, health care and social services, are as a result more vulnerable to the risk of infection and to the personal and social impact of the pandemic,

Alarmed at discriminatory laws and policies and the emergence of new forms of discriminatory practices which deny people living with HIV/AIDS, their families and associates, as well as high-risk groups, enjoyment of their fundamental rights and freedoms,

Concerned that the fear and ignorance surrounding HIV/AIDS are leading to increased stigmatization of and prejudice against people living with HIV/AIDS or presumed to be at risk of infection, sometimes resulting in intimidation, harassment or violence against such individuals, as well as to arbitrary detention and deportation,

Bearing in mind that, as recognized by the World Health Assembly in its resolution WHA 45.35, there is no public health rationale for any measures that limit the rights of the individual notably measures establishing mandatory screening,

Stressing that discrimination and stigmatization are counter-productive to measures to prevent and control HIV/AIDS, and that anti-discrimination measures form a component part of an effective public health strategy,

Emphasizing the responsibility of Governments, to take measures to counter social stigmatization of and discrimination against those affected by HIV/AIDS, and their commitment to strengthen national and international mechanisms that are concerned with HIV/AIDS-related human rights and ethics,

Recognizing that HIV transmission can be prevented through informed and responsible behaviour, and emphasizing the role and responsibility of individuals, groups and organs of society aimed at promoting, in a spirit of human solidarity and tolerance, a social environment supportive of the effective prevention and eradication of the root causes of the HIV/AIDS pandemic,

Welcoming the report by the Secretary-General on international and domestic measures taken to protect human rights and prevent discrimination in the context of HIV/AIDS (E/CN./4/1994/45) and his recommendations therein, but noting with concern that there is insufficient information about successful strategies for protecting human rights in the context of HIV/AIDS.

1. *Confirms* that discrimination on the basis of AIDS or HIV status, actual or presumed, is prohibited by existing international human rights standards, and that the term 'or other status' in non-discrimination provisions in international human rights texts can be interpreted to cover health status, including HIV/AIDS;
2. *Calls upon all* States to ensure, where necessary, that their laws, policies and practices, including those introduced in the context of HIV/AIDS respect human rights standards including the right to privacy and integrity of people living

with HIV/AIDS, prohibit HIV/AIDS-related discrimination and do not have the effect of inhibiting programmes for the prevention of HIV/AIDS and for the care of persons infected with HIV / AIDS;

3. *Also calls upon* all States to take all the necessary steps, including appropriate and speedy redress procedures and the introduction of protective legislation and appropriate education to combat discrimination, prejudice and stigma, to ensure the full enjoyment of civil, political, economic, social and cultural rights by people living with HIV/AIDS, their families and associates, and people presumed to be at risk of infection, with particular attention to women, children and vulnerable groups, and to address such concerns within their activities in the context of the International Year of Tolerance, 1995;
4. *Further calls upon* all States to strengthen their efforts to advance the legal, economic and social status of women children and vulnerable groups in order to render them less vulnerable to the risk of HIV infection and to the adverse socio-economic consequences of the AIDS pandemic;
5. *Recognizes* the need to protect women and girls from sexual abuse and violence and calls upon the Special Rapporteur on the sale of children, child prostitution and child pornography, the Committee on the Rights of the Child, the Commission on the Status of Women and the Working Group on Contemporary Forms of Slavery to pay sustained attention to the risk which the continuing exploitation of children, including child prostitution, poses for the transmission of HIV;
6. *Invites* States to involve non-governmental and community-based organizations and people living with HIV/ AIDS in the formulation and implementation of public policy including the support of participatory programme for prevention, care and social support among vulnerable and marginalized populations;
7. *Calls upon* States to take all necessary steps, in particular appropriate education and information measures, to facilitate informed and responsible behaviour;
8. *Invites* the Human Rights Committee, the Committee on Economic, Social and Cultural Rights and other similar bodies to give full attention to monitoring States parties' compliance with their commitments under the relevant

human rights instruments regarding the rights of people living with HIV/AIDS, their families and associates, or people presumed to be at risk of infection;

9. *Calls upon* the Sub-Commission on Prevention of Discrimination and Protection of Minorities to keep the issue of AIDS-related discrimination under continuous review under all relevant agenda items, as well as within the work of its relevant working groups and special rapporteurs;
10. *Calls upon* relevant professional bodies to re-examine their codes of professional practice with a view to strengthening respect for human rights dignity in the context of HIV/ AIDS, and calls upon the relevant authorities to develop training in this regard;
11. *Requests* the co-sponsors of the joint and co-sponsored United Nations programme on HIV/AIDS to integrate a strong human rights component throughout the strategies and work of the future programme;
12. *Requests* the High Commissioner for Human Rights to consider appropriate methods by which to keep under continuous review the protection of human rights in the context of the HIV/AIDS pandemic and to undertake with the Centre for Human Rights, in co-operation with the joint and cosponsored United Nations programme on HIV/AIDS, non-governmental agencies and other actors in the field, the task of elaborating guidelines on promoting and protecting respect for human rights in the context of HIV/ AIDS, and to reflect in this regard on the possibility of organizing a second international expert consultation on human rights and AIDS;
13. *Requests* the Secretary-General to consult with Governments, relevant United Nations bodies, specialized agencies and non-governmental organizations with a view to keeping under review the protection of human rights in the context of the HIV/AIDS pandemic and to prepare for the consideration of the Commission at its fifty-second session a progress report on the development of human rights component in the joint co-sponsored United Nations programme on HIV/AIDS and on the status of the guidelines mentioned in paragraph 12."

71

The United Nations Sub-commission on Prevention of Discrimination and Protection of Minorities Resolution on Discrimination in the context of HIV/AIDS

(Resolution 1995/21 Adopted on 24 August 1995)

The Sub-Commission on Prevention of Discrimination and Protection of Minorities

Recalling that respect for the principle of non-discrimination is the key to the protection and realization of fundamental human rights and freedoms as recognized and protected by international standards.

Convinced that discrimination against any person on the grounds of AIDS or HIV infection, actual or presumed, is a violation of fundamental rights and freedoms.

Recognizing that persons suffering from disadvantaged economic, social or legal status, such as women, street children and other children, indigenous people, minorities, migrants, refugees, commercial sex workers, injecting drug users, men who are homosexuals and others, are more vulnerable to the risk of HIV infection owing to the lack of full enjoyment of their fundamental rights owing to limited or no access to education, health care and social services, and that they suffer disproportionately from the economic and social consequences of HIV/AIDS.

Alarmed at the increasing rate of HIV infection among women and children,

Concerned that in spite of the intensive information campaigns that have been conducted, fear, ignorance and intolerance continue to cause stigmatization of and prejudice against people with HIV/AIDS, their families and associates, as well as those presumed to be infected or at risk of infection, resulting in discrimination in the areas of health care, employment, education, housing, social welfare and travel, as well as in arbitrary detention, deportation, violence and denial of asylum,

Noting with deep concern the lack of adequate international and domestic measures taken to combat HIV/AIDS-related discrimination and human rights violations, as indicated in the report of the Secretary-General to the Commission on Human Rights (E/CN.4/1995/45),

Recalling Commission on Human Rights resolution 1995/44 of 3 March 1995 in which the Commission called upon all States to take all the necessary steps, including appropriate and speedy redress procedures and the introduction of positive legislation and appropriate education to combat discrimination, prejudice and stigma, to ensure the full realization of civil, political, economic, social and cultural rights by people living with HIV/ AIDS and others affected by AIDS, and to address such concerns within their activities in the context of the United Nations Year for Tolerance, 1995,

Bearing in mind World Health Assembly resolution WHA 45.35 of 14 May 1992 in which the Assembly recognized that there was no public health rationale for any measures that limit the rights of the individual, notably measures establishing mandatory screening,

Welcoming progress made towards the establishment of the Joint United Nations Programme on HIV/AIDS (UNAIDS), which will come into full effect on 1 January 1996.

Welcoming also the Paris AIDS Summit held on 1 December 1994 and attended by representatives of 42 Governments, resulting in the adoption of the Final Declaration of the Paris AIDS Summit, in which it was reconfirmed, *inter alia.* that poverty and discrimination contribute to the spread of the pandemic and that the rights of people living with HIV/AIDS must be ensured,

1. *Reconfirms* that discrimination on the basis of HIV or AIDS status, actual or presumed, is prohibited by existing international human rights standards, and that the terms "or other status" in non-discrimination provisions in international human rights texts should be interpreted to cover health status, including HIV/AIDS,
2. *Calls upon* all States to continue to review their legislation, policies and practices in the context of HIV/AIDS in order to ensure that they respect human rights standards, including the prohibition of HIV/AIDS-related discrimination, and to take all the necessary steps, including the introduction of protective legislation and appropriate education, to combat discrimination and stigma, and to ensure the full enjoyment of human rights and freedoms by people with HIV/AIDS, their families and those associated with them;
3. *Also calls upon* all States to strengthen their efforts to advance the legal, economic and social status of women, children, minorities, migrants, and other groups suffering lack of full enjoyment of their rights, in order to render them less vulnerable to the risk of HIV infection and to the adverse socio-economic consequences of the AIDS pandemic;
4. *Commends* the Committee on the Rights of the Child, the Commission on the Status of Women, the Committee on the Elimination of Discrimination against Women, the Working Group on Contemporary Forms of Slavery, as well as relevant special rapporteurs and United Nations human rights bodies, to pay sustained attention to the risk which the continuing social, economic and sexual exploitation of women and children poses for the transmission of HIV;
5. *Requests* the Centre for Human Rights, through the Commission, to maximize its efforts in combating HIV/AIDS related discrimination and to build close links with the Joint United Nations Programme on HIV/AIDS (UNAIDS) for ongoing collaboration;
6. *Stresses* the importance of the organization of a second international expert consultation on human rights and HIV/AIDS, as requested in Commission on Human Rights resolution 1995/44 of 3 March 1995, by the High Commissioner for Human Rights, within existing resources of the Centre for Human Rights and in co-operation with UNAIDS, non-governmental agencies and people living with

HIV/AIDS, with a view to considering developments in the field, including the production of guidelines for the prevention of HIV/AIDS-related discrimination;

7. *Urges* the Commission on Human Rights to keep under review the issues of HIV/AIDS-related human rights violations and discrimination, including in the areas of health care, employment, education, housing, social welfare and travel, as well as in arbitrary detention, deportation, violence and denial of asylum;
8. *Reiterates its request* to UNAIDS to ensure the integration of a strong human rights component in all its activity areas;
9. *Encourages* the full implementation of the Paris Summit initiatives, including the use of an advisory council on human rights, ethical and legal issues in the context of HIV/ AIDS;
10. *Decides* to keep the issue of HIV/AID-related discrimination and human rights violations under continuous review, and to give consideration to this issue under all relevant items of its agenda, as well as in the work of its relevant working groups and special rapporteurs.

72

Guidance on Ethical Aspects of HIV Infection and AIDS Statement Issued by the General Medical Council of the United Kingdom

The following is the text of a May 1993 "Statement on HIV Infection and AIDS—The Ethical Considerations" (superseding an earlier Statement on the ethical implications of HIV and AIDS, issued by the GMC in August 1988):

Introduction

This paper brings together the Council's guidance to the medical profession on some of the ethical considerations which arise in relation to HIV infection and AIDS. It deals first with general principles and then discusses specific matters in relation to the duties of doctors towards infected persons, the duties of doctors who may themselves be infected, the need to obtain patients' consent to investigation or treatment and the need to observe the rules of professional confidence.

The Doctor/Patient Relationship

The doctor/patient relationship is founded on mutual trust, which can be fostered only when information is freely exchanged between doctor and patient on the basis of honesty, openness and understanding. Acceptance of that principle is, in the view of the Council, fundamental to the resolution of the questions which have been identified in relation to AIDS.

The Council has been impressed by the significant increase in the understanding of AIDS and AIDS-related conditions, both within the profession and by the general public, which appears to have occurred. It seems that most doctors are now prepared to regard these conditions as similar in principle to other infections and life-threatening conditions, and are willing to apply established principles in approaching their diagnosis and management, rather than treating them as medical conditions quite distinct from all others. The Council believes that an approach of this kind will help doctors to resolve many of the difficulties which have arisen hitherto.

In all areas of medical practice doctors need to make judgments which they may later have to justify. This is true both of clinical matters and of the complex ethical problems which arise regularly in the course of providing patient care, because it is not possible to set out a code of practice which provides solutions to every such problem which may arise. The Council would remind the profession of the statements of general principle which are set out for the guidance of doctors in its booklet, 'Professional Conduct and Discipline: Fitness to Practise.' In the light of that general guidance the Council has formed the following views on questions of particular significance in relation to HIV infection and the conditions related to it.

The Doctor's Duty Towards Patients

The Council expects that doctors will extend to patients who are HIV positive or are suffering from AIDS the same high standard of medical care and support which they would offer to any other patient. It has, however, expressed its serious concern at reports that, in a small number of cases, doctors have refused to provide such patients with necessary care and treatment.

It is entirely proper for a doctor who has a conscientious objection to undertaking a particular course of treatment, or who lacks the necessary knowledge, skill or facilities to provide appropriate investigation or treatment for a patient, to refer that patient to a professional colleague.

However, it is unethical for a registered medical practitioner to refuse treatment, or investigation for which there are appropriate facilities, on the ground that the patient suffers, or may suffer, from a condition which could expose the doctor to personal risk. It is equally unethical for a doctor to withhold treatment from any patient on the basis of a moral judgment that the patient's activities or lifestyle might have contributed to the condition for which treatment was being sought. Unethical behaviour of this kind may raise a question of serious professional misconduct.

Duties of Doctors Infected with the Virus

Considerable public anxiety has been aroused by suggestions that doctors who are HIV positive might endanger their patients. The risk is very small; to date there is only one known case anywhere in the world of HIV having been transmitted by a health care worker to patients, in the course of dental treatment. Nonetheless, it is imperative, both in the public interest and on ethical grounds, that any doctors who think they may have been infected with HIV should seek appropriate diagnostic testing and counselling and, if found to be infected, have regular medical supervision.

Doctors who are HIV positive should also seek specialist advice on the extent to which they should limit their practice in order to protect their patients. Such advice will usually be obtained locally from a consultant in occupational health, infectious diseases or public health, who may in turn seek guidance, on an anonymous basis, form the UK Advisory Panel of the Expert Advisory Group on AIDS. Doctors must act upon that advice which, in some circumstances, would include a requirement not to practise or to limit their practice in certain ways. No doctors should continue in clinical practice merely on the basis of their own assessment of the risk to patients. The principles underlying this advice are already familiar to the profession, which has well-established policies and procedures designed to prevent the transmission of infection from doctors to patients.

It is unethical for doctors who know or believe themselves to be infected with HIV to put patients at risk by failing to seek appropriate counselling or by failing to act upon it when given. Such behaviour may result in proceedings by the Council which could lead to the restriction or removal of a doctor's registration if this were necessary to protect patients or the doctor's own health. The Council has already given guidance, in paragraph 63 of the booklet 'Professional Conduct and Discipline: Fitness to Practise' on doctors duty to inform an appropriate person or authority about a colleague whose professional conduct or fitness to practise may be called into question. A doctor who knows that health care worker is infected with HIV and is aware that the person has not sought or followed advice to modify his or her professional practice, has a duty to inform the appropriate regulatory body and an appropriate person in the health care worker's employing authority, who will usually be the most senior doctor.

Rights of Doctors Infected with the Virus

Doctors who become infected with the virus are entitled to expect the confidentiality and support afforded to other patients. Only in the most exceptional circumstances, where the release of a doctor's name is essential for the protection of patients, may a doctor's HIV status be disclosed without his or her consent.

Consent to Investigation or Treatment

It has been long accepted, and is well understood within the profession, that a doctor should treat a patient only on the basis of the patient's informed consent. Doctors are expected in all normal circumstances to be sure that their patient's consent to the carrying out of investigative procedures involving the removal of samples or invasive techniques, whether those investigations are performed for the purposes of routine screening, for example in pregnancy or prior to surgery, or for the more specific purpose of differential diagnosis. A patient's consent may in certain circumstances be given implicitly, for example by agreement to provide a specimen of blood for multiple analysis. In other circumstances it needs to be given explicitly, for example before undergoing a specified operative procedure or providing a specimen of blood to be tested specifically for a named condition. As the expectations of patients, and consequently the demands made upon doctors, increase and develop, it is essential that both doctor and patient feel free to exchange information before investigation or treatment is undertaken.

Testing for HIV Infection: the Need to Obtain Consent

The Council believes that the above principle should apply generally, but that it is particularly important in the case of testing for HIV infection, not because the condition is different in kind from other infections but because of the possible serious social and financial consequences which may ensue for the patient from the mere fact of having been tested for the condition. These are problems which would be better resolved by a developing spirit of social tolerance than by medical action, but they do raise a particular ethical dilemma for the doctor in connection with the diagnosis of HIV infection or AIDS. They provide a strong argument for each patient to be given the opportunity, in advance, to consider the implications of submitting to such a test and deciding whether to accept or decline it. In the case of a patient presenting with certain symptoms which the doctor is expected to diagnose, this process should form part of the consultation. Where blood samples are taken for screening purposes, as in antenatal clinics, there will usually be no reason to suspect HIV infection but even so the test should be carried out only where the patient has given explicit consent. Similarly, those handling blood samples in laboratories, either for specific investigation or for the purpose of research, should test for the presence of HIV only where they know the patient has given explicit consent. Only in the most exceptional circumstances where a test is imperative in order to secure the safety of persons other than the patient, and where it is not possible for the prior consent of the patient to be obtained, can testing without explicit consent be justified.

A particular difficulty arises in cases where it may be desirable to test a child for HIV infection and where, consequently, the consent of a parent, or a person in loco parentis, would normally be sought. However, the possibility that the child may have been infected by a parent may, in certain circumstances, distort the parent's judgment so that consent is withheld in order to protect the parent's own position. The doctor faced with this situation must first judge whether the child is competent to consent to the test on his or her own behalf. If the child is judged competent in this context, then consent can be sought from the child. If, however, the child is judged unable to give consent the doctor must decide whether the interests of the child should over-ride the wishes of the parent. It is the view of the Council that it would not be unethical for a doctor to perform such a test without parental consent, provided always that the doctor is able to justify that action as being in the best interests of the patient.

Confidentiality

Doctors are familiar with the need to make judgments about whether to disclose confidential information in particular circumstances, and the need to justify their action where such a disclosure is made. The Council believes that, where HIV infection or AIDS has been diagnosed, any difficulties concerning confidentiality which arise will usually be overcome if doctors are prepared to discuss openly and honestly with patients the implications of their condition, the need to secure the safety of others, and the importance for continuing medical care of ensuring that those who will be involved in their care know the nature of their condition and the particular needs which they will have. The Council takes the view that any doctor who discovers that a patient is HIV positive or suffering from AIDS has a duty to discuss these matters fully with the patient.

Informing Other Health Care Professionals

When a patient is seen by a specialist who diagnoses HIV infection or AIDS, and a general practitioner is or may become involved in that patient's care, then the specialist should explain to the patient that the general practitioner cannot be expected to provide adequate clinical management and care without full knowledge of the patient's condition. The Council believes that the majority of such patients will readily be persuaded of the need for their general practitioners to be informed of the diagnosis.

If the patient refuses consent for the general practitioner to be told, then the doctor has two sets of obligations to consider: obligations to the patient to maintain confidence, and obligations to other carers whose own health may be put unnecessarily at risk. In such circumstances the patient should be counselled about the difficulties which his or her condition is likely to pose for the team responsible for providing continuing health care and about the likely consequences for the standard of care which can be provided in the future. If, having considered the matter carefully in the light of such counselling, the patient still refuses to allow the general practitioner to be informed, then the patient's request for privacy should be respected. The only exception to that general principle arises where the doctor judges the failure to disclose would put the health of any of the health care team at serious risk. The Council believes that, in such a situation, it would not be improper to disclose such information as that person needs to know. The need for such a decision is, in present circumstances, likely to arise only rarely, but if it is made the doctor must be able to justify his or her action.

Similar principles apply to the sharing of confidential information between specialists or with other health care professionals such as nurses, laboratory technicians and dentists. All persons receiving such information must of course consider themselves under the same general obligation of confidentiality as the doctor principally responsible for the patient's care.

Informing the Patient's Spouse or other Sexual Partner

Questions of conflicting obligations also arise when a doctor is faced with the decision whether the fact that a patient is HIV positive or suffering from AIDS should be disclosed to a third party, other than another health care professional, without the consent of the patient. The Council has reached the view that there are grounds for such a disclosure only where there is a serious and identifiable risk to a specific individual who, if not so informed, would be exposed to infection. Therefore, when a person is found to be infected in this way, the doctor must discuss with the patient the question of informing a spouse or other sexual partner. The Council believes that most such patients will agree to disclosure in these circumstances, but where such consent is withheld the doctor may consider it a duty to seek to ensure that any sexual partner is informed, in order to safeguard such persons from possibly fatal infection.

Conclusion

It is emphasized that the advice set out above is intended to guide doctors in approaching the complex questions which may arise in the context of this infection. It is not in any sense a code, and individual doctors must always be prepared, as a matter of good medical practice, to make their own judgments of the appropriate course of action to be followed in specific circumstances, and able to justify the decisions they make. The Council believes that the generality of doctors have acted compassionately, responsibly and in a well-informed manner in taking the especially sensitive problems with which the spread of this group of conditions has confronted society. It is confident that they will continue to do so."

73

International Ethical Guidelines for Biomedical Research Involving Human Subjects

[Prepared by the Council for International Organizations of Medical Sciences (CIOMS) in Collaboration with the World Health Organization (WHO), 1993]

The Guidelines

Informed Consent of Subjects

Guideline 1: Individual Informed Consent

For all biomedical research involving human subjects, the investigator must obtain the informed consent of the prospective subject or, in the case of an individual who is not capable of giving informed consent, the proxy consent of a properly authorized representative.

Guideline 2: Essential Information for Prospective Research Subjects

Before requesting an individual's consent to participate in research, the investigator must provide the individual with the following information, in language that he or she is capable of understanding:

— that each individual is invited to participate as a subject in research, and the aims and methods of the research;
— the expected duration of the subject's participation;
— the benefits that might reasonably be expected to result to the subject or to others as an outcome of the research;
— any foreseeable risks or discomfort to the subject, associated with participation in the research;
— any alternative procedures or courses of treatment that might be as advantageous to the subject as the procedure or treatment being tested;
— the extent to which confidentiality of records in which the subject is identified will be maintained;
— the extent of the investigator's responsibility, if any, to provide medical services to the subject;
— that therapy will be provided free of charge for specified types of research-related injury;
— whether the subject or the subject's family or dependents will be compensated for disability or death resulting from such injury; and
— that the individual is free to refuse to participate and will be free to withdraw from the research at any time without penalty or loss of benefits to which he or she would otherwise be entitled.

Guideline 3: Obligations of Investigators Regarding Informed Consent

The investigator has a duty to:
— communicate to the prospective subject all the information necessary for adequately informed consent;
— give the prospective subject full opportunity and encouragement to ask questions;
— exclude the possibility of unjustified deception, undue influence and intimidation;
— seek consent only after the prospective subject has adequate knowledge of the relevant facts and of the consequences of participation, and has had sufficient opportunity to consider whether to participate;
— as a general rule, obtain from each prospective subject a signed form as evidence of informed consent; and
— renew the informed consent of each subject if there are material changes in the conditions or procedures of the research.

Guideline 4: Inducement to Participate

Subjects may he paid for inconvenience and time spent, and should be reimbursed for expenses incurred, in connection with their participation in research; they may also receive free medical services. However, the payments should not be so large or the medical services so extensive as to induce prospective subjects to consent to participate in the research against their better judgment ("undue inducement"). All payments, reimbursements and medical services to be provided to research subjects should be approved by an ethical review committee.

Guideline 5: Research Involving Children

Before undertaking research involving children, the investigator must ensure that:

— children will not be involved in research that might equally well be carried out with adults;

— the purpose of the research is to obtain knowledge relevant to the health needs of the children;

— a parent or legal guardian of each child has given proxy consent;

— the consent of each child has been obtained to the extent of the child's capabilities;

— the child's refusal to participate in research must always be respected unless according to the research protocol the child would receive therapy for which there is no medically-acceptable alternative;

— the risk presented by interventions not intended to benefit the individual child-subject is low and commensurate with the importance of the knowledge to be gained; and

— interventions that are intended to provide therapeutic benefit are likely to be at least as advantage the individual child-subject as any available alternative.

Guideline 6: Research Involving Persons with Mental or Behavioural Disorders

Before undertaking research involving individuals who by reason of mental or behavioural disorders are not capable of giving adequately informed consent, the investigator must ensure that:

— such persons will not be subjects of research that might equally well be carried out on persons in full possession of their mental faculties;

— the purpose of the research is to obtain knowledge relevant to the particular health needs of persons with mental or behavioural disorders;
— the consent of each subject has been obtained to the extent of that subject's capabilities, and a prospective subject's refusal to participate in non-clinical research is always respected;
— in the case of incompetent subjects, informed consent obtained from the legal guardian or other duly authorized person;
— the degree of risk attached to interventions that are not intended to benefit the individual subject is low and commensurate with the importance of the knowledge to be gained, and
— interventions that are intended to provide therapeutic benefit are likely to be at least as advantageous to the individual subject as any alternative.

Guideline 7: Research Involving Prisoners

Prisoners with serious illness or at risk of serious illness should not arbitrarily be denied access to investigational drugs, vaccines or other agents that show promise of therapeutic or preventive benefit.

Guideline 8: Research Involving Subjects in Underdeveloped communities

Before undertaking research involving subjects in underdeveloped communities, whether in developed or developing countries, the investigator must ensure that:
— persons in underdeveloped communities will not ordinarily be involved in research that could be carried out reasonably well in developed communities;
— the research is responsive to the health needs and the priorities of the community in which it is to be carried out;
— every effort will be made to secure the ethical imperative that the consent of individual subjects be informed; and
— the proposals for the research have been reviewed and approved by an ethical review committee that has among its members or consultants persons who are thoroughly familiar with the customs and traditions of the community.

Guideline 9: Informed Consent in Epidemiological Studies

For several types of epidemiological research individual informed consent is either impracticable or inadvisable. In such cases the ethical review committee should determine whether it is ethically acceptable to proceed without individual informed consent and whether the investigator's plans to protect the safety and respect the privacy of research subjects and to maintain the confidentiality of the data are adequate.

Selection of Research Subjects

Guideline 10: Equitable Distribution of Burdens and Benefits

Individuals or communities to be invited to be subjects of research should be selected in such a way that the burdens and benefits of the research will be equitably distributed. Special justification is required for inviting vulnerable individuals and, if they are selected, the means of protecting their rights and welfare must be particularly strictly applied.

Guideline 11: Selection of Pregnant or Nursing (breast feeding) Women as Research Subjects

Pregnant or nursing women should in no circumstances be the subjects of non-clinical research unless the research carries no more than minimal risk to the fetus or nursing infant and the object of the research is to obtain new knowledge about pregnancy or lactation. As a general rule, pregnant or nursing women should not be subjects of any clinical trials except such trials as are designed to protect or advance the health of pregnant or nursing women or fetuses or nursing infants, and for which women who are not pregnant or nursing would not be suitable subjects.

Confidentiality of Data

Guideline 12: Safeguarding Confidentiality

The investigator must establish secure safeguards of the confidentiality of research data. Subjects should be told of the limits to the investigators' ability to safeguard confidentiality and of the anticipated consequences of breaches of confidentiality.

Compensation of Research Subjects for Accidental Injury

Guideline 13: Right of Subjects to Compensation

Research subjects who suffer physical injury as a result of their participation are entitled to such financial or other assistance as would compensate them equitably for any temporary or permanent impairment or disability. In the case of death, their dependents are entitled to material compensation. The right to compensation may not be waived.

Review Procedures

Guideline 14: Constitution and Responsibilities of Ethical Review Committees

All proposals to conduct research involving human subjects must be submitted for review and approval to one or more independent ethical and scientific review committees. The investigator must obtain such approval of the proposal to conduct research before the research is begun.

Externally Sponsored Research

Guideline 15: Obligations of Sponsoring and Host Countries

Externally sponsored research entails two ethical obligations:

- an external sponsoring agency should submit the research protocol to ethical and scientific review according to the standards of the country of the sponsoring agency, and the ethical standards applied should be no less exacting than they would be in the case of research carried out in that country.
- After scientific and ethical approval in the country of the sponsoring agency, the appropriate authorities of the host country, including a national or local ethical review committee or its equivalent, should satisfy themselves that the proposed research meets their own ethical requirements.

Note:

[Ed.: A commentary on the above guidelines can be found in Bankowski, Z. and Levine, R.J. *Ethics and Research on Human Subjects,* CIOMS, Geneva, 1993].

74

World Medical Association Declaration of Helsinki

Recommendations Guiding Physicians in Biomedical Research Involving Human Subjects

**Adopted by the 18th World Medical Assembly Helsinki, Finland, June 1964
And Amended by the 29th World Medical Assembly Tokyo, Japan, October, 1975 35th World Medical Assembly Venice, Italy, October 1983 and the 41st World Medical Assembly Hong Kong, September 1989**

Introduction

It is the mission of the physician to safeguard the health of the people. His or her knowledge and conscience are dedicated to the fulfillment of this mission.

The Declaration of Geneva of the World Medical Association binds the physician with the words, "The health of my patient will be my first consideration," and the International Code of Medical Ethics declares that, "A physician shall act only in the patient's interest when providing medical care which might have the effect of weakening the physical and mental condition of the patient."

The purpose of biomedical research involving human subjects must be to improve diagnostic, therapeutic and prophylactic procedures and the understanding of the aetiology and the pathogenesis of disease.

In current medical practice most diagnostic, therapeutic or prophylactic procedures involve hazards. This applies especially to biomedical research.

Medical progress is based on research which ultimately must rest in part on experimentation involving human subjects.

In the field of biomedical research a fundamental distinction must be recognized between medical research in which the aim is essentially diagnostic or therapeutic for a patient, and medical research, the essential object of which is purely scientific and without implying direct diagnostic or therapeutic value to the person subjected to the research.

Special caution must be exercised in the conduct of research which may affect the environment, and the welfare of animals used for research must be respected.

Because it is essential that the results of laboratory experiments be applied to human beings to further scientific knowledge and to help suffering humanity, the World Medical Association has prepared the following recommendations as a guide to every physician in biomedical research involving human subjects. They should be kept under review in the future. It must be stressed that the standards as drafted are only a guide to physicians all over the world. Physicians are not relieved from criminal, civil and ethical responsibilities under the laws of their own countries.

I. BASIC PRINCIPLES

1. Biomedical research involving human subjects must conform to generally accepted scientific principles and should be based on adequately performed laboratory and animal experimentation and a through knowledge of the scientific literature.
2. The design and performance of each experimental procedure involving human subjects should be clearly formulated in an experimental protocol which should be transmitted for consideration, comment and guidance to a specially appointed committee independent of the investigator and the sponsor, provided that this independent committee is in conformity with the laws and regulations of the country in which the research experiment is performed.
3. Biomedical research involving human subjects should be conducted only by scientifically qualified persons and under the supervision of a clinically competent medical person. The responsibility for the human subject must always rest

with a medically qualified person and never rest on the subject of the research, even though the subject has given his or her consent.

4. Biomedical research involving human subjects cannot legitimately be carried out unless the importance of the objective is in proportion to the inherent risk to the subject.
5. Every biomedical research project involving human subjects should be preceded by careful assessment of predictable risks in comparison with foreseeable benefits to the subject or to others. Concern for the interests of the subject must always prevail over the interests of science and society.
6. The right of the research subject to safeguard his or her integrity must always be respected. Every precaution should be taken to respect the privacy of the subject and to minimize the impact of the study on the subject's physical and mental integrity and on the personality of the subject.
7. Physicians should abstain from engaging in research projects involving human subjects unless they are satisfied that the hazards involved are believed to be predictable. Physicians should cease any investigation if the hazards are found to outweigh the potential benefits.
8. In publication of the results of his or her research, the physician is obliged to preserve the accuracy of the results. Reports of experimentation not in accordance with the principles laid down in this Declaration should not be accepted for publication.
9. In any research on human beings, each potential subject must be adequately informed of the aims, methods, anticipated benefits and potential hazards of the study and the discomfort it may entail. He or she should be informed that he or she is at liberty to abstain from participation in the study and that he or she is free to withdraw his or her consent to participation at any time. The physician should then obtain the subject's freely-given informed consent, preferably in writing.
10. When obtaining informed consent for the research project the physician should be particularly cautious if the subject is in a dependent relationship to him or her or may consent under duress. In that case the informed consent should be obtained by a physician who is not engaged in the investigation and who is completely independent of this official relationship.

11. In case of legal incompetence, informed consent should be obtained from the legal guardian in accordance with national legislation. Where physical or mental incapacity makes it impossible to obtain informed consent, or when the subject is a minor, permission from the responsible relative replaces that of the subject in accordance with national legislation.

Whenever the minor child is in fact able to give a consent, the minor's consent must be obtained in addition to the consent of the minor's legal guardian.

12. The research protocol should always contain a statement of the ethical considerations involved and should indicate that the principles enunciated in the present Declaration are complied with.

II. MEDICAL RESEARCH COMBINED WITH PROFESSIONAL CARE

(Clinical Research)

1. In the treatment of the sick person, the physician must be free to use a new diagnostic and therapeutic measure, if in his or her judgment it offers hope of saving life, re-establishing health or alleviating suffering.
2. The potential benefits, hazards and discomfort of a new method should be weighed against the advantages of the best current diagnostic and therapeutic methods.
3. In any medical study, every patient—including those of a control group, if any—should be assured of the best proven diagnostic and therapeutic method.
4. The refusal of the patient to participate in a study must never interfere with the physician-patient relationship.
5. If the physician considers it essential not to obtain informed consent, the specific reasons for this proposal should be stated in the experimental protocol for transmission to the independent committee (1, 2).
6. The physician can combine medical research with professional care, the objective being the acquisition of new medical knowledge, only to the extent that medical research is justified by its potential diagnostic or therapeutic value for the patient.

III. Non-Therapeutic Biomedical Research Involving Human Subjects

(Non-clinical Biomedical Research)

1. In the purely scientific application of medical research carried out on a human being, it is the duty of the physician to remain the protector of the life and health of that person on whom biomedical research is being carried out.
2. The subjects should be volunteers either healthy persons or patients for whom the experimental design is not related to the patient's illness.
3. The investigator or the investigating team should discontinue the research if in his/her or their judgment it may, if continued, be harmful to the individual.
4. In research on man, the interest of science and society should never take precedence over considerations related to the well being of the subject.

75

UNDP Intercountry Consultation on Law, Ethics and HIV

STATEMENT OF BELIEF

— We believe that every individual has a right to dignity, health and life. Public health and the interests of the community in the context of the HIV epidemic depend upon respect for individual rights and recognition of the worth of each member of our societies.

— We acknowledge that we are all likely to be affected by the HIV epidemic.

— We believe that the law must promote an environment that enables, encourages and sustains voluntary behaviour change and the care and support of those affected. This requires the empowerment of individuals and communities to protect themselves against HIV, and that people living with HIV remain integrated within society and free from all forms of discrimination.

— We affirm that it is the responsibility of each individual, community and nation to take up this cause through existing means of advocacy and by creating new ones. We must

---

This statement was drafted and endorsed by the participants at the "UNDP Intercountry Consultation on Law, Ethics, and HIV," held in Cebu, Philippines, 3-6 May 1993.

express and act upon a concern for ourselves and others.

— We recognise that the subordinate position of women within their families and communities makes them particularly susceptible to HIV infection. Social structures, laws and practices, as well as values and attitudes, must change to improve the status of women.

— We believe that the development of effective responses to the HIV epidemic requires, above all, the active participation of people affected by the epidemic, as well as the building of partnerships amongst communities, governments and the legal, health and other professions.

76

Behaviour Change: A Central Issue in Responding to the HIV Epidemic

Statement of Belief

We believe that individuals and whole communities have the inherent capacity to change attitudes and behaviours. The power to fulfill this capacity is often denied or is not exercised.

This power must now be recognised, called forth and supported from both within and without. This will enable people to initiate change and sustain behaviours that promote a healthy state of mind, body, spirit and environment. A critical component in this process is a supportive response to those living with HIV in the community.

We recognise that behaviour change at individual and community level in the present HIV pandemic is a complex and on-going process. It is inextricably linked to such basic human values as care, love, faith, family and friendship, respect for people and cultures, solidarity and support.

The present pandemic affects everyone. Our experience as affected and infected individuals proves that behaviour change is possible. We believe that behaviour change is the most essential strategy in overcoming the HIV pandemic.

77

African Network on Ethics, Law and HIV Dakar Declaration

RECOGNIZING the impact that the HIV epidemic is having on all aspects of human life;

RECOGNIZING the need for an urgent response;

RECOGNIZING that the fundamental value of respect for human rights, life and human dignity provides the foundation on which all is built,

WE, the participants at the Intercountry Consultation of the African Network on Ethics, Law and HIV. Affirm that any action, whether personal, institutional, professional or governmental, in response to the HIV epidemic should be guided by the following principles:

This Declaration was drafted and endorsed by participatns at the Intercountry Consultation of the African Network on Ethics, Law and HIV, organized Dakar Senegal from 27 June to 1st 1994, by the UNDP HIV and Development Programme (Dakar and New York). Participants came from Central African Republic. Cote d'Ivoire Ghana, Kenya, Rwanda, Senegal, South Africa, Uganda, Zambia, the Who Global Programme on AIDS, the WHO Regional Office for Africa the UNDP Management Development and Governance Division, the UNDP HIV Development Project in Asia and the Pacific, the Asian and Latin American Network on Law, Ethics and HIV, the African Council of AIDS Service Organizations (AFRICASO), the Association of African Jurists (AJA), ENDA Tiers Monde, the Network of African People Living with HIV AIDS (NAP+), the Organisation Pan-African de Lutte contre le SIDA (OPALS) and ORSTOM.

The Principle of Responsibility: Every person, government, community, institution, private enterprise and medium must be aware of his or her responsibility and must exercise it in an active and sustainable manner.

The Principle of Engagement: Every person is affected directly or indirectly and therefore should respond with commitment, concern, courage and hope for the future.

The Principle of Partnership and Consensus-Building: All persons, couples, families, communities and nations must work together with compassion to build and share a common vision. These partnerships must reflect and actively promote solidarity, inclusion, integration, dialogue, participation and harmony.

The Principle of Empowerment: The empowerment of every person but particularly women, the poor, the uneducated and children, is essential and must guide all action. Empowerment requires recognition of the right to knowledge, information and technology, freedom of choice and economic opportunity.

The Principle of Non-discrimination: Every person directly affected by the epidemic should remain an integral part of his or her community, with the right of equal access to work, housing, education and social services, with the right to marry, with freedom of movement, belief and association. With the right to counselling. Care and treatment, justice and equality.

The Principle of Confidentiality and Privacy: Every person directly affected by the epidemic has a right to confidentiality and privacy. It can only be breached in exceptional circumstances.

The Principle of Adaptation: Every person and community should change and adapt social and cultural conditions to the new challenges of the epidemic in order to respond effectively.

The Principle of Sensitivity In Language: Language should uphold human dignity, reflect inclusion, be gender sensitive accurate and understandable.

The Principle of Ethics Research: The interests of the research subjects or communities should be paramount. Research should be based on free and informed consent, be non-obtrusive and non-coercive, and the results should be made available to the community for timely and appropriate action.

The Principle of Prohibition of Mandatory HIV Testing: HIV testing without consent should be prohibited HIV testing should also not be a pre-requisite for access to work, travel or other services.

78

Beijing Training Workshop: HIV Law and Law Reform

(Report of the Proceedings of the UNDP Regional Project on HIV and Development Regional Training Workshop on HIV Law and Law Reform in the Asean, Greater Mekong Region and other Countries, 24-27 April 1995, Beijing, China)

Introduction

The regional training workshop on HIV Law and Law Reform in the ASEAN and Greater Mekong Region and other countries was held in Beijing from 24 to 27 April 1995. The workshop was co-sponsored by the UNDP Regional Project on HIV and Development and the Chinese Academy of Preventive Medicine. Participants from Australia, Cambodia, China, Hong Kong, India, Indonesia, Lao PDR, Malaysia, Mongolia, Myanmar, Philippines, Republic of Korea, Singapore, Sri Lanka, Thailand, United States of America and Vietnam attended the workshop.

Opening Session

Welcoming the participants to the workshop, Dr. D.C. Jayasuriya, Regional HIV and Development Adviser, UNDP Regional Project on HIV and Development, noted that the use of legislation in the field of public health is not new. Health legislation-as the branch of law dealing with medical or health matters is called - has a long history going back to several centuries. What is new, however, is the concern that legislative measures in this field must respect the dignity and the rights of the individual, whether infected or not. With countries around the world beginning to legislate on matters concerning HIV and AIDS, within two years of the reporting of the first AIDS cases, a movement has emerged which challenges the ways in which existing laws are reviewed or new laws are drafted and implemented. This approach of 'strategic questioning' is critical to the efforts to create and sustain an environment in which individual rights can be delicately balanced with those of society and the infected can live side by side with the uninfected, without being marginalized or discriminated against. Most importantly, such an approach enables all concerned to work together, in a spirit of co-operation and mutual respect, to minimize the risks of transmitting the causative virus underlying AIDS and mitigate the problems brought in the wake of the infection.

HIV-related legal, ethical and human rights issues, Dr. Jayasuriya pointed out, have been an integral part of the work of the United Nations Development Programme in the area of HIV and development. In this region, a major Regional Consultation on HIV Law and Ethics was held in Cebu in the Philippines in 1993. This consultation brought together jurists and service providers to examine HIV-related legal and ethical issues and develop approaches that are consistent with acceptable standards of law and ethics. A 'Statement of Belief' was adopted by the participants which states that *'the law must promote an environment that enables, encourages and sustains voluntary behaviour change and the care and support of those affected. This requires the empowerment of individuals and communities to protect themselves against HIV, and that people living with HIV remain integrated within society and free from all forms of discrimination.'*

The Cebu consultation, he noted, was followed by the Regional Project supporting a focal point for a regional network on law, ethics and human rights. This focal point, which is located within the Law Faculty of the University of Colombo in Sri Lanka, seeks to promote national networks and to facilitate the exchange of information on current and emerging legal, ethical and human rights issues.

Dr. Jayasuriya drew the attention of the participants to the three key projects, identified by the UNDP Regional Project on HIV and Development, to be undertaken during the course of this year. In the spirit of the new UNAIDS programme, these activities have not only been formulated, but will also be implemented, in consultation with other UN agencies.

The first project, conducting a series of regional training workshops on HIV law and law reform, is already underway. These workshops are intended to (a) create a better understanding and awareness of the scope, content and functional role of HIV law; (b) sharpen the focus on issues of critical importance, so that they receive due consideration when countries review existing laws or draft new ones; and (c) promote national and subregional activitie6 such as national networks, study and research groups, and legal assistance services.

The first in the series of three regional training workshops, Dr. Jayasuriya reminded the participants, was held in February, 1995 in Colombo, Sri Lanka, for participants from the SAARC countries. The current workshop in Beijing, for the ASEAN and the Greater Mekong Region countries, is the second in this series. The third final workshop will be held in Fiji in May 1995 for the South Pacific countries. These three workshops are intended for over 120 participants from some 30 countries in the Asia and Pacific region.

The second major activity being sponsored by the Regional Project this year is the compilation of a source book on HIV law ethics and human rights that can be used in legal practice and teaching. It is likely that the entire text or selected portions of it will be translated into major Asian languages for wider dissemination. This is particularly important for those countries where law teaching and court proceedings are conducted in one or more of the national languages. The third major activity is to promote national networking by offering technical and information backstopping services.

Finally, Dr. Jayasuriya informed the participants, that in order to accord more prominence to HIV related-legal, ethical and human rights issues, the Regional Project will co-sponsor will the Indian Law Institute a major international conference on AIDS law to be held in New Delhi in December 1995.

In his welcome address on behalf of the UNDP Resident Representative in China, Mr. He Jin, Social Development Division Chief, UNDP Beijing, noted that UNDP has always emphasized that AIDS is a medical as well as a social problem, one that encompasses all segments of society. Its prevention and control is the responsibility of not one ministry or agency, but of a diverse group of affected parties. There are many social, economic, political and legal implications of this incurable disease. That is why the acutely needed legislation on AIDS/HIV should address not only legal and ethical issues, but also drug abuse, health education, patient care and other such dimensions.

Mr. He Jin observed that while China has one of the lowest HIV/ AIDS incidence rates in the world, with its large population it cannot afford to be complacent or apathetic. There is an urgent need for more education and for greater exchange of experience and expertise between those countries which have suffered from this scourge. Australia, in particular, has gained valuable experience and achieved success in preventing the spread of the disease.

With the help of a US$ 1 million grant, Mr. He Jin pointed out, UNDP Beijing has provided technical assistance to China at three levels: at the central level, on policy research and advice; at the provincial level, on training; and at the community level, on demonstration projects on health education. Significant breakthroughs were made with the preparation of a National AIDS Strategy and the convening of a top-level policy seminar to discuss the strategy, at which state leaders actively participated and offered their strong support. The findings and recommendations of this seminar are presented in a policy booklet entitled *Beware of AIDS: For the Survival of the Chinese Nation.*

Mr. He Jin said that UNDP hoped to continue with its HIV/ AIDS prevention and control efforts, in consultation with its government counterparts. He noted that the UNDP, along with WHO and other international agencies, has a unique role in providing the international dimension to China's efforts in dealing with the disease. While there is still a window of opportunity to combat the disease effectively, it is growing smaller everyday. This calls for the intensification of all efforts and more effective collaboration to prevent and control the spread of HIV/AIDS in all countries.

He concluded with the hope that the exchange of information between the ASEAN and Greater Mekong Region countries on the issue of AIDS law reform, and the lessons drawn from each other, will bring them closer in their common campaign against AIDS.

The President of the Chinese Academy of Preventive Medicine, Prof. Zeng Yi, in his welcome address, noted that globally the AIDS epidemic has become one of the most severe public health problems of this century. While compared to the rest of the world China still has a low HIV infection rate, it has little reason to be optimistic in the long run. The following fastors predispose China to a largescale AIDS epidemic: a large, mobile workforce; a large sexually active population; and poor medical care in the rural areas. Thus, AIDS prevention here is an uphill task.

Prof. Zeng Yi stressed that advantage needs to be taken of the primary phase of the disease in China, characterized by a low incidence rate, to fully equip the country to cope with a potentially massive epidemic. It is important to not only strengthen sentinel surveillance and health education of the entire population in general and the high-risk population, in particular but also formulate new legislation and improve the existing laws and regulations on HIV/AIDS. The Beijing Workshop, with its focus on HIV related law, ethics and human rights, will definitely give an impetus to this process in China.

The Chinese Academy of Preventive Medicine, which was separated from the Chinese Academy of Medical Sciences and founded in 1983, is the only national preventive medicine research institution in China. It has eight institutes with a staff of more than 2,000 who are engaged in scientific and technological research in the fields of prevention and control of communicable and non-communicable diseases; inspection of food and environmental hygiene; health regulation standards, etc. Specifically with regard to AIDS prevention and control, the academy has set up two centers: one for AIDS research and detection, and another for AIDS surveillance.

Dr. Qi Xiaoqiu, Deputy Director of the Diseases Control Division of the Ministry of Public Health in Beijing, described in detail the evolution of the epidemic in China and the preventive measures in place.

Epidemiological Trends

In the first presentation, entitled 'HIV/AIDS: Modes of Transmission and Epidemiological Trends in Asia', Dr. James Mullaly of the World Health Organization stressed that it was important to dispel myths about the spread of HIV/AIDS. He identified global trends and noted that the projected figures for increased spread in Asia were a cause for alarm.

He argued that the universality of risks should not be stressed; instead, more specific arguments should be marshalled depending upon the target audience. He pointed out that human behaviour required a number of changes—new social and technical skills had to be developed and priorities judiciously chosen.

In the discussion that followed Dr. Mullaly's presentation, some participants questioned the wisdom of not stressing the universality of risks. Other issues that were highlighted were the impact of sex education in schools and the increasing prevalence of condom use in Thailand. Though considered undesirable in some countries, sex

education, it was pointed out, by highlighting risks, delayed the start
education, it was pointed out, by highlighting risks, delayed the start
of an active sex life. Regarding the prevalence of condom use in Thailand, it was pointed out that whilst this was the case for relationship within sex establishments, it was not so outside.

Public Health Aspects

In his presentation on 'HIV and STDs: Public Health Aspects', Dr. Zhang Konglai noted that with individuals and groups such as taxi-drivers and college students moving away from 'traditional culture' under the impact of economic liberalization, existing efforts to control the spread of HIV were coming under strain. He recommended that various categories of individuals should be targeted before they disperse throughout the country. Dr. Zhang ended with the question: What kind of law reform is possible?

Socio-Economic Aspects

In his presentation, 'The Socio-economic Impact of the HIV Epidemic in Asia', Dr. D. C. Jayasuriya drew attention to the fact that only US$ 200 million out of a total of US $1.5 billion was spent on AIDS prevention in the developing countries in 1993; and not surprisingly, there was little available data to make an assessment of the socio-economic impact of HIV/AIDS in the Asian region.

He went on to note that there are two dominant types of rhetoric on AIDS: the 'medical' model and the 'stigma' model. The focus of the former is organic, highlighting the body. Its principal mode of conceptualizing is scientific; it offers a biological explanation and relies on clinical methods of management. The 'stigma' model, on the other hand, is characterized in terms of a behavioural and lifestyle focus and a conceptual emphasis on the moral, political and theological. It advances explanations through the notions of sin, choice and responsibility and favours segregation, discrimination and exclusion as modes of management.

Dr. Jayasuriya pointed out that evidence suggested the emergence of a 'development model', which focusses on the individual and the community. He also cited a number of examples in support of the statement that there is a growing body of research on how sex is dealt with in society. He observed that more is known today than a decade ago on sexual networks and on the dynamics underlying recruitment to commercial sex.

He argued, through the enumeration of examples, that HIV/AIDS has deep ramifications for society. By virtue of its impact on demographic factors and key life cycle events, lifestyles and practices of discrimination, HIV/AIDS was an important issue for social scientists. Dr. Jayasuriya also highlighted the effect of structural adjustment policies on HIV/AIDS—especially the consequences of the withdrawal of subsidies; devaluation resulting in price increases of imported drugs; and privatization resulting in more limited access to health care services and facilities for persons with limited financial resources.

The Expanding Frontiers of HIV Law

Speaking on 'The Nature and Scope of HIV Law: The Expanding Frontiers', Dr. Jayasuriya noted that HIV-related pieces of legislation are to be found in over 180 legal jurisdictions. Adumbrating the functional role of HIV law, he mentioned monitoring; regulating human behaviour; the establishment of policy frameworks and institutional mechanisms; resource allocation and NGO recognition; standard setting, in terms of licensing and quality control of blood and blood products, condoms, organs, tissues; counselling and testing; and creating supportive and enabling environments.

Dr. Jayasuriya concluded his presentation with a discussion of the factors affecting policy and legal choices. These were identified as: the current state of knowledge; the experience with traditional public health control models; political expediency; conformity with constitutional or legal provisions and ethical practices; role of vested interests and interest groups; public opinion; religious and cultural acceptability; administrative and economic feasibility; and the role of the judiciary. Precedents set by other countries and resolutions adopted by the UN and other specialized agencies were also considered as additional factors.

HIV-Related Ethical Issues

Ms. Susan Timberlake of the Global Programme on AIDS made a presentation on 'HIV-Related Ethical issues'. It was structured around the general ethical principles of wellbeing or beneficence, justice and respect, professional ethics and legal obligations. She observed that ethical considerations have not characterized the response to the epidemic. The approach to such a complex and sensitive issue should be marked by a sense of compassion, solidarity, responsibility and tolerance and the obligation to inform and empower.

Privacy and Confidentiality Laws and HIV

Prof. Larry Gostin of the Georgetown University Law Center introduced his presentation by pointing out that privacy is one of the defining concepts of any system of law and ethics. He defined privacy as the right of an individual to limit access by others to a part of him or her. The concept of 'informational privacy' relates to information about the individual and is particularly important in the context of HIV.

In addition to the ethical justifications for privacy protection, including respect for autonomy, Prof. Gostin emphasized that privacy protection is good for public health. It encourages good partner notification in the context of the HIV epidemic and avoids driving the epidemic underground. In addition, disclosure of a person's HIV status without permission can lead to discrimination and other adverse consequences for the person involved. Protection of privacy is, therefore, both a personal and a collective good.

Difficult questions arise when there is a need to balance competing interests, namely the need for information gathering to serve a particular public objective and an individual's right to privacy. He argued that one must take privacy protection very seriously and uphold privacy unless there is clear evidence that withholding disclosure of information is causing direct and serious harm to others.

Prof. Gostin then discussed the issue of whether there may be a legal power or duty to warn other people about the risk of HIV infection, such as where a health worker knows that a person's sexual partner is being put at risk. He also discussed the issue of disclosure of HIV status in the case of sexual assault and also where a health care worker is infected with HIV. In both cases, he suggested an approach that first looks at what will be achieved by breaching privacy and whether there is an ethical or public health justification for doing so—will it prevent the spread of HIV? In the case of sexual assault, he pointed out, there is no public health benefit in disclosing the HIV status of the alleged perpetrator since the harm has already been done. Similarly, in the case of the HIV infected health care workers, the actual risk of HIV transmission to patients is so low that it is difficult to justify disclosure.

Prof. Gostin concluded by recommending that all countries should consider legislation to protect privacy in relation to HIV. Only where there is a clear and real danger to others should any encroachment on privacy be legally justified.

In the course of the discussion following Prof. Gostin's paper, it was pointed out that legislation cannot always solve the dilemmas surrounding privacy and HIV. Consideration needs to be given to the ethical principles that govern these dilemmas.

HIV-Related Human Rights Issues

Ms. Timberlake's presentation highlighted why human rights considerations are so critical in relation to the HIV epidemic. Indeed, she noted that the slogan for this year's World AIDS Day is 'Shared Rights, Shared Responsibilities'.

Ms. Timberlake also pointed out that the right to health has not yet been adequately defined in the international human rights arena. Very often, the notion of public health has been misused to justify other encroachments upon individual rights. This has led to blame, stigma and discrimination of people with HIV.

She pointed to the fact that HIV is different from other infectious diseases in that the primary intervention strategy is changing individual behaviour. With appropriate behavioural change, people can protect themselves from the risk of HIV infection, but appropriate social support is needed to facilitate this behavioural change.

She outlined the various recognized human rights that are relevant in the context of the HIV epidemic. These include the rights to life, the right to privacy, the right to education, the right to health and the right to human dignity. In addition, because many groups have been identified as having inadequate access to HIV prevention information (e.g., women, poor people, children), it is also relevant to consider access to available medical treatment.

Ms. Timberlake argued that whenever law reform is contemplated in response to the HIV epidemic, human rights considerations need to be brought into the debate to ensure that people have access to the necessary information to protect themselves and also have the means to act upon this information. Further, there is a need to address risk activities that are determined by other external factors, such as forced migration and poverty induced prostitution.

Ms. Timberlake concluded by emphasizing the importance of a close scrutiny of any attempt to justify infringements of human rights on grounds of public health. In all cases, a restriction of human rights can be justified only if it is proportional to the objective sought to be achieved, is the least restrictive means available for achieving that objective, and does actually achieve the objective. She pointed out that many so-called public health measures often fail to meet these criteria.

Country Status Reports

During the first three days of the workshop, the current situation in relation to the HIV epidemic in each of the participating countries was presented in the form of country reports, which were circulated to all the participants. A summary of selected reports is included in Part III of this publication.

Public Health Policy, HIV and the Law-Why Individual Rights Matter?

In her presentation, Ms. Julie Hambling from Australia argued that the traditional approach to HIV, which sought to 'balance' public health interests against individual rights, was fundamentally flawed. She argued that strategies in response to the HIV epidemic could be successful only if policy-makers strongly recognized that individual rights are an integral part of good public health policy. In other words, there is rarely a conflict between public health and individual rights; rather, the two interests are often complementary.

She pointed out that the notion of conflict between public health and individual rights rested upon an 'us and them' approach to the epidemic. Such an approach meant that policy-makers sought to deny the fact that everyone is likely to be touched by the HIV epidemic and that they must work together to deal with it rather than seek to punish certain groups perceived to be the only people at risk. Because it is now known as to what needs to happen in order to respond effectively to the HIV epidemic (i.e., personal behavioural change in a supportive social environment), the problem lies in finding ways of implementing these changes. Experience has shown that effective change can be brought about only through consultation, collaboration, and a sense of shared responsibility among all people within any community.

Ms. Hamblin argued that the essential principles that must underpin any effective response to the HIV epidemic are partnership and shared responsibility. Only if there is this recognition of common interests, will a country be able to support the necessary behavioural changes. Therefore, it is dangerous and wrong to analyze the issue in the context of a conflict between public health and individual rights.

In relation to the potential role of criminal law, Ms. Hamblin emphasized that the vast majority of cases of HIV transmission in the world today occur in circumstances where neither party knows that he or she is infected. Criminal law is not applicable to these cases. Where a person deliberately and knowingly causes harm to others, the already existing criminal law in most countries is adequate to deal with such a situation. However, this is not the central issue in the response to the HIV epidemic, and must not be allowed to divert attention from the real question, which is: How best can the necessary behavioural changes be encouraged and sustained? Certainly, punitive interventions that rely upon the use of criminal law are far more likely to obstruct appropriate behavioural changes than to support it.

The Status of Women—The Role of Law and Religion

Ms. Mehrun Siraj from Malaysia outlined the issues that are particularly relevant to the impact of the HIV epidemic upon women. In particular, she pointed out that women continue to be infected in large numbers even when their only sexual partner is their husband. Even where the law does not formally discriminate against women, their inferior social status often leaves them vulnerable to HIV infection. There are some countries, for example, where the offence of marital rape does not exist.

Ms. Siraj suggested that in times of crisis, it is necessary to go back to the religious foundations of a society. Otherwise, one risks 'pulling up the anchor' and losing the social stability that religion can provide.

Religious values and beliefs can be relied upon to address HIV in many different ways. Under Islamic law, for example, it is recognized that a wife can refuse sexual intercourse with her husband if there is a 'just cause'. Thus, the efforts of a wife whose husband is infected with HIV to protect herself can be interpreted to have religious sanction. However, this involves an increased emphasis on the importance of religious beliefs and practices.

Ms. Siraj believed that law had a limited role to play in changing the factors that place women at risk. She pointed out that women are often forced to take up prostitution because of poverty. In these circumstances, the solution is not to criminalize prostitution but to address the needs of women in other ways, such as providing skills training and alternative sources of income. She suggested that religion is a more effective way of bringing about behavioural change than is law.

Discrimination and Legal Protection

Mr. Manuel Goyena from the Philippines pointed out that the HIV epidemic is reflecting inequities already existing in many societies. Discrimination takes several forms. In addition to the long established patterns of discrimination, such as those based on race, HIV infection is now becoming a focus for discrimination.

He observed that discrimination against people on grounds of HIV infection is often not motivated by evil intent but by fear and ignorance. While many seek to justify discrimination by relying upon public health considerations, this is in fact an unjustifiable denial of human rights.

In looking at how the law can assist in addressing HIV-relates discrimination. Mr. Goyena suggested that legal measures should be directed towards developing an enabling environment for behavioural changes to deal with the impact of the HIV epidemic. Legal measures should be consistent with the principles of equality and human dignity, and should be implemented only after consultation with people with HIV.

Panel Discussion on the Role of Non-Government Organizations in HIV Law Review and Law Reform

Mr. Jon Ungphakorn from Thailand served as the moderator. Other members were Mr. Khim Chong Yee (Malaysia), Mr. Manuel Goyena (Philippines), Prof. Kyung-Kyoon Chung (Republic of Korea) and Ms. Lin-Oi-Chu (Hong Kong).

Panel members began by pointing out that the kind of NGOs that can effectively respond to the HIV epidemic are not limited to HIV service organizations. NGOs which work with affected communities, such as drug users and sex workers, also have a particular role to play.

The special role of NGOs in the response to the HIV epidemic stems from their concern for the rights of the affected people. Equally important, these organizations can speak on their behalf, express their particular needs and concerns, and enable them to have a role in articulating HIV policy. This is a critical element of any community's response to the epidemic, since in many countries there are very few people with HIV who are willing to talk publicly about their infection.

The main human rights issues identified by panel members were discrimination and equal opportunity, confidentiality, the problem of mandatory testing, and the need for greater empowerment of people with HIV. Because some governments tend to suppress public discussions on human rights issues, it is important that NGOs remain active and vocal.

A need to collaborate with other relevant individuals in groups was identified. For example, it was suggested that it is important for NGOs in Malaysia to work in partnership with religious leaders as far as possible. Only through these kinds of partnerships can effective change be brought about.

Panel members felt that NGOs could play a range of different roles in response to the HIV epidemic, including:

* Bringing together diverse groups to encourage dialogue and develop consensus.
* Promoting HIV education and prevention measures.
* Advocacy for people with HIV.
* Acting as a role model for collaboration and consultation.
* Recommending appropriate legislation and law reform.
* Raising awareness of the rest of the community, especially the media, about HIV.

Panel members felt that the law could be a useful tool for bringing about changes in the response to the HIV epidemic. However, for it to be effective, law reform must be concomitant with social activism and efforts to change social values. It was also pointed out that one of the biggest challenges facing NGOs is to take the discussion about law and ethics to the grassroots level, so that it reflects the real needs of the affected communities. This in turn emphasizes the importance for NGOs of maintaining close links with affected individuals and groups.

In the ensuing discussion, it was pointed out that there are many existing human rights NGOs which have not yet focussed upon HIV. It was agreed that efforts need to be made to draw these organizations into the response to the epidemic. However, it was recognized that many of them are already overstretched, making it difficult for them to focus on a whole new policy area.

Creating an Environment Supportive of Legal and Practice Changes

Dr. Jayasuriya spoke briefly about the elements that promote an environment which is supportive of the changes necessary to respond to the HIV epidemic. Among the factors he identified were:

* Capacity building
* Policy/legal practice reforms
* Existence of legal structures to determine complaints
* Facilitating access to legal and administrative remedies
* Current awareness/information sharing/strategic questioning

Models for A Consultative Process

Dr. Abdul Rasid of Malaysia described his country's experience in establishing a model for consultation and collaboration between the many government departments involved in responding to the HIV epidemic, the NGO community, and other relevant community sectors such as the media. The Ministry of Health in Malaysia, he pointed out, believed that effective government policies on HIV must take religious and cultural factors into account, and that effective responses, therefore, required consultation with the affected communities.

Dr. Rasid then described the process by which this consultation and collaboration had come about in Malaysia. His description of the Malaysian model is included in this publication.

Panel Discussion on National and Regional Networks on Ethics, Law and HIV

Dr. Paikiasothy Saravanamuttu from Sri Lanka served as the moderator. Other members were Mr. Manuel Goyena (Philippines), Ms. Mehrun Siraj (Malaysia), Ms. Julie Hamblin (Australia), Mr. Khim Chong Yee (Malaysia), and Dr. Herkutanto (Indonesia).

The panel discussed the initiatives taken so far to establish regional and national networks on ethics, law and HIV. Ms. Julie Hamblin outlined the process by which the UNDP had formed regional networks in Asia and the Pacific, Africa, Latin America and the Caribbean. Mr. Manuel Goyena and Mr. Khim Chong Yee described their experience with the APCASO Network, while Ms. Mehrun Siraj described the Malaysian HIV Legal Network. Ms. Hamblin also referred to a recent consultation held at the UNDP headquarters on networking.

Dr. Saravanamuttu then spoke about the regional focal point for the UNDP network based at the Centre for Policy Research and Analysis (CEPRA) at the University of Colombo in Sri Lanka. He pointed out that the role of CEPRA was to facilitate the consideration, within individual countries in the region, of ethical and legal issues relating to the HIV epidemic and encourage networking within and between countries. CEPRA brings out a regular newsletter to keep network members informed of relevant activities in the region.

Following the introductory presentation by the panel members, participants were divided into small groups to discuss questions associated with networking.

National Networking: Group Discussions

Groups were asked to consider the following four questions:

* Is there a need to address the legal and ethical issues relating to HIV/AIDS in your country?
* How can a network assist in this?
* How can national networks be launched and sustained? What are the obstacles to this?
* How can the UNDP Regional Project Focal Point on Law, Ethics and Human Rights located at CEPRA in Colombo help?

All the groups agreed that there was a need to address the legal and ethical issues relating to HIV/AIDS in countries of the region. It was pointed out, however, that each country needs to determine its own particular priorities.

The need for leadership within each country in order to establish a national network was emphasized, as was the need for funding to support and maintain the network.

It was felt that national networks could help bridge the communication gap by evolving a common language and approach to legal and ethical issues. The networks could also play an advocacy or lobbying role to bring about change. It was, therefore, important that the membership include both the 'unconverted' as well as those who are already sensitive and committed to these issues.

It was suggested that the national networks should be multisectoral even though this could give rise to differences of opinion that would need to be accommodated. It was also felt that countries should explore common subregional issues, such as the movement of sex workers between Thailand and Myanmar, which could lead to fruitful collaboration between their national networks.

The importance of involving the media in these networks was underlined by several participants.

It was agreed that before launching networks, it is important to identify people within each country who are committed to these issues. CEPRA could assist by providing information on networking and sharing knowledge and experience. Participants felt that the regional network could also provide facilitators to assist countries in addressing some of the more difficult issues.

Dr. Saravanamuttu on behalf of CEPRA, however, emphasized that the role of the Regional Focal Point was not to provide expertise to countries on a one-way basis; rather it was to facilitate the flow of information between individuals, organizations and countries in the region. He urged participants to keep CEPRA fully informed of their activities in the area of law, ethics and human rights, so that this information can be used to assist other networking activities in the region.

Analysis of Proposed Legislative Measures

Three discussion groups were formed for this session and they dwelt on legal, ethical and human rights issues raised by a list of proposed legislative measures. The legislative proposals are annexed.

Moot Court Hearing

A hypothetical legal problem resulting in litigation was distributed to various participants who were nominated to play the roles of legal counsel and others for the purposes of a moot court hearing. The case-study is reproduced below:

Moot Case (Trial)

The major exercise for Day 4 was a Moot Trial based on the following hypothetical case, *Chokchai* vs. *The Attorney-General and the District Medical Officer:*

Facts

> Thongchai regularly donates blood as a meritorious deed. He last donated blood two months ago. A few days later the public health officer of his village had come to his factory where he is the manager and had directed him to report to the general hospital. He had been taken away in a police jeep. He did not return home that day and his friend Vichit had informed Noi, his pregnant wife, that Thongshai has been taken away by the police. It was only after unsuccessfully trying to track him down for two days that Noi had come to know that Thongchai is being detained at the Infectious Diseases Hospital. On presenting herself at the hospital to see Thongchai, Noi had been asked as to when the baby is due. When she had replied that she was seven months pregnant, she too had been detained in another ward in the same hospital. Meanwhile Chockshai, Thongchai's father, had contacted the District Medical Officer for information about his son and daughter-in-law. The officer had refused to intervene on the ground that

under the new law on AIDS prevention, he cannot disclose any information concerning patients at the Infectious Diseases Hospital. This law provides for detention upto six months of persons engaging in 'high-risk' activities.

On returning home, Chockchai had informed his wife, Supnee, that there is nothing more that he can possibly do to help his son and daughter-in-law, but Supnee had disagreed. After consulting a lawyer action is eventually filed by Chockchai against:

1. The Attorney General as representing the gc /ernment (Defendant 1)
2. The District Medical Officer (Defendant 2)

The following participated in the Moot Trial:

* Judges	:	Professor Chao Tzee Cheng and Mr. D. Sugar.
* Counsel for Plaintiff	:	Atty. Antonio Dujua, Ms. Yeoh Wee Siam and Mr. Dang Thanh Son.
* Counsel for the first defendant	:	Dr. Herkutanto SH, Mr. Khamkong Liemphrachanh and Mr.Kranh Cheyleaphy Tony.
* Counsel for the second defendant	:	Mr. U Saw Soe Phone Myint and Mrs. Duk-Hyn Kim.
* Newspaper Reporters	:	Mr. Bhaskar Bhattacharji and Ms. Shiela Zhou.
* Human Rights Observers	:	Mr. Pipat Thongpadungrojana and Mr. Manuel Goyena.
* Court Registrar	:	Mr. S. Gurumurthy.

Panel Discussion on Legal, Ethical and Human Rights Issues from the Perspective of National AIDS Programme Managers

Dr. Evelyn Gacad from the Philippines served as the moderator. Other members were Dr. Tia Phalla (Cambodia), Dr. Wiput Phoolcharoen (Thailand), Mr. Dang Thanh Son (Vietnam), Dr. G. Dashzeveg (Mongolia), and Dr. Myo Aung (Myanmar).

The national programme managers represented on the panel agreed that there was a need to consider ethical issues when implementing policies on HIV. While in some of the countries represented little work had been done to date on HIV law, it was recognized that in any law reform process it was important to balance the advantages and disadvantages of each proposed change.

The importance of integrating the social and economic aspects with legal aspects was noted. Similarly, the benefits of exchange of information and expertise between national AIDS programme managers (who most commonly have a medical background) and lawyers were underlined. The involvement of NGOs in the policy process can also be helpful in creating a momentum for change.

The need to inform law-makers (lawyers, members of parliament, etc.), about HIV law, ethics and human rights was noted. One programme manager emphasized the need for financial assistance to enable countries to consider which law reforms might be appropriate.

In general, it was felt that national and international workshops on law, ethics and HIV can be of valuable assistance to HIV policy makers addressing these issues. Another useful approach is the setting up of subcommittees on legal and ethical issues to advise the national AIDS programmes.

Among the other points raised during this session were the importance of giving leadership on legal and ethical issues by the national AIDS programmes and the need to mobilize the support of prominent public figures outside the government to aid policy changes.

Development of Check-Lists to Facilitate the Law Review/Law Reform Process

Dr. D.C. Jayasuriya and Ms. Susan Timberlake presented to the workshop two proposed check-lists to assess the appropriateness of proposed legislative measures and their conformity with human rights requirements. The group made various suggestions, including amendments to incorporate matters that had emerged during the course of the workshop. In particular, it was suggested that the checklists should include the following questions:

* What further information is needed in order to assess the proposed legal measure?
* What objective is sought to be achieved by the measure?
* Is the measure effective in achieving that objective in the least restrictive way possible?

Session to Discuss Follow-up Activities

During the workshop, a form had been circulated among the participants to enable them to list further follow-up activities by the UNDP Regional Project which they participants considered would be useful. The suggestions made by participants include the following:

* Making available more publications on law, ethics and human rights.

* Preparing an inventory of existing laws.
* Undertaking a nationwide survey of the attitudes of lawyers to HIV.
* Preparation of a directory of HIV law, ethics and human rights experts in the region.
* Promoting national networking—if possible, with seed funding from UNDP.
* Encouraging CEPRA to be more pro-active in promoting national networks.
* Arranging further workshops on specific subject areas - e.g., HIV and criminal law; teaching of HIV law; the process of legal change etc.

On the question of funding, Dr. Jayasuriya indicated that the UNDP Regional Project in New Delhi would be contacting organizations to investigate possible funding for the regional and national networks. Participants would be informed of the outcome of these discussions.

Evaluation

A questionnaire was circulated to obtain feedback from the participants as to their views on the workshop - its scope and content, structure, working modalities, usefulness and relevance. Their overall impression was very positive, as exemplified by the following responses:

* Exceptionally good — 13
* Good — 16
* Satisfactory — 4
* Not very satisfactory — nil

Dr. Jayasuriya remarked that on the basis of this feedback, certain modifications would be mate to the agenda of the next workshop.

Closing Session

A highlight of the last day of the Training Workshop was the announcement made by Prof. Chen Chun Ming of the Chinese Academy of Preventive Medicine concerning its decision to serve as the focal point for a national network on HIV law in China. The participants congratulated the academy for taking this important and timely initiative.

Dr. Jayasuriya underlined the need for participants to follow the Chinese example by establishing similar networks for their respective countries.

In his closing remarks, Dr. Jayasuriya expressed the gratitude of the Regional Project to the Chinese Academy of Preventive Medicine for co-sponsoring the workshop. He also thanked the participants, the two consultants, the various service organizations that had nominated the participants, UNDP Beijing, other UNDP field offices and UNOPS for making it possible to orgariize and conduct this training workshop.

79

Colombo Training Workshop: On HIV Law and Law Reform

(Report of the Proceedings of the UNDP Regional Project on HIV and Development Training Workshop on HIV Law and Law Reform in SAARC Countries, 13-16 February 1995, Colombo, Sri Lanka)

OPENING SESSION

In his opening remarks, Dr. D.C. Jayasuriya, the Regional HIV and Development Adviser, UNDP Regional Project on HIV and Development in Asia and the Pacific, set out briefly the them of the regional training workshop: HIV-related laws and law reform. He pointed out that within two years of the outbreak of the pandemic, several countries had enacted HIV specific laws; some adopted an isolationist strategy while others sought to create supportive environments by avoiding discriminatory treatment of persons with HIV. At the interface between medical practices and legal measures relating to HIV and its management are issues of ethics, human rights, and social and individual responsibility. He spoke of the functional role of the law in monitoring HIV cases, protecting individuals who were known to be infected, and in regulating measures designed to slow down the spread of HIV.

In his welcome speech, Mr. Robert England, the Resident Representative of UNDP in Sri Lanka, emphasized the importance of viewing HIV/AIDS as a special development issue. The issue, he pointed out, is not only difficult to acknowledge, discuss, handle and confront openly, but also demands bringing together the distinct entities addressing it, be it the doctor and the community worker or the UNDP and WHO. The United Nations has now decided to launch an inter-agency initiative-UNAIDS to bring together the development perspectives and expertise of its various agencies to deal with what is now seen as the dominant development issue. He underlined the centrality of issues of governance—broadly defined as the relationships between the individual, community and society at large -and the participation of the people, in particular, the role of women, in the resolution of HIV-related problems.

In his keynote address, the Chief Guest, Mr. Justice Sarath Silva, President of the Court of Appeal in Sri Lanka, emphasized that in the absence of a cure or a vaccine for HIV/AIDS, social and administrative action and the establishment of a suitable legal machinery are the main strategies that can be deployed to arrest the spread of this deadly virus. There are two roles that law can play in relation to HIV/AIDS. First, punitive, i.e., the imposition of sanctions and mandatory requirements to prevent the spread of the virus. Second, protective, i.e., safeguarding the rights of those infected to ensure that they are not discriminated against and that they enjoy equal rights. However, to effectively contain the spread of the epidemic, the law should move beyond these two functions to play a more positive and pro-active role.

Justice Silva also underlined the importance of taking into account the socio-economic setting in reviewing and drafting laws. The broadly similar pattern in the South Asian region -small, fairly developed urban pockets with relatively good health infrastructure surrounded by large, backward rural areas with rudimentary health care systems -is highly conducive to the spread of HIV/AIDS. Laws should take into consideration this socio-economic context.

With regard to prevention, Justice Silva stressed that the most effective legal strategy is to devise a scheme of voluntary testing with legal safeguards, to preserve the anonymity, confidentiality and autonomy of the individual. While upholding human rights and fundamental freedoms, it was important, however, to have legal mechanisms, subject to safeguards and conditions, whereby mandatory testing can be permitted in extreme cases. Finally, Justice Silva underlined the need for a proper legal mechanism to protect society against the awesome fear and panic reaction that HIV/AIDS evokes in people.

MODES OF TRANSMISSION AND EPIDEMIOLOGICAL TRENDS IN THE SAARC REGION

In the first presentation entitled 'Modes of Transmission and Epidemiological Trends in Asia', Dr. J.P. Narain of the World Health Organization stressed the need for urgent action in South Asia. This is necessary if the horrendous consequences of AIDS, expected to peak in the region in the next few years, are to be minimized. He maintained that the number of AIDS cases officially reported in the region were not a reliable basis for planning because of gaps in testing, monitoring and reporting. For these reasons, WHO and other agencies work out informed guestimates. (For example, while the number of reported cases in India as of 1 January 1995 stood at 905, the estimated HIV infections were in the region of 1,500,000.) Such figures may be closer to the actual figure which cannot be ascertained accurately at present given the limitations of infrastructure, including facilities for voluntary testing. He emphasized the importance of a quick, broad consensus on the figures. He felt that there was no justification for the considerable time and effort wasted by different parties in some countries in defending the number of HIV cases.

There were, he said, worrying trends in terms of the considerable increase in the rate of infection amongst sex workers in Bombay and Madras and in the number of pregnant women who tested positive (between 1992 and 1994 their percentage doubled, from 0.06 to 0.12 per cent). An interesting feature of testing of pregnant women is the fact that it is anonymous, in the sense that neither the women's identities are known nor are they told about the tests since the testing is done only for epidemiological purposes.

PUBLIC HEALTH AND ETHICAL ISSUES IN HIV/STD PREVENTION AND CONTROL

In the next presentation, Dr. G. Jayakuru, the National AIDS Programme Manager in Sri Lanka, outlined a series of ethical and legal issues that he and his team faced in their work. Existing laws on infectious diseases appear to require the notification of AIDS to health authorities within 12 hours of detection. (Interestingly, under current Sri Lankan law only 'AIDS' is notifiable but not 'HIV'.) He wondered whether this requirement was at all relevant and useful when applied to AIDS. He felt that notification procedures have to be regulated by law because they can and do compromise confidentiality considerably. He pointed to the haphazard, inaccurate and inefficient methods of testing in private laboratories in Sri Lanka, a situation which he was anxious to see regulated through law. He recalled one or two instances when blood samples were mixed up and the wrong people informed of the wrong results, causing considerable anguish to some individuals and engendering a false sense of security in others. He was very concerned that the careless disposal of syringes and hospital wastes be stopped through the enforcement of proper legislation.

In Sri Lanka, there is a follow-up of those donors whose blood is found to be infected. Dr. Jayakuru observed that the doctors did not accept that informed consent was a necessary legal or ethical requirement in such cases of, what was really, mandatory testing. He wondered whether patients suffering from dementia or those who are unconscious can be tested without their consent or the consent of their guardians. He further raised issues of ethics and law in relation to filling out of death certificates. Should the doctor cite HIV-related causes as the actual causes of death or not? And, should persons who perform pre-burial embalming procedures be notified of infected individuals? He also said he found that infected patients who continued to engage in high-risk behaviour after knowing their HIV status could not be compelled to refrain from such behaviour because the authorities could not find any law that made such behaviour an offence.

THE SOCIO-ECONOMIC IMPACT OF THE EPIDEMIC

Discussing the socio-economic impact of the HIV epidemic in Asia, Dr. D.C. Jayasuriya pointed out that the Asian region was lagging behind in the quality and quantum of social research needed to discern trends and identify areas where the impact of HIV should be better understood. While the main source of risk behaviour in the Asian region is heterosexual, in a number of countries risk factors include a combination of both (a) homosexual behaviour and heterosexual behaviour; (b) heterosexual behaviour and IV drug use; and (c) homosexual behaviour and IV drug use. During the early years of the HIV epidemic two models—the "medical model" and the "stigma model"—influenced attitudes and the choice of preventive methods. It has taken time to realize that preventive methods must be based on a broader 'mix' of underlying causes that take into account the role of behavioural change and safety practices in slowing the pace of HIV transmission. Speaking on the sexual transmission of HIV, Dr. Jayasuriya drew attention to the social and cultural context of sex and the need to take a closer look at aspects such as cultural rules and norms regulating premarital and extramarital sex; gender imbalance; economic inequality; negotiating skills; and sexual networking.

With regard to the economic dimensions of the HIV epidemic, reference was made to a study done in Thailand which revealed that the aggregate direct and indirect costs of AIDS between the period 1991-2000 will reach US $ 8 billion. The study identified the negative effects on tourism, foreign investment and labour remittances from abroad. Dr. Jayasuriya also cited a number of economic impact studies conducted in other Asian countries with the support of the UNDP Regional Project and the Asian Development Bank.

NATURE AND SCOPE OF HIV LAW

Speaking on the evolution of HIV-related laws, Dr. D.C. Jayasuriya commented on the different functional roles of law:

1. Monitoring—case detection, reporting and surveillance.
2. Regulating conduct/behaviour
3. Establishing policy
4. Standard setting
5. Mandating interventions and programmes
6. Establishing services
7. Creating a supportive and enabling environment.

He also drew attention to the possible factors or considerations that influence policy and legal choices, namely: current state of medical knowledge; experience with traditional public health control models; political expediency; conformity with constitutional or other legal provisions and ethical practices; professional bias of policy - and law-makers; influence of vested interests/key groups; public opinion; perceived social, religious and cultural acceptability; administrative or economic feasibility; precedents in other countries or geopolitical groupings; resolutions of UN or specialized agencies; and, finally, the role of the judiciary.

ETHICAL PRINCIPLES

Ms. Susan Timberlake of the World Health Organization spoke on the general ethical principles that are relevant to HIV matters. Among these are:

* Informed consent : Benefits/risks/problems/alternatives are fully explained to the individual.
* Obligation to Treat : Health professionals must, to the best of their ability, treat all persons seeking their

medical attention without discrimination and without prejudice.

* Confidentiality : Professionals must maintain strict confidentiality concerning all personal information obtained from clients in the con text of their professional work.
* Respect for Persons : Individuals must have the capacity and right to make choices about their bodies, personal integrity and actions, as long as they do not diminish or violate the rights of others.
* Distributive Justice : The burdens and benefits of a policy should be distributed equitably among the population.

She maintained that ethical principles are important in yielding a supportive social response, which, in turn, helps affected individuals to assume responsibility for themselves and the community in which they live. She said that policy-makers need to ensure that no particular group or groups in society shoulder an undue share of the burden of general and specific policies adopted.

LAW AND POLICY ON HIV TESTING

In the final presentation on the first day, Dr. T.K.K. Iyer spoke on the theme of 'Law and Public Policy on HIV Testing'. He said that while it is important to note that a law is only as good as the extent of its enforcement, laws do enjoy a high profile in society insofar as they embody the highest and most authoritative declarations of social, ethical and political values. The role of law turns out to be more than just symbolic. It can generate public opinion where none exists. But the paths of law-making and law reform are difficult, even where the legislators can be successfully lobbied. In the area of HIV law reform, besides the parliamentarians and administrators, the other principal actors are, the medical community and the NGOs. There may be some advantages in lobbying the medical community to support specific legislative initiatives in the area of testing, consent and confidentiality. It is unlikely that Parliaments would ignore the views of the medical community in this matter; hence the need to lobby them first before approaching Parliaments or governments with proposals for law reform.

He noted that the inherent limitations of laws and legal systems should also be borne in mind. Laws can either be inadequate in their coverage or too technical, and legal processes can be costly and time-consuming. In South Asia, the legal systems have become overburdened with consequent delays and expenses. It is unlikely that indigent minorities can have ready access. Nevertheless, constitutional guarantees of personal liberty, including rights to privacy are well entrenched in countries such as India, constituting a jurisprudence of public law interpreted and upheld by a vibrant legal bench and the bar. Clearly there is scope in the future for developing rights and obligations in the health-care setting which may benefit HIV positive individuals.

Dr. Iyer pointed out that although testing has often been viewed from the standpoint of public health policies meant to stop the spread of HIV, testing should also be viewed from the individual's standpoint -as affording him or her an early start in learning to cope with the virus, securing family and community support, and generally organizing his or her life economically, professionally, and in other ways.

He then outlined the different public policy approaches to testing, ranging from the adoption of the ethically difficult mandatory testing, through the ethically neutral unlinked testing, to the ethically defensible voluntary testing. The list would include: (a) mandatory testing, (b) voluntary testing, (c) anonymous testing, (d) unlinked testing and (e) surreptitious testing.

He maintained that the presumption is in favour of individual privacy and choice in the matter of testing. Those who wish to impose testing should be asked to show which public interest would be served by such obligatory testing; and if shown, they should be asked to confine the testing and dissemination of the results strictly to that purpose or objective. He listed the following areas where some policy-makers have argued that public interest justified mandatory testing: (a) surgeries where the chances of prick injuries to the surgeon and other medical staff are said to be high; (b) recruitment to the defence forces where soldiers often live closely together and sexual contacts do occur, or where blood transfusions occur during emergencies with soldiers being required to donate blood; (c) immigration where the host country wishes to keep out HIV positive immigrants lest they become a burden on their health care systems; and (d) sex workers.

He then proceeded to list the more controversial areas where public interest is not so immediately obvious to justify mandatory testing: (a) pre-employment testing as part of the general medical examination given by an employer, who is concerned with i.e. medical bills that have to be settled; (b) insurance proposals involving life coverage; (c) prisons where voluntary and involuntary sexual contacts do occur; and (d) pregnant women who may have been IV drug users or sex workers.

He concluded by saying that testing cannot be viewed in isolation. It has to take place in the context of counselling, notification of partners, and helping the individual and his or her family to cope with the virus. He said that it would be difficult to pretend that there would be no imperatives to test for reason of public interest, including, in the South Asian context, for the protection of vulnerable groups such as women and children, especially in the rural areas.

INFORMED CONSENT AND CONFIDENTIALITY IN SOUTH

On the utility of HIV specific laws, Dr. P. Salil, from India's National AIDS Control Organization, cautioned that given the South

Asian setting where the medical profession and the patients are not yet used to observing and demanding confidentiality, any procedures specific to HIV patients may have the negative effect of making them stand out from other patients, and, thus isolating them even more than they are now. Thus, the negative externalities of well-intentioned laws must be carefully monitored, he said. It was noted by others that medical professionals in South Asia, as elsewhere, complained that given the pressures of medical practice and the numbers of patients they see daily, it would be unrealistic to insist on informed consent and strict confidentiality in medical situations.

HIV-RELATED HUMAN RIGHTS

The sessions of Day 2 began with Ms. Susan Timberlake speaking on the theme of 'HIV Related Human Rights Issues'. She said that there are three ways in which human rights relate to HIV. First, there are good reasons to urge that upholding basic rights is an optimally effective way of reducing the spread of HIV. As a historical footnote, she cited examples from the past when minority groups were readily blamed for the spread of infectious diseases when the truth of that spread lay in a much wider context which had nothing to do with the chosen scapegoats. In medieval Europe the plague was blamed on the Jews, while in the 1900s plague in Australia was blamed on the Chinese minority and 'their habits'. Secondly, the victims of HIV have hitherto been, and still largely are, minority groups already disadvantaged in society in terms of poverty, fewer opportunities of access to education and health facilities, and, above, all, outside the reach of preventive information programmes. The need seems to be, therefore, to give such groups more rights, and certainly, protect them from discriminatory exclusions. As a specific example, she cited the need to empower women to refuse unsafe sex with husbands or male companions. She felt that coerced, unsafe sex, even within marriage, was a problem that needs to be addressed quickly. Thirdly, discrimination against those who are already infected, or at times suspected of being infected, means that it is necessary to examine how best to preserve their rights in such life choices as marriage (in some jurisdictions which require a marriage licence, it may be denied because of positive HIV status), sterilization (evidence shows women with HIV might have been compelled to accept sterilization), emigration or asylum (mandatory tests for potential emigrants and asylum seekers).

She pointed out that international human rights laws have laid down guidelines as to how and when rights may be restricted on grounds of "public health". She emphasized that even where public health justifications are demonstrated, the restrictions must be imposed through democratically enacted laws that are proportional to the achievement of clearly stated and understood aims. It is important to review periodically such restrictive laws to establish that they do in fact achieve the intended objectives.

She circulated a tabulated sheet, *not* as an official document of WHO, showing the human rights applicable to HIV and public health.

In the ensuing discussions, it was agreed that principles of administrative law and not merely of constitutional law be invoked to review whether a particular legally enacted restriction of human rights of HIV positive persons is proportional to the objectives laid down in the law and whether in fact those objectives are met in the administration of that law. Some participants wondered whether the state can legitimately claim to restrict the reproductive rights of a woman who may be HIV positive when medical evidence suggests that AZT administered during pregnancy reduces further the 30 per cent natural chances of infection of the baby.

COUNTRY PRESENTATIONS

1. Sri Lanka

Ms. Charika Marasinghe of the Faculty of Law of the University of Colombo described HIV-related legal issues in Sri Lanka. She listed a number of laws, many going back to the last century, and pointed to the specific provisions which need urgent review and reform in the light of HIV and related matters. She said that despite the illegality of the activity, commercial sex work was widespread with nearly 4,500 street sex workers and another nearly 4,000 brothel workers in Sri Lanka. In addition, nearly 1,500 children are in the sex work trade in the country. She felt that current pressures for new legislation in other economic and commercial areas are so heavy that inevitably HIV law reform will be relegated to the background. Considerable lobbying is needed to move it to the top of the parliamentary legislative agenda.

Since the public health laws enacted by the British colonial administration in the last century are a common heritage of almost all the South Asian countries, the need for reform of these old laws in the Sri Lankan context will, in many ways, apply to others countries in the region. The Chairman, Dr. D.C. Jayasuriya, reminded the Workshop that participants needed to develop for their respective countries a checklist of laws that may require review and reform.

2. Bangladesh

Mr. Subhan, a retired judge from Bangladesh, speaking on the situation in his country remarked that there was a severe legal vacuum on the HIV/AIDS front. The legality of certain measures prescribed by Islamic religious courts presided over by mullahs is yet to be determined. These courts have sentenced women 'suspected of illicit sexual connections' to up to a 100 lashes. The infliction of this type of punishment has led to the death of several women. The legality of this punishment is debatable. He observed that the AIDS Council of Bangladesh has much work to do in its campaign on education and law reform.

3. India

Dr. Salil, Assistant Director of India's National AIDS Control Organization (NACO) said that to assist the process of reviewing existing laws or of proposing amendments and new laws, NACO has created a Technical Advisory Committee. Of its several subcommittees there is a Social, Legal and Ethical Subcommittee consisting of experts from the professions as well as from NGOs and community organizations. A review report by this sub-committee is under preparation. NACO has sought to minimize the conflict between human rights and requirements of public health. He was confident that with a partnership between the government authorities, hospitals and the activist NGOs, such conflicts in India can be minimized.

Dr. Salil remarked that NACO was mindful of the need to review the following laws and legal provisions in particular: (a) The Prevention of Immoral Traffic (in Women and Girls) Act (the Indian police has interpreted this law as one enabling them to arrest men and women found with condoms in their possession after 19:00 hours); (b) Narcotics and Psychotropic Drugs and Substances Act (some agencies think that this law makes it an offence to possess a syringe unless the person is a medical practitioner); and (c) Section 377 of the Indian Penal Code which makes homosexual acts an offence.

Through the efforts of NACO, the Drugs and Cosmetics Act has been amended to make blood testing mandatory prior to transfusions. But mandatory testing has been limited to specific situations and the general policy of the programme has been against mandatory testing. The single instance of a State law that provided for mandatory testing, the Goa Public Health Act, under which an HIV positive person was detained and which attracted litigation and adverse publicity in India, has now been repealed.

In the ensuing discussion, Mr. Pavan Duggal, an Indian lawyer, said that some hospitals in India were flouting the guidelines issued by the National AIDS Control Programme. He cited the example of a person in indigent circumstances who had paid Rs.10,000 to a hospital in the Indian state of Gujarat for an operation, but was removed by the hospital from its premises as soon as it was found out that he was HIV positive. There are still no guidelines for the media on how to raise and discuss HIV-related matters. Questions such as whether the HIV positive status of a spouse can be a ground for divorce under Indian law needed to be examined carefully.

4. Nepal

Ms. Shanta Dixit of Himal Association from Nepal said that it was still early days in her country for creating an adequate basis for HIV education and treatment of HIV infected persons, both in the medical and socio-legal senses. However, her country had a fairly successful needle exchange programme. In responding to queries from participants from India, she said that Nepal considered the problem of young Nepali girls being 'sold' or consigned to the red-light districts of Bombay and Calcutta in India to be serious enough to warrant a subregional convention on trafficking in minors and sex workers. There appeared to be a general consensus that this suggestion may well benefit if UNDP, WHO and UNICEF supported.

5. Pakistan

Mr. Shoukat Ali from Pakistan AIDS Prevention Society listed the following problems as demanding urgent attention in his country: (a) increasing drug addiction, (b) inadequate screening of blood, (c) inadequate levels of sex education, and finally (d) inadequate awareness and protection of human rights, largely because of Pakistan's political history of military regimes with the attendent suspension of fundamental rights. He also mentioned that matters such as the Hadood Ordinance and the punishment of 'illicit sex' would have to be examined in the HIV context to see how far they hinder the prevention of HIV. He pointed out that some provincial governments were in the process of preparing two bills, one for a new law to cover blood donations and screening and another on child abuse, including sexual abuse of children. Although some relaxation had taken place recently, considerable change was still needed, he said, with regard to media treatment of sexual information. He also noted that the monitoring of HIV cases needed to be improved. The figure of 802 HIV cases for the whole country, he felt, was a very rough, and far from accurate, estimate. He added that in recent years about 700 Pakistanis had been deported from Middle Eastern countries on account of their HIV positive status and at many foreign embassies in Pakistan now require 'HIV free certificates' from Pakistani applicants for visas.

6. Maldive Islands

Mr. Al-Su'ood from the Attorney General's Department in the Maldives said that his country has a small population of about 250,000 people and, as of 1994, there were only three reported cases of HIV infection. Steeped in Islamic religion and culture, the country has no HIV specific laws. However, the newly established National AIDS Council has taken many administrative steps to disseminate information and offer HIV tests. Although proposals have been mooted to compulsorily test visiting sailors and seamen, there is no compulsory testing mandated by law. Being a small community, persons are anxious not to be identified as HIV positive because of the quick and extensive ostracism that will inevitably follow. This anxiety has a bearing on testing and dissemination of the results. Those identified may also face prosecution for the use of narcotic drugs or for illicit 'immoral' behaviour, all of which are religious offences. In such prosecutions, there is no provision for defence lawyers even though the prosecutor is a lawyer. However, he pointed out, his country has sought to ensure, through administrative means, confidentiality for persons who are HIV positive. Given the small size of the community, it is going to be difficult to preserve confidentiality. All in all, developing a strategy of voluntary testing in his country will be difficult.

7. Other Countries

In a brief account of the history of HIV and AIDS measures in Australia, Mr. David Patterson of the Canadian AIDS Organization, highlighted the partnership that has been forged between the public health authorities on the one hand and activist groups such as gay and lesbian coalitions and a whole range of community based NGOs on the other, as the basis for the preventive measures in place to slow down the spread of HIV. In Canada, the community based organizations are just beginning to garner their efforts in improving matters relating to HIV prevention, such as outreach, counselling and preventive education.

CONFIDENTIALITY

Speaking on 'HIV, Confidentiality and the Process of Policy Development', Mr. David Patterson pointed out that confidentiality is a matter of process and not merely of stated policy. In developing processes that respect the right to privacy, a fundamental human right, the involvement of people living with HIV/AIDS is essential. There needs to be a process of professional and community consensus-building.

He said that the central fact of confidentiality is that disclosure may, and often does, lead to discrimination. Thus there are legal, social and other implications of unregulated disclosures of HIV information. On the question as to what is HIV-related information, he listed a number of situations prior to and after testing. He said that there are several situations that give rise to dilemmas in terms of disclosure. Some examples of these are: (a) workplace issues such as employees refusing to work with a person found to be HIV positive -what should the employer do? (b) A person who is HIV positive refuses to tell his or her sexual partner -what should the doctor or counsellor do? (c) A victim of sexual assault wants the alleged attacker tested for HIV -what should the medical authorities or courts do?

In approaching these issues, he said there is a need for:

1. Factual clarification (e.g., modes of transmission, degrees of risk).
2. Conceptual clarification (e.g., partner notification, HIV related information, whether private or confidential).
3. Agreement on ethical theory, moral principles or values (i.e., utilitarianism versus moral imperatives, right to privacy and so on).

He concluded by listing what he saw to be characteristics of good policies with reference to confidentiality:

1. *Preventive*: Policies should emphasize the prevention of breaches of confidentiality rather than focus on remedies after the fact.
2. *Simple:* Policies should be easily understood.
3. *Consistent:* Good codes of practice should be enforced and reflected, if necessary, in law.
4. *Holistic:* Policies should be integrated with and complement other aspects of the national HIV/AIDS strategy, such as epidemiological research, vaccine and drug trials, and the general civil and criminal law.
5. *Proactive:* Policies should anticipate developments in technology, such as the availability of cheap, rapid tests for HIV antibodies in saliva.
6. *Failsafe: Only* the minimum amount of data should be collected for the particular purpose. If there is a breach, minimal damage will be done.
7. *Bold:* We should not shy away from questioning assumptions (for example, notions of absolute freedom of contract that might allow employers to demand testing of employees for HIV) or the relevance of judicial decisions given before the onset of HIV and thus valid for a very different context.
8. *Flexible:* Where interests conflict, policies should adopt a 'harm reduction approach'. For example, there may be grounds for disclosing a person's HIV status if that person is knowingly placing another at risk, if the disclosur will reduce the risk of HIV transmission and if a less harmful alternative for reducing the risk is not available.

DISCRIMINATION AND LEGAL PROTECTION

In his presentation entitled 'Discrimination and Legal Protection', Mr. J. L. Ignacio, a lawyer working with ALTERLAW in the Philippines, pointed out that discrimination continues to be the main issue in this area. Attention has to be paid to the Universal Declaration of Human Rights to determine the basic parameters of equal treatment and protection under the law. Laws cannot be based solely on the health status of groups or their identification as 'high risk'.

In planning strategies to avoid discrimination, it may be necessary at times to think in terms of positive discrimination in favour of disadvantaged groups such as people living with AIDS. But it is very important to ensure that such positive discrimination laws do not become counter-productive. The cure should not become the poison, a point also made by Dr. Salil of India during his presentation. It is important, nevertheless, that laws be enacted to stop the vilification and incitement to hatred of people belonging to vulnerable groups.

STATUS OF WOMEN

Ms. V.S. Rekha, a lawyer from New Delhi spoke on 'HIV Epidemic and Law - Status of Women'. She said that women are, to a disproportionate extent, victims of HIV; in other words, that they suffered greater social and economic disabilities than male victims of HIV. They experience added difficulties because of prejudices inherent in society. The 'causative factors' affecting most of the HIV positive women centre around either economic dependence or ineffective and weak laws that deny them empowerment. From earlier Vedic times, India had known and often upheld the concept that a woman is an equal partner. That would have to be reclaimed and put into practice once again, she said.

Ms. Rekha outlined the history of the abortive attempt in 1989 to enact the AIDS Prevention Bill, by India's federal Parliament. Since the withdrawal of this bill, the prevention policy of the Indian health authorities, rested on IEC, i.e., information, education and communication.

Ms. Mehrun Siraj, a Malaysian lawyer said that adequate research has not been directed at questions as to how HIV affects women in particular: What happens to their reproductive physiology and the reproductive choices they can or cannot make once they are infected. Can they avoid forcible sterilization? There are even more basic questions: Are wives able to stop husbands from infecting them? Can a woman refuse sex if her husband refuses to use condoms? In Islamic law such refusal of sex is a valid ground for divorcing the wife, she said. Although Islamic religion has granted many rights to women, Islamic countries have not enforced these rights.

In the ensuing discussion, it was underlined that reproduction and sexual health are both women's issues as well as development issues. Joint responsibility lies with women and men for their family size and welfare. References were made to the Cairo Conference and to its recommendations on reproductive and sexual health.

PANEL DISCUSSION ON THE ROLE OF SERVICE ORGANIZATIONS IN LAW REVIEW AND LAW REFORM

Ms. Anjali Gopalan from NAZ, New Delhi, served as the moderator of this panel discussion. Several participants outlined the gaps and tasks which face service organizations in their respective countries. Discussions focussed on three issues: (a) Do we need new laws? (b) Can we enforce existing laws more effectively? (c) Are there matters that fall outside the purview of laws and legal mechanism?

Ms. Anjali Gopalan said that she was aware of laws that helped and those that hindered her work with HIV. An example of the latter was the absence of a legal provision requiring or accommodating the teaching of sex education in schools. Conversely, the existence of certain laws can act as a hindrance to other types of outreach programmes. For example, in public places such as parks, where men have sex with men, the distribution of condoms can be seen as an infringement of the existing laws against sodomy and homosexuality. Under the Prevention of Immoral Traffic Act in India, any woman outreach worker can be arrested by a policeman if he interprets her activity as 'soliciting'. For AIDS service organizations to be effective, they have to work with government organizations, hospitals, jails and other institutions. In the case of hospitals they are expected to comply with the guidelines issued by the National AIDS Control Organization on how to treat HIV infected persons. Pre-and post-test counselling are not provided by many hospitals, which is contrary to the guidelines issued by NACO. Contrary to government policy against mandatory testing, most hospitals test patients undergoing surgery without their consent. They deny services to those infected. In prisons too, Section 337 of the Indian Penal Code, which makes sodomy punishable, is being interpreted to make it impossible to conduct prevention activities; making condoms available is seen as promoting homosexual acts which, according to the authorities, in any case 'does not exist in prisons.'

Another concern for AIDS service organizations is that blood is not always screened. There is a law which mandates testing of all blood, but there are several unlicensed blood banks using unhygienic methods.

Ms. Gopalan said that her organization would wish to urge the following reforms: (a) mandating health education in schools, including HIV/AIDS education; (b) stronger enforcement of anti-discriminatory laws; (c) mandating all medical colleges to address social, legal and ethical aspects of HIV; (d) encouraging medical professionals to look at HIV/AIDS as an integral part of their work instead of seeing it as falling outside the scope of their particular specialties; (e) training for teachers to include sex education; (f) mandating an interministerial approach in dealing with the HIV; and (g) the creation of a body to monitor discrimination against people who are infected.

Following on, Ms. Mehrun Siraj said that although NGOs working at the grassroots level in Malaysia are failiar with the problems faced by the target groups, they cannot by themselves identify the legal issues involved. They need to work in partnership with lawyers to ascertain whether the problems they face arise from: (a) a lack of laws (including the absence of regulations and administrative directions); (b) inappropriate laws; (c) poor enforcement of existing laws; or (d) infringement of existing laws (e.g., exercise of powers .in excess of that provided for by the law).

In turn, lawyers need to work closely with service organizations to know what is needed by way of law reform. Concerned organizations should be requested to comment on proposals for reform as they are better placed to assess the impact of the proposed legal provisions on those most likely to be affected by the law.

Service organizations must be involved in every stage of the law review and reform process. The monitoring of problems and difficulties by these organization, Mr. Siraj pointed out, was an essential first step. Service organizations in Malaysia have also gained valuable experience in lobbying ministry officials.

Mr. Ignacio said that service organizations in Philippines were the leading source of information on HIV. They were also more effective in identifying the needs and problems of those affected by HIV. Thus, NGOs in his country, by acting as information purveyors, performed an essential role.

Mr. Shoukat Ali said that the NGOs in Pakistan faced a difficult task in that they had very little lobbying power to persuade the authorities to help people with HIV or AIDS. NGOs in his country, he felt, should create networks of professionals' and employers' organizations to increase their lobbying power. The other major task of NGOs was to continue to provide the type of essential information that the media in Pakistan did not or could not provide.

Mr. Shirley Tissera of Sri Lanka spoke of the strengths and weaknesses of NGOs. They can count amongst their strengths flexibility in operations; strong and committed membership; and ability to render help at short notice. A major weakness is the absence of unity of purpose among NGOs working in the same field. Co-ordination can be difficult because many are inflexible and tend to hold on to their perceptions of issues as unique and always valid.

TOWARDS AN ENABLING AND SUPPORTIVE ENVIRONMENT

Day 3 began with Dr. D.C. Jayasuriya speaking on 'Creating an Environment Supportive of Legal and Practice Changes'. He said that awareness campaigns in the media, including education programmes, should avoid implying that particular groups in society were responsible for the spread of HIV. He elaborated that an enabling and supportive environment should include the following elements:

1. Building the capacity of individuals, service organizations and NGOs in a range of HIV-related matters such as monitoring laws and policies.
2. Legal and policy reforms.
3. Existence of legal structures—not just the regular courts and tribunals, but also non-judicial avenues of redress such as ombudsman arrangements and hospital complaints and ethical committees. While the complaints committees can entertain individual grievances, ethical committees can influence the formulation of general policies towards HIV-related matters.
4. Facilitating access to legal and administrative remedies. As part of this effort, NGOs and service organizations should establish contacts with legal aid committees and alert them to the needs of persons with HIV/AIDS.
5. Information sharing, current awareness and resource centres for information dissemination.

Following Dr. Jayasuriya's presentation, Mr. N.J. Abeysekera, the Chief Legal Draftsman of the Government of Sri Lanka, pointed out that questions of whom and when to consult and the extent of such consultations are important to the administration when formulating laws. He outlined the various consultative mechanisms and processes that come into play when before laws are made:

1. Although consultations with groups outside of government is often discretionary, there are some laws in Sri Lanka which provide a standard machinery for consultation through standing advisory committees.
2. Governments use 'green' or 'white' papers as a means of wider consultation with several interested members and groups in the community. The added advantage of this mechanism is that the underlying assumptions and difficulties of the proposed law may be better understood. For example, HIV-related laws may in the first instance be seen as issues of law and order, but on consultation they may turn out to be issues of social and economic significance.
3. Commissions of inquiry in Sri Lanka are of two types: (a) departmental commissions and (b) special presidential commissions. The former are very easily set up through administrative fiat; and with a floating membership and their informal procedures, they are very flexible and useful instruments of consultation in the law-making process. The latter are rather more formal, presided over by sitting judges of the high courts of Sri Lanka.
4. Law commissions are very useful for extensive reform of existing laws as well as for proposing new laws.

NATIONAL AND REGIONAL NETWORKING

The panel discussion on 'National and Regional Networks on HIV-Related Law, Ethics and Human Rights' was moderated by Dr. P. Saravanamuttu of CEPRA, Sri Lanka. It focussed on the challenges of and opportunities for establishing and sustaining national networks in the Asia—Pacific region, and the facilitating role of a regional focal point in this respect.

The varying degrees of awareness of in this region of the legal, human rights and ethical dimensions of HIV/AIDS were clearly brought out in the general discussion. In addition, the need to target groups who are key opinion-makers and are directly responsible for law reform, such as politicians and media persons, was emphasized.

The interactive character of the CEPRA Focal Point was also stressed. The importance of the regular receipt of material to the information dissemination activities of the Focal Point was reiterated.

The Focal Point would attain its full potential with the active co-operation of interested organizations and persons in the region.

The general discussion, in which Mr. J. Ignacio, Ms. Mehrum Siraj, Mr. David Patterson and several others participated, also focussed on the financial requirements for setting up national networks. The participants were informed that while the Regional Project is not equipped at present to provide financial assistance to maintain the operations of national networks, the project will be prepared to consider providing other forms of support.

PROPOSED (HYPOTHETICAL) LEGISLATIVE MEASURES

The participants were divided into two groups, A and B, for purposes of discussing and commenting on the following hypothetical problem:

You are the Minister of Health. A committee headed by the Minister of Justice has prepared a draft HIV/AIDS Prevention and Control Bill. The other members of the committee are the Attorney-General, the Director-General of Health, the Director-General of Social Services, the Chief of Police, a senior judge of the Supreme Court, and representatives of associations of lawyers, doctors, social workers and non-governmental organizations. At a Cabinet meeting, you are asked by the Prime Minister to express your views on the desirability of including the following provisions proposed unanimously by the committee:

1. A requirement to subject to compulsory testing for HIV any person whom a police officer or public health inspector suspects to be a 'drug addict', a 'homosexual' or a 'sex worker'.
2. A requirement for foreign visitors intending to reside for more than two weeks to be tested for HIV within ten days of their arrival, and thereafter at intervals of six months.
3. A requirement to quarantine all nationals who are HIV seropositive and to deport all seropositive foreign nationals.
4. A requirement to prohibit nationals from marrying foreigners.
5. A requirement to provide free needles, syringes and condoms to all drug addicts who are registered with the police.
6. A requirement to permit commercial sex establishments to employ as sex workers only those in possession of a HIV-free certificate issued by a government doctor during the past six months.
7. A requirement to compulsorily pre-screen for HIV all jobs

applicants and new university entrants.

8. A requirement for the compulsory teaching of sex education from the primary school level upwards.
9. A requirement to make the presence of infection with HIV or STD a ground for divorce.
10. A requirement for the compulsory use of condoms in all commercial sex encounters.

Group A was asked to consider questions '1' to '5', and Group B the remaining questions. At the end of the deliberations of the two groups, a report from each group was presented to all the participants.

SYNTHESIS OF THE REPORT OF GROUP A

1. It is doubtful if compulsory testing can be justified, either on financial grounds or on moral grounds. By what criteria can a police officer identify persons in the high risk groups? There is too much power vested in police officers, which cannot be supported by any public health rationale.
2. There is no justification for singling out foreigners for testing.
3. Quarantine, in the HIV context, serves no useful purpose and there is no justification either for this or for deportation. The proposed measures will only serve to stigmatize a whole group and deny them their basic human rights. Dissenting note by one member: While there may not be compulsory testing of tourists, long-term residents, such as contract workers, should be tested in order to contain the spread of HIV over international borders.
4. The group disagreed with this requirement although one member felt that the state should be able to advise citizens wishing to marry foreign nationals to arrange for the individuals concerned to be voluntarily tested.
5. Some countries, Muslim countries in particular, may not accept these measures. By a majority, the group agreed with the needle exchange measures because such schemes in place elsewhere were not known to promote drug use. The minority view was that drug abuse was a bigger problem than HIV; therefore, any hasty measures that perpetuated the drug problem should be avoided. With the exception of a few, the rest of the group felt that there was an urgent need to stop the spread of HIV by distributing condoms.

SYNTHESIS OF THE REPORT OF GROUP B

6. The group disagreed with the proposal for the following reasons: These certificates can be misleading if one takes into account the 'window period' and the fact that false certificates may be obtained. It is far more important to educate clients and encourage the voluntary use of condoms. Government and community organizations should provide social support for sex workers.
7. The group saw no reason why HIV should be singled out for screening when there are many other similar viruses leading to various life-threatening diseases.
8. The group agreed in principle with the proposal, although it was underlined that attention should be accorded to the following matters: Are there qualified teachers? Which age groups of children will receive this information? Would there be any religious sensitivities involved, especially in Islamic countries? Perhaps, this should not be called 'sex education' but 'population education' or 'family life education'. It is necessary to rely on the experience of family planning NGOs in developing the curriculum.
9. The group disagreed with this proposal because the more relevant approach is to promote the 'safe sex' norm. Moreover, there are some issues relating to the human rights of the HIV affected spouse which appear to have been ignored.
10. There was a divergence of views on this matter. Some felt that for economic reasons some sex workers may not use condoms if so instructed by their clients. Others pointed out the difficulty in monitoring this requirement. Still others favoured this requirement as a clear message that the law and the community wish to promote the 'safer sex' norm.

MOOT CASE (TRIAL)

The major exercise for Day 4 was a Moot Trial based on the following hypothetical case, *Chokchai* vs. *The Attorney-General and the District Medical Officer:*

Facts

Thongchai regularly donates blood as a meritorious deed. He last donated blood two months ago. A few days later the public health officer of his village came to his factory where he was the manager and directed him to report to the General Hospital. He was taken away in a police jeep. He did not return home that day and his friend Vichit informed Noi, his pregnant wife, that Thongchai had been taken away by the police. It was only after unsuccessfully trying to track him down for two days that Noi came to know that Thongchai was being detained at the Infectious Diseases Hospital.

On presenting herself at the hospital to see Thongchai, Noi was asked as to when the baby was due. When she replied that she was seven months pregnant, she too was detained in another ward in the same hospital. Meanwhile Chockchai, Thongshai's father, contacted the district medical officer for information about his son and daughter-in-law. The officer refused to intervene on the ground that under the new law on AIDS prevention, he could not disclose any information concerning patients at the Infectious Diseases Hospital. This law provides for detention upto six months of persons engaging in 'high-risk' activities.

On returning home, Chockchai informed his wife, Supnee, that there was nothing more that he could possibly do to help his son and daughter-in-law; but Supnee disagreed. After consulting a lawyer, a case is eventually filed by Chockshai against:

1. The Attorney-General as representing the government (Defendant 1)
2. The district medical officer (Defendant 2)

Mr. Subhan was designated as the Presiding Judge, and the following counsel were nominated to represent the Plaintiff and the two Defendants:

* Counsel for plaintiff: Mr. Pavan Duggal and Mr. Husnu Al-Su'ood
* Counsel for the first defendant: Mr. Samith Silva and Ms. Malkanthie Wickremasinghe
* Counsel for the second defendant: Ms. V.S. Rekha and Dr. Hemalal Jayawardena

In addition, the following were also nominated:

* Human rights observer: Mr. J. Ignacio
* Newspaper journalist: Mr. David Patterson
* Court Registrar: Mr. S. Gurumurthy

For the Plaintiff: The counsel raised a preliminary objection to the presence of a press photographer in the court room. He argued that the right to privacy was an important right recognized in the International Covenant on Civil and Political Rights. In view of the sensitive and stigmatizing nature of HIV, the court should order the photographer to leave the court premises and bar him from publishing the names of the plaintiff and his family members.

For the Photographer: It was argued that the principle of trial in an open court is a fundamental one, and in the matter of HIV a responsible press person would seek to educate the public—an important function of the press which should not be underestimated.

Order: On this preliminary issue, the court ruled that the press person could not take photographs, much less print them; nor could he publish or otherwise reveal the names of the parties. He could, however, report the case with regard to other matters. The judge said that donating infected blood was a serious matter that was newsworthy.

Plaintiff's Arguments

1. The law provides for six months' detention for 'engaging in high-risk activities', but it does not indicate through definitions or guidelines what 'engaging in' or 'high-risk activities' are. Given the period of detention and the deprivation of human rights it entails, the law is bad for vagueness.
2. The purpose of the law is not obvious. Even if the court is willing to assume certain purposes behind this law, it is contended that the law overreaches those purposes.
3. The law is not for 'prevention'; 'punishment' seems to be the primary purpose of this law.
4. The law imposes unreasonable and discriminatory restrictions.
5. It is conceded that blood donation is an important activity of considerable public interest but, it is argued, infected blood can be eliminated through proper screening procedures. This law suffers from wrong emphasis.
6. The district medical officer cannot refuse basic information to which close relatives are entitled. They have a right to such information as part of their basic human rights.

Attorney-General's (Defendant 1) Arguments

1. This law provides for ascertaining whether a person whose blood has been found to be infected engages in highrisk activities or not.
2. There is no punitive detention. The plaintiff's son and daughter-in-law are patients in the hospital for treatment and counselling.
3. The six months' detention caters for the 'window period' during which time the patients may not show any signs of infection.
4. The purpose of the law is patent and obvious - to prevent the spread of HIV.
5. When the above factors are taken into account, the court will see that the law imposes reasonable and necessary restrictions, justifiable in the public interest and in the interest of the relatives of the plaintiff.
6. It should be borne in mind that the screening procedures of blood banks in the country are still inadequate; hence, this law attempts to prevent individuals suspected of being HIV infected from contaminating the blood supply or otherwise spreading HIV.

District Medical Officer's (Defendant 2) Arguments

1. Confidentiality is an important principle, both of law and medical ethics.
2. No information which may reveal that the patients may be HIV infected can be disclosed, not even to close relatives, without special justification.
3. Even the patients themselves cannot authorize such disclosure, when it is not certain that they are infected.
4. The law imposes a duty on the medical officer to maintain confidentiality. The plaintiff has no legal basis to characterize this as an 'abuse of power'.

Judgment

The authorities have the power under this law to oblige those whose blood has been found to be infected to submit to further medical examination and counselling. In this case, the authorities had good reason to ask the plaintiff's son and daughter-in-law to submit to further medical examinations. On the last occasion that blood was donated by the son, they found it to be infected.

But the law does not empower the police or the medical authorities to withhold information as to the whereabouts of detained patients or the general reasons for their detention from them or their relatives or guardians. If the law is thought to bestow such a power, then it is a violation of both international and national laws guaranteeing basic human rights. So the police and the medical authorities acted illegally, insofar as they failed to provide information both to the patients themselves and their close relatives. The court will grant a writ of habeas corpus for the immediate release of the plaintiff's son and dauqhter-in-law.

Comments on the Judgment

A brief discussion followed the moot session. Many participants felt that the law was not well-thought-out from the human rights standpoint. While there was appreciation of the need to protect the blood supply system, it was felt that this could have been done without violating so many of the basic rights of the plaintiff and his relatives. There was general agreement that the judgment was sound and balanced.

RELATIONSHIP BETWEEN 'LAW', 'LEGISLATION' AND 'POLICY'

Dr. D.C. Jayasuriya made a presentation on the relationship between law, legislation and policy. He said that it was important to recognize, on the one hand, the rules of law embodied in statutes and judicial decisions and, on the other, in policy documents and declarations. The latter often contained strategies to be adopted, while laws need not be explicit on these matters. However, laws may incorporate national policies. It was worth examining laws to see how far they expressed those declared national policies. Court decisions often have policy implications. It is not unknown for legislatures to seek to reverse, through amendments to laws, the effects of judicial decisions that may have interferred with the policy laid down by the government.

With respect to a given policy, he suggested that the following questions be asked to identify whether a legislative basis was required: Which components of the policy must be reflected in legislation since without a legal basis the policy components cannot be translated into action? Which component need not be reflected in new legislation but which may be dealt with administratively with such a simple device as a departmental circular? The easier path is often to enact subsidiary legislation instead of a new law. As for departmental circulars, which are even easier than subsidiary legislation to draft, they may bind government doctors, but where those circulars appear to lack any statutory authority they will not be binding on private doctors. He urged national AIDS committees to identify laws in their respective countries that prevent the introduction of basic sex education and dissemination of AIDS education materials. Particularly in the South Asian region, there are some laws that had been enacted in the previous century and which need to be reviewed. At times one ministry may announce a policy, but another ministry of the same government may, without being aware of the implications, enact a new law running counter to the policy of the first ministry. National AIDS committees should help in monitoring such contradictions because often the ministries themselves may not be aware of such anomalies.

PANEL DISCUSSION OF NATIONAL AIDS MANAGERS ON HIV-RELATED LEGAL, ETHICAL AND HUMAN RIGHTS

The moderator of this panel discussion was Ms. Husna Razee from the Maldive Islands. Others panel members were Dr. Salil (India), Dr. Jayakuru (Sri Lanka) and Dr. Fernando (Sri Lanka).

Dr. Salil from India said that the laws and the system of justice in India had helped in some ways. He cited two examples of the country's developing 'public interest litigation'. In a hearing taking place before the Supreme Court of India, the petitioners have prayed that the court issue an order to the Government of India obliging it to provide proper organizational infrastructure to screen all blood used in transfusions. The second example of such litigation is a petition to the Delhi High Court for an order that the authorities should make condoms available to prisoners. His organization, NACO, which is part of the Ministry of Health, had submitted affidavits supportive of the petition in the first case. Whatever the outcome of these litigation, the publicity they have provided for HIV-related issues has been invaluable. Moreover, the respondents in cases such as these are not only the central government, but also all the state governments and prison authorities in the country. The awareness amongst these numerous government agencies on the issues raised will be of considerable benefit.

On confidentiality, Dr. Salil pointed out that there was no specific law in India, but the position in the English common law respecting medical confidentiality may well apply. In any event, the declared policy of the health authorities was that there should be no testing without informed consent. It might help clarify matters further if there was a law on confidentiality. Meanwhile, NACO had conducted a number of training workshops for doctors. Indian law requires foreigners staying in the country beyond one year to be tested for HIV. A committee of NACO had recommended that this requirement be reviewed. However, Dr. Salil pointed out, in India HIV/AIDS was not notifiable but only a reportable disease. The latter implies reporting only for epidemiological purposes; thus the identity of the individual is always kept confidential. He said that NACO was actively seeking the support of NGOs, with up to 15 per cent of its funding allocated for NGO projects. NACO was in the process of consulting NGOs in formulating a five-year strategic plan. He also mentioned the formation of PAMS, Physicians Responsible for AIDS Management - an entity representing doctors both from the private and public sectors.

Dr. Gamini Jayakuru from Sri Lanka drew the attention of the participants to the controversy generated in his country, largely by the strong negative stance of the media over surgery done on a patient with HIV at the Colombo General Hospital. He felt that if there had been a law which made it unlawful to deny treatment to HIV positive patients, the doctors might have been spared a great deal of agony caused by the ill-informed, strong public criticism of their actions in this case. The media alleged that the patient was treated in secret in return for a lucrative fee. The patient's name, they pointed out, was not entered in the hospitals records. Dr. Jayakuru said that this sort of criticism rested on ignorance of the need to respect the confidentiality and privacy of the patient in question. In many countries, it is an offence to reveal the names of HIV patients. So the Sri Lankan doctors in this case were right not to record the name in the public records of the hospital. The next example he gave was of the difficulties caused by lack of legislation relating to standards that must be met by test kits marketed by different pharmaceutical concerns. Recently, he said, some test kits were withdrawn in Sri Lanka by the companies themselves, implying that the kits were defective. This caused considerable concern to AIDS managers like himself about the hundreds of tests that had already been done. How many cases of HIV infection might have slipped through? Neither any licensing machinery existed nor were there any standards of quality for laboratories in place. A law was needed requiring all laboratories to maintain standards and quality. With advancing technology, the soon-to-be available saliva test kits for example, new problems may arise - for instance, individuals testing themselves in secret, well away from HIV counsellors. Legal regulation of these matters would be necessary.

This was followed by a short presentation by Dr. Manil Fernando from Sri Lanka on 'Notification to Third Parties'. Under the country's Quarantine and Prevention of Diseases Ordinance, AIDS is a notifiable disease. This means that doctors treating such patients are obliged to inform the public health authorities the name, race and place of residence of the infected persons. This raises certain problems with 'confidentiality'. Several health care officials would be privy to these particulars. In addition, some clerical staff might also have access to them. Confidentiality wears thin under these circumstances. But certain steps taken in the interest of confidentiality could cause problems too. He cited the example of writing death certificates. In Sri Lanka it is the practice not to mention in such certificates AIDS as the cause of death. This means that the statistics compiled by the Registrar-General will not reflect the figures for deaths attributable to AIDS.

Ms. Husna Razee from Maldives said that contrary to official policy, mandatory testing did take place. There was no legislation prohibiting such testing. In the absence of any express prohibition, therefore, some medical staff felt justified in performing mandatory and surreptitious testing. It is often difficult to find out which doctor might have ordered the HIV test. On confidentiality, she said that since religious law in her country made it an offence for counsellors of IV drug users not to notify the authorities, they found it difficult to uphold confidentiality. Furthermore, being a small community, just turning up at an HIV clinic or testing centre is enough to put the concerned person under a cloud. A major obstacle to prevention is the fact that condoms can be imported only by the government and not by private or commercial entities. Under existing law it is far easier for a husband to divorce his wife than *vice versa.* Lack of child support and maintenance is another problem for the divorced or deserted wives with young children. The teaching of sex education is not possible due to strong religious sentiments. She concluded that legal support was necessary to uphold the declared policies of the government. Otherwise, policies cannot be easily translated into action.

THE STRUCTURE AND FUNCTIONS OF NATIONAL AIDS COMMITTEES

Dr. Jayasuriya pointed out that the following organizational features would have to be considered in formulating the structure and functions of a national AIDS committee (NAC):

* *Terms of Reference of the NAC:* Is it merely advisory, or is it charged with monitoring tasks? Can it be pro-active in terms of policy initiatives?
* *The Appointing Authority: Is it* the Minister of Health? Is the NAC under ministerial supervision or is there a degree of autonomy, notwithstanding the nature of the appointing authority?
* *Composition of the NAC:* Are all the members government officials or civil servants? Are some members representatives of community organizations or social groups or other interest groups?
* *Channels of Communication:* Is the NAC obliged to use the channels of the Ministry of Health? If so, can it access the Minister of Health directly?
* *Budgetary Provisions:* Who allocates funds? Are there any restrictions attached?
* *Status of Decisions or Recommendations:* Do the recommendations made by the NAC carry any weight?
* *Degree of Independence and Autonomy:* Who has the power and authority to appoint staff, exercise supervision, monitor and evaluate, etc.
* *Official Level at which the NAC Functions:* What is the rank of the Chairperson of the NAC? In the organizational structure, where is the NAC placed?
* *Oversight:* The nature and scope of the supervisory arrangements.

It is necessary to focus on the above issues in determining the nature, profile and status of a NAC.

FOLLOW-UP ACTIVITIES

It was proposed that a SAARC HIV Law Study Group should be formed. Other proposals included the following:

1. Study groups should be formed in each of the SAARC countries to focus on their individual legal, ethical and human rights issues, needs and problems.
2. Specific legal areas that need further examination are (a) the provision of free legal aid to the indigent, in general, and to HIV positive persons, in particular, with a view to strengthening existing legal aid services so that persons

with HIV/AIDS can access such services; and (b) review of the laws and regulations impacting education, with a view to promoting legal reforms to facilitate awareness about AIDS/HIV.

3. A model curriculum-cum-manual for the teaching HIV-related legal, ethical and human rights issues in the law schools of SAARC countries should be compiled.
4. A list of laws requiring review and reform in the light of the special circumstances of HIV should be drawn up by each country.
5. National level seminars for parliamentarians to inform them of HIV - related legal and administrative issues should be organized. In some countries where laws and customs based on religion play an important role, the ethics of dealing humanely with persons with HIV/AIDS should be raised with parliamentarians, religious leaders, community groups, etc.
6. With the help of the participants in this workshop, national networks should be formed.

Several participants from the region indicated their interest in co-ordinating the above activities and related follow-up activities. Accordingly, the following were assigned the tasks of coordinating the activities listed against their names:

1. Ms. Anjali Gopalan: Comparative study of legislation in SAARC countries on the teaching of sex education and the dissemination of AIDS/HIV materials.
2. Mr. Pavan Duggal: Promotion of national networks in SAARC countries.
3. Ms. V.S. Rekha: Comparative study of free legal aid schemes in SAARC countries.
4. Mr. Subhan: Promotion of research on HIV law, ethics and human rights.
5. Ms. Charika Marasinghe: Promotion of the teaching of HIV law, ethics and human rights in law schools.
6. Ms. V.S. Rekha: Fund raising to support HIV-related legal, ethical and human rights activities.
7. Ms. Charika Marasinghe: Development of resource materials for the teaching of human rights relevant to HIV/AIDS.

Dr. Jayasuriya indicated that the funds required for some of the above activities will be identified in due course. Participants were also encouraged to approach funding agencies with a view to mobilizing the resources necessary to undertake the above activities.

EVALUATION

A questionnaire was circulated to obtain feedback from the participants as to their views on the workshop—its scope and content, structure, working modalities, usefulness and relevance. Their overall impression was very positive, as exemplified by the following responses:

1. Exceptionally good	—	11
2. Good	—	09
3. Satisfactory	—	nil
4. Not very satisfactory	—	nil
5. Did not reply	—	01

CLOSING REMARKS

Being the first in the series of three workshops, Dr. Jayasuriya remarked that he was very pleased with the way the training workshop had been received by the participants and the active interactions that had taken place during the four days. He thanked CEPRA; the participants; the NGOs and service organizations that nominated representatives; UNDP Colombo and other UNDP field offices; and UNOPS for the support that was extended to make the workshop a success.

80

Nadi Training Workshop: HIV Law and Law Reform

(Report of the Proceedings of the UNDP Regional Project on HIV and Development Regional Training Workshop on HIV Law and Law Reform in the South Pacific and other countries, 22-25 May 1995, Nadi, FIJI)

The workshop was attended by 40 participants from the following countries: Fiji, Australia, New Zealand, Sri Lanka, Cook Islands, Kiribati, Papua New Guinea, Solomon Islands, Nauru, Tonga, Vanuatu, Western Samoa, and Nuie. Participants from the Federated States of Micronesia, Marshall Islands and Tuvalu could not attend.

OPENING SESSION

Dr. D. C. Jayasuriya, Regional HIV and Development Adviser, UNDP Regional Project on HIV and Development briefly explained the background to the workshop. It is the third such workshop to be held; previous ones were held in Colombo in February 1995 and in Beijing in April 1995.

The UNDP is concentrating on three main activities in its regional programme:

1. Holding training workshops designed to sharpen the focus on, and promote better awareness and understanding of, HIV-related legal, ethical and human rights issues.
2. Assisting countries to review and draft HIV-related, legislation.

3. Promoting national and regional networking, studies and research.

The regional training workshops, which have the following objectives, are a critical element of the response of the Regional Project to promote capacity-building:

1. Create a better understanding of the nature, scope and content of HIV-related law, ethics and human rights.
2. Sharpen the focus of legal ethical and human rights considerations in reviewing and formulating laws.
3. Consider the legal, ethical and human rights responses required by national programme managers.
4. Identify the role of service organizations in facilitating HIV law reform.
5. Consider the mechanics of promoting national and regional networking.

Encouraging follow-up action has been reported by some countries that attended the Colombo and Beijing workshops. Both China and Sri Lanka have established a national focal point on HIV law and arrangements for national seminars are in place in several countries.

In his welcome address Mr. Somsey Norindr, UNDP Resident Representative, remarked that the evolution of HIV law has been piecemeal, without a holistic approach. In the South Pacific, only French Polynesia had AIDS—related legislation. Other countries such as Vanuatu and Kiribati were only now reviewing public health legislation drafted in colonial times. There are three different ways in which law can incorporate policy:

1. Prescriptive and punitive laws, e.g., criminal law. However, prohibiting certain activities, such as homosexual acts and prostitution, can be counter-productive because of the obstacles placed in the way of effective strategies and the inadequate recognition given to their indirect impact.
2. Protective laws which uphold the rights of People Living with AIDS (PLWA), such as anti-discrimination legislation. Their philosophical basis is positive and constructive.
3. Proactive laws which can change patterns of social interaction. Currently, there are over 7 million infected people in developing countries, mainly poor women. In the USA, Afro-American and Hispanic people are disproportionately affected. In sub-Saharan Africa, three times as many women are infected as men. By limiting access to information or preventive measures, socio-

economic inequalities increase the vulnerability of certain population sub-groups to HIV. Laws which entrench the economic dependence of women prohibit independent ownership of property, or even paid employment. Traditional patterns of behaviour have to change, and law reform has the potential to change such cultural values in the South Pacific.

Justice Daniel Fatiaki, in his Keynote Address, highlighted the risk of complacency in the South Pacific region because of its relative isolation from the HIV/AIDS epidemic, notwithstanding the recent increase in the cases reported. He confirmed that little action had been taken in relation to law reform, which remained largely untapped as a catalyst for social change. Public health legislation in Fiji bears the stamp of its colonial origins in the 1930's. Fortunately, HIV/AIDS has not been included in traditional measures, such as isolation and quarantine. Also HIV/AIDS has not been included in immigration legislation, as is the case in some other countries of the region in order to authorize mandatory testing and exclude positive cases.

Justice Fatiaki examined six areas in terms of law reform implications for HIV/AIDS. Firstly, he thought privacy is imperative in a small society such as Fiji, even if it seems to run counter to the accepted cultural norm. Secondly, he suggested that the public health of the wider community is dependent on the recognition of the rights of the affected community. There is no inevitable conflict which requires sacrifice of individual rights. Thirdly, it is important to recognize that beliefs, traditions and laws cannot by themselves alter behaviour which is the product of individual decision-making. The cornerstones of law reform should be non-judgmental attitudes and cultural sensitivity. Fourthly, the importance of the family as a support mechanism, in the absence of a state welfare system, should be underlined. Urbanization, however, has led to a shift from extended networks to a more nuclear family structure. Fifthly, testing should be examined in relation to the need for counselling and informed consent, screening of donated blood, and the existence of discrimination, even where negative results are concerned (e.g., insurance). Finally, Justice Fatiaki emphasized the need to identify high-risk factors rather than groups for prevention programmes. The challenge is to formulate a strategy for the less heterogenous groups of women, children and infants who can become the passive and involuntary recipients of infection in the heterosexual population.

MODES OF TRANSMISSION AND EPIDEMIOLOGICAL TRENDS

Dr. Govind of the Ministry of Public Health, Fiji gave a basic outline of the modes of transmission (sex, perinatal, tissue transplant, infected blood donation/injection) and methods for prevention (celibacy, mutual monogamy, safe sex and clean injecting). He explained the differences between testing positive for HIV-antibodies testing and AIDS as a clinical entity, characterized by opportunistic infections. Confirmatory tests are not available in the region as the nearest reference laboratory is Fairfield Hospital in Melbourne, Victoria which takes four to six weeks to convey results. He outlined the exposure categories of the 28 positive cases found in Fiji, out of 100,000 tests. Dr.Govind spoke of the high rate of STDs, e.g., genital ulcers in Fiji, which could be a co-factor in transmission rather than an indicator of promiscuity. He explained the emerging patterns of the epidemic. Half of those affected are in their most productive years.

SOCIO-ECONOMIC IMPACT OF THE HIV EPIDEMIC IN ASIA

Dr.D.C.Jayasuriya identified the main source of risk behaviour in three different groups of countries: heterosexual and IVDU (intravenous drug use); homosexual and IVDU; heterosexual and homosexual. He compared the 1992 worldwide expenditure on prevention (US$ 1 billion) with the small amount spent in developing countries (US$ 200 million) where 85 per cent-of the new infections occur. There is a dearth of research data in developing countries. It is expected that 5.5 million children will become orphans in the 1990s. In the USA, 90 per cent of the cases are in the productive age group (20 - 49 years). The epidemic affects key life cycle events such as family formation, employment and national development. It is necessary to look at broader social and cultural contexts. In Asia, projects looking at sexual networking in Thailand have commenced.

Speaking on the economic impact, Dr. Jayasuriya said that a study done in Thailand showed a cost of US$ 8 billion up to the year 2000 if 3.5 million new infections are not prevented. A joint UNDP and Asian Development Bank study has shown a 40 per cent reduction in consumption/income of half the affected Thai households. Structural readjustment programmes can have negative implications for HIV/AIDS: withdrawal or restriction of subsidies will increase drug costs and health care fees; devaluation will also increase the cost of imported drugs; health services will be privatized; civil services would be pruned and vulnerable subgroups can fall through existing safety nets.

THE NATURE AND SCOPE OF HIV LAW

Dr.D.C.Jayasuriya gave a comprehensive overview of the possible functions of HIV/AIDS law:

1. Monitoring, e.g., case reporting (usually the first legal response).
2. Regulating behaviour, e.g., restricting blood and tissue donation, prostitution.
3. Establishing a policy framework, e.g., institutionalizing national AIDS committees.
4. Standard setting and quality control, e.g., importation of condoms.
5. Mandating, interventions and programmes, e.g., needle and syringe exchanges, counselling.
6. Establishing services, e.g., free AZT treatment.
7. Creating a supportive and enabling environment, e.g., free legal aid.

He also outlined 12 factors that could influence policy and legal choices. One is the current state of medical knowledge—early on in the epidemic quarantine is usually suggested. Political expediency is another factor, e.g., the existence of the epidemic is sometimes denied because it can affect the tourism industry. The influence of key groups can be important, e.g., community based service organizations in Australia. Traditionally, public health has not been a hotly debated area. However, the opposite occurred in Thailand where draconian measures prompted pro-democratic public opinion.

HIV-RELATED ETHICAL ISSUES

Ms. Timberlake explained ethics as principles which guide moral decisions and behaviour, what individuals and society as a whole believe, e.g., religion, culture.

There are three levels of ethics:

1. Individual responsibility.
2. Professional codes, e.g., health care workers' duty to treat.
3. Legal obligations.

People with HIV have been shunned, ostracized, harassed, arrested, attacked and even killed. The potent combination of blood, sex, disease and death had resulted in fear, blame and discrimination. There was a need for compassion, solidarity, responsibility, tolerance, information, and empowerment to protect the infected.

There are three main themes of professional codes:

1. Beneficence or wellbeing - weighing the harms and benefits of measures.
2. Equitable and distributive justice-groups should not be signalled out or discriminated against, e.g., testing of captive populations.
3. Respect for persons. In relation to medical interventions this means that:
   (a) Persons have the capacity and right to make choices about the integrity of their bodies.
   (b) Persons should be free from unjustified interference.
   (c) Those with diminished autonomy (dependent and vulnerable) needed protection from harm.

The right to confidentiality affects the quality of service. If clients do not trust their health care provider, then they will not accept advice. Informed consent is critical for HIV testing drugs, treatment and participation in research. It needs to be explicit rather than implied to prevent covert activities.

The professional/client relationship has undergone a radical change from paternalism to equal partnership. One participant noted that expatriate doctors still tend to be treated like 'gods' and patients need to be educated about their rights. There is also the problem in small societies of group rights taking priority over individual rights. Ms. Timberlake noted that it was critical for society to outline what is important for itself. She then explained the legal elements of informed consent: competence, provision of necessary information (benefits vs. risk, freedom to withdraw without penalty, confidentiality), lack of coercion, provision of an authorized representative for incompetent people.

HIV/AIDS DISCRIMINATION AND PRIVACY

Ms. Watchirs emphasized the positive use of anti-discrimination laws and privacy protection for PLWAs in order to facilitate participation, co-operation and trust. She explained the basic elements of such laws: educative rather than punitive, but with remedies if conciliation fails; applicable to public rather than private acts; and enforceable through complaints to independent agencies such as equal opportunity bodies and privacy commissioners. Western models could be adapted for use in the South Pacific. She highlighted the close relationship between discrimination and privacy: the pre-requisite for unfair treatment is usually knowledge of the other's HIV status; therefore the need for confidentiality is based on fear of discrimination. The essential features of disability discrimination laws are:

- HIV infection as well as AIDS must be covered.
- Carers, associates and families of HIV infected people, as well as those perceived to be infected, need to be included.
- Direct and indirect discrimination must be included.
- Exceptions need to be narrowly framed, e.g., reasonable obligations should be placed on employers to accommodate HIV infected employees, such as having flexible working hours, but not where it would cause unreasonable hardship.
- Affirmative action should be allowed, e.g., AIDS councils preferring HIV infected employees.
- Proving discrimination should be simplified and vilification covered.
- Administrative procedures should be effective, e.g. streamlined mechanisms and representative complaints.

Legislative protection of privacy needed to clarify the following issues:

- When HIV related information should be collected.
- Security measures required to protect it.
- Entitlement of individuals to see their own records.
- Exceptions to further use or disclosure, e.g., informed consent, criminal proceedings and needlestick injuries, specific legal requirements or court orders, and partner notification (with detailed protocols being applicable).

Groundswell support for law reform, backed up by education campaigns, are necessary for changing attitudes, as well as behaviour.

HIV RELATED HUMAN RIGHTS ISSUES

Mr. Timberlake gave a comprehensive list of human rights enshrined in international instruments relevant to HIV/AIDS and explored their application in practice:

- Non-discrimination and equality before the law.
- Life, e.g., perinatal transmission.
- Health, e.g., denial of treatment.
- Liberty and security of person, e.g., isolation of HIV positive people.
- Free expression, e.g., censorship of explicit HIV/AIDS educational materials.

- Freedom from inhuman and degrading treatment or punishment, e.g., coerced, unsafe sex.
- Free movement, e.g., HIV testing of tourists.
- Privacy, e.g., confidentiality of HIV test results.
- Marriage and forming a family, e.g., banning marriage of HIV positive people, or coerced abortions.
- Education, e.g., exclusion from universities of HIV positive students.
- Work, e.g., dismissing HIV positive workers.
- Adequate standard of living.
- Social security assistance and welfare.
- Asylum, e.g., excluding HIV positive refugees.
- Scientific advancement.
- Participation in public and cultural life, e.g., formulate and implement AIDS policy.

It was important, she pointed out, that public health exceptions to these rights not be abused by governments to justify ineffective traditional approaches to infectious diseases. She formulated the following criteria for a justifiable restriction:

- Prescription by law.
- Necessity.
- Democratic processes followed.
- Legitimate aim.

Further the restriction must be proportional to achieving the aim, be the least restrictive means available, and effectively achieve the aim. It is tragic that the epidemic disproportionately affects those who are already vulnerable, whose basic human rights have never been fully respected, e.g., migrant workers, refugees, IVDUs, gays, women, children, poor and sex workers. It is debateable whether all rights are equal or can be prioritized. The developing world has serious endemic health problems, 90 per cent of which are easily and inexpensively treatable.

COUNTRY CASE-STUDIES

Country profiles were discussed in three group sessions and a report from each group was presented to the plenary. Copies of selected country papers are reproduced in Part III of this publication.

1. New Zealand, Papua New Guinea, Nuie

The reported case numbers for New Zealand were 953 HIV and 451 AIDS, for Papua New Guinea 236 HIV and 87 AIDS, and nil for Nuie.

A comprehensive country report for New Zealand described the current risk factors as male homosexual acts, heterosexual acts (both sexes), and unsafe injecting drug use. There have been no new cases of medically acquired HIV since 1985, and only one case of perinatal transmission. New Zealand has a large tourist population and a high migration rate, especially of refugees; but there is no mandatory HIV testing. While HIV infection is not notifiable, AIDS is. The Health Act, 1956, is being reviewed with a view to moving away from the communicable diseases model to a health promotion model. Needle and syringe exchanges have been legally protected since 1987. While homosexual acts have been decriminalized since 1986, prostitution related offences still exist (some businesses operate under the pretext of being massage parlours rather than brothels). The Human Rights Act 1993, prohibits discrimination on the basis of physical illness (widely defined to include HIV infection) and sexual orientation. The Privacy Act, 1993, and Health Information Privacy Code 1994 are both relevant to HIV/AIDS privacy protection. A complementary policy paper is currently being prepared on STDs by the Public Health Commission's Advisory Committee on STDs/HIV/AIDS (soon to be renamed).

Papua New Guinea is vulnerable in terms of the high rate of STDs and incidence of genital ulcers. Urban drift is a factor, along with large employment groups in the mining and timber industries. Women are not empowered to make decisions about safe sex and polygamy is common. Fear has been engendered by rumours of AIDS rapists and needle bandits. The Law Reform Commission is looking critically at relevant legislation.

Nuie had a very small gay population, no injecting drug use or sex industry. Also, tourism and immigration are limited. No information is available on the legal framework applicable to HIV/AIDS.

2. Western Samoa, Tonga, Solomon Islands, Vanuatu, Nauru, Tuvalu

The only countries with reported cases are Tonga with five AIDS and six HIV, and Solomon Islands with one HIV.

The risk factors described in country reports are as follows:

Western Samoa has a small transsexual population; drug and alcohol use are on the increase, along with teenage pregnancies, tattooing, and prostitution. The Solomon Islands has high STD rates, some unscreened blood and high mobility of the population. Tattooing is also a traditional practice, but homosexuality does not have cultural and religious sanctions. Vanuatu likewise has increasing teenage pregnancies, gonococcal infections, mobility of population and tourism. Sex education has been approved for schools but has not yet begun, as is the case in Tuvalu.

Western Samoa's public health legislation is a remnant of colonial times. Only AIDS is notifiable, as it will also be under the Health of the People Bill, 1995-96 . A HIV positive tourist was recently deported under the Immigration Act, 1966, but mainly because he and his partner were in possession of drugs. In Tonga, HIV is notifiable and there is power to isolate under public health legislation, but it has never been exercised. In the Solomon Islands, HIV is not notifiable under the Public Health Act, 1970. There is no law reform commission body, but human rights are enshrined in the Constitution. In the one case of HIV infection which occurred, there was public demand to breach confidentiality, but an education campaign quelled these fears. In Vanuatu, HIV and AIDS are notifiable under the Public Health Act, 1994 and human rights are protected under the Constitution. In Nauru, foreign workers will be screened for HIV.

3. Australia, Fiji, Cook Islands, Kiribati

The reported case numbers for Australia are 5,324 AIDS and 18,530 HIV; Fiji 7 AIDS and 21 HIV; Kiribati 2 HIV; and, nil for Cook Islands.

In Australia, risk factors are homosexual and heterosexual sex, and small numbers of infections through infected blood, perinatal route and unsafe injecting. New seroconversions are declining to 450 cases per year. Sex workers have been the focus of good education campaigns. There is high usage of condoms. In Fiji, the risk factors are similar to those in Australia. Further, there is a high prevalence of STDs, problems with condoms (no vending machines and poor quality control), and increasing use of alcohol. Sentinel surveillance of hotel employees has not shown tourism to be a risk factor. In Kiribati, the two cases of infection occurred when locals travelled abroad. There is no drug abuse, but there were alcohol problems. STD rates vary. The sex industry is not visible and condom usage has improved with outreach work. In the Cook Islands, there is considerable population movement (more people live abroad than locally) and tourism, but STDs are declining. Condoms are free to the public and are available in pharmacies and prisons; the Rotary is going to pay for five public vending machines. Sex education is included in the curriculum of all these countries.

In Australia, HIV/AIDS is notifiable in most states and territories under the public health legislation. An ambitious programme of law reform has been launched by the Commonwealth government including representatives from the Health and Attorney-General's Departments on a body created by the First National Strategy, called the Legal Working Party of the Intergovernmental Committee on AIDS. It has issued nine discussion papers on the following topics: public health; anti-discrimination laws; homosexuality; injecting drug use; prostitution; employment law; civil liability for HIV transmission; media law; and therapeutic goods. Following public consultation and submissions, a final report was issued in 1992, of which about half has been implemented. In 1992, the Privacy and HIV/AIDS Working Party also released a final report. NGOs have been pleased with the progress on discrimination laws, needle and syringe exchange, and decriminalition of homosexuality, but more needs to be achieved with prostitution, prison, and voluntary euthanasia.

In Fiji HIV along with STDs is notifiable under the Public Health Act. There have been cases of discrimination by health care workers and employers. The government has used the moral (rather than legal) force of resolution 41.24 of the World Health Assembly on the avoidance of HIV/AIDS discrimination. The national AIDS committee is likely to have a lawyer from the Law Reform Commission or from the office of the Director of Public Prosecutions. In Kiribati, there are no HIV specific laws, but public health legislation is being reviewed. In the Cook Islands, the situation is similar, except that there is a constitutionally entrenched Bill of Rights. There had been a rumour that a local young man returning from abroad had been HIV infected, and there was pressure on the health officials to disclose details. Education about the need for voluntary testing and modes of transmission had quelled these fears. It was observed that most South Pacific countries criminalize homosexual acts and prostitution.

CRIMINAL LAW AND HIV

Ms. Shameem described the three possible roles of law-making:

1. Punitive, e.g., criminalizing prostitution, drug use and acts of homosexuality. Fiji had only used these types of laws, e.g., section 193 of the Criminal Code—for negligently spreading disease, and section 177 of the Criminal Code—dealing with male gross indecency.
2. Protective, e.g., Bill of Rights. The only protection given to

confidentiality in Fiji is under the common law which has never been tested.

3. Instrumental - changing the structure of society itself. In Africa, the Carribbean and South-East Asia, the HIV epidemic disproportionately affects poor women. Socioeconomic nomic dependency makes women powerless to negotiate in sexual matters, and limits access to information and prevention strategies. Examples of the pivotal role of law are:
   - Rape law—corroboration is required for a conviction, and rape in marriage is not recognized.
   - Prostitution law - focusses on the worker and not the client.
   - Reconciliation - in rape cases victims are not consulted and they are under pressure to withdraw charges.
   - Abortion—only lawful for necessary medical reasons, and no regulation of procedures.

NGOs in Fiji have been active in lobbying for law reform in the areas of rape, abortion, incest, and sexual abuse of children. A Children's Co-ordinating Committee has been established with a legal subcommittee; and the police has set up a Child Protection Unit.

THE STATUS OF WOMEN

Ms. Jalal gave an exhaustive analysis of the legal situation of South Pacific women. Women are the largest risk group vulnerable to HIV infection. Law can play a positive role in addressing the problem of lack of control over bodily integrity (e.g., rape), access to land and property, and freedom of movement. Some rights pass patrilineally, not matrilineally, e.g., citizenship, primogeniture. Customary laws tend to be glamorized in the West, but in fact it can entrench class and gender inequalities. Family law, with its emphasis on fault, tends to make it difficult for women to leave unhappy marriages, e.g., if a husband is HIV infected. Only in the Cook Islands is a right to share matrimonial property recognized. As distribution is not based on equal contribution, women tend to get only one-third of the matrimonial property. Sexual fidelity is one-way, and virility is admired in men. Double standards are evident in cases of adultery. No recognition is given to *de facto* spouses or illegitimate children. Domestic violence, marital rape and incest are rife, but not taken seriously by the police. Judicial attitudes are sexist as evidenced by sentencing practices for rape cases, as opposed to crimes again property.

EDUCATION AND INFORMATION LAWS

Mr.Alexander presented his experiences from Australia and invited participation from other country members. He emphasized that the role of law-makers is to enhance and not impede educators, whose work is central to prevention programmes. Behavioural change can only be achieved by giving accurate information about the virus and modes of transmission. Law is only one factor in education, a complex phenomenon which needs to take into account various issues and questions—Who is the target group? Will they be shocked or offended by the material? Will commercial advertisers be happy with the material? Will the churches (who usually have the final word regarding childrens' education) or school principals object? Obscenity laws have their origin in colonial times. Participants from Fiji and Papua New Guinea gave examples of instructions inserted into condom packaging being removed completely by censors. In Australia an unrestricted classification has been given to explicit photographs showing how to put on a condom, because the AIDS Council of NSW has given an undertaking to only circulate them in the target group of gay men. With activities such as prostitution and drug use criminalised, educators risked prosecution for aiding and abetting offences.

PANEL DISCUSSION—THE ROLE OF SERVICE ORGANISATIONS IN HIV LAW REVIEW REFORM

The Moderator of this discussion was Dr. Sainath. Other members were Dr. Tabana, Mr. Alexander, Mr. Buchanan, Ms. Tyler, Ms. Smith and Rev. Tu'uholoaki.

Dr. Tebana described her work with the South Pacific Alliance for Family Health consisting of 10 member countries in the South Pacific, which project officers and managers visit. In the areas of family planning and health (HIV and STDs), information workshops are held to provide education and training. Legal barriers to public distribution of condoms, for example, are identified. As treatment is not available except for care by hospitals and relatives, integration into home-life and community-life is encouraged, to increase privacy and decrease discrimination.

Mr. Alexander outlined the ongoing role of the Australian Federation of AIDS Organizations (an apex body of NGOs) in law reform. His position, which involved advocating on behalf of people with HIV, was funded by the government. The law reform process of the Legal Working Party described elsewhere has been surprisingly progressive, notwithstanding the lack of NGO representation (but not consultation). The Implementation Working Group which is now operating does, however, have NGO representation.

Mr. Buchanan described the activities of the AIDS Council of NSW (ACON) in achieving law reform. The best way for service organizations to work out strategies for action was to identify the needs of its constituency. ACON did this by collecting data on legal complaints which highlighted existing problems, and then using the data for campaigns, such as amendments to the Anti-Discrimination Act 1977 (NSW).

Ms. Taylor outlined her work with the AIDS Taskforce in Suva which began in March 1994. It is staffed by youth and concentrates on outreach and peer education in bars and nightclubs. Soon, rural areas, will be included and later, the tourist and business sectors. Its strength is its ability to access groups which the government cannot reach. Likewise, the Taskforce collects data on matters such as the quality of condoms. Its role in care and support is important in the area of discrimination.

Ms. Smith described the work of the Fiji Women's Crisis Centre which was established 10 years ago. Counsellors are trained to provide information and raise community awareness in the areas of domestic violence and sexual assault, including child abuse. HIV is important because of the high rate of heterosexual transmission and the resulting risk to women with HIV.Reverent Tu'uholoaki from the Fiji Council of Churches emphasized the role of advocacy in creating attitudes within a cultural setting. Education structures are important at the school and family levels.

CREATING AN ENVIRONMENT SUPPORTIVE OF LEGAL AND PRACTICE CHANGES

Elements of an enabling and supportive environment were described by Dr. Jayasuriya:

1. Capacity building - developing skills and interest in the area of HIV law, ethics and human rights. In addition to the three training workshops, the UNDP Regional Project will be supporting a two-week training course on health legislation co-sponsored by WHO (Manila) and the University of New South Wales in Sydney.
2. Encouraging policy, legal and practice reforms.
3. Developing structures such as the institution of ombudsmen or hospital complaints committees to determine complaints.

4. Facilitating access to legal and administrative remedies, e.g., providing free legal aid services to persons with HIV/AIDS.
5. Current awareness, information sharing and strategic questioning, e.g., selected individuals and institutions are being provided with various publications.

PANEL DISCUSSION ON NATIONAL AND REGIONAL NETWORKS

The Moderator of the discussion was Dr. Saravanamuttu. Others members were Mr. Alexander, Ms. Tyler, Ms. Smith, Professor Skegg, Mr. Singin and Ms. Timberlake.

Dr. Saravanamuttu outlined the activities of CEPRA, including information collection, compilation of a mailing list, and interactive sharing of critical information. It has also succeeded in providing a forum for the discussion of ideas. An International Advisory Board is being established to provide information and expertise. There are varying degrees of awareness in the region and sensitivity is needed to gauge what is possible or feasible. Key target groups are politicians and the media. There is the possibility of providing technical support to the setting up of national networks, e.g. among NGOs, academics and policy and research experts.

Mr. Alexander described the formal and informal networking of NGOs in Australia. All AIDS Councils have legal working groups attached to them and are influential in formulating laws and policies and in educating the community about their rights (e.g., through pamphlets). Laws vary between jurisdictions within the country, and volunteers are spread out geographically. The apex body which advises the Australian Federation of AIDS Organizations (AFAO), the National Legal Working Group, is difficult to organize and can meet only infrequently. Without financial resources, it is difficult to involve mainstream lawyers. While it is important to include other professions (e.g., doctors, academics, social workers, public servants etc.), it is difficult to find people who were interested in legal issues.

Ms. Tyler emphasized the importance of establishing and utilizing existing networks; e.g., the Fijian AIDS Task Force has recently used AFAO trainers in towns and villages. This was an extremely successful experiment, despite some criticisms that this may have been inappropriate. It is important to have an open mind about what a larger developed country might have to offer smaller countries such as Fiji. A multisectoral and united approach is essential to face the enormous problems involved in transmission through illegal activities.

Ms. Smith described the long and successful history of formal and informal (e.g. support) networking by women's groups. A wealth of experience can be shared by getting to know each other and tapping into expertise which is sensitive and specialized.

Professor Skegg said that although the role of the law is important, it should not be exaggerated. Too legalistic an approach can be counter-productive. A collaborative approach, not in isolation from the broader educational and public policy aspects, is necessary. HIV/AIDS should not be separated from STDs; measures taken should not be HIV specific, but address general social, medical and ethical issues. It is important that smaller countries in the South Pacific decide for themselves what networking is appropriate, taking into account the size, values, resources and legal traditions of a country.

Mr. Singin emphasized that HIV touched on many aspects of law, such as human rights enshrined in the Constitution. Legal policy needs direction from AIDS experts rather than lawyers. It is important to tap into existing groups (e.g., NGOs) rather than create new institutions. The UNDP Regional Project can help in drafting model legislation, which smaller countries can adapt to their own situation.

Ms. Timberlake spoke of the difficulties in defining the amorphous concept of 'networking', and identifying what keeps members together to make them accomplish various tasks. AIDS service organizations with experienced activists need to integrate legal and ethical issues into their other work. In order to get governments to respond it is critical to know what is happening at the grass-roots level, e.g., monitoring abuses.

A lively discussion ensued among participants as to whether this workshop was premature, as not enough bodies existed yet to network. Mr. Alexander responded that people still can contribute individually to a newsletter on what was happening in their country. Ms. Roth said that a UNDP study of legal and ethical issues in the South Pacific is being prepared and a draft would be available at the end of July. Mr. Buchanan emphasized the importance of involving the affected community. A debate followed about whether NGOs or government agencies are more stable. If there is sustained funding, NGO staff are committed and tend to stay in positions, whereas there can be a high turnover of staff in the public service. On the other hand, government agencies may have better resources. A role was suggested for the South Pacific Commission.

Proposed (Hypothetical) Legislative Measures

The participants were divided into various groups for purposes of discussing and commenting on the following hypothetical problem:

> You are the Minister of Health. A committee headed by the Minister of Justice has prepared a draft HIV/AIDS Prevention and Control Bill. The other members of the committee are the Attorney-General, the Director-General of Health; the Director-General of Social Services, the Chief of Police, a senior judge of the Supreme Court, and representatives of associations of lawyers, doctors, social workers and non-governmental organizations. At a Cabinet meeting, you are asked by the Prime Minister to express your views on the desirability of including the following provisions proposed unanimously by the committee:
>
> 1. A requirement to subject to compulsory testing for HIV any person whom a police officer or public health inspector suspects to be a 'drug addict', a 'homosexual' or a 'sex worker'.
> 2. A requirement for foreign visitors intending to reside for more than two weeks to be tested for HIV within ten days of their arrival, and thereafter at intervals of six months.
> 3. A requirement to quarantine all nationals who are HIV seropositive and to deport all seropositive foreign nationals.
> 4. A requirement to prohibit nationals from marrying foreigners.
> 5. A requirement to provide free needles, syringes and condoms to all drug addicts who are registered with the police.
> 6. A requirement to permit commercial sex establishments to employ as sex workers only those in possession of a HIV-free certificate issued by a government doctor during the past six months.
> 7. A requirement to compulsorily pre-screen for HIV all jobs applicants and new university entrants.
> 8. A requirement for the compulsory teaching of sex education from the primary school level upwards.
> 9. A requirement to make the presence of infection with HIV or STD a ground for divorce.

10. A requirement for the compulsory use of condoms in all commercial sex encounters.
11. A requirement that medical practitioners who are HIV seropositive must inform all patients with whom they come into physical contact their HIV status at the earliest possible opportunity.
12. A requirement to prohibit newspapers from reporting the names of persons with HIV or AIDS.

The consensus of the groups in relation to the twelve proposals is summarized below:

1. Rejected the proposal for compulsory testing of drug users, homosexuals and sexworkers on suspicion by police or public health inspectors. The real issue was dangerous behaviour, which does not automatically follow from membership of these groups. Testing is not reliable, treatment is not available for cases found this way, and it would induce a false sense of security in the population. Police had no public health training, and it would drive these three groups underground or marginalize them even further.
2. Testing foreigners is not cost - effective and will adversely affect tourism. There is no public health benefit in the proposal; therefore it was rejected.
3. The proposal to quarantine HIV positive nationals was rejected on grounds of costs and the public health problem of driving people into hiding, where it would be impossible to access them for education and prevention campaigns. Likewise, the proposal to deport HIV positive foreigners was rejected because it is unfair and prejudicial - it assumes irresponsible behaviour rather than consider cases on individual merit.
4. Most participants rejected the proposal to prohibit marriage to foreigners. It was noted this is the current legal situation in Nauru. The risk behaviour is 'sex' and not 'marriage', and the legal provision will have no impact on HIV prevention.
5. The proposal to supply free needles, syringes and condoms was supported, but not the registration of drug addicts with the police, as this will make people reluctant to come forward for HIV/AIDS education. Also, free supplies should be given to others who need them, such as diabetics. Accompanying the proposal should be an exchange/ disposal programme so that used needles and syringes

are not dangerously disposed of in public places. The police should be educated on the public health/harm minimization rationale of the programme. Cost factors and the image of promoting drug taking were considered. The proposal to provide needles and syringes was rejected. However, condoms may be sold in bulk at cost prices (rather than given free) to commercial sex establishments .

6. The proposal for HIV free certificates for sex workers was rejected as unreliable, both in terms of forgeries and the timeliness of HIV testing, i.e., window period, subsequent exposures, etc.
7. The proposal to compulsorily test job applicants and university students was rejected because of costs, and the very low risk of infection at the work-place.
8. The proposal to mandate sex education in schools was supported with several amendments: the terminology should be "family life education" and parents should be able to conscientiously object and remove their children from such classes. It was noted that in some countries education is not compulsory for children.
9. No fault divorce instead of HIV infection was proposed as a ground for divorce. HIV-infection does not necessarily imply adultery, and 'irretrievable breakdown of the relationship' is the relevant criterion.
10. The proposal to mandate the use of condoms in commercial sex establishments was supported, but with some concern about enforcement, e.g., need for occupational health and safety inspectors to inspect such establishments.
11. The proposal for HIV positive doctors to self-declare to patients was rejected, because it does not respect privacy or the right to work where there was little risk of infection. Instead, it was proposed that universal infection control measures be codified.
12. The proposal to prohibit newspapers from publishing the names of HIV positive persons was supported with the additional criterion of lack of written consent, as some activists may want to publicize their own cases in the media.

CASE-STUDIES

1. Political will and the Legislative Process

Dr. Saravanamuttu emphasized the importance of appealing

to politicians; it should be in their self-interest to push- for law reform, as there is no political capital in the issue by itself. It is easier to influence the law-making process where there are well-developed institutions and channels to feed information to legislators, such as non-partisan professional organizations and NGOs. The onus and responsibility for lobbying are on civil society, which have competing interests for funding resources and priorities. A coherent political coalition should be formed to pool resources once differences have been resolved. A delicate balance has to be reached between drafting less contentious proposals which have more chances of success, and comprehensive reform which can be delayed. Key individuals should be targeted and their favourite subjects identified. Party functionaries can be more effective than government officials. The objective is to change minds and perspectives.

2. Legal Drafting in Countries with Limited Legal Manpower

Ms. Fenton described the process for setting a legislative agenda. The responsible minister puts a policy paper through the Cabinet (strong ministers are rare in the health portfolio) and once approval in principle is received, detailed drafting instructions are prepared. The bill then goes through a Cabinet subcommittee before being introduced or tabled in Parliament. Because of the scarcity of draftsmen in the region, often overseas consultants are used, but they were not sensitive to existing laws (e.g. customary); also, funding is usually not sufficient to complete the work, and local agencies have to pick up the pieces. Law reform commissions existed in Fiji and Papua New Guinea. Resources for research is a problem and overseas precedents tend to be used inappropriately. Select committees and committees of inquiry tend to be ineffectual as their reports are often shelved. Sometimes administrative practice notes can be used effectively in the interim. Participants from the region actively participated in this session, describing their own experiences.

3. Experience of the Australian Legal Working Party (LWP)

Ms. Watchirs outlined the history of the production of the LWP Final Report, the green and white papers (National HIV/AIDS Strategy), the Report of the Working Panel on Discrimination and other Legal Issues, LWP discussion papers (nine papers with 13,000 copies circulated)—all of which involved broad community consultation, resulting in 300 submissions from 111 individuals and organizations. The LWP is a unique body: intergovernmental but also multisectorial (medical and legal expertise). Work was expedited by forming subcommittees for different subject matters. Model legislation was not drafted because of the time and expense involved, and uncertainty of implementation. The text of the Final Report identified problem in individual jurisdictions, but recommendations did not single out any state or territory. Sometimes softer options were included for practical reasons, in areas such as prostitution and injecting drugs. The Minister for Health launched the discussion papers and final report, indicating maximized public interest and political commitment. It is essential that NGOs are funded in order to be in a position to respond adequately; e.g., AFAO had an advocate under the First National Strategy, and a legal policy analyst under the Second National Strategy. Complementary projects are funded to educate the affected community and lawyers. The Implementation Working Group was formed in September 199 to facilitate the implementation of recommendations of the LWP.

EXPERIENCE WITH THE AUSTRALIAN DISABILITY DISCRIMINATION ACT (DDA)

Mr. Buchanan illustrated the law reform process in the enactment of the DDA, and the difficulty in generating the necessary impetus from eight provinces within Australia. Essentially, anti-discrimination legislation prevents decision-makers from using irrelevant and unfair criteria. The classic features of this legislation are: a legal definition of what discrimination is; the attributes which are covered, e.g., disability, race, sex, etc.; declaration of unlawfulness of the activity; deeming indirect discrimination to be included; defining public, rather than private, areas of life as being covered; providing for defences and exceptions, e.g., reasonable accommodation, *bona fide* occupational qualification, affirmative action, religion, public health, etc.; and including harassment, incitement and vilification. He gave examples of several reported HIV-related cases in Australia.

AUSTRALIAN DEVELOPMENTS ON EDUCATION AND INFORMATION LAWS

Mr. Alexander spoke of the importance of positive protection by the law; e.g., public health legislation can prevent untrue advertisements for products professing to cure AIDS. Codes of ethics for journalists to prevent them from identifying HIV positive people without their consent, for example, are not always effective.

In Australia a Media Information Handbook had been very educative, e.g., removing inappropriate terminology such as "AIDS victims". The Legal Working Party has recommended that the media law be amended to require broadcasters to publish some public health promotions free of charge.

THE NEW ZEALAND HUMAN RIGHTS ACT

Professor Skegg described the evolution of the legislation. The original 1977 legislation was broadened in 1994 to include illness (widely defined to include HIV-infection) and sexual orientation. It operates by conciliation and mediation, but with damages being available in recalcitrant cases. It needs some fine tuning and more resources, but the system is working well in terms of its educative effect, rather than merely in individual cases. There are three other relevant commissioners: Privacy; Health and Disability; and the Ombudsman (Parliamentary Commissioner). It is important that legislation not be HIV specific, nor should it be presumed that law reform is enough by itself. Other measures, e.g., needle and syringe exchanges, are also necessary.

THE ROLE OF WHO RESOLUTIONS AND RECOMMENDATIONS

Ms. Timberlake explained that international instruments are documents emanating at the international level which can either be legally binding or statements/declarations of principles. There are sufficient human rights instruments to cover HIV/AIDS, but what is unclear is their application in certain situations, i.e., the public health exceptions. WHO is trying to utilize the UN system to integrate and mainstream HIV, by holding briefing sessions and writing letters and trying to convince various bodies (e.g. Commission on Human Rights) to put HIV/AIDS on their agenda. It has been difficult to make any significant progress became of competing priorities. In the last few years WHO has been successful in persuading CHR to have a HIV Resolution, but this is not binding. The input of NGOs can be improved by gaining consultative status. WHO has the power to make rules which are legally binding on the members, but technical guidance at high government levels is currently thought to be more appropriate. Consensus statements on a range of issues such as testing, prisons, partner notification, travel, sports etc., have been produced after broad consultation with governments, NGOs and PLWAs. There is an on-going process of consultation with the creation of the new UNAIDS programme. Participants were invited to contribute their views on how UNAIDS may operate.

MOOT TRIAL

A moot trial based on the following facts was held:

Johnny regularly donates blood as a meritorious deed. He last donated blood two months ago. A few days later the public health officer of his village had come to his factory where he is the manager and had directed him to report to the general hospital He had been taken away in a police jeep. He did not return home that day and his friend had informed Mary, his pregnant wife, that Johnny has been taken away by the police. It was only after unsuccessfully trying to track him down for two days that Mary had come to know that Johnny is being detained at the Infectious Diseases Hospital.

On presenting herself at the hospital to see Johnny, Mary had been asked as to when the baby is due. When she had replied that she was seven months pregnant, she too had been detained in another ward in the same hospital. Meanwhile Jimmy, Johnny's father, had contacted the District Medical Officer for information about his son and daughter-in-law. The officer had refused to intervene on the ground that under the new law on AIDS prevention, he cannot disclose any information concerning patients at the Infectious Diseases Hospital. This law provides for detention upto six months of persons engaging in 'high-risk' activities. On returning home, Jimmy had informed his wife that there is nothing more that he can possibly do to help his son and daughter-in-law, but his wife had disagreed. After consulting a lawyer action is eventually filed by Jimmy against:

1. The Attorney-General as representing the government (Defendant 1)
2. The District Medical Officer (Defendant 2)

HIV-Related Specific Laws

The only statute in the country specific to HIV is the new AIDS Prevention Law. This law has only two provisions. Section 1 empowers the health authorities to detain upto six months any person engaging in "highrisk" activities. Section 2 states that no information can be provided to any member of the public concerning person detained at the infections Diseases Hospital.

General Law

Under the general law an action can be instituted against the Attorney general for any legal complaint against the Government. The Constitution provides for the validity of laws to be challenged even after the law has come into operation. In addition to the remedy for damages, the law provides for the following actions:

1. writ of habeas corpus (for the release of persons held illegally or without authority);
2. declaration of 'right' or 'status';
3. writ of mandamus to compel a public authority to perform a duty; and
4. an injunction to restrain from performing any act.

Admissions

The Counsel for the Plaintiff must set out the facts, the reliefs claimed and the law applicable. All parties admit the facts stated on page 1, but the Counsel for the 1st and 2nd Defendants do not agree that there has been any violation of the law or any irregular or unauthorized act.

On the day of hearing, a newspaper reporter is present in the court premises and threatens to publish the names and photographs of Johnny and his wife, Mary.

The following participants participated in the Moot Trial:

Judges	:	Ms. Kathy Ettershank
		Mr. Fagaloa Tufuga
		Mr. Primo Afeau
Counsel for Plaintiff	:	Ms. Florence Fenton
Counsel for the first defendant	:	Ms. Imrana Jalal
		Mr. Togia Sioneholo
Counsel for the second defendant	:	Mr. Alan Marsh
		Ms. Linda Folaumoetu'i
Journalist	:	Mr. Michael Alexander
Human Rights Observers	:	Professor Peter Skegg
		Mr. Tingika Elikana

The Supreme Court of Mocambo gave Jimmy Johnny's father) standing as next friend or guardian. It ordered the release of Johnny and Mary from detention and damages of $2000 each to be paid, as there was no evidence under section 1 of the AIDS Prevention

Law that either had engaged in "high risk activities—both were respected community members; Johnny had merely donated blood and Mary was pregnant. A declaration was made that the legislation is not *ultra virus* the Constitution (rights to privacy and freedom of movement, but with exceptions for public health). The court, however, recommended that section 2 be amended to make the intention of the legislature clear—information about a person's detention at the infectious Diseases Hospital is prohibited from being publicly divulged, but not in a closed court. An interim ruling was made that test results be revealed to the court by the District Medical Officer. An interim finding was that the DMO is not vicariously liable and can be struck out as a party. Also the press were able to remain in court, except for in-camera proceedings, upon giving an undertaking to neither release photographs of the plaintiffs, nor to publish their identities.

Participants discussed the judgment in terms of protection of privacy and civil liberties. Of particular concern was any interference with pregnant women who are HIV infected - even if AZT does reduce the risk of perinatal transmission, it is too expensive to be freely available in the region.

PANEL DISCUSSION ON HIV-RELATED LEGAL, ETHICAL AND HUMAN RIGHTS RESPONSES AS PERCEIVED BY NATIONAL AIDS PROGRAMME MANAGERS

Lady Keith was the moderator of this Panel Discussion. Panel members included Dr. Salik Ram Govind, Dr. Takeieta Kienene, Ms. Mayriam Abel, Mr. Kamuta Seuseu, Dr. Sitaleki A. Finau, Ms. Elizabeth Amram, Dr. F. Sipeli and Ms. Neti Tamarua Hermánn.

Dr. Govind remarked that law has a very useful role to play in relation to HIV/AIDS, and that, therefore, there is a need to educate legislators. Supportive legislation, such as those dealing with anti-discrimination is preferable to hasty, restrictive measures which could be counter-productive. It is important that governments coordinate these efforts, because the mix of NGOs looking at these issues tends to keep changing; however, their views should definitely be taken into account.

Dr. Kienene emphasized the importance of controlling Hepatitis B. Ms. Abel was concerned about the instability of politics; the training and education of politicians would be wasted, given their high turnover. Mr. Seuseu stressed the importance of including lawyers at the planning stages and working together with other groups such as churches and women. Mr. Finau saw a role for lawyers in HIV education, but was concerned that by promoting privacy and confidentiality in small societies, individualism had been preferred to extended family values. He thought that the risk behaviour of HIV positive people demonstrated that they are not always rational and responsible. Ms. Amram spoke of what she had learned at this workshop, but emphasized that Nauru is at a different stage from other countries, as it has no HIV cases yet. Dr. Specific was also concerned about Hepatitis B. It is important that small island countries watch and observe what is happening in the region. Ms. Hemann said that the Cook Islands did not have any HIV specific laws, but public health and criminal laws could impact on HIV/AIDS (although their efficacy in this respect had not yet been tested). Positive steps should be taken to collaborate in law reform, e.g.., having Crown Law Office representatives on national AIDS committees.

A heated discussion ensued between the participants. Ms. Jalal said that the law can be a catalyst for change and it symbolizes a society's values. Even if bills are defeated, at least legislators are forced to deal with the issues. On the duty to care for HIV infected patients, medical practitioners expressed concern about needle stick injuries. Mr. Finau highlighted the inappropriateness of having foreigners draft local laws without asking what the fundamental effects would be e.g., the distinction between discrimination and social sanction. Ms. Timberlake thought that it was important that the region's low prevalence of HIV remains that way; opening up a dialogue on taboo subjects is a good way to achieve this, even if some countries are not yet ready for law reform. Mr. Singin thought the workshop was timely; it is up to individual countries to decide if or when to adopt legal measures.

CHECKLIST TO FACTUALITY THE LAW REVIEW/REFORM PROCESS

Dr. Jayasuriya presented a matrix to facilitate the consideration of issues relevant to law review/law reform. This is reproduced in Part IV of this publication. Ms. Timberlake presented a checklist on human right issues. Concerns were expressed that this checklist may not necessarily be relevant to South Pacific countries. Since a detailed discussion of the checklist was not possible, participants were invited to send their written comments to Dr. Jayasuriya.

EVALUATION

A questionnaire was administered to elicit the views of the

participants with regard to the structure, content and organization of the workshop. On the last question as to the 'overall impression' the following responses were recorded:

Exceptionally good	-	5
Good	-	18
Satisfactory	-	4
Not very satisfactory	-	1

CLOSING SESSION

Dr. Jayasuriya remarked that this workshop was timely because most South Pacific nations were at the very ea 'y stages in adding the HIV law, ethics and human rights dimension to their national AIDS programmes. He said mat he was impressed by the statements of many participants who regarded this workshop as the begging of a process of talking a closer look at these issues from a national perspective. The Regional Project as well as UNDP field offices will take note of the calls for support to organize national level workshops where these issues can be discussed more fully, having regard to local conditions and needs. The need for training in health legislation, including HIV law, and for the development of a model law on HIV prevention that countries with lived resources for le gal drafting can use as the basis for discussions, and possibly for the development of their own legislation, were also noted.

The Regional Project was delighted to learn from the Director of Public Prosecutions in Fiji as well as from the Programme Manager of the National AIDS Programme that a national focal point will be created shortly. UNDP Suva will be requested to provide seed funding to launch this national network as well as to organize a national workshop on HIV law, ethics and human rights. Dr. Jayasuriya hoped that other countries will Saw suit.

Finally, Dr. Jayasuriya expressed his gratitude to the participants, the key-note speaker, the consultant, the NGOs *which* nominated various representatives, CEPRA and to the representatives of UN and other international and regional agencies for their active participation. The Regional Project, he said, is grateful to the Governments of Australia and New Zealand for meeting the expenses of the participants nominated by these governments. On behalf of the Regional Project he also thanked the various UNDP field offices and UN-OPS for facilitating the nomination of participants and for arranging the logistics. Finally, a special word of thanks was extended to the UNDP Representative, Fiji and his staff for making every effort to make the workshop a success.